Oligodendrocyte Physiology and Pathology Function

Oligodendrocyte Physiology and Pathology Function

Editor

Markus Kipp

MDPI • Basel • Beijing • Wuhan • Barcelona • Belgrade • Manchester • Tokyo • Cluj • Tianjin

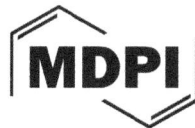

Editor
Markus Kipp
Rostock University Medical Center
Germany

Editorial Office
MDPI
St. Alban-Anlage 66
4052 Basel, Switzerland

This is a reprint of articles from the Special Issue published online in the open access journal *Cells* (ISSN 2073-4409) (available at: https://www.mdpi.com/journal/cells/special_issues/oligodendrocyte_function).

For citation purposes, cite each article independently as indicated on the article page online and as indicated below:

LastName, A.A.; LastName, B.B.; LastName, C.C. Article Title. *Journal Name* **Year**, *Article Number*, Page Range.

ISBN 978-3-03943-689-7 (Hbk)
ISBN 978-3-03943-690-3 (PDF)

Cover image courtesy of Markus Kipp.

© 2020 by the authors. Articles in this book are Open Access and distributed under the Creative Commons Attribution (CC BY) license, which allows users to download, copy and build upon published articles, as long as the author and publisher are properly credited, which ensures maximum dissemination and a wider impact of our publications.

The book as a whole is distributed by MDPI under the terms and conditions of the Creative Commons license CC BY-NC-ND.

Contents

About the Editor vii

Markus Kipp
Oligodendrocyte Physiology and Pathology Function
Reprinted from: *Cells* **2020**, *9*, 2078, doi:10.3390/cells9092078 1

Sarah Joost, Stefan Mikkat, Michael Wille, Antje Schümann and Oliver Schmitt
Membrane Protein Identification in Rodent Brain Tissue Samples and Acute Brain Slices
Reprinted from: *Cells* **2019**, *8*, 423, doi:10.3390/cells8050423 7

Zihao Yuan, Peipei Chen, Tingting Zhang, Bin Shen and Ling Chen
Agenesis and Hypomyelination of Corpus Callosum in Mice Lacking Nsun5,
an RNA Methyltransferase
Reprinted from: *Cells* **2019**, *8*, 552, doi:10.3390/cells8060552 21

**Emanuela Nocita, Alice Del Giovane, Marta Tiberi, Laura Boccuni, Denise Fiorelli,
Carola Sposato, Elena Romano, Francesco Basoli, Marcella Trombetta, Alberto Rainer,
Enrico Traversa and Antonella Ragnini-Wilson**
EGFR/ErbB Inhibition Promotes OPC Maturation up to Axon Engagement by Co-Regulating
PIP2 and MBP
Reprinted from: *Cells* **2019**, *8*, 844, doi:10.3390/cells8080844 37

**Tanja Hochstrasser, Sebastian Rühling, Kerstin Hecher, Kai H. Fabisch, Uta Chrzanowski,
Matthias Brendel, Florian Eckenweber, Christian Sacher, Christoph Schmitz and
Markus Kipp**
Stereological Investigation of Regional Brain Volumes after Acute and Chronic Cuprizone-
Induced Demyelination
Reprinted from: *Cells* **2019**, *8*, 1024, doi:10.3390/cells8091024 59

**Marina Khodanovich, Anna Pishchelko, Valentina Glazacheva, Edgar Pan, Andrey Akulov,
Mikhail Svetlik, Yana Tyumentseva, Tatyana Anan'ina and Vasily Yarnykh**
Quantitative Imaging of White and Gray Matter Remyelination in the Cuprizone Demyelination
Model Using the Macromolecular Proton Fraction
Reprinted from: *Cells* **2019**, *8*, 1204, doi:10.3390/cells8101204 77

**Assia Tiane, Melissa Schepers, Ben Rombaut, Raymond Hupperts, Jos Prickaerts,
Niels Hellings, Daniel van den Hove and Tim Vanmierlo**
From OPC to Oligodendrocyte: An Epigenetic Journey
Reprinted from: *Cells* **2019**, *8*, 1236, doi:10.3390/cells8101236 95

**Stella Nyamoya, Julia Steinle, Uta Chrzanowski, Joel Kaye, Christoph Schmitz,
Cordian Beyer and Markus Kipp**
Laquinimod Supports Remyelination in Non-Supportive Environments
Reprinted from: *Cells* **2019**, *8*, 1363, doi:10.3390/cells8111363 115

**Meray Serdar, Annika Mordelt, Katharina Müser, Karina Kempe, Ursula Felderhoff-Müser,
Josephine Herz and Ivo Bendix**
Detrimental Impact of Energy Drink Compounds on Developing Oligodendrocytes
and Neurons
Reprinted from: *Cells* **2019**, *8*, 1381, doi:10.3390/cells8111381 131

Sarah Kuhn, Laura Gritti, Daniel Crooks and Yvonne Dombrowski
Oligodendrocytes in Development, Myelin Generation and Beyond
Reprinted from: *Cells* **2019**, *8*, 1424, doi:10.3390/cells8111424 147

**Lukas S. Enz, Thomas Zeis, Annalisa Hauck, Christopher Linington and
Nicole Schaeren-Wiemers**
Combinatory Multifactor Treatment Effects on Primary Nanofiber Oligodendrocyte Cultures
Reprinted from: *Cells* **2019**, *8*, 1422, doi:10.3390/cells8111422 171

**Jiangshan Zhan, Vladislav Yakimov, Sebastian Rühling, Felix Fischbach, Elena Nikolova,
Sarah Joost, Hannes Kaddatz, Theresa Greiner, Julia Frenz, Carsten Holzmann and
Markus Kipp**
High Speed Ventral Plane Videography as a Convenient Tool to Quantify Motor Deficits during
Pre-Clinical Experimental Autoimmune Encephalomyelitis
Reprinted from: *Cells* **2019**, *8*, 1439, doi:10.3390/cells8111439 185

**Florian J. Raabe, Lenka Slapakova, Moritz J. Rossner, Ludovico Cantuti-Castelvetri,
Mikael Simons, Peter G. Falkai and Andrea Schmitt**
Oligodendrocytes as A New Therapeutic Target in Schizophrenia: From Histopathological
Findings to Neuron-Oligodendrocyte Interaction
Reprinted from: *Cells* **2019**, *8*, 1496, doi:10.3390/cells8121496 207

**Ina Schäfer, Johannes Kaisler, Anja Scheller, Frank Kirchhoff, Aiden Haghikia and
Andreas Faissner**
Conditional Deletion of LRP1 Leads to Progressive Loss of Recombined NG2-Expressing
Oligodendrocyte Precursor Cells in a Novel Mouse Model
Reprinted from: *Cells* **2019**, *8*, 1550, doi:10.3390/cells8121550 223

Laura Reiche, Patrick Küry and Peter Göttle
Aberrant Oligodendrogenesis in Down Syndrome: Shift in Gliogenesis?
Reprinted from: *Cells* **2019**, *8*, 1591, doi:10.3390/cells8121591 247

**Gábor Kriszta, Balázs Nemes, Zoltán Sándor, Péter Ács, Sámuel Komoly, Zoltán Berente,
Kata Bölcskei and Erika Pintér**
Investigation of Cuprizone-Induced Demyelination in mGFAP-Driven Conditional Transient
Receptor Potential Ankyrin 1 (TRPA1) Receptor Knockout Mice
Reprinted from: *Cells* **2020**, *9*, 81, doi:10.3390/cells9010081 267

Erik Nutma, Démi van Gent, Sandra Amor and Laura A. N. Peferoen
Astrocyte and Oligodendrocyte Cross-Talk in the Central Nervous System
Reprinted from: *Cells* **2020**, *9*, 600, doi:10.3390/cells9030600 281

**Stefan Gingele, Florian Henkel, Sandra Heckers, Thiemo M. Moellenkamp,
Martin W. Hümmert, Thomas Skripuletz, Martin Stangel and Viktoria Gudi**
Delayed Demyelination and Impaired Remyelination in Aged Mice in the Cuprizone Model
Reprinted from: *Cells* **2020**, *9*, 945, doi:10.3390/cells9040945 303

About the Editor

Markus Kipp
Universitätsmedizin Rostock
Instituts für Anatomie
Gertrudenstrasse 9
18057 Rostock
Germany
Tel/Fax: +49 (0) 381 494 8400
markus.kipp@med.uni-rostock.de
https://anatomie.med.uni-rostock.de/

Education

Approbation Human Medicine..2006
Faculty of Medicine
Rheinisch-Westfälische Technische Hochschule Aachen
Doctorate as Dr. Med..2008
Faculty of Medicine
Rheinisch-Westfälische Technische Hochschule Aachen
Doctorate as Dr. Rer. Nat..2011
Faculty of Natural Sciences
Rheinisch-Westfälische Technische Hochschule Aachen

Work Experience

Scientific employee, Anatomy, RWTH Aachen..2006–2010
DFG Research Scholarship; VU medical center Amsterdam.............................2010–2012
Appointment for W1-professorship for Cellular Neurodegeneration RWTH Aachen University, Faculty of Medicine..2012–2015
Appointment for W2-professorship for Neuroanatomy and Histology LMU Munich University, Faculty of Medicine..2015–2018
Appointment for W3-professorship for Anatomy University Rostock, Faculty of Medicine...2018–present

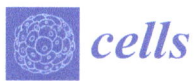

Editorial

Oligodendrocyte Physiology and Pathology Function

Markus Kipp [1,2]

1. Institute of Anatomy, Rostock University Medical Center, Gertrudenstrasse 9, 18057 Rostock, Germany; markus.kipp@med.uni-rostock.de; Tel.: +49-381-494-8401
2. Center for Transdisciplinary Neurosciences Rostock (CTNR), Rostock University Medical Center, Gelsheimer Strasse 20, 18147 Rostock, Germany

Received: 4 September 2020; Accepted: 9 September 2020; Published: 11 September 2020

Introduction

The adult vertebrate central nervous system (CNS) mainly consists of neurons, astrocytes, microglia cells and oligodendrocytes. Oligodendrocytes, the myelin-forming cells of the CNS, are subjected to cell stress and subsequent death in a number of metabolic or inflammatory disorders, among which is multiple sclerosis (MS) [1–5]. This disease is associated with the development of large demyelinated plaques, oligodendrocyte destruction and axonal degeneration [6,7], paralleled by the activation of astrocytes and microglia as well as the recruitment of peripheral immune cells to the site of tissue injury. Of note, viable oligodendrocytes and an intact myelin sheath are indispensable for neuronal health. For example, it has been shown that oligodendrocytes provide nutritional support to neurons [8], that fast axonal transport depends on proper oligodendrocyte function [9] and that mice deficient in mature myelin proteins eventually display severe neurodegeneration [10].

Due to the presence of multifocal white and grey matter demyelination in the CNS of MS patients, any pathogenetic concept has to provide an explanation for the highly specific destruction of myelin and oligodendrocytes. While several treatment options are currently available to dampen the peripheral, T- and B-cell driven inflammatory activity in MS patients, treatment options to ameliorate oligodendrocyte pathology and strengthen neuronal health are, unfortunately, limited. For the development of such novel therapies, a basic understanding of oligodendrocyte development, maintenance, destruction and regeneration is needed as well as novel tools to precisely monitor neuronal and functional deficits during pre-clinical studies. This Special Issue collects articles that address ongoing research into promoting myelin repair, address our understanding of the physiology and pathology of oligodendrocytes, summarize the interaction of oligodendrocytes with central and peripheral immune cells and introduce novel models that allow us to study oligodendrocyte physiology and pathology.

Therefore, various animal models exist with key characteristic features. In experimental autoimmune encephalomyelitis (EAE), the active or passive immunization with CNS-related antigens results in multifocal inflammatory CNS lesions with secondary oligodendrocyte injury and demyelination to a variable extent. Toxin models, such as the cuprizone model, are characterized by a primary oligodendrocyte degeneration leading to demyelination, axonal degeneration and reactive gliosis. The cuprizone model has become increasingly popular in recent years to study key pathological events during MS lesion development and progression. This Special Issue includes six articles using the cuprizone model to understand underlying MS pathologies.

To investigate mechanisms operant during de- and regeneration of the axon-oligodendrocyte-myelin compartment, and to develop effective MS treatment options, the following are required: (i) novel, dynamic technical platforms to investigate complex cell–cell interactions in a CNS-like microenvironment such as the oligodendrocyte-nanofiber platform described by Enz and colleagues [11]; (ii) unbiased evaluation systems to monitor disease progression and successful therapeutic interventions in pre-clinical models such as those described by Zhan an colleagues [12], Joost and colleagues [13], and Hochstrasser and colleagues [14]; and (iii) novel imaging modalities which would allow longitudinal studies as described by Khodanovich and colleagues [15]. Of note, a better understanding of the axon-oligodendrocyte-myelin compartment might lead to restorative therapies not just in MS but also other neuronal disorders such as Down Syndrome (reviewed by Reiche and colleagues [16]) or schizophrenia (reviewed by Raabe and colleagues [17]).

In this Special Issue, two papers address key regulators of oligodendrocyte development. Nocita and colleagues demonstrate, by using oligodendrocyte cell lines in combination with electrospun polystyrene microfibers as synthetic axons, that the pro-myelinating drugs Clobetasol and Gefitinib promote oligodendrocyte differentiation by G-protein-coupled seven-pass transmembrane receptor Smoothened (Smo) and EGFR/ErbB inhibition [18]. Another paper focuses on a rare genetic disorder called Williams–Beuren syndrome, which is caused by the deletion of genetic material from a specific region of chromosome 7. The deleted region includes up to 28 genes among the *Nsun5* gene, encoding a cytosine-5 RNA methyltransferase. This condition is characterized by mild to moderate intellectual disability or learning problems, unique personality characteristics, distinctive facial features and heart and blood vessel (cardiovascular) problems. The brains of patients suffering from Williams–Beuren syndrome show several oligodendrocyte-myelin abnormalities including a reduced myelin thickness, lower mature oligodendrocyte cell numbers and reduced mRNA levels of myelination-related genes. Yuan and colleagues report that a single-gene knockout of *Nsun5* in mice results in a reduced volume of the corpus callosum, paralleled by a decline in the number of myelinated axons and ultrastructural abnormalities of the myelin sheath [19]. Beyond this, the authors found that *Nsun5* was highly expressed in oligodendrocyte progenitor cells and *Nsun5*-KO mice show reduced oligodendrocyte progenitor cell proliferation, suggesting that *Nsun5* regulates the cell cycle in developing oligodendrocytes.

Another protein highly expressed during oligodendrocyte development is the low-density lipoprotein receptor-related protein 1 (LRP1), a transmembrane receptor, mediating endocytosis and activating intracellular signaling cascades. Schäfer and colleagues generated a novel inducible conditional knockout mouse model, which enabled an NG2-restricted LRP1 deficiency [20]. Although the underlying pathways are not yet characterized, LRP1 appears to be a regulator of oligodendrocyte progenitor cell survival.

The mechanisms underlying the progressive neurodegeneration in MS are currently unknown, but failure of remyelination appears to play a major role. Remyelination is a very complex biological process and can be classified, at the cellular level, as four consecutive steps: (i) proliferation of oligodendrocyte progenitor cells; (ii) oligodendrocyte progenitor cell migration towards the demyelinated axons; (iii) oligodendrocyte progenitor cell differentiation; and, finally, (iv) interaction of the premature oligodendrocyte with the naked axon (i.e., axon wrapping) [21]. The existence of so-called "shadow plaques" in post-mortem brains of MS patients, representing remyelinated lesions, clearly demonstrates that complete repair of MS plaques is principally possible, although it is more common to observe only limited repair at the edge of lesions [22,23]. It is not clear why in some patients remyelination is widespread while in others it is sparse, but aging might well play an important role. Gingele and colleagues demonstrate in their work, using the cuprizone model, that myelin repair and the repopulation of oligodendrocytes is less effective in aged compared to young mice [24], implicating that the regenerative potential of the CNS decreases during aging. Beyond this, this work provides a protocol to induce reproducible demyelination in aged mice, allowing the development of remyelination-promoting therapies in a disease-relevant experimental setting. By using the same model, Nyamoya and colleagues demonstrate that laquinimod, a substance previously shown to protect mature oligodendrocytes against metabolic insults, supports myelin repair in a non-supportive environment [25]. There is a growing list of drugs for relapsing remitting MS, and most of these drugs act by reducing the adaptive immune system. Treatments which promote remyelination would offer the potential to delay, prevent or reverse disability, and numerous pre-clinical as well as clinical studies currently focus on this highly relevant topic.

To understand the physiology and pathology of the oligodendrocyte-myelin unit needs, on the one hand, a better understanding of the oligodendrocyte-intrinsic regulative pathways. On the other hand, cell–cell communication pathways are equally important. While two review articles of this Special Issue focus on the intrinsic regulatory networks of oligodendrocytes [26,27], Erik Nutma's work focuses on the astrocyte–oligodendrocyte crosstalk [28]. In this review article, the authors nicely point out that communication occurs via direct cell–cell contact as well as via secreted cytokines, chemokines, exosomes and signaling molecules. Understanding the pathways involved in this crosstalk will reveal important insights into the pathogenesis and treatment of CNS diseases. One candidate protein implicated in this cell–cell communication network might be the Transient receptor potential ankyrin 1 (TRPA1) receptor, as described by Krizta and colleagues in this Issue [29]. The conditional deletion of *Trpa1* in *Gfap*-expressing astrocytes delayed toxin-induced demyelination in the cuprizone model.

Currently, MS is considered a multifactorial disorder, with substantial evidence for a role of both genetic and environmental factors. Several lifestyle changes might help to ameliorate the MS disease course, of which are physical and mental exercise [30], which can induce remyelination, or quitting smoking to ameliorate oxidative and nitroxidative stress [31]. In this context, the work published by Serdar and colleagues is of interest. The authors were able to demonstrate that caffeine and taurine, ingredients of energy drinks, induce degeneration of the axon-oligodendrocyte-myelin unit [32]. Considering the continuously rising number of children and adolescents consuming energy drinks, and the fact that brain development is vulnerable in this phase of life, a closer look at particular lifestyle changes might tell us a lot about MS and other neuronal disorders.

The disease which comes first to our minds when thinking about oligodendrocyte pathology is, quite often, multiple sclerosis. As outlined, the destruction of the axon-oligodendrocyte-myelin unit is the key pathological feature of MS. However, several other diseases can be linked to oligodendrocyte pathology. Primarily, these are the leukodystrophies, a group of usually inherited disorders characterized by degeneration of the white matter in the brain. Examples are metachromatic leukodystrophies, Canavan disease or X-linked adrenoleukodystrophy. Beyond this, the de- and regeneration of oligodendrocytes appears to be an important pathological aspect of many other neuronal disorders including spinal cord injury, where remyelination improves functional recovery [33], Alzheimer's disease, where myelination-related processes are recurrently perturbed in multiple cell types, suggesting that myelination has a key role in Alzheimer's disease pathophysiology [34], or stroke, where it is believed that oligodendrocyte progenitor cells can promote angiogenesis [35]. Beyond this, it has recently been suggested that cells of the oligodendrocyte lineage can transform, under specific conditions, into antigen-presenting cells, suggesting that oligodendrocytes can act as active immunomodulators [36].

In summary, this Special Issue adds to our understanding of a central CNS cell population: oligodendrocytes.

References

1. Armati, P.; Mathey, E. *The Biology of Oligodendrocytes*; Cambridge University Press: Cambridge, UK, 2010.
2. Jäkel, S.; Dimou, L. Glial cells and their function in the adult brain: A journey through the history of their ablation. *Front. Cell. Neurosci.* **2017**, *11*, 24. [CrossRef] [PubMed]
3. Bradl, M.; Lassmann, H. Oligodendrocytes: Biology and pathology. *Acta Neuropathol.* **2010**, *119*, 37–53. [CrossRef] [PubMed]
4. Caprariello, A.V.; Mangla, S.; Miller, R.H.; Selkirk, S.M. Apoptosis of oligodendrocytes in the central nervous system results in rapid focal demyelination. *Ann. Neurol.* **2012**, *72*, 395–405. [CrossRef] [PubMed]
5. Traka, M.; Podojil, J.R.; McCarthy, D.P.; Miller, S.D.; Popko, B. Oligodendrocyte death results in immune-mediated CNS demyelination. *Nat. Neurosci.* **2016**, *19*, 65–74. [CrossRef]
6. Popescu, B.F.G.; Pirko, I.; Lucchinetti, C.F. Pathology of multiple sclerosis: Where do we stand? *CONTIN. Lifelong Learn. Neurol.* **2013**, *19*, 901. [CrossRef]

7. DeLuca, G.; Williams, K.; Evangelou, N.; Ebers, G.; Esiri, M. The contribution of demyelination to axonal loss in multiple sclerosis. *Brain* **2006**, *129*, 1507–1516. [CrossRef]
8. Funfschilling, U.; Supplie, L.M.; Mahad, D.; Boretius, S.; Saab, A.S.; Edgar, J.; Brinkmann, B.G.; Kassmann, C.M.; Tzvetanova, I.D.; Mobius, W.; et al. Glycolytic oligodendrocytes maintain myelin and long-term axonal integrity. *Nature* **2012**, *485*, 517–521. [CrossRef]
9. Edgar, J.M.; McLaughlin, M.; Yool, D.; Zhang, S.C.; Fowler, J.H.; Montague, P.; Barrie, J.A.; McCulloch, M.C.; Duncan, I.D.; Garbern, J.; et al. Oligodendroglial modulation of fast axonal transport in a mouse model of hereditary spastic paraplegia. *J. Cell Biol.* **2004**, *166*, 121–131. [CrossRef]
10. Uschkureit, T.; Sporkel, O.; Stracke, J.; Bussow, H.; Stoffel, W. Early onset of axonal degeneration in double (plp-/-mag-/-) and hypomyelinosis in triple (plp-/-mbp-/-mag-/-) mutant mice. *J. Neurosci.* **2000**, *20*, 5225–5233. [CrossRef]
11. Enz, L.S.; Zeis, T.; Hauck, A.; Linington, C.; Schaeren-Wiemers, N. Combinatory Multifactor Treatment Effects on Primary Nanofiber Oligodendrocyte Cultures. *Cells* **2019**, *8*, 1422. [CrossRef]
12. Zhan, J.; Yakimov, V.; Rühling, S.; Fischbach, F.; Nikolova, E.; Joost, S.; Kaddatz, H.; Greiner, T.; Frenz, J.; Holzmann, C.; et al. High Speed Ventral Plane Videography as a Convenient Tool to Quantify Motor Deficits during Pre-Clinical Experimental Autoimmune Encephalomyelitis. *Cells* **2019**, *8*, 1439. [CrossRef] [PubMed]
13. Joost, S.; Mikkat, S.; Wille, M.; Schümann, A.; Schmitt, O. Membrane Protein Identification in Rodent Brain Tissue Samples and Acute Brain Slices. *Cells* **2019**, *8*, 423. [CrossRef] [PubMed]
14. Hochstrasser, T.; Rühling, S.; Hecher, K.; Fabisch, K.H.; Chrzanowski, U.; Brendel, M.; Eckenweber, F.; Sacher, C.; Schmitz, C.; Kipp, M. Stereological Investigation of Regional Brain Volumes after Acute and Chronic Cuprizone-Induced Demyelination. *Cells* **2019**, *8*, 1024. [CrossRef]
15. Khodanovich, M.; Pishchelko, A.; Glazacheva, V.; Pan, E.; Akulov, A.; Svetlik, M.; Tyumentseva, Y.; Anan'ina, T.; Yarnykh, V. Quantitative Imaging of White and Gray Matter Remyelination in the Cuprizone Demyelination Model Using the Macromolecular Proton Fraction. *Cells* **2019**, *8*, 1204. [CrossRef]
16. Reiche, L.; Küry, P.; Göttle, P. Aberrant Oligodendrogenesis in Down Syndrome: Shift in Gliogenesis? *Cells* **2019**, *8*, 1591. [CrossRef] [PubMed]
17. Raabe, F.J.; Slapakova, L.; Rossner, M.J.; Cantuti-Castelvetri, L.; Simons, M.; Falkai, P.G.; Schmitt, A. Oligodendrocytes as A New Therapeutic Target in Schizophrenia: From Histopathological Findings to Neuron-Oligodendrocyte Interaction. *Cells* **2019**, *8*, 1496. [CrossRef] [PubMed]
18. Nocita, E.; Del Giovane, A.; Tiberi, M.; Boccuni, L.; Fiorelli, D.; Sposato, C.; Romano, E.; Basoli, F.; Trombetta, M.; Rainer, A.; et al. EGFR/ErbB Inhibition Promotes OPC Maturation up to Axon Engagement by Co-Regulating PIP2 and MBP. *Cells* **2019**, *8*, 844. [CrossRef]
19. Yuan, Z.; Chen, P.; Zhang, T.; Shen, B.; Chen, L. Agenesis and Hypomyelination of Corpus Callosum in Mice Lacking Nsun5, an RNA Methyltransferase. *Cells* **2019**, *8*, 552. [CrossRef]
20. Schäfer, I.; Kaisler, J.; Scheller, A.; Kirchhoff, F.; Haghikia, A.; Faissner, A. Conditional Deletion of LRP1 Leads to Progressive Loss of Recombined NG2-Expressing Oligodendrocyte Precursor Cells in a Novel Mouse Model. *Cells* **2019**, *8*, 1550. [CrossRef]
21. Kipp, M.; Amor, S. FTY720 on the way from the base camp to the summit of the mountain: Relevance for remyelination. *Mult. Scler. J.* **2012**, *18*, 258–263. [CrossRef]
22. Prineas, J.W.; Connell, F. Remyelination in multiple sclerosis. *Ann. Neurol.* **1979**, *5*, 22–31. [CrossRef] [PubMed]
23. Prineas, J.W.; Barnard, R.O.; Kwon, E.E.; Sharer, L.R.; Cho, E.S. Multiple sclerosis: Remyelination of nascent lesions. *Ann. Neurol.* **1993**, *33*, 137–151. [CrossRef] [PubMed]
24. Gingele, S.; Henkel, F.; Heckers, S.; Moellenkamp, T.M.; Hümmert, M.W.; Skripuletz, T.; Stangel, M.; Gudi, V. Delayed Demyelination and Impaired Remyelination in Aged Mice in the Cuprizone Model. *Cells* **2020**, *9*, 945. [CrossRef] [PubMed]
25. Nyamoya, S.; Steinle, J.; Chrzanowski, U.; Kaye, J.; Schmitz, C.; Beyer, C.; Kipp, M. Laquinimod Supports Remyelination in Non-Supportive Environments. *Cells* **2019**, *8*, 1363. [CrossRef]
26. Kuhn, S.; Gritti, L.; Crooks, D.; Dombrowski, Y. Oligodendrocytes in Development, Myelin Generation and Beyond. *Cells* **2019**, *8*, 1424. [CrossRef]
27. Tiane, A.; Schepers, M.; Rombaut, B.; Hupperts, R.; Prickaerts, J.; Hellings, N.; van den Hove, D.; Vanmierlo, T. From OPC to Oligodendrocyte: An Epigenetic Journey. *Cells* **2019**, *8*, 1236. [CrossRef]

28. Nutma, E.; van Gent, D.; Amor, S.; Peferoen, L.A.N. Astrocyte and Oligodendrocyte Cross-Talk in the Central Nervous System. *Cells* **2020**, *9*, 600. [CrossRef]
29. Kriszta, G.; Nemes, B.; Sándor, Z.; Ács, P.; Komoly, S.; Berente, Z.; Bölcskei, K.; Pintér, E. Investigation of Cuprizone-Induced Demyelination in mGFAP-Driven Conditional Transient Receptor Potential Ankyrin 1 (TRPA1) Receptor Knockout Mice. *Cells* **2019**, *9*, 81. [CrossRef]
30. Jensen, S.K.; Michaels, N.J.; Ilyntskyy, S.; Keough, M.B.; Kovalchuk, O.; Yong, V.W. Multimodal Enhancement of Remyelination by Exercise with a Pivotal Role for Oligodendroglial PGC1α. *Cell Rep.* **2018**, *24*, 3167–3179. [CrossRef]
31. Tobore, T.O. Oxidative/Nitroxidative Stress and Multiple Sclerosis. *J. Mol. Neurosci.* **2020**, 1–9. [CrossRef]
32. Serdar, M.; Mordelt, A.; Müser, K.; Kempe, K.; Felderhoff-Müser, U.; Herz, J.; Bendix, I. Detrimental Impact of Energy Drink Compounds on Developing Oligodendrocytes and Neurons. *Cells* **2019**, *8*, 1381. [CrossRef]
33. Nagoshi, N.; Khazaei, M.; Ahlfors, J.E.; Ahuja, C.S.; Nori, S.; Wang, J.; Shibata, S.; Fehlings, M.G. Human Spinal Oligodendrogenic Neural Progenitor Cells Promote Functional Recovery After Spinal Cord Injury by Axonal Remyelination and Tissue Sparing. *Stem Cells Transl. Med.* **2018**, *7*, 806–818. [CrossRef] [PubMed]
34. Mathys, H.; Davila-Velderrain, J.; Peng, Z.; Gao, F.; Mohammadi, S.; Young, J.Z.; Menon, M.; He, L.; Abdurrob, F.; Jiang, X.; et al. Single-cell transcriptomic analysis of Alzheimer's disease. *Nature* **2019**, *570*, 332–337. [CrossRef] [PubMed]
35. Kishida, N.; Maki, T.; Takagi, Y.; Yasuda, K.; Kinoshita, H.; Ayaki, T.; Noro, T.; Kinoshita, Y.; Ono, Y.; Kataoka, H.; et al. Role of Perivascular Oligodendrocyte Precursor Cells in Angiogenesis After Brain Ischemia. *J. Am. Heart Assoc.* **2019**, *8*, e011824. [CrossRef]
36. Falcão, A.M.; van Bruggen, D.; Marques, S.; Meijer, M.; Jäkel, S.; Agirre, E.; Samudyata; Floriddia, E.M.; Vanichkina, D.P.; Ffrench-Constant, C.; et al. Disease-specific oligodendrocyte lineage cells arise in multiple sclerosis. *Nat. Med.* **2018**, *24*, 1837–1844. [CrossRef]

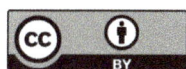

© 2020 by the author. Licensee MDPI, Basel, Switzerland. This article is an open access article distributed under the terms and conditions of the Creative Commons Attribution (CC BY) license (http://creativecommons.org/licenses/by/4.0/).

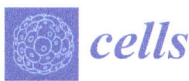

Article

Membrane Protein Identification in Rodent Brain Tissue Samples and Acute Brain Slices

Sarah Joost [1], Stefan Mikkat [2], Michael Wille [1], Antje Schümann [1] and Oliver Schmitt [1,*]

[1] Institute of Anatomy, University Medical Center Rostock, 18057 Rostock, Germany; Sarah.Joost@med.uni-rostock.de (S.J.); michael-wille@gmx.de (M.W.); antje.schuemann@uni-rostock.de (A.S.)
[2] Core Facility Proteome Analysis, University Medical Center Rostock, 18057 Rostock, Germany; stefan.mikkat@med.uni-rostock.de
* Correspondence: schmitt@med.uni-rostock.de

Received: 11 April 2019; Accepted: 8 May 2019; Published: 8 May 2019

Abstract: Acute brain slices are a sample format for electrophysiology, disease modeling, and organotypic cultures. Proteome analyses based on mass spectrometric measurements are seldom used on acute slices, although they offer high-content protein analyses and explorative approaches. In neuroscience, membrane proteins are of special interest for proteome-based analysis as they are necessary for metabolic, electrical, and signaling functions, including myelin maintenance and regeneration. A previously published protocol for the enrichment of plasma membrane proteins based on aqueous two-phase polymer systems followed by mass spectrometric protein identification was adjusted to the small sample size of single acute murine slices from newborn animals and the reproducibility of the results was analyzed. For this, plasma membrane proteins of 12 acute slice samples from six animals were enriched and analyzed by liquid chromatography-mass spectrometry. A total of 1161 proteins were identified, of which 369 were assigned to membranes. Protein abundances showed high reproducibility between samples. The plasma membrane protein separation protocol can be applied to single acute slices despite the low sample size and offers a high yield of identifiable proteins. This is not only the prerequisite for proteome analysis of organotypic slice cultures but also allows for the analysis of small-sized isolated brain regions at the proteome level.

Keywords: plasma membrane proteins; liquid chromatography-mass spectrometry; murine acute brain slices; reproducibility; rat cerebellum

1. Introduction

Acute brain slices are an important sample format in neuroscience [1]. The 300–500 μm thick acute slices of rodent brains are the basis, among other things, for organotypic slice cultures [2], electrophysiological applications [3], as well as functional local synaptic circuitry analyses. Organotypic brain slice cultures are an ex vivo model for maintaining the three-dimensional structure of rodent brain tissue in culture over weeks [4]. They can be easily manipulated, and neuronal as well as glial cell types are available for almost all commonly used analytical options in these cultures. An exception is mass spectrometry (MS)-based proteome analyses, which are hardly ever applied to single brain slices, probably due to the small sample mass of one single acute slice or even a subregion of an acute slice. However, MS-based protein identification and quantification allows for the determination of complex quantitative protein profiles for differential or explorative analyses. Only a few studies were performed on the proteome of single slices. Bowling and colleagues [5] analyzed the stimulus-triggered protein synthesis in acute hippocampal slices. In different studies, plasma membrane proteins were extracted by biotinylation and streptavidin-pulldown and subsequently identified by MS in proof-of-principle approaches from slices of the visual cortex [6] and the hippocampus [7].

Plasma membrane proteins turn out to be of special interest in neuroscience as they comprise ion channels, neurotransmitter receptors, ion transporters, and many more sizeable protein classes with particular importance on neuronal functions [8,9]. Furthermore, the myelin sheaths in the central nervous system are formed by the differentiated plasma membrane of a myelinating glial cell, the oligodendrocyte, which is involved in many pathological processes, including immune-mediated destruction or metabolic-induced cell stress. For the specific enrichment of plasma membrane proteins, several methods were reported that are either based on chemical labeling of membrane proteins or on macromolecular and physicochemical properties of the plasma membrane itself [10]. In the first case, different labeling strategies with biotin followed by streptavidin-pulldown are widely employed [11,12]. Particular plasma membrane properties allow for their isolation by differential and density gradient centrifugation [10] and by aqueous polymer two-phase enrichment [13]. This method uses a mixture of dextran and polyethylene glycol (PEG) for the separation of a homogenized cell extract. After mixing, phases settle and thereby separate the different components of the cell extract on the basis of their affinity for either of the two phases, resulting in partition of the plasma membrane to the hydrophobic PEG-enriched top phase [14]. This protocol is efficient in regards to membrane protein enrichment, technical requirements, and costs. However, it is unclear if the protein yield after plasma membrane enrichment from single acute brain slices allows for liquid chromatography (LC)-MS-driven reproducible protein identification and quantification.

In this study, we demonstrate that the enrichment and identification of membrane proteins is feasible and reproducible in single acute brain slices despite the small sample mass.

2. Material and Methods

2.1. Animals

For this study, male adult Wistar rats (P40) and postnatal wild-type C57BL/6 mice (P5) were used. Day of birth was designated P0. Animals were kept at 22 ± 2 °C under a 12 h light/dark cycle with free access to water and standard diet. For rats, each cage (825 cm^2) contained one or two animals, depending on the animal weight. For mice, each cage (363 cm^2) contained one mother with litter. All cages were provided with bedding and nesting material. All animal-related procedures were conducted in accordance with the local ethical guidelines and the German federal animal welfare law (approval number 74.02-kau).

2.2. Tissue Preparation

For dissection of the rat cerebellum, adult rats were euthanized and transcardially perfused with 250 mL sodium chloride solution (0.9%). The cerebellum was dissected, weighed, and shock frozen in liquid nitrogen. Tissue was stored at −80 °C until further use.

For preparation of murine brain slices, postnatal C57BL/6 mice (P5) were decapitated and brains were quickly dissected. The tissue was embedded in 4% agarose and cut in sagittal orientation with a McIllwain tissue chopper (Ted Pella, Redding, CA, USA) into 350 μm thick slices as described in [4]. The cutting planes of all slices were documented and slices were weighed before shock freezing in cryovials in liquid nitrogen. Slices were stored at −80 °C until further use. All slices used in this study originated from the same cutting plane.

2.3. Sample Preparation for Whole Protein Analysis

For homogenization of tissue samples, the following solutions were added to the frozen samples: lysis buffer (9 μL/μg sample, 7 M urea, 2 M thiourea, 65 mM CHAPS hydrate, 70 mM dithiothreitol), 15% ampholytes (40%, Fluka, 39878), protease inhibitor cocktail (cOmplete™, Roche 11836153001, 0.4 μL/μg sample), PepstatinA (0.1 μL/μg sample, 0.1 mg/mL, solved in ethanol), and phenylmethanesulfonyl fluoride (0.1 μL/μg sample, 0.1 M, solved in ethanol). Samples were thawed, shock frozen, rethawed, and homogenized with a hand homogenizer (Wheaton potter and mortar, 2 mL, neolab). Afterwards, samples underwent the following circle five times: 20 s vortexing, 20 s ultrasonic bath, 20 s slewing. By then, the samples should have changed from yellow to transparent. Samples were shock frozen again, rethawed, vortexed for 30 s, and stirred on ice water for 15 min. After vortexing for another 30 s, samples were centrifuged at 17,860× g for 20 min at 4 °C (OptimaTM TLX, rotor TLA 110, Beckman, Brea, CA, USA). Pellet was discarded and the supernatant was stored at −80 °C until further use.

2.4. Plasma Membrane Enrichment

Plasma membrane protein enrichment was performed in accordance with [13]. In brief, an aqueous polymer two-phase system containing polyethylene glycol, dextrane, and Tris (tris(hydroxymethyl)aminomethane) was used for plasma membrane protein enrichment. After thawing, brain tissue was added to the two-phase system and homogenized with a homogenizer (Wheaton potter and mortar, 10 mL, neolab) and by sonification. Afterwards, phase separation was accelerated by centrifugation for 5 min at 1089× g and the resulting top phase was transferred to a fresh bottom phase. To enhance protein yield, the bottom phase was mixed with new top phase, then both phase systems were thoroughly mixed and again separated by centrifugation. These steps were conducted eight times in total. The top phases G and F were pooled. The resulting top phases were diluted 2:1 with 1 M KCl and 15 mM Tris (pH 7.4) and the membrane fraction was sedimented at 233,000× g for 1 h at 4 °C. After washing (twice with 1 M KCl/15 mM Tris (pH 7.4), thrice with 0.2 M Na_2CO_3), pellets were solved in lysis buffer (7 M urea, 2 M thiourea, 32.5 mM CHAPS hydrate, 5 mM dithiothreitol).

2.5. Measurement of Protein Concentration

For measuring protein concentrations, 4 μL of sample (in lysis buffer, see above), protein assay standard for calibration curve (Thermo Scientific, 23208, prediluted 1:5 in lysis buffer, Waltham, MA, USA), or albumin standard as a control (Thermo Scientific, 23210, prediluted 1:5 in lysis buffer) were mixed with 60 μL Pierce 660 nm protein assay reagent (Thermo Scientific, 22660). After incubation for 1 min shaking and 5 min without movement in the dark at room temperature, absorbance at 660 nm was measured in cuvettes for small volumes (Eppendorf Uvette 50–2000 μL) in a UV spectrophotometer (Ultrospec 1100pro, Amersham Bioscience, expanded by Ultrospec adapter, Amersham, UK). The calibration curve was prepared for a protein range of 0.025–0.4 μg/μL. All samples were measured in triplicates. Independent controls (0.08 μg/μL, 0.16 μg/μL, and 0.35 μg/μL albumin standard) were measured repeatedly.

2.6. Two-Dimensional (2D) Gel Electrophoresis

Two-dimensional gel electrophoresis was performed as previously described [15,16]. In brief, for the first dimension, the samples were diluted with rehydration buffer (6 M urea, 2 M thiurea, 32.5 mM CHAPS hydrate, 16.2 mM dithiothreitol (DTT), 2.5% ampholytes (Biochemika, 39878)). A protein mass of 8 μg in 125 μL buffer was added to Immobiline DryStrips (pH 3-10NL, 7 cm, GE Healthcare 17-6001-12). After active rehydration at 20 °C for 12 h, isoelectric focusing was performed in a Protean IEF Cell (Biorad) as follows: linear voltage rise to 300 V for 30 min, hold at 300 V for 30 min, slow voltage rise to 1000 V in 30 min, linear voltage rise to 5000 V in 90 min, hold at 5000 V for 8000 Vh.

Afterwards, stripes were rehydrated in equilibration buffer (4.4 M urea, 50.5 mM sodium dodecyl sulfate (SDS), 25 Vol% glycerol, 2.4 Vol% Tris-HCl buffer pH 8.8) containing 10 mg/mL DTT for 45 min and another 45 min in equilibration buffer with 40 mg/mL iodacetamide. Rehydrated strips were placed on precast stain-free electrophoresis gels (Mini Protean Stain free Gels 12%, BioRad, 4568041), marker (Full Range Rainbow Marker, GE Healthcare, RNP800E) was added, and stripes were overlayed with agarose solution (1% agarose, 30% glycerol, 3.4% separation gel buffer (1.5 M Tris, 14 mM SDS, pH 8.8), 55.5 mM SDS) to improve protein transfer from strip to gel. An electrophoresis chamber (Mini Protean Tetra Cell, Biorad) was filled with running buffer (TGS buffer, Biorad 161-0732) and electrophoresis was performed for 150–180 min at 100 V.

2.7. Silver Staining of 2D Gels

Following electrophoresis, gels were fixated in fixation solution (50% ethanol, 5% acetic acid) for 30 min. Gels were washed twice for 20 min in 50% ethanol and twice in ultrapure water for 5 min. Gels were bathed in sodium thiosulfate solution (2 mg/mL) for 1 min and washed in ultrapure water for 1 min. Afterwards, gels were incubated in silver nitrate solution (1.5 mg/mL) for 20 min and were washed for 1 min in ultrapure water. Then, gels were bathed in developer solution (0.04% formaldehyde 37%, 20 mg/mL sodium carbonate for approx. 1–10 min) until spots were detectable and reaction was stopped with 5% acetic acid. After washing in ultrapure water, gels were digitized with a ProXima 2850 imaging system.

2.8. In-Solution Digestion of Proteins

Samples were reduced with 10 mM DTT, subsequently sonicated for 10 min using a bath sonicator, and loaded onto Microcon YM-30-filter devices (Millipore) to perform filter-aided sample preparation (FASP) according to [17]. The processing steps for detergent removal, alkylation, buffer exchange, and protein digestion comprised two initial washes with urea solution (UA) followed by incubation with 50 mM iodoacetamide (IAA) in UA for 20 min, two washes with UA to deplete IAA, and finally three washes with 50 mM ammonium bicarbonate (ABC), before digestion with trypsin was performed at an enzyme-to-protein ratio of 1:25 in 40 µL of 50 mM ABC at 37 °C for 16 h. Peptides were collected by centrifugation and fresh trypsin solution was added onto the filter for a second digestion for 2 h. After centrifugation, the combined digests were acidified with trifluoroacetic acid (final concentration 0.25%), concentrated by use of a centrifugal evaporator and diluted to a final volume of 20 µL with a solution containing 2% acetonitrile and 0.1% formic acid (FA) in water. Peptide concentration was measured using the Qubit protein assay (Thermo Fisher Scientific, Waltham, MA, USA).

2.9. Analysis by nanoLC-HDMS^E

Liquid chromatography-mass spectrometry analyses were carried out using a nanoAcquity UPLC system (Waters, Manchester, UK) coupled to a Waters Synapt G2-S mass spectrometer as described before by [18]. Mobile phase A contained 0.1% FA in water, and mobile phase B contained 0.1% FA in acetonitrile. Peptide samples corresponding to approximately 200 ng of digested protein were trapped and desalted using a precolumn (nanoAcquity UPLC Symmetry C18, 5 µm, 180 µm × 20 mm, Waters) at a flow rate of 10 µL/min for 4 min with 99.9% A. Peptides were separated on an analytical column (ACQUITY UPLC HSS T3, 1.8 µm, 75 µm × 250 mm, Waters) at a flow rate of 300 nL/min using a gradient from 3% to 32% B over 120 min for mouse samples and a gradient from 3% to 35% B over 90 min for rat samples. The column temperature was maintained at 35 °C. The SYNAPT G2-S instrument was operated in data-independent mode with ion-mobility separation as an additional dimension of separation (referred to as HDMS^E). By executing alternate scans at low and elevated collision energy (CE) of each 0.6 s, information on precursor and fragment ions, respectively, was acquired. In low-energy MS mode, acquisitions were performed at a constant CE of 4 eV, whereas drift time-dependent CE settings [19] were applied in elevated-energy MS mode. As a reference compound, 100 fmol/µL [Glu1]-fibrinopeptide B was delivered at 500 nL/min to the reference sprayer of the NanoLockSpray source. Lock spray was acquired once every 30 s for a 1 s period. Samples were measured once without technical replication.

2.10. NanoLC-HDMS^E Data Processing, Protein Identification, and Quantification

Progenesis QI for Proteomics version 2.0 and 4.1 (Nonlinear Dynamics, Newcastle upon Tyne, UK) was used for raw data processing, protein identification, and label-free quantification of HDMS^E data from rat and mouse samples, respectively. Alignment was performed to compensate for between-run variation in the LC separation. Peak picking parameters included (i) sensitivity set to automatic, and (ii) a maximum ion charge of +4. Peptide and protein identifications were obtained by searching against databases containing 29,799 protein sequences of the *Rattus norvegicus* proteome (UniProt release 2017_03) and 16,970 reviewed protein sequences from *Mus musculus* (UniProt release 2018_04), respectively. Precursor and fragment ion mass tolerances were automatically determined. Two missing cleavage sites were allowed, oxidation of methionine residues was considered as variable modification, and carbamidomethylation of cysteines as fixed modification. The false discovery rate was set to 1%. Peptides were required to be identified by at least three fragment ions and proteins by at least six fragment ions and two peptides. Subsequently, peptide ion data were filtered to retain only peptide ions that met the following criteria: (1) identified at least two times within the dataset (only applied to the mouse data set), (2) ion score greater than or equal to 5.4 and 5.6 for mouse and rat data, respectively, (3) mass error below 13.0 ppm, (4) at least six amino acid residues in length. Only proteins identified by at least two unique peptides were included in the quantitative analysis of the mouse data set. Proteins were quantified by the Hi3 method [20], which uses the sum of signal intensities of the three most intense tryptic peptides of any protein. To estimate the final rate of false peptide identifications, the search was repeated using a shuffled target-decoy database applying identical peptide filtering criteria. Comparing the number of decoy peptides to those identified with the target sequences resulted in a false positive rate of 0.08%. Moreover, the search did not result in any protein identification based on more than one peptide.

The subcellular locations of identified proteins were assigned to their accession numbers using the Uniprot database. For exact reproduction of the analysis of the rat cerebellum [13], information on the subcellular localization of proteins was additionally extracted from the database Genecards.

2.11. Statistical Analysis

Data organization was performed in spreadsheet applications. Statistical analysis was done in SPSS25. ANOVA testing and a Mann–Whitney test were applied to determine sample variances and differences.

3. Results

3.1. Reproducibility of Plasma Membrane Enrichment Protocol

To ensure technical reproducibility of plasma membrane separation and identification of the Schindler protocol [13], the whole procedure was performed using the cerebella of two adult Wistar rats. By means of LC-MS, 1378 proteins were identified by at least one unique peptide (Table S1). The subcellular localizations of these proteins were assigned using the database Genecards (Figure 1). Of the total 1378 proteins, 804 (58%) were assigned to membranes, and 522 proteins (38%) were not assigned to membranes. For 52 proteins (4%), no information on the subcellular localization was available. For comparison, Schindler et al. [13] identified 586 proteins, of which 191 (33%) were assigned to membranes by the use of Genecards. In their original article, Schindler et al. defined a list of selected plasma membrane proteins with neurobiological relevance. Almost all of these proteins were also found in our analysis, as demonstrated in Table 1. Six proteins (Dihydropyridine-sensitive L-type, calcium channel alpha-2/delta subunits, Potassium voltage-gated channel subfamily C member 3, Sodium channel protein type 1 subunit alpha, Sodium bicarbonate cotransporter 3, Electrogenic sodium bicarbonate cotransporter 1, Plasma membrane calcium-transporting ATPase 3) reported in [13] were not shown in Table 1 because they were associated with a protein group and not confirmed by unique peptides in our analysis. In addition, typical membrane proteins that were identified here, but were not described in [13], are introduced in the following. The adhesion G protein-coupled receptor L3 (ADGRL3), which has functions in cell–cell adhesion as well as neuron guidance and is necessary for the development of glutamatergic synapses in the cortex, was identified in different samples. A further example is the ciliary neurotrophic factor receptor subunit alpha (CNTFR), which binds the neurotrophin CNTF. CNTF promotes neurotransmitter synthesis and neurite outgrowth in certain neural populations. Beyond this, four gamma-aminobutyric acid (GABA) and glycine transporter proteins were identified. These are sodium- and chloride-dependent GABA transporter 1, sodium- and chloride-dependent GABA transporter 3, sodium- and chloride-dependent glycine transporter 1, and sodium- and chloride-dependent glycine transporter 2. Again, these four transmembrane proteins were not identified by Schindler et al. [13].

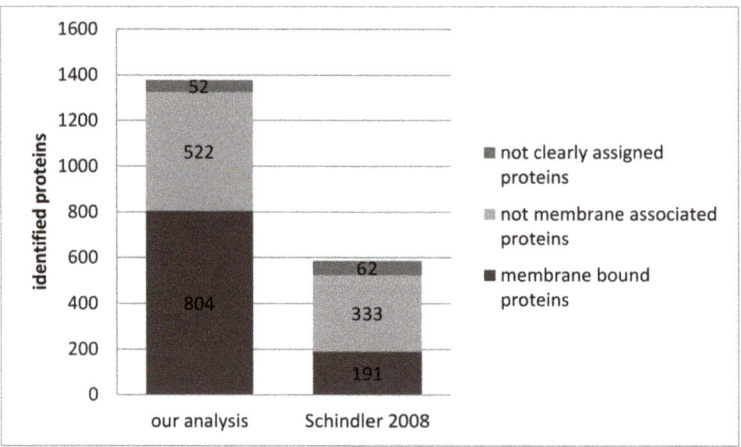

Figure 1. The number of protein identifications in plasma-membrane-enriched samples of rat cerebellum. Plasma membrane proteins were enriched in samples of adult rat cerebellum. Proteins were identified with LC-MS. Subcellular protein localization was assigned with aid of the database Genecards.

Excerpt of identified membrane proteins from Schindler et al. [13]. The Swiss-Prot primary accession number, protein names, the number of transmembrane helices (TMH), and the number of identified peptides per protein in Schindler's analysis (pep) [13] and in our analysis (A/B: sample A/B) are listed. Seven proteins that were identified in Schindler et al. have not been identified in our samples and, therefore, are not shown in this table. Six proteins that were associated with a protein group but not confirmed by unique peptides in our analysis were also not included.

3.2. Protein Analysis in Single Acute Slices

For all subsequent experiments, acute slices were prepared from 5-day-old C57BL/6 mice (Figure 2A). As our group strives for analyses of the proteome of organotypic slices during culture, slices for this study were prepared in the very same way as slices for organotypic culturing. Slices were cut sagittally at a thickness of 350 μm and weighed between 9 and 19 mg. To ensure that the protein mass of one single slice is sufficient for protein-based analysis approaches, we performed 2D gel electrophoresis of the whole protein fraction of single slices (Figure 2B). It turned out that the protein mass of a single slice is sufficient to perform a 2D gel electrophoresis. The distribution of protein spots in the resulting gels demonstrated the availability of proteins over the complete isoelectric point (pI) range from 3 to 11 as well as the protein size range from 10 kDa to 225 kDa.

Table 1. Comparison of cerebellar protein identifications.

Accession		TMH	Schindler et al.	Our Analysis	
	Neurotransmitter Release		pep	A	B
P61765	Syntaxin-binding protein 1	0	30	43	43
Q9WU70	Syntaxin-binding protein 5	1	1	4	4
P32851	Syntaxin-1A	1	6	4	4
P61265	Syntaxin-1B2	1	21	17	16
P60881	Synaptosomal-associated protein 25	0	19	19	19
	Neurotransmitter Receptors				
P19490	Glutamate receptor 1	5	3	9	9
Q63226	Glutamate receptor delta-2 subunit	3	6	28	29
P23385	Metabotropic glutamate receptor 1	8	6	23	17
Q9Z0U4	Gamma-aminobutyric acid type B receptor, subunit 1	8	3	8	6
O88871	Gamma-aminobutyric acid type B receptor, subunit 2	8	2	10	10
P62813	Gamma-aminobutyric-acid receptor alpha-1 subunit	5	5	4	4
P30191	Gamma-aminobutyric-acid receptor alpha-6 subunit	4	0	8	7
P63138	Gamma-aminobutyric-acid receptor subunit beta-2	5	5	3	3
P18506	Gamma-aminobutyric-acid receptor delta subunit	5	2	3	3
P18508	Gamma-aminobutyric-acid receptor gamma-2 subunit	5	3	0	1
	Neurotransmitter Reuptake				
P31662	Orphan sodium- and chloride-dependent neurotransmitter transporter NTT4	11	12	5	5
P23978	Sodium- and chloride-dependent GABA transporter 1	12	5	5	7
P31647	Sodium- and chloride-dependent GABA transporter 3	11	8	6	5
P28572	Sodium- and chloride-dependent glycine transporter 1	12	4	4	4
P24942	Excitatory amino acid transporter 1	10	14	8	7
P31596	Excitatory amino acid transporter 2	11	12	9	7
O35921	Excitatory amino acid transporter 4	8	7	7	6
	Ion Channels				
Q9Z2L0	Voltage-dependent anion-selective channel protein 1	0	9	12	11
P10499	Potassium voltage-gated channel subfamily A member 1	6	4	1	1
P25122	Potassium voltage-gated channel subfamily C member 1	7	4	3	3
P04775	Sodium channel protein type 2 subunit alpha	24	8	3	3
Q00954	Sodium channel beta-1 subunit	2	1	2	2
P54900	Sodium channel beta-2 subunit	2	5	4	5
	Transporters				
Q9JHZ9	System N amino acid transporter 1	10	2	0	1
P11167	Solute carrier family 2, facilitated glucose transporter member 1	11	3	3	2
Q8VII6	Choline transporter-like protein 1	10	1	1	0
Q63016	Large neutral amino acids transporter small subunit 1	14	3	5	5
Q63633	Solute carrier family 12 member 5	12	12	17	15
P11505	Plasma membrane calcium-transporting ATPase 1	9	23	13	19
P11506	Plasma membrane calcium-transporting ATPase 2	9	36	2	3
Q64542	Plasma membrane calcium-transporting ATPase 4	11	13	10	9
P06685	Sodium/potassium-transporting ATPase alpha-1 chain	8	42	29	28
P06686	Sodium/potassium-transporting ATPase alpha-2 chain	8	48	28	28
P06687	Sodium/potassium-transporting ATPase alpha-3 chain	8	50	32	32
P07340	Sodium/potassium-transporting ATPase subunit beta-1	1	14	15	15
P13638	Sodium/potassium-transporting ATPase subunit beta-2	1	10	8	9
Q63377	Sodium/potassium-transporting ATPase subunit beta-3	1	5	7	7
P53987	Monocarboxylate transporter 1	12	2	4	5
Q01728	Sodium/calcium exchanger 1	11	3	4	4
P48768	Sodium/calcium exchanger 2	11	11	14	15

Single acute slices were then processed for plasma membrane enrichment following the protocol of Schindler et al. [13]. Performing this protocol with single slice samples proved to be challenging because pellets after ultracentrifugation of the enriched membrane fraction were not visible due to their small size. Furthermore, protein concentration measurements had to be adjusted to small sample sizes and low protein concentrations. As illustrated in Figure 3A, protein concentrations of processed samples ranged between 0.04 and 0.09 µg/µL, corresponding to an available protein amount of about 3–6 µg for subsequent MS analyses. Accuracy of the protein concentration measurements was ensured by determining the protein concentration of every sample three times. The standard error of the mean of protein concentration measurements from the same samples was considerably small and did not exceed 0.007. For visualization of protein content of the processed slice samples, 2D gel electrophoresis was performed (Figure 3B). Protein spots were distributed over the complete analyzed pI and protein size range. However, the 2D gel also showed that samples after plasma membrane enrichment contained a significant amount of proteins not intrinsic to membranes because hydrophobic membrane proteins are typically not resolved by 2D gel electrophoresis.

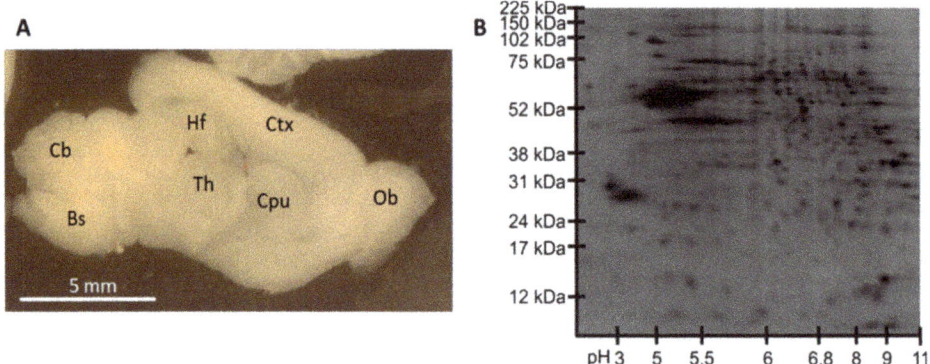

Figure 2. Protein analysis in single acute slices. (**A**) Acute slices were prepared from 5-day-old C57BL/6 mice. Sagittally cut slices contained cortex (Ctx), hippocampal formation (Hf), thalamus (Th), caudate–putamen complex (Cpu), olfactory bulb (OB), cerebellum (Cb), and brain stem (Bs). (**B**) Two-dimensional protein separation of the whole-protein fraction of one single acute slice demonstrated abundance of various proteins over a large protein weight and pI range.

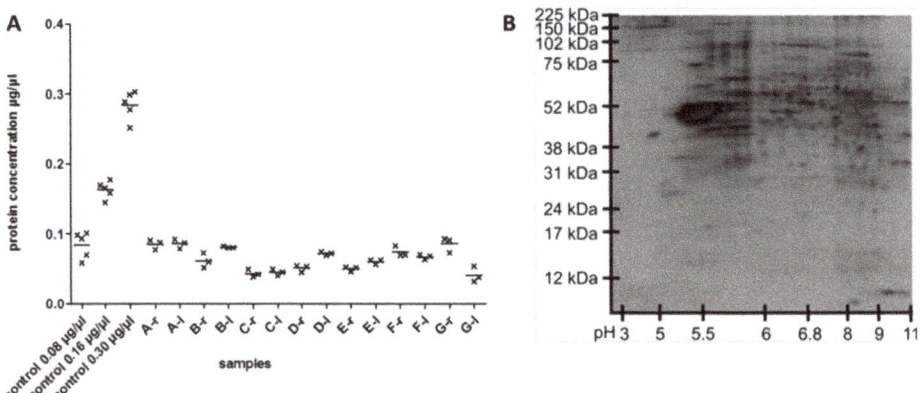

Figure 3. Protein content after membrane protein enrichment in single acute slices. (**A**) Protein concentrations after membrane protein enrichment in single slice samples. Samples were termed after the animal (letter) and originate from right or left hemispheres (r or l). Protein concentration was determined three times per sample. (**B**) Two-dimensional protein separation after membrane protein enrichment of one single acute slice demonstrated abundance of various proteins over a large protein weight and pI range.

3.3. Plasma Membrane Protein Separation in Single Acute Slices

For evaluation of the reproducibility of the plasma membrane separation protocol in single slices, acute slices from seven animals were chosen for MS analysis. Per animal, one slice per hemisphere from the same cutting plane was processed. By means of LS-MS, an average of 8000 peptides was identified. A total of 1161 proteins was identified by at least two peptides (Table S2), while 248 proteins were identified by only one peptide and, therefore, were excluded from analysis due to insufficient specificity of identification and quantification. One sample showed considerably lower protein concentration (sample G-l in Figure 3A) and peptide as well as protein identifications. This sample and the corresponding sample from the same animal were excluded from analysis.

Protein localizations were assessed with the aid of Uniprot. A total of 369 proteins (32%) were assigned to membranes, 612 proteins (53%) were assigned to other subcellular compartments, while no localization information was available in Uniprot for 180 proteins (16%) (Figure 4).

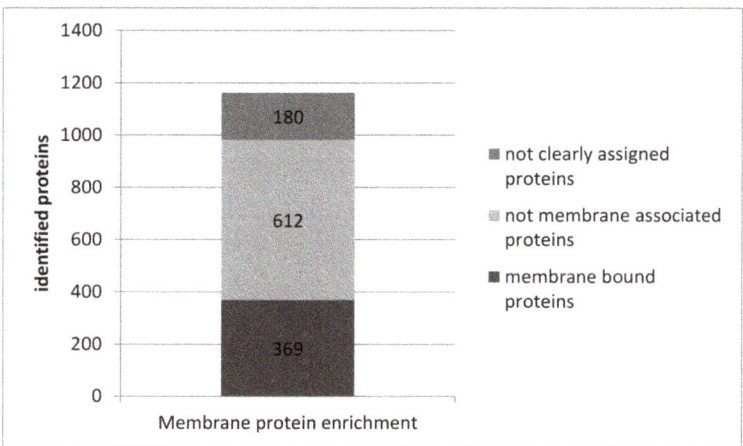

Figure 4. The number of protein identifications in plasma-membrane-enriched samples of single acute slices. Plasma membrane proteins were enriched in samples of single murine acute slices. Proteins were identified with LC-MS. Subcellular protein localization was assigned with aid of the database Uniprot.

For evaluation of constancy of abundance measurements in the 12 samples, the difference between the minimal and maximal mean abundance per animal was calculated for each protein and expressed as fold-change (Table S2). Furthermore, ANOVA testing was performed to analyze if abundances of all samples were significantly different. For 164 proteins, the fold change between maximal and minimal abundance was larger than 2. Seventy-eight of these proteins also had a p-value < 0.05 and therefore were supposed to be significantly different. Regarding all proteins, 762 out of 1161 showed a p-value > 0.05 after ANOVA and therefore showed no significant variability (Table S2).

We hypothesized that the amounts of identified proteins were comparable in all samples since they all originated from comparable animals and the same cutting planes. So, the variance of abundances from all 12 samples was calculated for every identified protein. Variances of single slice samples were 0.091 ± 0.053 on average. Furthermore, we assumed that, due to interindividual differences between the animals, slices from different animals would vary more in their protein amounts than slices from the same animal. Hence, the mean abundance from both samples of an animal was determined and then the variances of these means for every identified protein were calculated. The overall average variance of single animal protein amounts was 0.168 ± 0.095 on average. This analysis demonstrated that variance of the samples from individual animals was significantly higher than variance of all samples ($p < 0.0001$, Figure 5A).

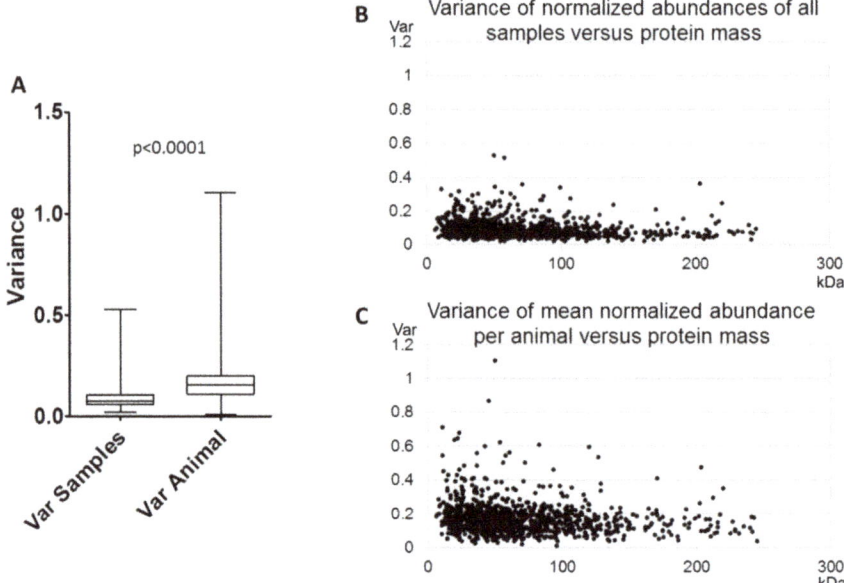

Figure 5. Variance of normalized protein abundance in single acute slices. (**A**) For each identified protein, the variance of normalized abundances for all samples was calculated (Var Samples) as well as the variance of the mean protein abundances per animal (Var Animal). (**B**) The variances of normalized abundances of all samples were plotted against the weight of the respective protein. No correlation was found (r = −0.14744). (**C**) The variances of the mean normalized abundances per animal were plotted against the weight of the respective protein. No correlation was found (r = 0.13419).

Furthermore, variances were plotted against the protein weight of the respective proteins. The distribution of variances between samples showed a lower variability (Figure 5B) than between (Figure 5C) animals. No correlation was found between variances of single samples and protein mass nor between variances of animals and protein mass (Pearson correlation test, r = −0.14744, respectively r = 0.13419, Figure 5B).

The identified proteins of the membrane protein enrichment procedure in the rat cerebellum were compared with the myelin proteome of Jahn et al. [21] to prove coincidence with proteins of the myelin proteome, respectively, oligodendrocyte compartment. Interestingly, we found 35 proteins in our membrane protein enrichment samples of the rat cerebellum that were also described in the myelin proteome: 14-3-3 protein epsilon, 14-3-3 protein eta, 14-3-3 protein gamma, 14-3-3 protein theta, annexin A6, calnexin, clathrin heavy chain, cofilin 2, destrin, elongation factor 2, gelsolin, glial fibrillary acidic protein, glucose-6-phosphate isomerase, glutamine synthetase, heat shock 70 kDa protein 1B, heat shock 70 kDa protein 4, macrophage migration inhibitory factor, moesin, myelin basic protein, myelin proteolipid protein, myelin-associated glycoprotein, neural cell adhesion molecule 1, neural cell adhesion molecule 1, neurofascin, neurotrimin, nucleoside diphosphate kinase A, nucleoside diphosphate kinase B, phosphoglycerate mutase 1, prohibitin, septin 4, synaptophysin, transketolase, triosephosphate isomerase, and vimentin.

4. Discussion

4.1. Reproducibility of the Plasma Membrane Enrichment Protocol

The protocol of Schindler et al. [13] was successfully reproduced with material of the cerebellum of adult Wistar rats (Figure 1, Table S1). A large number of proteins was identified by LC-MS, and more than half of them are assigned to plasma membranes in the database Genecards. In Schindler's original analysis, only half as many proteins could be identified in the same sample tissue, and a considerably smaller amount of them were assigned to membranes. This notable increase in protein identification efficiency most certainly is due to advances in MS technology and the expanded scope of database content during the last decade. The successful reproduction of plasma membrane protein enrichment and identification is the prerequisite for applying the protocol to the small sample volume of single acute murine slices.

4.2. Protein Analysis in Single Acute Slices

Protein-based analyses of single slices are rarely executed due to their small sample volume. We were able to demonstrate that one single acute murine slice provides enough protein for two-dimensional gel electrophoresis. The whole protein fraction of one single slice contains a broad range of sufficiently separable protein spots, indicating the suitability of the sample format of acute slices for protein-based analyses (Figure 2).

Based on this result, plasma membrane protein enrichment was performed on single acute murine slices. We anticipated a considerable loss of protein content due to the high number of processing steps in the protocol (eightfold repetition of phase separation), but the separation of the enriched membrane protein fraction in two-dimensional gel electrophoresis demonstrated a remarkable number of distinct protein spots (Figure 3B).

Since the sample preparation for MS requires the measurement of protein concentration, the protocol for protein measurements needed to be optimized for low sample volumes. Despite the use of small volumes for protein measurement and a comparably low protein concentration range of the standard curve, measurements of protein concentrations were reproducible for all samples measured. The protein concentration of every sample was measured in triplicates, and the low variability of the resulting protein concentrations for each sample proved the applicability of our optimized protein measurement protocol (Figure 3A).

4.3. Membrane Proteins in Single Acute Slices

The MS-based protein identification of membrane protein-enriched single murine slice samples resulted in the identification of 1161 proteins (Table S2). By using the database Uniprot, 369 of these proteins (31.8%) were allocated to membranes (Figure 4). For comparison, the enrichment of membrane proteins in whole rat cerebellum resulted in 804 membrane protein identifications (58.3% of all identified proteins, Figure 1), a remarkably higher yield. However, comparability of both analyses is limited due to samples from different species and different brain regions. Therefore, we consider the yield of membrane proteins from single acute slices as sufficient for further analyses.

The most important prerequisite for the use of MS-based analysis approaches on single slices is reliable reproducibility of the results. For evaluation of this subject, we analyzed slices from seven mice from one litter, two slices per animal, all from the same cutting levels. Out of the 14 samples, one sample yielded insufficient protein concentrations and was excluded from further analysis. We therefore consider the probability of extensive sample loss during membrane protein enrichment as acceptable given the sophisticated enrichment protocol.

For evaluation of reproducibility of MS protein quantification, the variance of normalized abundances of all samples (sample variance) was compared with the variance of the mean normalized abundances per animal (animal variance) (Figure 5). The results show that the animal variance is considerably higher than the sample variance. We conclude that (i) slices from the same animal reliably have comparable protein abundances and that (ii) our method is sensitive enough to detect interindividual differences of protein abundances in single slice samples.

To further evaluate the constancy of protein quantifications in samples from different animals, the fold change between highest and lowest mean abundance per animal for every protein identified was calculated (Table S2). For 14.1% of all identified proteins, a fold change larger than 2 was found. ANOVA testing proved that only 78 of these proteins (6.7% of all identified proteins) showed significant variability of abundances and, therefore, can be considered to be differential. This amount of differentially expressed proteins appears to be realistic because interindividual differences of protein profiles between individuals of inbred mice of the same strain and age physiologically exist.

Taken together, our results prove that the membrane protein profile of single slice samples can be analyzed by LC-MS. The small sample volume constitutes no restriction for reproducible and reliable protein identification and quantification. Since acute brain slices can be analyzed with this method, it can be assumed that cultured organotypic slices also are a suitable sample format for MS-based analysis. This enables studies on the changes of protein profiles over the course of organotypic slices propagation as well as protein expression analyses in various lesion or intoxication models of organotypic slice cultures [22,23]. However, the application of the method is not restricted to slice preparations. Also, small dissected brain areas with minor sample weight can probably be employed for enrichment of plasma membrane proteins and MS protein identification.

The technique of plasma membrane protein enrichment and MS protein identification is now ready for specific differential analyses in neuroscientific research. One example is the investigation of differential protein abundances in models of de- and remyelination in the context of multiple sclerosis. It was shown that 35 proteins of the myelin proteome [21] were also identified by the plasma membrane enrichment approach. Both organotypic slice culture models with demyelinating lesions [24,25] and single topographic regions dissected from murine brains (corpus callosum, cerebellum, spinal cord [26,27]) are difficult to analyze due to their small sample volume and protein mass. However, by the use of our protocol presented in this study, these samples are now accessible for proteome-based investigation.

Supplementary Materials: The following are available online at http://www.mdpi.com/2073-4409/8/5/423/s1. Table S1: Identified proteins after membrane protein enrichment in rat cerebellum, 1378 proteins were identified. Proteins were sorted with regard to number of membrane descriptions. mem: number of words "membrane" in localization description of proteins. Table S2: Identified proteins after membrane protein enrichment in single acute murine slices, 1161 proteins were identified. Proteins were sorted by descending p-values of ANOVA testing for homogeneity between all samples. p: probability error ANOVA testing, Change: fold change between smallest and highest measured mean abundance per animal, mem: number of words "membrane" in localization description of proteins. Samples were named after the animal (letter) and origin from the right or the left hemisphere (r or l).

Author Contributions: Conceptualization, O.S.; Formal Analysis, S.J., S.M., M.W., O.S., and A.S.; Investigation, S.J., S.M., and A.S.; Resources, S.J., O.S.; Data Curation, M.W., O.S.; Writing—Original Draft Preparation, S.J.; Writing—Review & Editing, S.J., S.M., and O.S.; Visualization, S.J. and O.S.; Project Administration, O.S.

Funding: We acknowledge financial support by Deutsche Forschungsgemeinschaft and Universität Rostock/Universitätsmedizin Rostock within the funding programme Open Access Publishing. No further external funding was received.

Conflicts of Interest: The authors declare no conflict of interest.

References

1. Lossi, L.; Merighi, A. The Use of ex Vivo Rodent Platforms in Neuroscience Translational Research with Attention to the 3Rs Philosophy. *Front. Vet. Sci.* **2018**, *5*, 164. [CrossRef] [PubMed]
2. Humpel, C. Organotypic brain slice cultures: A review. *Neuroscience* **2015**, *305*, 86–98. [CrossRef] [PubMed]
3. Phillips, W.S.; Herly, M.; Del Negro, C.A.; Rekling, J.C. Organotypic slice cultures containing the preBötzinger complex generate respiratory-like rhythms. *J. Neurophysiol.* **2016**, *115*, 1063–1070. [CrossRef] [PubMed]
4. Joost, S.; Kobayashi, K.; Wree, A.; Haas, S.J.-P. Optimisation of murine organotypic slice culture preparation for a novel sagittal-frontal co-culture system. *J. Neurosci. Methods* **2017**. [CrossRef]
5. Bowling, H.; Bhattacharya, A.; Zhang, G.; Lebowitz, J.Z.; Alam, D.; Smith, P.T.; Kirshenbaum, K.; Neubert, T.A.; Vogel, C.; Chao, M.V.; et al. BONLAC: A combinatorial proteomic technique to measure stimulus-induced translational profiles in brain slices. *Neuropharmacology* **2016**, *100*, 76–89. [CrossRef] [PubMed]

6. Smolders, K.; Lombaert, N.; Valkenborg, D.; Baggerman, G.; Arckens, L. An effective plasma membrane proteomics approach for small tissue samples. *Sci. Rep.* **2015**, *5*, 10917. [CrossRef] [PubMed]
7. Qiao, R.; Li, S.; Zhou, M.; Chen, P.; Liu, Z.; Tang, M.; Zhou, J. In-depth analysis of the synaptic plasma membrane proteome of small hippocampal slices using an integrated approach. *Neuroscience* **2017**, *353*, 119–132. [CrossRef] [PubMed]
8. Grant, K.J.; Wu, C.C. Advances in neuromembrane proteomics: Efforts towards a comprehensive analysis of membrane proteins in the brain. *Brief. Funct. Genom. Proteom.* **2007**, *6*, 59–69. [CrossRef] [PubMed]
9. Volknandt, W.; Karas, M. Proteomic analysis of the presynaptic active zone. *Exp. Brain Res.* **2012**, *217*, 449–461. [CrossRef]
10. Vuckovic, D.; Dagley, L.F.; Purcell, A.W.; Emili, A. Membrane proteomics by high performance liquid chromatography-tandem mass spectrometry: Analytical approaches and challenges. *Proteomics* **2013**, *13*, 404–423. [CrossRef] [PubMed]
11. Weekes, M.P.; Antrobus, R.; Lill, J.R.; Duncan, L.M.; Hör, S.; Lehner, P.J. Comparative Analysis of Techniques to Purify Plasma Membrane Proteins. *J. Biomol. Tech.* **2010**, *21*, 108–115. [PubMed]
12. Hörmann, K.; Stukalov, A.; Müller, A.C.; Heinz, L.X.; Superti-Furga, G.; Colinge, J.; Bennett, K.L. A Surface Biotinylation Strategy for Reproducible Plasma Membrane Protein Purification and Tracking of Genetic and Drug-Induced Alterations. *J. Proteome Res.* **2016**, *15*, 647–658. [CrossRef] [PubMed]
13. Schindler, J.; Lewandrowski, U.; Sickmann, A.; Friauf, E. Aqueous polymer two-phase systems for the proteomic analysis of plasma membranes from minute brain samples. *J. Proteome Res.* **2008**, *7*, 432–442. [CrossRef]
14. Schindler, J.; Nothwang, H.G. Aqueous polymer two-phase systems: Effective tools for plasma membrane proteomics. *Proteomics* **2006**, *6*, 5409–5417. [CrossRef] [PubMed]
15. Wille, M.; Schumann, A.; Wree, A.; Kreutzer, M.; Glocker, M.O.; Mutzbauer, G.; Schmitt, O. The Proteome Profiles of the Cerebellum of Juvenile, Adult and Aged Rats—An Ontogenetic Study. *Int. J. Mol. Sci.* **2015**, *16*, 21454–21485. [CrossRef]
16. Wille, M.; Schumann, A.; Kreutzer, M.; Glocker, M.O.; Wree, A.; Mutzbauer, G.; Schmitt, O. The proteome profiles of the olfactory bulb of juvenile, adult and aged rats—An ontogenetic study. *Proteome Sci.* **2015**, *13*, 8. [CrossRef] [PubMed]
17. Wiśniewski, J.R.; Zougman, A.; Nagaraj, N.; Mann, M. Universal sample preparation method for proteome analysis. *Nat. Methods* **2009**, *6*, 359–362. [CrossRef] [PubMed]
18. Pappesch, R.; Warnke, P.; Mikkat, S.; Normann, J.; Wisniewska-Kucper, A.; Huschka, F.; Wittmann, M.; Khani, A.; Schwengers, O.; Oehmcke-Hecht, S.; et al. The Regulatory Small RNA MarS Supports Virulence of *Streptococcus pyogenes*. *Sci. Rep.* **2017**, *7*, 12241. [CrossRef]
19. Distler, U.; Kuharev, J.; Navarro, P.; Levin, Y.; Schild, H.; Tenzer, S. Drift time-specific collision energies enable deep-coverage data-independent acquisition proteomics. *Nat. Methods* **2014**, *11*, 167–170. [CrossRef]
20. Silva, J.C.; Gorenstein, M.V.; Li, G.-Z.; Vissers, J.P.C.; Geromanos, S.J. Absolute quantification of proteins by LCMSE: A virtue of parallel MS acquisition. *Mol. Cell Proteom.* **2006**, *5*, 144–156. [CrossRef]
21. Jahn, O.; Tenzer, S.; Werner, H.B. Myelin proteomics: Molecular anatomy of an insulating sheath. *Mol. Neurobiol.* **2009**, *40*, 55–72. [CrossRef]
22. Lenz, M.; Galanis, C.; Kleidonas, D.; Fellenz, M.; Deller, T.; Vlachos, A. Denervated mouse dentate granule cells adjust their excitatory but not inhibitory synapses following in vitro entorhinal cortex lesion. *Exp. Neurol.* **2019**, *312*, 1–9. [CrossRef] [PubMed]
23. Tan, G.A.; Furber, K.L.; Thangaraj, M.P.; Sobchishin, L.; Doucette, J.R.; Nazarali, A.J. Organotypic Cultures from the Adult CNS: A Novel Model to Study Demyelination and Remyelination Ex Vivo. *Cell Mol. Neurobiol.* **2018**, *38*, 317–328. [CrossRef] [PubMed]
24. Birgbauer, E.; Rao, T.S.; Webb, M. Lysolecithin induces demyelination in vitro in a cerebellar slice culture system. *J. Neurosci. Res.* **2004**, *78*, 157–166. [CrossRef] [PubMed]
25. Llufriu-Dabén, G.; Carrete, A.; Chierto, E.; Mailleux, J.; Camand, E.; Simon, A.; Vanmierlo, T.; Rose, C.; Allinquant, B.; Hendriks, J.J.A.; et al. Targeting demyelination via α-secretases promoting sAPPα release to enhance remyelination in central nervous system. *Neurobiol. Dis.* **2018**, *109*, 11–24. [CrossRef] [PubMed]

26. Nyamoya, S.; Leopold, P.; Becker, B.; Beyer, C.; Hustadt, F.; Schmitz, C.; Michel, A.; Kipp, M. G-Protein-Coupled Receptor Gpr17 Expression in Two Multiple Sclerosis Remyelination Models. *Mol. Neurobiol.* **2018**. [CrossRef] [PubMed]
27. Kipp, M.; Nyamoya, S.; Hochstrasser, T.; Amor, S. Multiple sclerosis animal models: A clinical and histopathological perspective. *Brain Pathol.* **2017**, *27*, 123–137. [CrossRef]

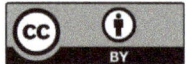

© 2019 by the authors. Licensee MDPI, Basel, Switzerland. This article is an open access article distributed under the terms and conditions of the Creative Commons Attribution (CC BY) license (http://creativecommons.org/licenses/by/4.0/).

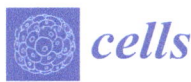

Article

Agenesis and Hypomyelination of Corpus Callosum in Mice Lacking Nsun5, an RNA Methyltransferase

Zihao Yuan [1,2,†], Peipei Chen [1,2,†], Tingting Zhang [1,2], Bin Shen [1,*] and Ling Chen [1,2,*]

1. State Key Laboratory of Reproductive Medicine, Department of Physiology, Nanjing Medical University, Nanjing 211166, China; 15250963556@yeah.net (Z.Y.); 15720803023@163.com (P.C.); ztt19921004@163.com (T.Z.)
2. Department of Physiology, Nanjing Medical University, Nanjing 211166, China
* Correspondence:binshen@njmu.edu.cn (B.S.); lingchen@njmu.edu.cn (L.C.); Tel./Fax: +86-25-86869441 (B.S. & L.C.)
† These authors contributed equally to this work.

Received: 19 May 2019; Accepted: 4 June 2019; Published: 6 June 2019

Abstract: Williams-Beuren syndrome (WBS) is caused by microdeletions of 28 genes and is characterized by cognitive disorder and hypotrophic corpus callosum (CC). *Nsun5* gene, which encodes cytosine-5 RNA methyltransferase, is located in the deletion loci of WBS. We have reported that single-gene knockout of *Nsun5* (*Nsun5*-KO) in mice impairs spatial cognition. Herein, we report that postnatal day (PND) 60 *Nsun5*-KO mice showed the volumetric reduction of CC with a decline in the number of myelinated axons and loose myelin sheath. Nsun5 was highly expressed in callosal oligodendrocyte precursor cells (OPCs) and oligodendrocytes (OLs) from PND7 to PND28. The numbers of OPCs and OLs in CC of PND7-28 *Nsun5*-KO mice were significantly reduced compared to wild-type littermates. Immunohistochemistry and Western blot analyses of myelin basic protein (MBP) showed the hypomyelination in the CC of PND28 *Nsun5*-KO mice. The *Nsun5* deletion suppressed the proliferation of OPCs but did not affect transition of radial glial cells into OPCs or cell cycle exit of OPCs. The protein levels, rather than transcriptional levels, of CDK1, CDK2 and Cdc42 in the CC of PND7 and PND14 *Nsun5*-KO mice were reduced. These findings point to the involvement of *Nsun5* deletion in agenesis of CC observed in WBS.

Keywords: Nsun5; Williams-Beuren syndrome (WBS); corpus callosum (CC); oligodendrocyte (OL); myelination

1. Introduction

Williams-Beuren syndrome (WBS; MIM 194,050) is a rare (7.5–10/100,000) and complex neuro-developmental disorder with multisystemic manifestations [1]. WBS is caused by 26 to 28 contiguous gene deletions [2] on human chromosome 7q11.23 [1]. These microdeletions have been detected in 90–99% of individuals with WBS [3].

The corpus callosum (CC) is the largest interhemispheric commissure known to modulate cerebral specialization and interhemispheric communication. During brain development, midline structures, including the CC, are the most vulnerable to the influence of complex mechanical and genetic factors [4]. Previous studies that analyzed the CC in WBS reported morphologic abnormalities and volumetric reductions. Luder et al. [5] found a significantly thinner callosal region in patients with WBS. In close agreement with the observation, the CC in WBS patients has been observed to be shorter and less curved [6]. Moreover, callosal midline lengths were found to be reduced and the callosal bending angles were enlarged [7,8]. A recent study reported the neuroradiological features in the brains of 12 WBS patients and showed several structural abnormalities of the central nervous system, for example, a hypotrophic CC and hypoplastic temporal lobes [9]. A shorter, less curved and thinner posterior callosal region might be associated with the unique cognitive and behavioral profile of WBS patients [5]. Thus, the abnormal shape of CC is an attractive candidate for exploring the pathological mechanisms underlying the cognitive aspects associated with WBS.

The *Nsun5* gene, which encodes a cytosine-5 RNA methyltransferase, is deleted in WBS [1,10]. Nsun5 is deleted in about 95% patients with WBS [11]. Nsun5 can directly methylate cytosine 2278 of 25S ribosomal RNA (rRNA) [11,12]. The lack of this methylation has been demonstrated to alter the structural conformation of the ribosome and to reduce the translational fidelity [13]. We have recently reported that Nsun5 was selectively expressed in the oligodendrocyte precursor cells (OPCs) of adult hippocampal gray matter [14]. The single-gene *Nsun5* knockout (*Nsun5*-KO) in mice impairs the development of OPCs [14].

Although the majority OPCs appear in early neonatal rodent brains, the maturation and myelination of oligodendrocytes (OLs) occur largely between postnatal day (PND) 7 and PND28 [15]. During CC development, OPCs proliferate and differentiate from PND7 to become mature OLs [16]. OPCs exit the cell cycle, become postmitotic OLs and further mature into myelinating OLs. The formation of myelin provides essential trophic support for CC axonal development during the developmental growth windows and mediates the fast conduction of neuronal information [17,18]. The Nsun5 transcript is enriched in the developing mouse brain. Nsun5 deficiency has been found to reduce the proliferation of OPCs in the adult hippocampus [14]. Therefore, it is of great interest to investigate whether the Nsun5 deficiency affects the development of CC.

To this end, we employed *Nsun5*-KO mice and observed their midline structures of the CC and axonal myelination. To explore the underlying molecular mechanisms, we further examined the proliferation and differentiation of OPCs and the maturation and myelination of OLs during CC development of *Nsun5*-KO mice. The results indicate that Nsun5 is required for the development of the CC by regulating the proliferation of OPCs and myelination of OLs. This finding points to the Nsun5 deficiency is associated with the agenesis of CC observed in WBS patients.

2. Materials and Methods

2.1. Generation and Identification of Nsun5-null Mice

All animals were treated according to the guidelines of Animal Care by the Institutional Animal Care and Ethical Committee of Nanjing Medical University (No. 2014-153). The generation of *Nsun5*-KO mice was performed by CRISPR/Cas9 genome editing. The in vitro transcription and microinjection of CRISPR/Cas9 has been previously described [19]. Two sgRNAs were designed to target exon 3 of the *Nsun5* gene. The oligos for the generation of sgRNA expression plasmids were annealed and cloned into the BsaI sites of pUC57-sgRNA (Addgene 51,132). Oligo sequences are sgRNA1-sense: TAGGCCCAGCAGAGCCTTCCAT; sgRNA1-antisense: AAACATGGAAGGCTCTGCTGGG; sgRNA2-sense: TAGGCTGAGCTGGCCCGACTCA; sgRNA2-antisense: AAACTGAGTCGGGCCAGCTCAG. The *Nsun5*-KO mice were backcrossed with C57BL/6 background mice for over 10 generations. The homozygous *Nsun5*-KO mice used in the present study were obtained by mating between heterozygous *Nsun5* mice. Genotyping was determined by polymerase chain reaction (PCR) examination using the genomic DNA obtained from tail biopsies [14]. The genotyping primers were: 5'-CTGTCCAGGTGCTAGTGTATG-3' and 5'-GGTCCTCATTTCGGCTCAC-3'. The mice were maintained under constant conditions (temperature of 23 ± 2 °C, humidity of 55 ± 5% and a 12:12-h light/dark cycle) with free access to food and water.

Postnatal day (PND) 3 WT mice ($n = 12$), PND7 WT mice ($n = 36$) and *Nsun5*-KO mice ($n = 36$), PND14 WT mice ($n = 24$) and *Nsun5*-KO mice ($n = 24$), PND28 WT mice ($n = 18$) and *Nsun5*-KO mice ($n = 18$), PND60 WT mice ($n = 24$) and *Nsun5*-KO mice ($n = 24$) were used in the preset study. The mice were randomly divided into 4 experimental groups. In the first group, the samples of CC were harvested from PND3 ($n = 6$) WT mice, PND7 ($n = 12$), PND14 ($n = 12$), PND28 ($n = 6$) and PND60 ($n = 6$) WT mice and *Nsun5*-KO mice, to examine the expression of Nsun5, MBP, CDK1, CDK2,

Cdc42 and RhoA by real-time PCR and Western blot analysis. In the second group, PND60 ($n = 18$) WT mice and *Nsun5*-KO mice were required for Luxol fast blue (LFB) staining of mid-sagittal CC ($n = 6$) or coronal CC sections ($n = 6$) and ultrastructural examination of myelin ($n = 6$). In the third group, PND3 ($n = 6$) WT mice, PND7 ($n = 12$), PND14 ($n = 12$) and PND28 ($n = 12$) WT mice and *Nsun5*-KO mice were used in experiments of immunohistochemistry. In the fourth group, PND7 ($n = 12$) WT mice and *Nsun5*-KO mice were treated with the injection of BrdU to label 2 h ($n = 6$) and 24 h ($n = 6$) proliferating cells, respectively.

2.2. Antibodies

The following antibodies were used for immunohistochemistry or western blot analyses: rabbit anti-Nsun5 (15449-1-AP, Proteintech Group Inc., Wuhan, China; Western blot,1:300; IF,1:100), rat anti-MBP (MAB386, Millipore, Billerica, MA, USA; Western blot,1:500; IF,1:600), rabbit anti-PDGFRα (ab203491, Abcam, Cambridge, UK, 1:500), mouse anti-BrdU (MAB4072, Millipore, 1:1000), rabbit anti-NG2 (AB5320, Millipore, 1:200), rabbit anti-BLBP (ab32423, Abcam, 1:1000), mouse anti-CC1 (OP80, Millipore, 1:200), rabbit anti-Ki67 (ab16667, Abcam, 1:500), mouse anti-olig2 (MABN50, Millipore, 1:300), rat anti-NG2 (MAB6689-SP, Millipore, 1:400), rabbit anti-CDK2 (ab32147, Abcam, 1:5000), rabbit anti-CDK1 (19532-1-AP, Proteintech, 1:1000), rabbit anti-cleaved caspase-3 (ab2302, Abcam; 1:300) and rabbit anti-RhoA (10749-1-AP, Proteintech, 1:1000). The secondary antibodies-donkey anti-mouse or anti-rat-conjugated to either Alexa Fluor 488 (Jackson ImmunoResearch, West Grove, PA, USA, 1:500) or 555 (Jackson ImmunoResearch; 1:500) and the biotinylated goat anti-mouse secondary antibody (Santa Cruz Biotechnology, Santa Cruz, CA, USA, 1:200) was directed against the primary IgG antibody species.

2.3. Histology Analyses

The mice were injected with pentobarbital (50 mg/kg) and were transcardially perfused with cold PBS followed by 4% paraformaldehyde. For the analysis of OPC proliferation, mice were injected intraperitoneally (i.p.) with the thymidine analogue BrdU (Sigma-Aldrich, St. Louis, MO, USA) at a concentration of 50 mg/kg body weight [20]. Two hours later, the perfused brains were removed. For examination of cell cycle exit, the mice were injected with BrdU (50 mg/kg, i.p.) and were sacrificed 24 h later [21].

The brains were removed, and dissected brains were post-fixed in 4% paraformaldehyde overnight at 4 °C. For frozen sections, the brains were transferred into 15% and 30% sucrose. After the brains completely sank to the bottom in 30% sucrose, the sagittal sections (30 µm) or coronal sections (10 µm) were cut using a cryostat (Leica CM3050S; Leica Microsystems, Heidelberg, Germany). The coronal sections were cut continuously from the rostral to caudal CC and then were divided equally into 7 parts.

Luxol Fast Blue staining: The mid-sagittal CC sections and coronal CC sections were immersed in 0.1% Luxol Fast Blue solution at 37 °C for 12–16 h and then in 95% ethanol for 5 min. These sections were incubated in 0.05% lithium carbonate solution for 1 min and then were washed with 70% ethanol and distilled water. After crystal violet counterstaining, the sections were sealed for microscopic observation.

Immunohistochemistry: The coronal sections were incubated in 3% hydrogen peroxide for 30 min and were subsequently treated with 1% bovine serum albumin (BSA, Sigma Chemical Co.) for 60 min to block nonspecific binding. After blocking, sections were incubated with the primary antibodies overnight at 4 °C. The primary antibodies were visualized by incubating the sections with the appropriate fluorophore-conjugated secondary antibodies or biotinylated IgG antibodies for 2 h at room temperature. The immunoreactivities were visualized using an avidin biotin horseradish peroxidase complex (Vector Laboratories, Burlingame, CA, USA). Sections were counterstained with DAPI (1:1000; Sigma) and mounted with mounting medium (Vector Laboratories). The immunoreactivities were visualized using fluorescence microscopy (DP70; Olympus, Tokyo, Japan) or a conventional light microscope (DP70; Olympus). For double immunofluorescence staining, the sections were simultaneously incubated with two primary antibodies that were developed in different species and diluted in 1% BSA, overnight at 4te. Primary antibodies were detected with appropriate secondary antibodies for 2 h at room temperature. Images of stained sections were observed using a fluorescence microscope.

Transmission electron microscopy (TEM): The brains were immersed in 2.5% glutaraldehyde and 2% paraformaldehyde. After overnight fixation, a block ($1 \times 1 \times 2$ mm^3) was dissected from the CC at the level of the anterior-dorsal hippocampus under a Leica stereomicroscope (MZ 6; Leica Pte, Leica, Heidelberg, Germany). The samples were post-fixed in 1% osmium tetroxide and then dehydrated and embedded in Epon-Araldite. Ultrathin sections were cut and stained with uranyl acetate and lead citrate. The samples were observed and photographed using a JEM-1400 Transmission Electron Microscope (JEOL USA, Peabody, MA, USA).

Morphometric analysis and quantization: (1) The areas of mid-sagittal CC (3 sections/mouse) and coronal CC (2 sections per segment, total 7 segments/mouse; Figure 1E) were measured using digital photographs with a semiautomated image analysis system (ImagePro Plus V. 4.5, CyberneticsMedia, Silver Spring, MD, USA). The measurements were repeated 3 times for each sample to obtain an average value; (2) The mid-sagittal CC and coronal CC sections stained with LFB were scanned using a Leica scanner. Images from at least 6 sections were collected and quantitative image analysis was performed using ImageJ software package (National Institutes of Health) as described previously [22]. The intensity of LFB staining in each experimental group were normalized to controls and presented as bar graphs; (3) At least 6 sections for each mouse and each experimental condition were analyzed and counted. An average of 6 sections was quantified to obtain the number of positive cells per mouse. Cell counting was performed blindly; (4) The number of Ki67-/BrdU+ cells (cell cycle) was divided by total number of BrdU+ cells in the CC to obtain the cell-cycle exit index [21]; and (5) The myelinated axons were calculated from at least 10 sections for each mouse. The thickness of myelination was quantified by G ratio (the numerical ratio of the axonal diameter divided by the diameter of the myelinated fiber) [23]. Approximately 120 myelinated axons per block were randomly selected for a detailed morphometric analysis using ImageJ software (http://rsb.info.nih.gov/ij/). The cases were coded to facilitate blind quantification.

2.4. Western Blot Analysis

Each CC was dissected under a Leica stereomicroscope (MZ 6; Leica Pte) and was sonicated in 200 µL of Tris buffer (pH 7.4) containing 10% sucrose, phosphatase inhibitors and protease inhibitors (Complete; Roche Diagnostics). The protein concentrations were quantified by a Bio-Rad Protein Assay Kit (Bio-Rad, Rockford, IL, USA) according to the manufacturer's protocol. Equal amounts of proteins were separated by SDS-polyacrylamide gel electrophoresis and were transferred to PVDF membranes. The membranes were blocked with 5% nonfat milk in Tris-buffered saline/Tween-20 (TBS-T) and were then incubated with antibodies against CDK1, CDK2, Cdc42 and RhoA at 4 °C overnight. The appropriate horseradish peroxidase (HRP)-conjugated secondary antibodies were incubated with the membranes for 1 h at room temperature. The signals were visualized using an enhanced chemiluminescence detection kit (ECL, Millipore). Following visualization, the blots were stripped with stripping buffer for 15 min and were then incubated with the antibodies against the protein at 4 °C overnight. The Western blot bands were scanned and analyzed using the ImageJ software package.

2.5. Reverse Transcription-Polymerase Chain Reaction (RT-PCR)

The CC was immediately transferred to TRIzol Reagent (Invitrogen, Camarillo, CA, USA) and was processed for total RNA isolation according to the manufacturer's protocol and was quantified by spectrophotometry. Then, the RNA was reverse-transcribed into cDNAs using a Prime Script RT reagent kit (Takara, Japan) for quantitative PCR (ABI Step One Plus, Foster City, CA, USA) in the presence of a fluorescent dye (SYBR Green I; Takara, Japan). The relative expression of the genes was calculated using the $2^{-\Delta\Delta ct}$ method with normalization to the *GAPDH* expression level. The primer sequences were designed based on published sequences of mouse genes listed in Table 1 [24,25].

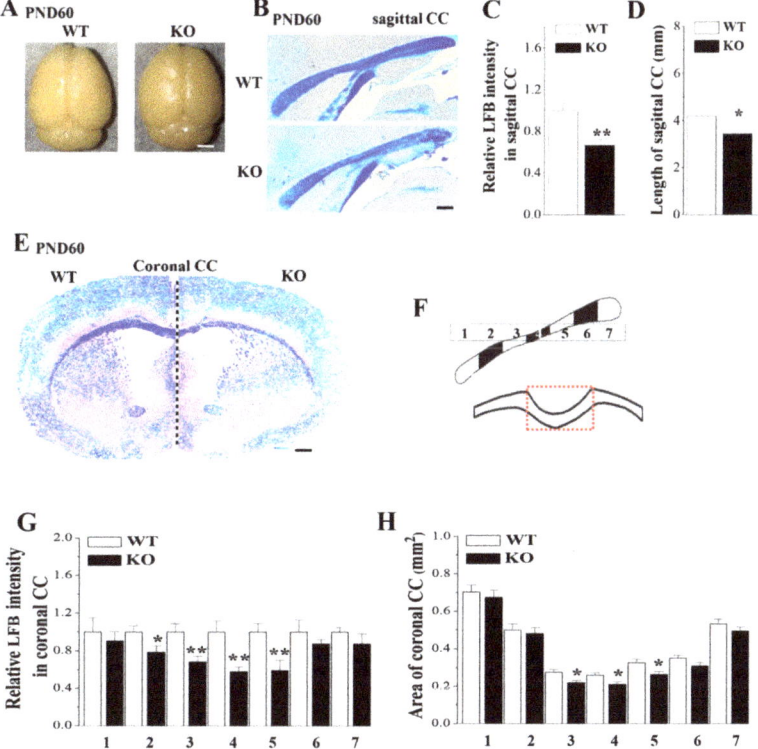

Figure 1. Loss of Nsun5 causes corpus callosum (CC) agenesis with hypomyelination. (**A**) Pictures of entire brain of PND60 WT mice (WT) and *Nsun5*-KO mice (KO). Scale bar = 0.25 cm. (**B**) Representative images of mid-sagittal CC stained with Luxol Fast Blue (LFB). Scale bar = 100 µm. (**C**, **D**) Bar graphs show the intensity of LFB staining and lengths of mid-sagittal CC in WT mice and *Nsun5*-KO mice. * $p < 0.05$, ** $p < 0.01$ vs. WT ($n = 6$). Error bars represent the mean ± SEM. (**E**) Representative images of the coronal CC of WT mice (left side) and *Nsun5*-KO mice (right side). Scale bar = 500 µm. (**F**) Schematic diagram of coronal sections from rostral to caudal CC divided equally into 7 segments (upper panel) and measured region in coronal CC (red dashed box). (**G**, **H**) Bar graphs represent the intensity of LFB staining and areas of coronal CC obtained from 7 segments, respectively. * $p < 0.05$, ** $p < 0.01$ vs. WT (one-way ANOVA, $n = 6$).

2.6. Data Analysis/Statistics

The data were processed with Origin 9.1 software (Origin Lab Corp., Northampton, MA, USA). The group's data were expressed as the mean plus or minus the standard error of the mean (SEM). All statistical analyses were performed using SPSS software, version 20.0 (SPSS Inc., Chicago, IL, USA). The differences between the means were analyzed using Student's t test or one-way analysis of variance (ANOVA), followed by the Bonferroni post hoc analysis to determine the significance of specific comparisons. The differences were considered statistically significant at $p < 0.05$.

Table 1. Primers for quantitative real-time polymerase chain reaction (PCR).

Gene	Forward	Reverse
Nsun5	GAGGGAAGGGTGGATAAGG	GGCACGATGCGGATGTAG
CDK2	GTTGGTGATGGTGCTGTTG	CTGTGGATAACTTAGCGGTCG
CDK1	AAAGCGAGGAAGAAGGAG	GGACAGGAACTCAAAGATGA
Cdc42	GTTGGTGATGGTGCTGTTG	CTGTGGATAACTTAGCGGTCG
RhoA	CATTGACAGCCCTGATAGTT	TCGTCATTCCGAAGGTCCTT
GAPDH	TGGGTGTGAACCACGAG	ACCACAGTCCATGCCATCAC

3. Results

3.1. Loss of Nsun5 causes CC Agenesis

The overall brain sizes of PND60 *Nsun5*-KO mice did not differ roughly from those of the littermate WT mice (Figure 1A). To investigate the possible role of Nsun5 in the development of CC, we performed Luxol Fast Blue (LFB) staining, a commonly used technique for detecting myelin sheaths [26], on the mid-sagittal CC and coronal CC sections from PND60 *Nsun5*-KO mice and wild-type (WT) mice ($n = 6$ per experimental group). As shown in Figure 1B,E the intensities of LFB staining in the mid-sagittal CC sections and the coronal CC sections were reduced in *Nsun5*-KO mice compared to WT littermates, indicating a decline in the myelin density. Notably, not only the intensity of LFB staining ($p < 0.01$; Figure 1C) but also the straight length of the mid-sagittal CC ($p < 0.05$; Figure 1D) in *Nsun5*-KO mice were less than those in WT mice. Subsequently, the coronal sections obtained from the rostral to caudal CC were divided equally into 7 segments (upper panels; Figure 1F) to measure the areas of the coronal CC (red dashed box) in different regions and the myelin density. In comparison with WT mice, the areas of the coronal CC in the 3rd–5th segments were significantly reduced in *Nsun5*-KO mice ($p < 0.05$; Figure 1H), while in other segments, there were no significant differences ($p > 0.05$). Similarly, the decline in the intensity of LFB staining was observed in the coronal CC of *Nsun5*-KO mice (2nd segment: $p < 0.05$; 3rd–5th segments: $p < 0.01$; Figure 1G). Although the intensity of LFB staining in other segments of *Nsun5*-KO mice had a decreasing tendency but the group when compared with WT mice failed to reach significance ($p > 0.05$). The results indicate that the loss of Nsun5 causes the volumetric reduction of CC with a decline of the myelin density.

3.2. Loss of Nsun5 Results in Myelination Defects of CC

To further determine whether the deletion of Nsun5 causes the ultrastructural alteration of callosal myelin, the cross-sections of CC (4th segment; Figure 2A) were examined by transmission electron microscopy (TEM, $n = 6$ per experimental group). As shown in Figure 2B. PND60 *Nsun5*-KO mice revealed structure turbulence and were missing the myelin sheath. The number of CC myelinated axons was significantly reduced in *Nsun5*-KO mice ($p < 0.01$; Figure 2C). Although G ratio analysis (the numerical ratio of the axonal diameter divided by the diameter of the myelinated axons) revealed that the myelin sheath thickness had no significant difference between the both groups ($p > 0.05$; Figure 2D), the myelination arrangement disorder and the loose myelin sheath were observed in the CC of *Nsun5*-KO mice (Figure 2E). The results indicate that the loss of Nsun5 leads to deficits in callosal myelination formation.

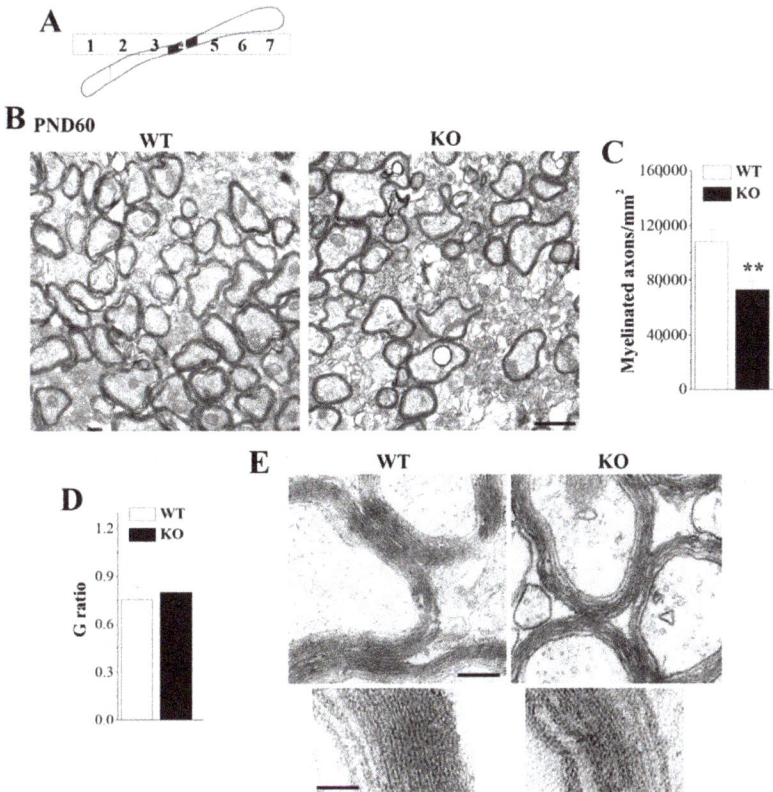

Figure 2. Loss of Nsun5 results in myelination defects in the CC. (**A**) Schematic diagram of coronal sections for TEM. (**B**) Representative transmission electron microscopy (TEM) images from 4th segment of CC (black region) in PND60 WT mice (WT) and *Nsun5*-KO mice (KO). Scale bar = 1 µm. (**C**) Number of myelinated axons in CC. ** $p < 0.01$ vs. WT ($n = 6$). (**D**) G ratio (numerical ratio of axonal diameter divided by the diameter of myelinated axons) in CC of PND60 WT mice and *Nsun5*-KO mice. (**E**) Representative higher power views of CC. Scale bar = 250 nm (upper); Scale bar = 100 nm (bottom).

3.3. Nsun5 is Expressed in the OL Lineage of the Developing CC

During the development of the CC, the OPCs proliferate and differentiate to become mature OLs, generating myelin. To explore the mechanisms underlying the impaired myelination formation in *Nsun5*-KO mice, we first examined the dynamic level of Nsun5 expression in the CC of PND3-60 WT mice (Figure 3A, $n = 6$ per experimental group) since the proliferation and differentiation of OPCs on PND7-14 and the initiation of myelination on PND14-28 are the most active [15]. Real-time PCR analysis revealed the peak of Nsun5 expression between PND7-28 (vs. PND3, PND7-14: $p < 0.01$; PND28: $p < 0.05$; Figure 3B), which was well matched with the developmental period of the CC.

To further identify the characteristics of cells expressing Nsun5 during the development of the CC, we performed a double immunohistochemistry analysis by using Nsun5 with the OPC markers (NG2 and PDGFRα), the OL lineage marker (Olig2) and the mature OL markers (CC1 and MBP). On PND3, Nsun5 was expressed in NG2 positive (NG2+) OPCs (Figure 3C). The NG2+ OPCs revealed a biphasic pattern along the axon tracts of the CC. On PND7, we also found that Nsun5 could be detected in PDGFRα positive (PDGFRα+) OPCs (Figure 3D) and Olig2 positive (Olig2+) OLs (Figure 3F). Nsun5 resided in the cytoplasm and was involved in the processes of OPCs and OLs. This anti-Nsun5 antibody was highly specific, because no signal was detected in the CC of PND7 *Nsun5*-KO mice (Figure 3E). It is noteworthy that CC1-positive (CC1+) OLs on PND14 display Nsun5 positivity (Figure 3G). Consistently, the amount of Nsun5 protein in OPCs and OLs was progressively elevated from PND3 to PND7-14. On PND28, the Nsun5 protein was detected in the myelin sheath formed by mature OLs expressing MBP (Figure 3H). There were some Nsun5+/MBP- cells that showed the morphological features of OPCs (arrowhead), termed white matter OPCs in the CC. The expression of Nsun5 in the OPCs and mature myelinating OLs further supports the notion that Nsun5 can regulate the development of the CC.

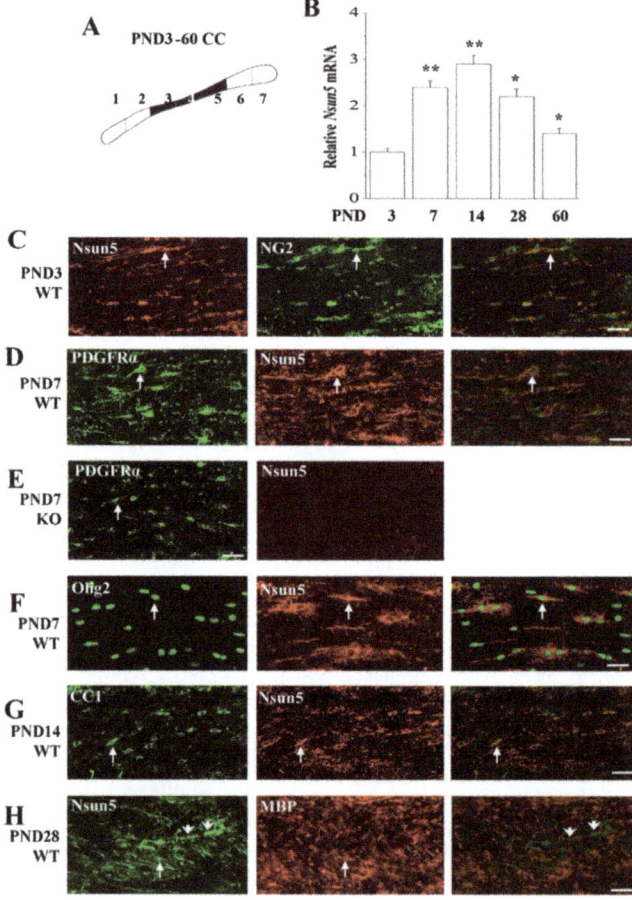

Figure 3. Nsun5 is expressed in oligodendrocyte (OL) lineage of developing CC. (**A**) Schematic diagram of CC obtained from wild-type (WT) mice. (**B**) Bar graphs show the levels of *Nsun5* mRNA obtained from 3rd to 5th segments (black region) of CC in PND3-60 WT mice. * $p < 0.05$ and ** $p < 0.01$ vs. PND3 mice (one-way ANOVA, $n = 6$). Representative images of double immunostaining for Nsun5 (green) and NG2 (red) in CC of PND3 WT mice, Scale bars = 30 μm (**C**); PDGFRα (green) and Nsun5 (red) in PND7 WT mice, Scale bars = 25 μm (**D**) and *Nsun5*-KO mice, Scale bars = 40 μm (**E**); Olig2 (green) and Nsun5 (red) in PND7 WT mice, Scale bars = 20 μm (**F**); CC1 (green) and Nsun5 (red) in PND14 WT mice, Scale bars = 25 μm (**G**); Nsun5 (green) and MBP (red) in PND28 WT mice. Scale bars = 30 μm (**H**).

3.4. Loss of Nsun5 Reduces OPCs and OLs Leading to Hypomyelination of CC

To further determine if the expression of Nsun5 is required for the proliferation and differentiation of OPCs, we quantified the total numbers of OPCs and OLs in the CC (red dashed box; Figure 4A) of PND7, PND14 or PND28 WT mice and *Nsun5*-KO mice ($n = 6$ mice per experimental group). As shown in Figure 4B, PDGFRα+ cells in the CC of PND7 *Nsun5*-KO mice was reduced. Quantitative measurement confirmed the decrease in the numbers of PDGFRα+/DAPI+ cells in PND7 ($p < 0.05$; Figure 4C) and PND14 ($p < 0.05$) *Nsun5*-KO mice compared to WT mice. We observed a significant reduction in the number of cells expressing the OL maturation marker CC1 in the CC of PND14 *Nsun5*-KO mice (Figure 4D). The numbers of CC1+/DAPI+ cells in PND14 ($p < 0.05$; Figure 4E) and PND28 ($p < 0.05$) *Nsun5*-KO mice were lower than those in WT mice. Next, we performed cleaved caspase-3 immunostaining to test whether the deletion of Nsun5 causes the apoptosis of OPC and OL. As shown in Figure 4F, the number of cleaved caspase-3 positive cells did not increase in PND28 *Nsun5*-KO mice. In addition, the hypomyelination in the CC of PND28 *Nsun5*-KO mice was observed by immunohistochemistry of myelin basic protein (MBP), a marker for mature OLs and myelin (Figure 4G). Furthermore, Western blot analysis showed an obvious reduction in the MBP protein level in *Nsun5*-KO mice compared with WT mice ($p < 0.05$; Figure 4H).

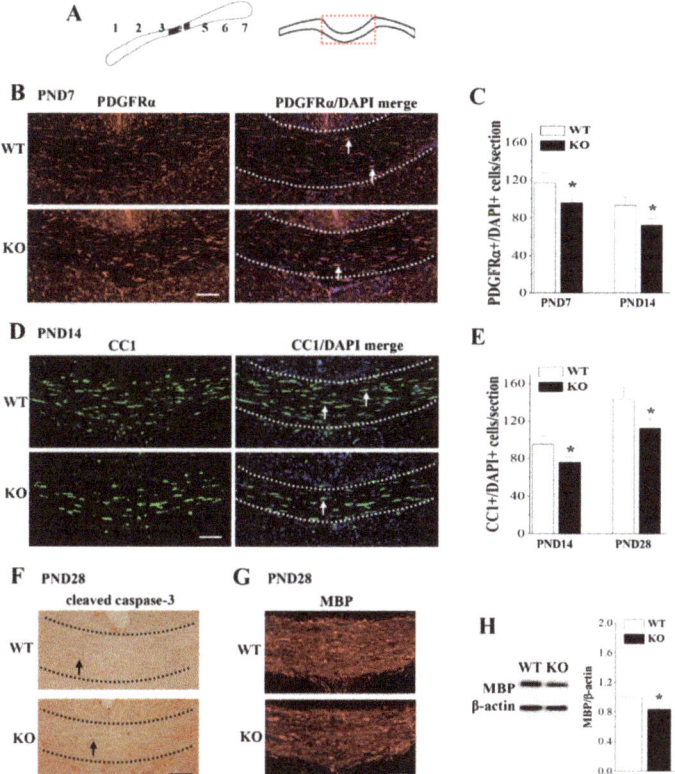

Figure 4. Loss of Nsun5 reduces OPCs and OLs leading to hypomyelination of CC. (**A**) Oligodendrocyte precursor cells (OPCs) and OLs were count in 4th segment of coronal CC (black region). (**B**) Representative images of immunohistochemistry for PDGFRα and PDGFRα/DAPI merge in PND7 WT mice (WT) and *Nsun5*-KO mice (KO). Scale bar = 35 μm. Arrows indicate PDGFRα+/DAPI+ cells.

(**C**) Bar graph indicates the number of PDGFRα+/DAPI+ cells per section of CC (as shown in **A**; red dashed box) in PND7 and PND14 WT mice and *Nsun5*-KO mice. * $p < 0.05$ vs. WT ($n = 6$). (**D**) Representative images of immunohistochemistry for CC1 and CC1/DAPI merge in PND14 WT mice and *Nsun5*-KO mice. Scale bar = 25 μm. Arrows indicate CC1+/DAPI+ cells. (**E**) Bar graph indicates the number of CC1+/DAPI+ cells per section of CC in PND14 and PND28 WT mice and *Nsun5*-KO mice. * $p < 0.05$ vs. WT ($n = 6$). (**F**) Immunohistochemistry of caspase-3 in CC of PND28 WT mice and *Nsun5*-KO mice. Scale bars = 20 μm. (**G**) Representative images of immunohistochemistry for MBP. Scale bars = 20 μm. (**H**) The levels of MBP protein in CC of PND28 WT mice and *Nsun5*-KO mice. * $p < 0.05$ vs. WT ($n = 6$).

3.5. Loss of Nsun5 Suppresses the Proliferation of OPCs

To test whether the reduced OPCs in *Nsun5*-KO mice are due to deficits in OPC proliferation, we performed double immunostaining of PDGFRα with BrdU to label the proliferating OPCs in the CC of *Nsun5*-KO mice and their littermate controls (Figure 4A) ($n = 6$ mice per experimental group). We chose to examine PND7 CC based on our observation that Nsun5 was highly expressed and that OPCs were decreased in *Nsun5*-KO mice at this stage. Two hours after BrdU injection, the number of BrdU-positive (BrdU+) cells in *Nsun5*-KO mice was reduced by approximately 35% compared to the number in WT mice ($p < 0.01$; Figure 5A-i). In particular, the number of PDGFRα+/BrdU+ cells in *Nsun5*-KO mice showed an approximately 42% decline ($p < 0.01$; Figure 5A-ii), indicating that Nsun5 deficiency suppresses OPC proliferation.

BrdU is known to label a cohort of cells in the S phase, while Ki67 is expressed in proliferating cells throughout all phases of the cell cycle. Thus, the BrdU+/Ki67+ cells are thought to represent the proportion of cycling cells, whereas the remaining BrdU+/Ki67− cells exit from the cell cycle. To examine the cell cycle dynamics of proliferating OPCs, a cell cycle exit experiment was performed by quantifying the proportion of BrdU+/Ki67+ cells ($n = 6$ mice per experimental group). In comparison with that in WT mice, the number of Ki67+/BrdU+ cells was reduced in *Nsun5*-KO mice ($p < 0.05$; Figure 5B-i). However, the cell cycle exit index of OPCs (BrdU+/Ki67− cells divided by the total population of BrdU+ cells) in the CC of *Nsun5*-KO mice did not differ from that in WT mice ($p > 0.05$; Figure 5B-ii).

To exclude whether the reduced BrdU+ cells are due to the reduced transition of radial glial cells (RGCs) into OPCs, immunostaining of brain lipid-binding protein (BLBP), a reliable marker of RGC, was used. The number of BLBP+ cells ($p > 0.05$; Figure 5C-i) or BLBP+/PDGFRα+ cells ($p > 0.05$; Figure 5C-ii) in *Nsun5*-KO mice was unchanged compared to those in WT mice.

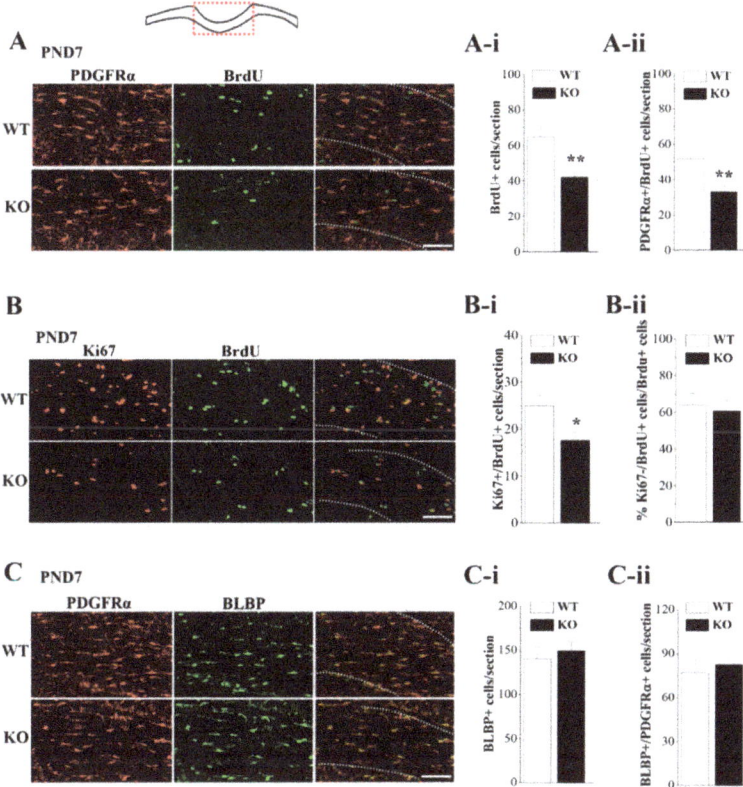

Figure 5. Nsun5 is required for the proliferation of OPCs. (**A**) Representative images of double immunostaining for PDGFRα (red) and Brdu (green) in CC of PND7 WT mice (WT) and *Nsun5*-KO mice (KO). Scale bar = 25 μm. Bar graphs indicate the number of BrdU+ cells (**A-i**) and PDGFRα +/BrdU+ cells (**A-ii**). ** $p < 0.01$ vs. WT ($n = 6$). (**B**) Representative images of double immunostaining for Ki67 (red) and BrdU (green) in PND7 WT mice and *Nsun5*-KO mice. Scale bar = 30 μm. Bars show the number of Ki67+/BrdU+ cells (**B-i**) and Ki67−/BrdU+ cells (**B-ii**). * $p < 0.05$ vs. WT ($n = 6$). (**C**) Representative images of double immunostaining for PDGFRα (red) and BLBP (green). Scale bar = 25 μm. Bars show the number of BLBP+ cells (**C-i**) and PDGFRα+/BrdU+ cells (**C-ii**).

3.6. Loss of Nsun5 Suppresses CDK1/2 Expression

Cyclin-dependent kinase 1 (CDK1) and CDK2 have been demonstrated to regulate cell proliferation [27]. CDK2 controls OPC cell cycle progression [27,28]. To further explore the mechanisms underlying the reduced proliferation of OPCs in *Nsun5*-KO mice, we examined the expression levels of CDK1 and CDK2 in isolated PND7 CC (Figure 6A, $n = 6$ mice per experimental group). The levels of *CDK1* ($p > 0.05$; Figure 6B) and *CDK2* mRNA ($p > 0.05$) in the CC of *Nsun5*-KO mice failed to be altered compared to those in WT mice. Interestingly, the western blot analysis showed a notable reduction in the level of the CDK1 protein ($p < 0.05$; Figure 6C) and the CDK2 protein ($p < 0.01$; Figure 6D).

Rho family GTPases, Cdc42 and RhoA, play an essential role in controlling the differentiation and processes of OLs [29]. The levels of *Cdc42* and *RhoA* mRNA in PND14 *Nsun5*-KO mice did not differ from that in WT mice ($p > 0.05$). The level of Cdc42 protein was lower in the CC of PND14 *Nsun5*-KO mice than it was in WT mice ($p < 0.05$; Figure 6E), whereas the RhoA protein did not decrease in *Nsun5*-KO mice ($p > 0.05$; Figure 6F).

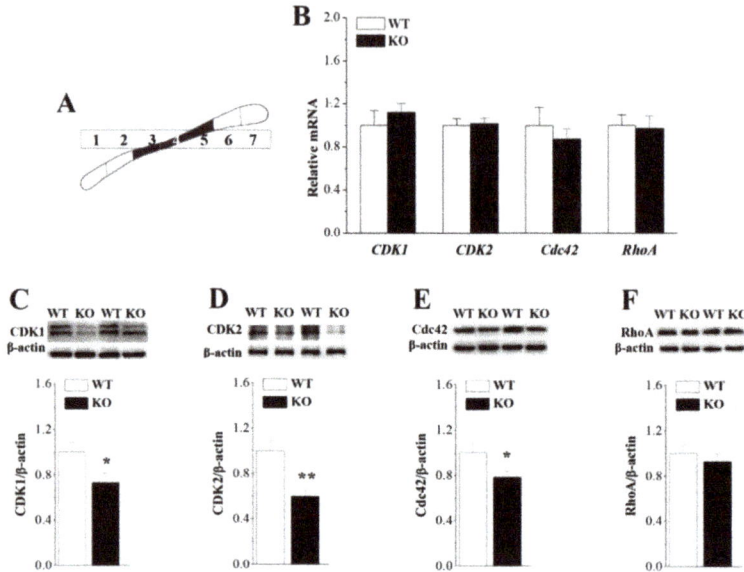

Figure 6. Loss of Nsun5 suppresses CDK1/2 and Cdc42 expression. (**A**) Schematic diagram of CC obtained from WT mice and *Nsun5*-KO mice. (**B**) Bar graphs show the levels of the *CDK1*, *CDK2*, *Cdc42* and *RhoA* mRNA in CC of WT mice (WT) and *Nsun5*-KO mice (KO). Bars represent the levels of the CDK1 (**C**), CDK2 (**D**), Cdc42 (**E**) and RhoA proteins (**F**) in CC of WT mice and *Nsun5*-KO mice. * $p < 0.05$, ** $p < 0.01$ vs. WT ($n = 6$).

4. Discussion

In the current study, we provided the first in vivo evidence that the loss of Nsun5 results in the agenesis of CC with postnatal hypomyelination of axons. This conclusion is deduced mainly from the following observations: the deletion of Nsun5 caused a decrease in the length of the sagittal CC (midline) and the area of the coronal CC (mid-segments), which was associated with fewer myelinated axons and the loose myelin sheath.

Nsun5 was highly expressed in OPCs during CC development. Notably, the number of OPCs (PDGFRα+ cells) was reduced in the CC of PND7 and PND14 *Nsun5*-KO mice. The size of the progenitor pool (the number of BLBP+ RGCs and BLBP+/PDGFRα+ cells) was unchanged in PND7 *Nsun5*-KO mice. Consistent with the report by Zhang et al. [14], the number of BrdU+/PDGFRα+ cells was lower in the CC of PND7 *Nsun5*-KO mice, indicating that the loss of Nsun5 suppresses the proliferation of OPCs. A principal finding in this study is that the expression of CDK1 and CDK2 was down-regulated in the CC of PND7 *Nsun5*-KO mice. The CDK2 activity has been reported to play a pivotal role in OPC cell cycle decisions occurring at G1/S checkpoint [28]. During the early G1 phase of proliferation, the pairing of CDK2 with cyclin E promotes entry into the S phase of the cell division cycle [30]; then CDK2 switches to partner with cyclin A to drive the cell though S phase [31]. CDK2 deletion in mouse embryo fibroblasts causes a delay in S phase entry [32]. The CDK1-cyclin B complex is thought to regulate the G2-M transition and progression through mitosis [33]. Although there are no reports of CDK1 mutant mice, mice lacking cyclin B2 do not show OPC cell cycle defects [34]. Thus, it is proposed that the Nsun5 deficiency may impede the S phase entry of OPCs [35]. The exclusion of exon 5 from the CDK2 transcription dramatically represses the expression of the CDK2 protein with a corresponding perturbation in cell cycle kinetics [36]. Caillava et al. [37], however, reported that the OPC proliferation in the CC during the early postnatal stages is CDK2-independent and that the CDK2 deficiency enhances the cycle exit of premature OPCs. Inconsistently, we observed that the proportion of exited cell cycle (percentage of Ki67−/BrdU+ cells against total BrdU+ cells) in PND7 *Nsun5*-KO mice was unchanged, indicating that the reduced proliferation of OPCs do not seem to be due to the prematurely exited cell cycle of OPCs. In Cdk2-deficient mice, CDK1 was found to compensate for the loss of CDK2 function by binding to cyclin E and regulating the G1/S transition [38]. Thus, one possible explanation is that the decline of CDK1/2 expression in *Nsun5*-KO mice is responsible for the reduced OPC proliferation.

Interestingly, the decrease in the CDK1/2 proteins in *Nsun5*-KO mice was not associated with transcription level changes in the *CDK1/2* mRNA. Nsun2, a tRNA methyltransferase, induces the methylation of tRNA to stabilize the tRNA and promote the protein synthesis [39]. An earlier study reported that the expression level of Nsun2 is cell cycle-dependent, with the highest expression in the S phase [40]. Nsun2 enhances CDK1 translation by methylating the CDK1 3′UTR at C1733 (m5C) without altering the *CDK1* mRNA level [41]. Sharma et al. [11] and Gigova et al. [12] have found that Rcm1—the yeast homologue of Nsun5—directly methylates 25S rRNA at cytosine 2278. Nsun5 ablation alters the structural conformation of the ribosome and the translational fidelity [13]. The Nsun5 deficiency is highly likely to affect the CDK1/2 expression at the translational level. Therefore, additional experiments will be needed to fully elucidate the mechanisms underlying the Nsun5 deletion-reduced CDK1/2 expression.

Notably, the number of OLs (CC1+ cells) was obviously reduced in the CC of PND14-28 *Nsun5*-KO mice. The OLs highly expressed Nsun5 during CC development, thus strongly indicating that Nsun5 is required for generating effective numbers of OLs. The apoptotic cells were not increased in the CC of PND28 *Nsun5*-KO mice, indicating that Nsun5 insufficiency does not impair OL survival. The OPCs generate the majority of myelinating OLs during the early postnatal period [42]. Although we cannot rule out the possibility that the deletion of Nsun5 may alter OPC differentiation, the reduced proliferation of OPC may be responsible for the decline of OLs.

We observed an obvious decline in the myelinated axons and hypomyelination in the CC of PND60 *Nsun5*-KO mice. Myelination occurs in a stepwise process where the OPCs proliferate and mature to become functional myelinating OLs. Olig2 ablation caused a nearly complete absence of myelination in the cortex during the early postnatal stages and severe dysmyelination, even in adulthood [43,44], suggesting that OPCs are a critical source for OL myelination in the developing cortex. On the other hand, Nsun5 is expressed in the process of mature OLs, implying its possible role in myelinogenesis. Our experimental data support this idea, because the deletion of Nsun5 was found to not only reduce the level of the MBP protein but also cause the myelination arrangement disorder and the loose myelin sheath in PND60 CC. Importantly, the expression level of Cdc42 was lower in the CC of PND14 *Nsun5*-KO mice, while no decrease was observed in the expression level of RhoA. Cdc42 activity is important for myelination when the OL processes ensheath the axons to form compacted myelin sheaths [45]. Cdc42 is thought to act as a positive regulator of OL process extension and branching [46]. The ablation of Cdc42 does not affect OPC proliferation or differentiation but it does lead to the extraordinary enlargement of the OL process and the abnormal accumulation of cytoplasmin [47]. Furthermore, the ablation of Cdc42 causes the widespread formation of aberrant myelin outfoldings through the abnormal accumulation of cytoplasm in the inner tongue of the oligodendrocyte process.

5. Conclusions

Pober reported that the *Nsun5* gene, a member of the NOL1/Nop2/sun protein family, is deleted in approximately 95% of patients with WBS. In this study, we determined that the loss of Nsun5 leads to the agenesis of CC with the postnatal hypomyelination of axons. The abnormal patterns of CC morphology and shape in the *Nsun5*-KO mice were similar to those in WBS individuals. The formation of myelin provides essential signals for the growth of axons as well as long-term structural integrity [48]. The agenesis of CC in *Nsun5*-KO mice suggests that the deletion of Nsun5 in WBS may play an important role in CC axonal growth and function. The fibers of the CC are implicated in a wide range of cognitive abilities [5,49]. Of note, the cognitive functions have been found to be affected in WBS [50]. Nsun5 is heterozygous in WBS patients [51]. *Nsun5*-KO mice and heterozygous *Nsun5* mice show the cognitive disorder phenotype [14], which is companied by the CC agenesis and hypomyelination (in this study). Although the single-gene knockout phenotype observed in the *Nsun5*-KO mice may not be relevant to the human deletion syndrome at all, these observed structural alterations in the CC might be associated with the cognitive behavioral profile of WBS patients.

Author Contributions: Individual contributions are as follows: conceptualization, Z.Y., P.C. and L.C.; methodology, Z.Y., P.C., B.S. and L.C.; formal analysis, Z.Y., P.C. and T.Z.; investigation, Z.Y., P.C., T.Z., B.S. and L.C.; writing of original draft preparation, L.C.; writing of review and editing, B.S. and L.C.; visualization, Z.Y.; supervision, B.S. and L.C.; funding acquisition, L.C.

Funding: This work was supported by the National Natural Science Foundation of China (81671253; 81471157), the Jiangsu Provincial Natural Science Foundation of China (BE2016765) and the National 973 Basic Research Program of China (2014CB943303).

Conflicts of Interest: The authors declare no conflict of interest.

References

1. Pober, B.R. Williams-Beuren syndrome. *N. Engl. J. Med.* **2010**, *362*, 239–252. [CrossRef] [PubMed]
2. Ewart, A.K.; Morris, C.A.; Atkinson, D.; Jin, W.; Sternes, K.; Spallone, P.; Stock, A.D.; Leppert, M.; Keating, M.T. Hemizygosity at the elastin locus in a developmental disorder, Williams syndrome. *Nat. Genet.* **1993**, *5*, 11–16. [CrossRef] [PubMed]
3. Mila, M.; Carrio, A.; Sanchez, A.; Gomez, D.; Jimenez, D.; Estivill, X.; Ballesta, F. Clinical characterization, molecular and FISH studies in 80 patients with clinical suspicion of Williams-Beuren syndrome. *Med. Clin. (Barc)* **1999**, *113*, 46–49. [PubMed]
4. Van Essen, D.C.; Drury, H.A. Structural and functional analyses of human cerebral cortex using a surface-based atlas. *J. Neurosci.* **1997**, *17*, 7079–7102. [CrossRef] [PubMed]
5. Luders, E.; di Paola, M.; Tomaiuolo, F.; Thompson, P.M.; Toga, A.W.; Vicari, S.; Petrides, M.; Caltagirone, C. Callosal morphology in Williams syndrome: A new evaluation of shape and thickness. *Neuroreport* **2007**, *18*, 203–207. [CrossRef] [PubMed]
6. Torniero, C.; Dalla Bernardina, B.; Novara, F.; Cerini, R.; Bonaglia, C.; Pramparo, T.; Ciccone, R.; Guerrini, R.; Zuffardi, O. Dysmorphic features, simplified gyral pattern and 7q11.23 duplication reciprocal to the Williams-Beuren deletion. *Eur. J. Hum. Genet.* **2008**, *16*, 880–887. [CrossRef] [PubMed]
7. Schmitt, J.E.; Eliez, S.; Warsofsky, I.S.; Bellugi, U.; Reiss, A.L. Corpus callosum morphology of Williams syndrome: Relation to genetics and behavior. *Dev. Med. Child. Neurol.* **2001**, *43*, 155–159. [CrossRef] [PubMed]
8. Tomaiuolo, F.; Worsley, K.J.; Lerch, J.; di Paola, M.; Carlesimo, G.A.; Bonanni, R.; Caltagirone, C.; Paus, T. Changes in white matter in long-term survivors of severe non-missile traumatic brain injury: A computational analysis of magnetic resonance images. *J. Neurotrauma* **2005**, *22*, 76–82. [CrossRef] [PubMed]
9. Castiglia, L.; Husain, R.A.; Marquardt, I.; Fink, C.; Liehr, T.; Serino, D.; Elia, M.; Coci, E.G. 7q11.23 microduplication syndrome: Neurophysiological and neuroradiological insights into a rare chromosomal disorder. *J. Intellect Disabil. Res.* **2018**, *62*, 359–370. [CrossRef]
10. Schubert, C. The genomic basis of the Williams-Beuren syndrome. *Cell Mol. Life Sci.* **2009**, *66*, 1178–1197. [CrossRef]
11. Sharma, S.; Yang, J.; Watzinger, P.; Kotter, P.; Entian, K.D. Yeast Nop2 and Rcm1 methylate C2870 and C2278 of the 25S rRNA, respectively. *Nucleic Acids Res.* **2013**, *41*, 9062–9076. [CrossRef] [PubMed]
12. Gigova, A.; Duggimpudi, S.; Pollex, T.; Schaefer, M.; Kos, M. A cluster of methylations in the domain IV of 25S rRNA is required for ribosome stability. *RNA* **2014**, *20*, 1632–1644. [CrossRef] [PubMed]
13. Schosserer, M.; Minois, N.; Angerer, T.B.; Amring, M.; Dellago, H.; Harreither, E.; Calle-Perez, A.; Pircher, A.; Gerstl, M.P.; Pfeifenberger, S.; et al. Methylation of ribosomal RNA by NSUN5 is a conserved mechanism modulating organismal lifespan. *Nat. Commun.* **2015**, *6*, 6158. [CrossRef] [PubMed]
14. Zhang, T.; Chen, P.; Li, W.; Sha, S.; Wang, Y.; Yuan, Z.; Shen, B.; Chen, L. Cognitive deficits in mice lacking Nsun5, a cytosine-5 RNA methyltransferase, with impairment of oligodendrocyte precursor cells. *Glia* **2018**. [CrossRef] [PubMed]

15. Baumann, N.; Pham-Dinh, D. Biology of oligodendrocyte and myelin in the mammalian central nervous system. *Physiol. Rev.* **2001**, *81*, 871–927. [CrossRef] [PubMed]
16. Levine, J.M.; Reynolds, R.; Fawcett, J.W. The oligodendrocyte precursor cell in health and disease. *Trends Neurosci.* **2001**, *24*, 39–47. [CrossRef]
17. Emery, B. Regulation of oligodendrocyte differentiation and myelination. *Science* **2010**, *330*, 779–782. [CrossRef]
18. Nave, K.A. Myelination and the trophic support of long axons. *Nat. Rev. Neurosci.* **2010**, *11*, 275–283. [CrossRef]
19. Shen, B.; Zhang, W.; Zhang, J.; Zhou, J.; Wang, J.; Chen, L.; Wang, L.; Hodgkins, A.; Iyer, V.; Huang, X.; et al. Efficient genome modification by CRISPR-Cas9 nickase with minimal off-target effects. *Nat. Methods* **2014**, *11*, 399–402. [CrossRef]
20. Giera, S.; Deng, Y.; Luo, R.; Ackerman, S.D.; Mogha, A.; Monk, K.R.; Ying, Y.; Jeong, S.J.; Makinodan, M.; Bialas, A.R.; et al. The adhesion G protein-coupled receptor GPR56 is a cell-autonomous regulator of oligodendrocyte development. *Nat. Commun.* **2015**, *6*, 6121. [CrossRef]
21. Zou, Y.; Jiang, W.; Wang, J.; Li, Z.; Zhang, J.; Bu, J.; Zou, J.; Zhou, L.; Yu, S.; Cui, Y.; et al. Oligodendrocyte precursor cell-intrinsic effect of Rheb1 controls differentiation and mediates mTORC1-dependent myelination in brain. *J. Neurosci.* **2014**, *34*, 15764–15778. [CrossRef] [PubMed]
22. Deshmukh, V.A.; Tardif, V.; Lyssiotis, C.A.; Green, C.C.; Kerman, B.; Kim, H.J.; Padmanabhan, K.; Swoboda, J.G.; Ahmad, I.; Kondo, T.; et al. A regenerative approach to the treatment of multiple sclerosis. *Nature* **2013**, *502*, 327–332. [CrossRef] [PubMed]
23. Jacobs, E.C.; Pribyl, T.M.; Feng, J.M.; Kampf, K.; Spreur, V.; Campagnoni, C.; Colwell, C.S.; Reyes, S.D.; Martin, M.; Handley, V.; et al. Region-specific myelin pathology in mice lacking the golli products of the myelin basic protein gene. *J. Neurosci.* **2005**, *25*, 7004–7013. [CrossRef]
24. Martinez-Montemayor, M.M.; Otero-Franqui, E.; Martinez, J.; de la Mota-Peynado, A.; Cubano, L.A.; Dharmawardhane, S. Individual and combined soy isoflavones exert differential effects on metastatic cancer progression. *Clin. Exp. Metastasis* **2010**, *27*, 465–480. [CrossRef] [PubMed]
25. Lavine, J.A.; Raess, P.W.; Davis, D.B.; Rabaglia, M.E.; Presley, B.K.; Keller, M.P.; Beinfeld, M.C.; Kopin, A.S.; Newgard, C.B.; Attie, A.D. Overexpression of pre-pro-cholecystokinin stimulates beta-cell proliferation in mouse and human islets with retention of islet function. *Mol. Endocrinol.* **2008**, *22*, 2716–2728. [CrossRef]
26. Choi, C.I.; Yoo, K.H.; Hussaini, S.M.; Jeon, B.T.; Welby, J.; Gan, H.; Scarisbrick, I.A.; Zhang, Z.; Baker, D.J.; van Deursen, J.M.; et al. The progeroid gene BubR1 regulates axon myelination and motor function. *Aging (Albany NY)* **2016**, *8*, 2667–2688. [CrossRef] [PubMed]
27. Jablonska, B.; Aguirre, A.; Vandenbosch, R.; Belachew, S.; Berthet, C.; Kaldis, P.; Gallo, V. Cdk2 is critical for proliferation and self-renewal of neural progenitor cells in the adult subventricular zone. *J. Cell Biol.* **2007**, *179*, 1231–1245. [CrossRef] [PubMed]
28. Belachew, S.; Aguirre, A.A.; Wang, H.; Vautier, F.; Yuan, X.; Anderson, S.; Kirby, M.; Gallo, V. Cyclin-dependent kinase-2 controls oligodendrocyte progenitor cell cycle progression and is downregulated in adult oligodendrocyte progenitors. *J. Neurosci.* **2002**, *22*, 8553–8562. [CrossRef] [PubMed]
29. Wolf, R.M.; Wilkes, J.J.; Chao, M.V.; Resh, M.D. Tyrosine phosphorylation of p190 RhoGAP by Fyn regulates oligodendrocyte differentiation. *J. Neurobiol.* **2001**, *49*, 62–78. [CrossRef]
30. Morgan, D.O. Cyclin-dependent kinases: Engines, clocks and microprocessors. *Annu. Rev. Cell Dev. Biol.* **1997**, *13*, 261–291. [CrossRef]
31. Ortega, S.; Prieto, I.; Odajima, J.; Martin, A.; Dubus, P.; Sotillo, R.; Barbero, J.L.; Malumbres, M.; Barbacid, M. Cyclin-dependent kinase 2 is essential for meiosis but not for mitotic cell division in mice. *Nat. Genet.* **2003**, *35*, 25–31. [CrossRef] [PubMed]
32. Aleem, E.; Kiyokawa, H.; Kaldis, P. Cdc2-cyclin E complexes regulate the G1/S phase transition. *Nat. Cell Biol.* **2005**, *7*, 831–836. [CrossRef] [PubMed]
33. Nigg, E.A. Mitotic kinases as regulators of cell division and its checkpoints. *Nat. Rev. Mol. Cell Biol.* **2001**, *2*, 21–32. [CrossRef] [PubMed]
34. Brandeis, M.; Rosewell, I.; Carrington, M.; Crompton, T.; Jacobs, M.A.; Kirk, J.; Gannon, J.; Hunt, T. Cyclin B2-null mice develop normally and are fertile whereas cyclin B1-null mice die in utero. *Proc. Natl. Acad Sci. USA* **1998**, *95*, 4344–4349. [CrossRef] [PubMed]

35. Jablonska, B.; Gierdalski, M.; Chew, L.J.; Hawley, T.; Catron, M.; Lichauco, A.; Cabrera-Luque, J.; Yuen, T.; Rowitch, D.; Gallo, V. Sirt1 regulates glial progenitor proliferation and regeneration in white matter after neonatal brain injury. *Nat. Commun.* **2016**, *7*, 13866. [CrossRef] [PubMed]
36. Ji, X.; Humenik, J.; Yang, D.; Liebhaber, S.A. PolyC-binding proteins enhance expression of the CDK2 cell cycle regulatory protein via alternative splicing. *Nucleic. Acids Res.* **2018**, *46*, 2030–2044. [CrossRef] [PubMed]
37. Caillava, C.; Vandenbosch, R.; Jablonska, B.; Deboux, C.; Spigoni, G.; Gallo, V.; Malgrange, B.; Baron-Van Evercooren, A. Cdk2 loss accelerates precursor differentiation and remyelination in the adult central nervous system. *J. Cell Biol.* **2011**, *193*, 397–407. [CrossRef]
38. Berthet, C.; Aleem, E.; Coppola, V.; Tessarollo, L.; Kaldis, P. Cdk2 knockout mice are viable. *Curr. Biol.* **2003**, *13*, 1775–1785. [CrossRef]
39. Tuorto, F.; Liebers, R.; Musch, T.; Schaefer, M.; Hofmann, S.; Kellner, S.; Frye, M.; Helm, M.; Stoecklin, G.; Lyko, F. RNA cytosine methylation by Dnmt2 and NSun2 promotes tRNA stability and protein synthesis. *Nat. Struct. Mol. Biol.* **2012**, *19*, 900–905. [CrossRef]
40. Frye, M.; Watt, F.M. The RNA methyltransferase Misu (NSun2) mediates Myc-induced proliferation and is upregulated in tumors. *Curr. Biol.* **2006**, *16*, 971–981. [CrossRef]
41. Xing, J.; Yi, J.; Cai, X.; Tang, H.; Liu, Z.; Zhang, X.; Martindale, J.L.; Yang, X.; Jiang, B.; Gorospe, M.; et al. NSun2 Promotes Cell Growth via Elevating Cyclin-Dependent Kinase 1 Translation. *Mol. Cell Biol.* **2015**, *35*, 4043–4052. [CrossRef] [PubMed]
42. Yuen, T.J.; Silbereis, J.C.; Griveau, A.; Chang, S.M.; Daneman, R.; Fancy, S.P.J.; Zahed, H.; Maltepe, E.; Rowitch, D.H. Oligodendrocyte-encoded HIF function couples postnatal myelination and white matter angiogenesis. *Cell* **2014**, *158*, 383–396. [CrossRef] [PubMed]
43. Lu, Q.R.; Sun, T.; Zhu, Z.; Ma, N.; Garcia, M.; Stiles, C.D.; Rowitch, D.H. Common developmental requirement for Olig function indicates a motor neuron/oligodendrocyte connection. *Cell* **2002**, *109*, 75–86. [CrossRef]
44. Yue, T.; Xian, K.; Hurlock, E.; Xin, M.; Kernie, S.G.; Parada, L.F.; Lu, Q.R. A critical role for dorsal progenitors in cortical myelination. *J. Neurosci.* **2006**, *26*, 1275–1280. [CrossRef] [PubMed]
45. Rajasekharan, S.; Baker, K.A.; Horn, K.E.; Jarjour, A.A.; Antel, J.P.; Kennedy, T.E. Netrin 1 and Dcc regulate oligodendrocyte process branching and membrane extension via Fyn and RhoA. *Development* **2009**, *136*, 415–426. [CrossRef] [PubMed]
46. Liang, X.; Draghi, N.A.; Resh, M.D. Signaling from integrins to Fyn to Rho family GTPases regulates morphologic differentiation of oligodendrocytes. *J. Neurosci.* **2004**, *24*, 7140–7149. [CrossRef] [PubMed]
47. Thurnherr, T.; Benninger, Y.; Wu, X.; Chrostek, A.; Krause, S.M.; Nave, K.A.; Franklin, R.J.; Brakebusch, C.; Suter, U.; Relvas, J.B. Cdc42 and Rac1 signaling are both required for and act synergistically in the correct formation of myelin sheaths in the CNS. *J. Neurosci.* **2006**, *26*, 10110–10119. [CrossRef] [PubMed]
48. Lee, Y.; Morrison, B.M.; Li, Y.; Lengacher, S.; Farah, M.H.; Hoffman, P.N.; Liu, Y.; Tsingalia, A.; Jin, L.; Zhang, P.W.; et al. Oligodendroglia metabolically support axons and contribute to neurodegeneration. *Nature* **2012**, *487*, 443–448. [CrossRef] [PubMed]
49. Paul, L.K.; van Lancker-Sidtis, D.; Schieffer, B.; Dietrich, R.; Brown, W.S. Communicative deficits in agenesis of the corpus callosum: Nonliteral language and affective prosody. *Brain Lang.* **2003**, *85*, 313–324. [CrossRef]
50. Karmiloff-Smith, A.; Grant, J.; Ewing, S.; Carette, M.J.; Metcalfe, K.; Donnai, D.; Read, A.P.; Tassabehji, M. Using case study comparisons to explore genotype-phenotype correlations in Williams-Beuren syndrome. *J. Med. Genet.* **2003**, *40*, 136–140. [CrossRef]
51. Segura-Puimedon, M.; Sahun, I.; Velot, E.; Dubus, P.; Borralleras, C.; Rodrigues, A.J.; Valero, M.C.; Valverde, O.; Sousa, N.; Herault, Y.; et al. Heterozygous deletion of the Williams-Beuren syndrome critical interval in mice recapitulates most features of the human disorder. *Hum. Mol. Genet.* **2014**, *23*, 6481–6494. [CrossRef] [PubMed]

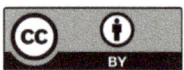 © 2019 by the authors. Licensee MDPI, Basel, Switzerland. This article is an open access article distributed under the terms and conditions of the Creative Commons Attribution (CC BY) license (http://creativecommons.org/licenses/by/4.0/).

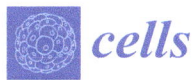

Article

EGFR/ErbB Inhibition Promotes OPC Maturation up to Axon Engagement by Co-Regulating PIP2 and MBP

Emanuela Nocita [1,†], Alice Del Giovane [1,†], Marta Tiberi [1], Laura Boccuni [1,‡], Denise Fiorelli [1,§], Carola Sposato [1], Elena Romano [2], Francesco Basoli [3], Marcella Trombetta [3], Alberto Rainer [3], Enrico Traversa [4] and Antonella Ragnini-Wilson [1,*]

1. NeurotechIT Laboratory, Department of Biology, University of Rome "Tor Vergata", 00133 Rome, Italy
2. Advanced Microscopy Center, Department of Biology, University of Rome "Tor Vergata", 00133 Rome, Italy
3. Department of Engineering, Università Campus Bio-Medico di Roma, 00128 Rome, Italy
4. School of Materials and Energy, University of Electronic Science and Technology of China, Chengdu 611731, China
* Correspondence: antonella.ragnini@uniroma2.it; Tel.: +39-0672594785
† These authors contributed equally to this work.
‡ Department of Microbiology, Immunology and Genetics, Max F. Perutz Laboratories, Dr. Bohr-Gasse 9, 1030 Wien, Austria.
§ Laboratory of Synaptic Immunology, University of Rome "Tor Vergata", 00133 Rome, Italy.

Received: 5 June 2019; Accepted: 5 August 2019; Published: 6 August 2019

Abstract: Remyelination in the adult brain relies on the reactivation of the Neuronal Precursor Cell (NPC) niche and differentiation into Oligodendrocyte Precursor Cells (OPCs) as well as on OPC maturation into myelinating oligodendrocytes (OLs). These two distinct phases in OL development are defined by transcriptional and morphological changes. How this differentiation program is controlled remains unclear. We used two drugs that stimulate myelin basic protein (MBP) expression (Clobetasol and Gefitinib) alone or combined with epidermal growth factor receptor (EGFR) or Retinoid X Receptor gamma (RXRγ) gene silencing to decode the receptor signaling required for OPC differentiation in myelinating OLs. Electrospun polystyrene (PS) microfibers were used as synthetic axons to study drug efficacy on fiber engagement. We show that EGFR inhibition per se stimulates MBP expression and increases Clobetasol efficacy in OPC differentiation. Consistent with this, Clobetasol and Gefitinib co-treatment, by co-regulating RXRγ, MBP and phosphatidylinositol 4,5-bisphosphate (PIP2) levels, maximizes synthetic axon engagement. Conversely, RXRγ gene silencing reduces the ability of the drugs to promote MBP expression. This work provides a view of how EGFR/ErbB inhibition controls OPC differentiation and indicates the combination of Clobetasol and Gefitinib as a potent remyelination-enhancing treatment.

Keywords: remyelination; EGFR inhibitor; smoothened agonist; microfibers; drug screening

1. Introduction

The myelin sheath insulates axons of the central nervous system (CNS), allowing neural impulses to be transmitted rapidly along axons. Remyelination is the natural process that restores damaged myelin and thereby neuronal function in the adult brain. This ability declines as a consequence of aging or during the progressive phases of multiple sclerosis (MS) [1–3]. Pharmacologically-induced remyelination has been envisaged in co-therapies with disease modifying agents for relapsing remitting and secondary progressive MS (RRMS and SPMS, respectively), not only to restore neuronal function, but also for its protective potential on neurodegeneration [1–4].

A number of bioactive drugs, such as Clobetasol, Gefitinib, Miconazole and Benztropine, have been successfully repositioned by screening FDA-approved compound libraries for their ability to promote myelin basic protein (MBP) expression in cell-based assays that employed either primary murine Oligodendrocyte Precursor Cells (OPCs) [5–7], mouse OPC cell lines such as Oli-neuM [8] or Epiblast-derived OPCs (EpiSC-OPC) [9]. However, a rational use of such drugs in remyelination therapies awaits the clarification of their molecular targets [1–10].

Remyelination essentially relies on two separate developmental steps: Oligodendrogenesis and Oligodendrocyte Precursor Cell (OPC) differentiation into myelinating OLs [1,3]. Promyelinating drugs can act either by promoting oligodendrogenesis and/or by enhancing OPC differentiation into mature OLs [1]. Oligodendrogenesis consists in neuronal precursor cell (NPC) differentiation into the OPC lineage [11] that involves the upregulation of Sonic Hedgehog (Shh) and mitogenic factors, including epidermal growth factor (EGF) [3,10,12–14]. Canonical Shh signaling leads to the activation of the G-protein-coupled seven-pass transmembrane receptor Smoothened (Smo) that binds to the transcription factors Gli1-3, thus promoting Shh-mediated gene transcription. For unclear reason, Shh upregulation does not result in Gli1 upregulation after remyelination stimuli, with the consequence that NPCs are fated to the OPC lineage [10,12–17]. The expression of myelin regulatory factor (Myrf) marks the entrance of OPCs into the second phase of differentiation. Upon Myrf expression, OPCs mature into premyelinating OLs (Pre-OLs) that are characterized by a transcriptional profile that only partially overlaps with that of OPCs. Pre-OLs begin to express myelin proteins, one of the most abundant being the cytosolic MBP [3,18–20]. The observation that Myrf is poorly expressed in chronic MS lesions suggests that OPC maturation might be defective in SPMS patients [21].

The final step of OL maturation is axon engagement. At the peak of MBP expression, the OL membrane enlarges and flattens in a process that requires phosphatidylinositol 4,5 bisphosphate (PIP2) binding to MBP. This triggers the release of cofilin and gelsolin, two actin-binding proteins that regulate cytoskeleton depolymerization [22–24]. The observation that OPCs readily recognize inert polystyrene (PS) microfibers of the appropriate diameter (2–4 μm, i.e., similar to axons) opened the way to study the physical and molecular cues required for axon engagement in vitro and the efficacy of promyelinating drugs in the process of axon engagement [25–29]. How OLs recognize the presence of fibers in the three-dimensional (3D) space and how OL membrane rolling on fibers is stimulated remains a field of active study [23,24,30].

To investigate the signals promoting OPC differentiation into myelinating OLs and how axon engagement is stimulated in the absence of neuronal feedback, here we used as a toolkit Clobetasol and Gefitinib, two drugs that have been shown to promote remyelination in vitro and/or in vivo [8,9,31]. Molecular studies have shown that Clobetasol acts essentially via the glucocorticoid receptor (GR) [9] and the Smo receptor [8,32] to promote MBP expression during OPC to OL differentiation, while Gefitinib is an epidermal growth factor receptor (EGFR) tyrosine kinase inhibitor (EGFR-TKI) potentially acting on multiple receptors of the EGFR/ErbB family [33].

Several studies have indicated that EGFR/ErbB antagonists promote OPC differentiation in a demyelination environment but, due to the complex regulation of the EGFR/ErbB family of receptors at different steps of OL formation and under remyelination stimuli, they have not clarified how these compounds promote remyelination [8,34–39].

Using Gefitinib, EGFR gene silencing, alone or in combination with Clobetasol treatment and chambers containing PS microfibers (synthetic axons) to simulate OPC differentiation in vitro in a 3D environment, we show that Gefitinib, by inhibiting EGFR, promotes MBP expression and by inhibiting the PI3K/AKT pathway causes PIP2 re-localization to membranes, thereby initiating the events that lead to membrane expansion at the peak of MBP expression. Gefitinib in combination with Clobetasol, by co-regulating multiple receptors involved in remyelination, greatly increases single drug activity, providing the basis to develop remyelination therapies based on a combination of these drugs.

2. Materials and Methods

2.1. Cell Culture

The Oli-neuM line (Cellosaurus ExPASy CVCL_VL76) was obtained and cultured as previously described [8] and routinely tested for contamination. Briefly, cells were expanded (six to eight passages) in growth medium (GM) composed of DMEM (Corning Inc., New York, NY, USA) supplemented with 10% fetal bovine serum (FBS, Corning), 2 mM L-glutamine (Gibco™, Thermo Fisher Scientific, Waltham, MA, USA), 1% pen-strep (Gibco™), 1 mM sodium pyruvate (Gibco™), and 15 mM HEPES (Sigma-Aldrich, Merck KGaA, Darmstadt, Germany) at 37 °C in 5% CO_2. Cells were grown until 80% confluence (approximately 3×10^6 cells in a 100 mm dish), then detached using Trypsin/EDTA (0.5%, Sigma-Aldrich) and centrifuged for 5 min at 132× g. The pellet was resuspended in fresh GM and placed in new sterile dishes. Differentiation medium (DM) was GM supplemented with 1% N2-supplement (175020–01, Gibco™), 60 nM triiodothyronine (T3, Sigma-Aldrich), and 53.7 ng/mL progesterone (Sigma-Aldrich). Oli-neuM cells were maintained under antibiotic selection with 500 µg/mL geneticin (G418, Gibco™), which was added to both GM and DM.

2.2. Compound Treatments

Clobetasol (Prestw-781), Gefitinib (Prestw-1270) were purchased from Prestwick Chemical Library® (http://www.prestwickchemical.com/prestwick-chemical-library.html). Drug stocks (100 mM) were pre-diluted to a concentration of 10 mM or 5 mM in dimethyl sulfoxide (DMSO) for Clobetasol and Gefitinib, and added at a final concentration of 5 µM or 1 µM in DM, respectively, so that final DMSO concentration did not exceed 0.5%. Optimal final concentrations were previously established according to MBP levels in titration experiments [8]. 5 µM Forskolin (F6886, Sigma-Aldrich), 1 µM Wortmannin [40,41] and 5 µg/mL insulin [42] were used dissolved in DMSO (0.5%). Unless otherwise stated, drug treatments were administrated in differentiation media (DM) after 24 h from Oli-neuM seeding. We refer to "vehicle treatment" as the combination of DM plus 0.5% DMSO max (DM + DMSO). Culturing and time of drug treatments (48 h) were previously established to be optimal for MBP expression in Oli-neuM [8]. Unless otherwise described, Oli-neuM cells were treated with 1 µM Gefitinib, 5 µM Clobetasol or drug vehicle (0.5% max DMSO) for 48 h in parallel experiments and cultured in 6–12 for biochemical assays or in 96-well plates for immunofluorescence studies or Real Time PCR (qPCR) studies.

2.3. Gene Silencing and Transfection

Retinoid X Receptor gamma (RXRγ) and Epidermal Growth Factor Receptor (EGFR) gene silencing was performed using MISSION® esiRNA Technology (Sigma-Aldrich; https://www.mpi-cbg.de/esiRNA/), which increases specificity due to the complexity of each MISSION® esiRNA pool that shares the same on-target but differs in the sequence-dependent off-target signatures. Specifically, we used EMU004971 (RXRγ; CAT n. ENSMUSG00000015843, 200 ng/µL, Sigma-Aldrich) and EMU075311 (EGFR; Cat n. ENSMUSG00000020122, 200 ng/µL, Sigma-Aldrich). Two Scramble siRNAs (Scramble7 n:4234503 and Scramble2 n:4234507; Sigma-Aldrich), were used as silencing controls for all analyses. siRNA Scramble 2 and/or 7 were run along with the EGFR esiRNA treatment. Mean data for siScramble were obtained from at least n ≥ 3 biological replicates. Silencing was performed using a Reverse protocol: 3 µg of esiRNA per well were diluted in 200 µL of Opti-MEM® (31985-070, 1X, Gibco™) and after 5 min combined with Lipofectamine® 2000 reagent (11668-09, Invitrogen™, Thermo Fisher Scientific) diluted in Opti-MEM®. The combined mixture was added after 20 min. Thereafter, 2.6×10^5 Oli-neuM cells were seeded in 6-well plates in GM media and cells were grown and differentiated in DM after 24 h with or without treatment. Plasmid Transfection: Oli-neuM cells were seeded in growth chamber containing PS fibers for 24 h, treatment with indicated drugs and transfected with the PH-PLCδ-pEGFP plasmid [43] using Lipofectamine® DNA Transfection Reagent Protocol (Invitrogen, Thermo Fisher Scientific). Plasmid amplification was performed as previously described [44] using GeneElute™

Plasmid Miniprep Kit (PLN70-1KT, Sigma-Aldrich) and the manufacture protocols. After extraction the plasmid were digested to confirm the presence of the specific insert described above.

2.4. Crude Extract Preparation and Immunoblot Analysis

Typically, 2.75×10^5 Oli-neuM cells were seeded in 6-well plates in GM media and cells were grown to 70% confluence. Treatments, unless otherwise specified, were performed as indicated in the text, as previously described. For immunoblot analyses, the following antibodies were used: Cell Signaling Technology (Danvers, MA, USA): anti-phospho-p44/42 MAPK (Erk1/2Thr202/Thr204: #9101, 1:5000), anti-p44/42 MAPK (Erk1/2: #1240, 1:3000), anti-Phospho AKT (Ser473: #4060, 1:2500); anti-AKT (pan: #4691, 1:2000). Sigma-Aldrich: anti-actin (2066, 1:2000). AbD Serotec (Bio-Rad Laboratories, Hercules, CA, USA): anti-MBP (MCA409S, 1:200). Proteintech® (Proteintech Group, Rosemont, IL, USA): anti-RXRγ (11129-1-AP,1:600). GeneTex (GeneTex, Inc., Irvine, CA, USA): anti-EGFR (GTX132810, 1:1000). Cell extract (CE) preparation and immunoblot analyses were performed as previously described [8]; briefly, bands signal intensity was estimated using ImageJ software (version 1.8.0), and data were plotted using GraphPad Prism 7.0 (GrahPad Software, San Diego, CA, USA) as the fold change versus vehicle, arbitrarily set to 1.

2.5. Quantitative Immunofluorescence Analysis and Confocal Microscopy

For IF quantitative analyses, Oli-neuM cells were plated in 96-well plates (655090, Greiner Bio-One, Kremsmünster, Austria), pre-coated with fibronectin from human plasma (Sigma-Aldrich) as previously described [44]. After 24 or 48 h (to obtain about 60% confluence), GM was removed and DM was added containing the indicated drug treatments or drug vehicle (0.5% DMSO). Unless otherwise specified, cells were further incubated for 48 h prior to fixation and processing for IF as previously described [8,44]. Acquisition was performed at 20× magnification (HCX PL FLUOTAR 20× NA 0.4) using a Leica DMI6000 B epifluorescence inverted microscope (Leica Microsystems, Wetzlar, Germany) equipped with Leica Application Suite X and Matrix Screener software (version 3.0) for automated image acquisition. Plate Array: vehicle-treated samples were spotted appropriately in different positions and acquired along with single drug treatments. Vehicle data (DM + DMSO 0.5%) of each plate was used to normalize signal intensity in the different channels in order to compare plate replicates. A minimum number of 1000 cells per sample was considered for mean intensity data evaluation of each treatment. Micrographs were analyzed with Scan^R (version 2.1; Analysis software version 1.1.0.6, Olympus, Tokyo, Japan) for quantification and statistical analyses as previously described [8,45]. Hoechst 33,342 (Invitrogen, Thermo Fisher Scientific) staining was used for nucleic acid quantification and nuclei detection. Rat anti-MBP (MCA409S; Serotec, 1:100), Rabbit anti-actin (A2066 Sigma-Aldrich, 1:80) primary antibodies and the respective Alexa Fluor 488 or Alexa Fluor 546 conjugated secondary antibodies (Thermo Fisher Scientific) were used as indicated in the text. Immunofluorescence (IF) and data quantification were performed as previously described [8,45]. Protein quantification in IF images was performed using the INTENSITY module of Scan^R analysis software: typically, the mean intensity FITC or TRITC values (±SEM) were detected on the mask MAIN of three biological replicates. One experimental replicate was constituted by 25 image/well, taken blindly by the acquisition software based on a 5 × 5 acquisition mask. Each sample was spotted in triplicate in each plate. Biological replicates that contained data from at least 1000 cells per sample were considered for statistical analyses. Quantitative morphological analysis was performed by using either EDGE or INTENSITY module of Scan^R analysis software (Olympus). We then calculated the percentage of the cell population with a higher membrane area using the Max Feret Diameter parameter of Scan^R software. The maximum Feret's diameter is a measure of an object size along its maximal axis. By plotting the Max Feret Diameter along one axis (y) and the Mean Intensity FITC on the other axis (X) of a scattered plot it is possible to visualize the cell distribution accordingly. Specifically, the following parameters were used for gating the cell population of interest: Max Feret Diameter > 70 (y)/Mean Intensity FITC (MBP) > 300 (x), using Scan^R analysis software. This gate identifies the cell population that has higher membrane extension as well as higher MBP levels (FITC or TRITC channel according to the secondary antibody used). Three wells per sample of three biological replicates were acquired for each experimental condition and tested for statistical significance using Student's *t* test vs. vehicle and one-way ANOVA for drug treatment comparisons.

To detect co-localization of MBP and PIP2, a LSM Fluoview 1000 confocal microscope (Olympus) equipped with an Olympus IX-81 inverted microscope was used. Microscopy inspection was performed at 48 h. Typically, Oli-neuM cells were seeded and treated on glass coverslips as indicated. After fixation, cells were alternatively incubated with FITC-conjugated anti-PIP2 (AC14-0106-12; Abcore, Ramona, CA, USA) or anti-MBP antibody, and stained with Hoechst 33342 to detect nuclei. Glass coverslips were mounted on a microscope slide using Fluoromount™ Aqueous Mounting Medium (Sigma-Aldrich). Micrographs were captured with a 20× UPLSAPO (NA 0.75, WD 0.65 mm) objective. For co-localization analysis, data were processed for 2D and 3D reconstruction using the isosurface tool of Imaris software (version 6.2.1, Bitplane, Zurich, Switzerland). Statistical coefficients (Pearson's Correlation Coefficient; Mander's Overlap Coefficient; Mander's Co-localization Coefficient) were calculated for each region of interest (ROI) and then expressed as mean ± Standard Deviation (SD). PLCδ1PH-GFP was acquired using 488 nm laser line.

2.6. Evaluation of Cell Engagement on PS Microfibers

Cell culture chambers containing electrospun fibers were prepared as follows. Fibers were electrospun on 22 × 22 mm glass coverslips placed on a lab-built cylindric rotating collector (diam. 200 mm, linear velocity 12 m/s), starting from a 30% polystyrene (PS, MW 280 kDa, Sigma-Aldrich) solution in 1:1 tetrahydrofuran/dichloromethane (Sigma-Aldrich), using a flow rate of 0.5 mL/h from a 23G needle placed at a distance of 22 cm from the collector, and with a voltage of +15kV and −1 kV (CZE-2000, Spellman High Voltage, Hauppauge, NY, USA) applied to the needle and to the collector, respectively. Following electrospinning, PS fibers were immobilized using rectangular PDMS gaskets obtained as replicas from PMMA micromachined molds, and irreversibly bonded to glass coverslip surface following oxygen plasma activation (FEMTO plasma cleaner, Diener, Ebhausen, Germany). Chambers were UV-sterilized before use and pre-treated with 10 μg/mL fibronectin (F0895, Sigma-Aldrich). 90,000 Oli-neuM cells were seeded in growth medium and, after 24 h, medium was exchanged with either differentiation medium (DM) supplemented with 0.5% DMSO (vehicle) or with the indicated treatment(s). Cells were grown for 72 h at 37 °C in 5% CO_2. After fixation, chambers were processed for immunofluorescence using the antibody indicated in the text. Acquisition was performed using a Leica DMI6000 automated microscope (Leica Microsystems) equipped with LAS-X Matrix Screener acquisition software (v. 3.0). Three positions per sample and 25 images (5 × 5 mosaic) for each position were considered for statistical analyses (n = 3). Engagement analyses were performed as described by Bechler et al., [25] with the following minor modification: nuclei located on fibers within a range of 86 μm around the fibers were considered engaged. The range of 86 μm was empirically chosen as it allows to distinguish cells occasionally near to fibers from those that effectively engage fibers, characterized also by MBP expression and elongated nuclei as described in the text. Images were visualized and analyzed with Scan^R (Olympus) or ImageJ [8,44] software tools as indicated above.

2.7. Total RNA Extraction and qPCR

Following drug administration, total RNA was extracted using TRI Reagent® (T9424, Sigma-Aldrich) according to the manufacturer's instructions. Typically, 2 μg of RNA sample were retro-transcribed using the High-capacity cDNA Reverse Transcription kit (4368814, Thermo Scientific) according to the manufacturer's instructions. qPCR was performed using either SYBR Green- or TaqMan-based technology and the StepOne™ Real-Time PCR System (Applied Biosystems®, Thermo Fisher Scientific). Primer pairs used with StoS Quantitative Master Mix 2X SYBR Green-ROX (GeneSpin Srl, Milan, Italy) are reported in Table S2. Predesigned primer sets were used with TaqMan™ Gene expression MasterMix (4369016, Thermo Fisher Scientific): RXRγ (Mm00436411_m1), Glyceraldehyde

3-phosphate dehydrogenase (GAPDH) (Mm99999915_g1). GAPDH was used as endogenous control. Typically, 50 ng of cDNA per sample were used per reaction. qPCR was performed in triplicate in MicroAmp Fast Optical 48-Well Reaction Plate (Applied Biosystems®), n = 3. The ΔΔCT method of relative quantification was used to determine the fold change in expression. This was done by normalizing the resulting threshold cycle (CT) values of the target mRNAs to the CT values of the endogenous control GAPDH in the same samples (ΔCT = CT_{target} − CT_{GAPDH}), and by further normalizing to the control (ΔΔCT = ΔCT − $ΔCT_{vehicle}$). Fold change in expression was then obtained ($2^{-ΔΔCT}$) and represented in the plots using a log_2 scale for ease of visualization of up/down-regulated genes.

2.8. Bioinformatics and Statistical Methods

Chemical-protein network analysis was performed using STITCH software (http://stitch.embl.de/) using ver. 3.0 software and high score cut-off settings. Drug list used as input is shown in Table S1 and base on Najm et al. [9] and Porcu et al. [8]. In studies performed in multiwell plates (immunofluorescence and qPCR), three replicates per sample were spotted in each plate and the mean values obtained from the three samples were considered as one biological replicate. The mean values ±SEM obtained from at least three biological replicates were considered for statistical analyses. Statistical analyses were performed using GraphPad Prism. Effects of each drug treatment versus its internal control (vehicle) in immunofluorescence experiments, WB and qPCR data were analyzed using paired two-tailed Student's *t* test, while one-way analysis of variance (ANOVA) with Tukey's or Holm-Sidak post hoc tests (as indicated in figure legends) were used to determine statistically significant differences among multiple single or combined treatments.

3. Results

3.1. Gefitinib Promotes MBP Expression and Oli-neuM Differentiation in Myelinating OLs

Four main pharmacological classes have been identified in phenotypical screens for promyelinating agents based on MBP upregulation: glucocorticoids, EGFR/ErbB inhibitors, Benztropine/Bromocriptine and antifungal drugs such as Miconazole and Clotrimazole. We established a chemical–protein network using STITCH ver. 3.0 software (www.stitch.embl.de), using a high score cut-off setting. This analysis indicated the membrane-associated ATP-binding cassette (ABC) transporter ABCB1A (MDR) at the hub of all selected drug classes (Figure 1A; Table S1). As expected, the glucocorticoid receptor GR/NR3C1 was found at the node of the glucocorticoid group of compounds [8] and the EGFR/ErbB receptors at the node of Gefitinib and Erlotinib drug action. Surprisingly, Benztropine and Bromocriptine form a group with DRD2/3 dopaminergic receptors as common targets (Figure 1A, Table S1). Previous work associated the effect of Benztropine on OPC differentiation with its activity on the M1/M2 muscarinic receptor [5]. More recently, the effects of Miconazole, Clotrimazole and Benztropine action on MBP expression has been attributed to their common ability to inhibit two key enzymes of the cholesterol biosynthetic pathway leading to 8,9-unsaturated sterol accumulation [46]. How these different observations can be reconciled remains to be investigated [47].

Here, we focused on validating the predicted role of the EGFR/ErbB antagonists in OPC maturation up to the stage of axon engagement. Gefitinib is a well-characterized anticancer agent that targets multiple membrane receptors of the EGFR/ErbB family, with a higher affinity for the ATP binding pocket of the EGFR receptor [33,48]. The glucocorticoids Clobetasol, Fluorandrenolide, Halcinonide, Amcinonide and Medrisone are characterized by agonistic activity on the Hedgehog pathway via Smo [32], in addition to their activity on the glucocorticoid receptor [49]. The requirement of Smo activation for MBP expression in Clobetasol-treated Oli-neuM cells was previously confirmed experimentally [8].

To compare the effects of Gefitinib and Clobetasol on MBP expression in Oli-neuM, we performed quantitative immunofluorescence microscopy (IF) and qPCR analyses (Figure 1B). Treatment of

Oli-neuM cells with either Gefitinib or Clobetasol confirmed that they are similar in their ability to increase MBP levels compared to the vehicle control (Figure 1B). Given that MBP mRNA is co-transported with ribonucleic particles to endosomes prior to being translated locally [50,51], we tested whether MBP upregulation was due to increased gene transcription and/or increased translation. Using qPCR, we observed that Clobetasol or Gefitinib treatment also enhances MBP gene transcription in addition to increasing MBP protein expression (Figure 1B, right panel).

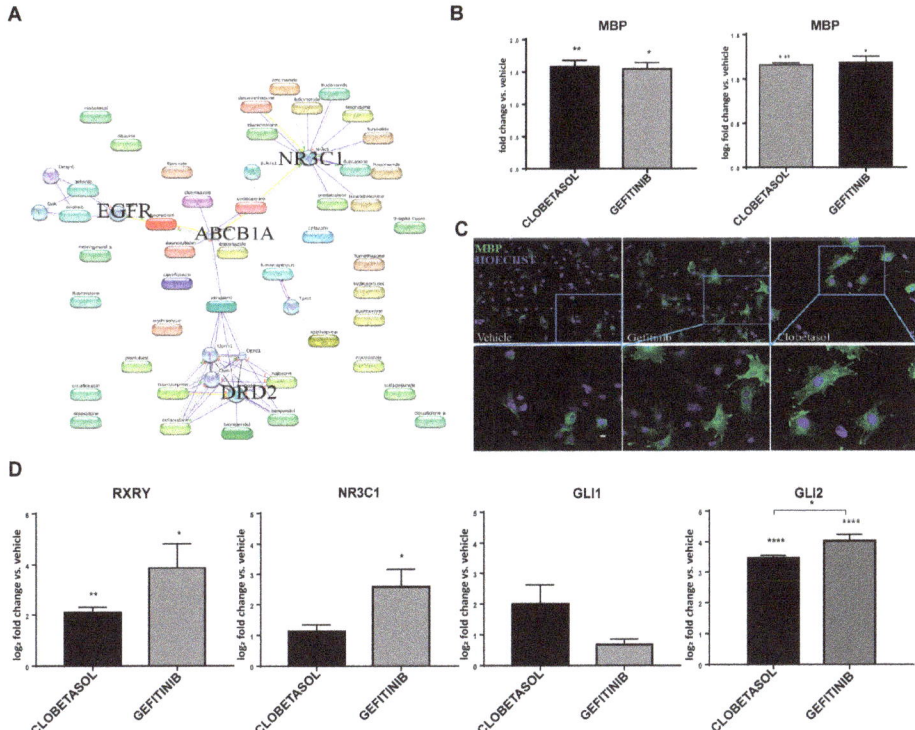

Figure 1. Gefitinib and Clobetasol stimulate MBP, RXRγ and Gli2 expression and Oli-neuM differentiation (**A**) STITCH Confidence view. Chemical-network analysis of drugs promoting MBP expression in OPC cell lines. Thicker lines indicate stronger associations; grey lines: protein-protein interactions. Green: chemical-protein interactions; red: interactions between chemicals. See Table S1 for chemical list and details. (**B**) MBP expression analysis of Oli-neuM treated for 48 h with 5 μM Clobetasol or 1 μM Gefitinib. Left panel: immunofluorescence quantitative analysis; Right panel: qPCR expression analyses. Data were normalized to vehicle, and are expressed as mean ± SEM (n = 3). Statistical significance: two-tailed paired Student's t test was used for treatment versus vehicle. (**C**) Representative images of cells quantified in the left panel in B. The bottom images show enlargements of the boxed areas. Scale bar, 10 μm. (**D**) qPCR expression analysis of Oli-neuM treated with the indicated drugs. qPCR was performed using oligos indicated in Table S2. Oli-neuM cells were treated as in (**B**). Data were normalized to an internal control (GAPDH) and plotted as log$_2$ fold change vs. vehicle, ±SEM using GraphPad Prism (n = 3). Log$_2$-fold changes were used to show graphically the positive and negative changes in expression in a symmetrical manner. The level of expression in the control (which equals 1) is represented as 0. Statistical significance: two-tailed Student's t test was used for treatment versus vehicle, ANOVA one-way with Tukey's multiple comparison test was used to determine significance among different treatments. * $p < 0.05$, ** $p < 0.01$, *** $p < 0.001$, **** $p < 0.0001$.

To test if this increase in MBP was paralleled by a progression in the differentiation of the cells to an OL-like stage, we monitored the morphology of Oli-neuM cells after Gefitinib or Clobetasol treatment using immunofluorescence microscopy. Differentiated OLs have enlarged and flattened membranes filled with MBP (Figure 1C) [24,50,51]. Oli-neuM cells pass from a triangular or round shape, typical of pre-OLs, to an enlarged and flattened morphology, typical of myelinating OLs. In cells with enlarged membranes, MBP filled the cytosol as well as the digit processes where the brightest spots of MBP were visualized, indicating that the protein accumulates at these sites (Figure 1C and see below for quantitative morphological analyses).

We concluded that Gefitinib and Clobetasol similarly promote MBP expression and Oli-neuM differentiation from a pre-myelinating stage to a differentiated morphology typical of myelinating OLs.

3.2. Gefitinib and Clobetasol Treatment Upregulate RXRγ and Gli2 Expression

The essential players required for pre-OL differentiation into mature OLs are poorly understood [3]. Oli-neuM express Myrf [8,19,52]; thus, we concentrated our attention on nuclear factors acting downstream of Myrf expression. Of these, the 9-cis retinoic acid-responsive element RXRγ is known to be upregulated at the transition from NPCs to the OPC lineage [53], as well as at lesions in the lysolecithin-induced murine demyelination model [54]. Furthermore, we have previously shown that the RXRγ inhibitor UV3003 downregulates MBP expression upon Clobetasol or Halcinonide treatment of Oli-neuM [8]. This indicates that the OPC transition to myelinating OLs is recapitulated in Oli-neuM under Clobetasol treatment via RXRγ expression. However, the signal that promotes RXRγ expression under remyelination stimuli or Clobetasol treatment remained to be determined [54,55].

To determine if RXRγ expression is similarly regulated under Gefitinib or Clobetasol treatment, we measured the expression of RXRγ along with that of Smo effectors Gli1 and Gli2 [56] or the GR NR3C1 [8] using qPCR and the oligos indicated in Table S2.

We confirmed that Clobetasol stimulates RXRγ expression without significantly altering Gli1 or NR3C1 expression (Figure 1D, respective panels) as previously reported [8]. Gefitinib treatment significantly up-regulates both RXRγ and NR3C1, but not Gli1 (Figure 1D, respective panels). Of note, either Gefitinib or Clobetasol treatment potently enhance Gli2 gene transcription (Figure 1D, respective panels).

Thus, Gefitinib and Clobetasol share the ability to promote expression not only of MBP, but also of Gli2 and RXRγ, while they poorly affect the expression of the canonical Smo target, Gli1. Since Gefitinib treatment has not been previously associated with RXRγ or Gli2 expression, we hypothesized that this is a specific function that the EGFR/ErbB inhibitor exerts in developing OPCs that might be required to promote their transition to myelinating OLs.

To determine the importance of RXRγ for Gefitinib- or Clobetasol-mediated MBP and/or Gli2 expression, we performed epistatic studies by silencing RXRγ expression using esiRNA (see Materials and Methods and Table S2) and measuring Gli2 and MBP expression in RXRγ-silenced cells after drug treatment. All data were evaluated against treated siScramble-transfected cells as control (Figure 2). RXRγ silencing completely abrogated the stimulatory effects of Clobetasol or Gefitinib on RXRγ gene transcription (Figure 2A, RXRγ panel). Furthermore, we observed that Clobetasol or Gefitinib treatment of RXRγ-silenced cells significantly reduced MBP expression over the siScramble control as determined by qPCR (Figure 2A; MBP panel), immunoblot (Figure S1, respective panels) and immunofluorescence analyses (Figure 2B, panels Clobetasol and, 2C, panels Gefitinib, respectively). Despite RXRγ being heavily down-regulated upon silencing (average silencing was about 80%, Figure S1), the reduction in Gli2 expression levels was statistically significant only for Clobetasol-treated but not for Gefitinib-treated cells, compared to controls (Figure 2A panel Gli2).

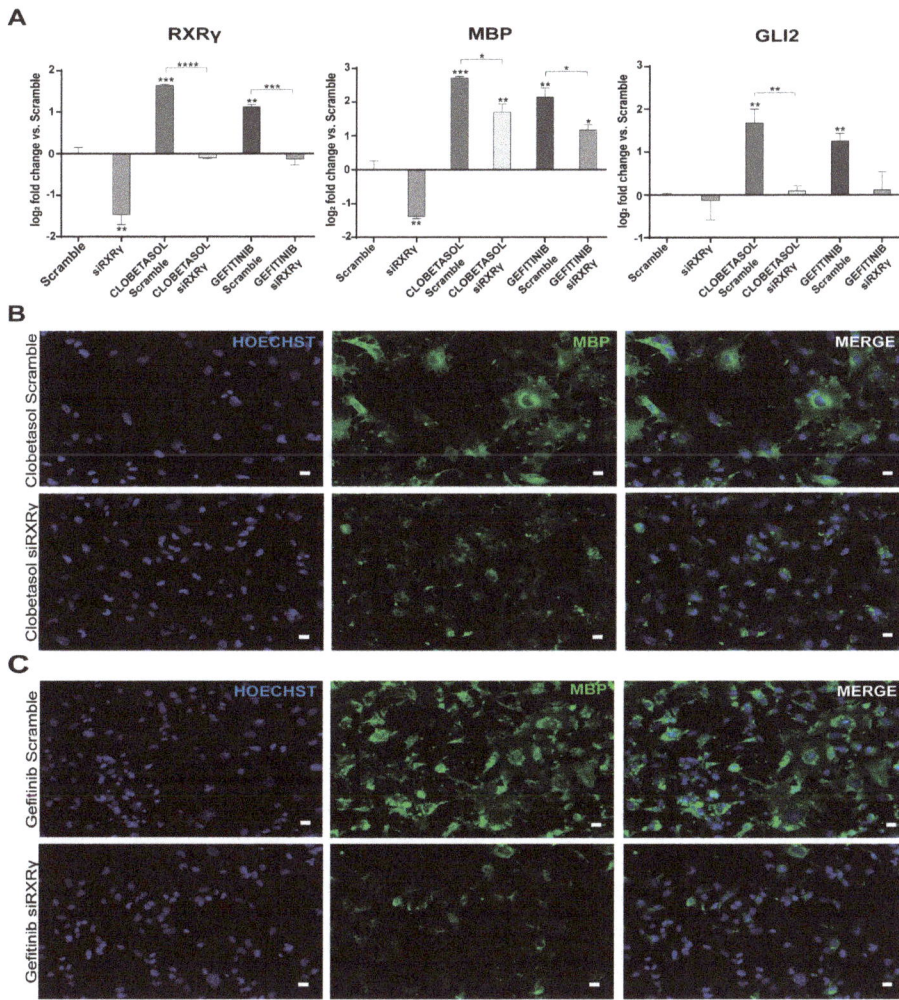

Figure 2. RXRγ gene silencing reduces MBP expression under Clobetasol or Gefitinib treatment. (**A**) qPCR analyses of RXRγ, MBP, and Gli2 gene expression in Scramble-silenced (Scramble) or RXRγ-silenced (siRXRγ) Oli-neuM cells. Cells were seeded and treated as indicated in Materials and Methods. After 48 h mRNA was extracted and processed for qPCR using oligos indicated in Table S2. Data were normalized to an internal control (GAPDH) and plotted as log$_2$ fold change vs. control (mean of siScramble 2 + 7) ± SEM (n ≥ 4) using GraphPad Prism. Log$_2$ fold changes were used to show graphically the positive and negative changes in expression in a symmetrical manner. The level of expression in the control (which equals 1) is represented as 0. Statistical significance: two-tailed paired Student's t test was used for treatment versus control. One-way ANOVA with post-hoc Tukey was used for comparing multiple treatments. * $p < 0.05$, ** $p < 0.01$, *** $p < 0.001$, **** $p < 0.0001$. (**B**) Representative images of siScramble-silenced or siRXRγ Oli-neuM cells treated for 48 h with Clobetasol or (**C**) Gefitinib. Immunofluorescence analyses were performed with anti-MBP and nuclei were stained with HOECHST (Blue) as indicated in Materials and Methods. Scale bar: 10 μm.

We concluded that MBP upregulation requires RXRγ expression after Clobetasol or Gefitinib treatment, and thus RXRγ expression is an essential component of the signaling that leads to MBP expression in Oli-neuM under these treatments. The requirement of RXRγ for Clobetasol-mediated Gli2 expression supports the view that Clobetasol treatment acts through multiple receptors in Oli-neuM differentiation, one of which is Smo, as we previously suggested [8].

3.3. EGFR/ErbB Inhibition Promotes MBP Expression and Gefitinib or siEGFR Silencing Combined with Clobetasol Treatment Potently Stimulates MBP Expression and Oli-neuM Differentiation

Since Gefitinib has a higher affinity for the ATP pocket of EGFR compared to other targets in the EGFR/ErbB family [33,48], we wondered if inhibition of this specific receptor regulates MBP and/or RXRγ expression. For this we used EGFR esiRNA (siEGFR; see Materials and Methods) and found that MBP gene transcription is significantly upregulated by EGFR silencing compared to siScramble-transfected cells (Figure 3A). While a slight increase in RXRγ gene expression and a slight reduction in Gli2 gene expression compared to controls were observed in EGFR silenced cells, these effects were not statistically significant (Figure 3A respective panels). These data are consistent with the idea that EGFR inhibition per se favors MBP expression, but that co-regulation of multiple receptors is at the basis of RXRγ and Gli2 gene expression under Gefitinib treatment.

These observations suggested that MBP expression might be further increased relative to other treatments by appropriately co-regulating EGFR (inhibition) and the Clobetasol receptor targets. Cooperative signaling responding to Smo and EGFR receptor co-activation was previously observed in medulloblastoma cells treated with Gefitinib [57] and Clobetasol action on MBP has been attributed to Smo [8] and/or GR [9] activation. Therefore, we wondered if the Clobetasol promyelinating activity could be further enhanced by EGFR gene silencing. To validate this idea, we treated EGFR silenced Oli-neuM cells with Clobetasol and measured MBP expression after 48 h by qPCR. Confirming a potential crosstalk between Smo and EGFR signaling pathways, silencing of EGFR under Clobetasol treatment potently stimulated MBP compared to controls (Figure 3A).

These data prompted us to evaluate the efficacy of the combinatorial treatment of Clobetasol and Gefitinib on MBP expression and on Oli-neuM differentiation.

Oli-neuM cells were treated with Clobetasol and Gefitinib (CLOB + GEF), with each drug alone, or with vehicle controls for 48 h and the effects on MBP expression were determined using qPCR (Figure 3B), by immunoblot analyses (Figure 3C), and by quantitative immunofluorescence microscopy (Figure 3D). Clearly, MBP expression is significantly enhanced at both the mRNA and protein level in co-treated cells compared with single treatments or vehicle controls. Accompanying the MBP increase, as expected, cells maximize their membrane size (Figure 3E), as determined by quantitative morphological analyses of the Max Feret Diameter of cells expressing high amounts of MBP (Figure 3F).

Collectively, these data show that EGFR inhibition per se stimulates MBP and partially RXRγ expression in pre-myelinating Oli-neuM. Importantly, when combined with Clobetasol treatment, potently stimulates not only MBP expression but also OPC differentiation by unlocking the events that lead to membrane expansion. Independently confirming this view, Gefitinib, which inhibits EGFR but also other members of this receptor family, not only promotes MBP expression and membrane expansion but also up-regulates RXRγ and Gli2 gene transcription.

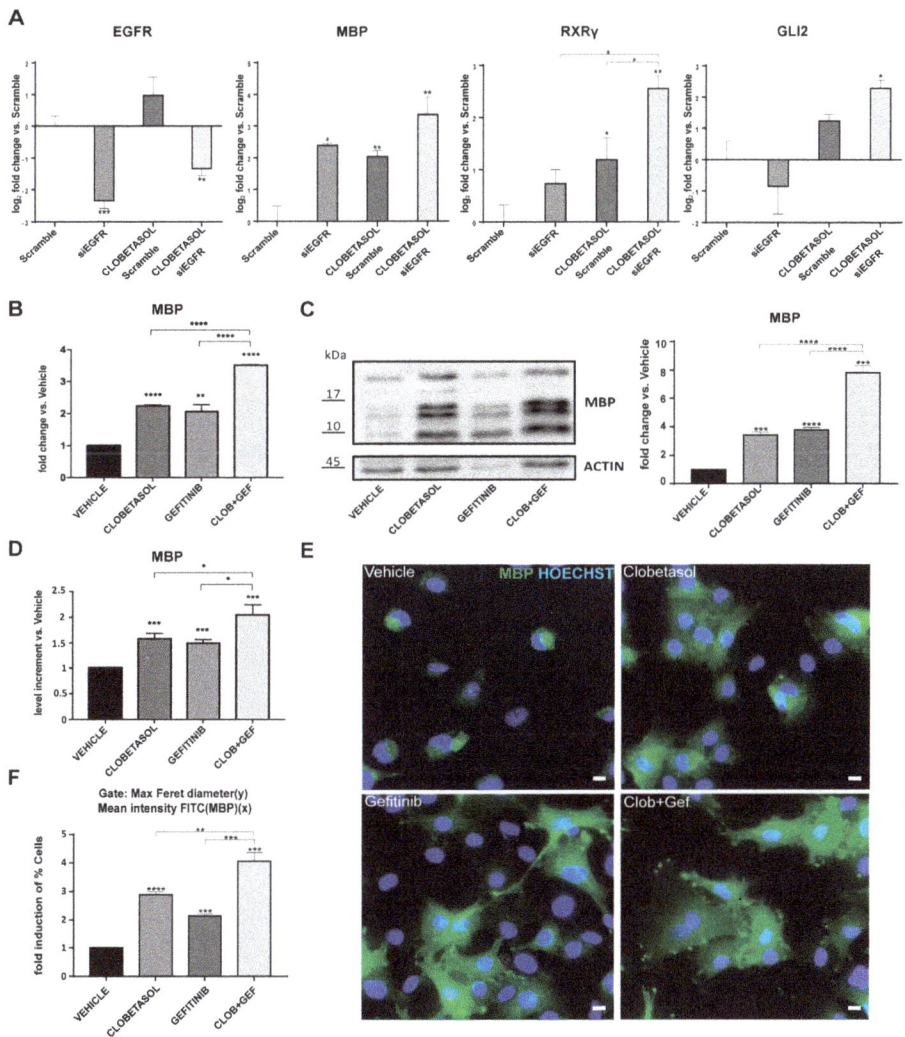

Figure 3. Epidermal growth factor receptor (EGFR) gene silencing upregulates MBP expression and increases Clobetasol-mediated Oli-neuM differentiation. (**A**) qPCR analysis of siEGFR Oli-neuM cells versus control (siScramble) in untreated or Clobetasol-treated Oli-neuM. The graphs show gene expression levels of EGFR, MBP, RXRγ and Gli2 (respective panels) after 48 h treatment. Data were plotted as $\log_2$ fold change versus control (siScramble) ± SEM (n ≥ 4) $\log_2$-fold changes were used to show graphically the positive and negative changes in expression in a symmetrical manner. The level of expression in the control (which equals 1) is represented as 0. (**B–F**) Comparison of 1 µM Gefitinib or 5 µM Clobetasol single or combinatorial drug effects: (**B**) qPCR analyses of MBP gene expression under the indicated treatments versus vehicle (DM + DMSO). Data were normalized to an internal control (GAPDH) and plotted as fold change induction above vehicle arbitrarily set as 1. Data are mean ± SEM (n = 3). (**C**) Immunoblot analyses of MBP expression with the indicated treatment. Left panel: Representative immunoblot analysis using anti-MBP or anti-Actin antibody as indicated in Material and Methods; right panel: quantification of bands detected in immunoblots (n = 3 ± SEM) using ImageJ tools. Data are plotted as fold induction versus vehicle arbitrarily set at 1; (**D**) Immunofluorescence

quantitative analyses of images of Oli-neuM cells treated as indicated. Mean intensity FITC (MBP) was plotted as mean ± SEM (n = 5). Data were normalized to vehicle, arbitrarily set to 1, and plotted as fold induction versus vehicle. (**E**) Representative images of Oli-neuM vehicle-treated cells stained with α-MBP primary and Alexa 488 secondary antibodies (FITC); HOECHST (Blue) = nuclei. Scale bar, 10 µm. (**F**) Quantitative morphological analysis was performed using Scan^R software (Olympus) using maxFeretDiameter and Mean Intensity FITC parameters. Data were plotted in a graph by Scan^R software and the mean % population within the gate MaxFeretDiameter > 70 (y)/MeanFITC (MBP) (x) comparatively evaluated to identify the treatment promoting higher MBP expression and larger membrane expansion. Data are shown as fold induction versus vehicle arbitrarily set at 1. Statistical significance was calculated using GraphPad: two-tailed Student's *t* test versus control (siScramble Figure 3A) or versus Vehicle (Figure 3B–F). One-way ANOVA with Tukey's correction was used for multiple treatment comparison. * $p < 0.05$, ** $p < 0.01$, *** $p < 0.001$, **** $p < 0.0001$.

3.4. Clobetasol and Gefitinib Co-Treatment Enhances Oli-neuM Differentiation by Co-Regulating PIP2 Availability with MBP Expression

It is well-described that Gefitinib inhibits the phosphatidylinositol-3-kinase (PI3K) signaling pathway and impairs proliferation in tumor cells [51]. PI3K uses PIP2 as a substrate to produce phosphatidylinositol (3,4,5)-trisphosphate (PIP3) [58], which is required to activate the AKT-dependent axis, which, when activated, promotes cell proliferation. However, how Gefitinib might promote membrane enlargement in OPCs by downregulating the PI3K/PIP3/AKT axis remains to be established. We reasoned that if Gefitinib downregulates the PI3K/PIP3/AKT signaling axis, it could (indirectly) favor an increase in PIP2 levels and/or its re-localization at OL membranes. Such an event could promote membrane enlargement by promoting PIP2/MBP complex formation [23,24]. Alternatively, Gefitinib treatment could promote differentiation by downregulating Ras/MAPK/ERK pathways.

We first asked if the PI3K/PIP3/AKT or Ras/MAPK/ERK pathways are affected under our experimental conditions. Oli-neuM cells were treated with Gefitinib alone or in combination with Clobetasol and the ratio of phospho-ERK1/2 (pERK) versus ERK or phospho-AKT (pAKT) versus AKT levels was determined by Western blot analysis. Forskolin was used as a positive control for MAPK/ERK activation [59], insulin as a positive control for PI3K/PIP3/AKT activation [42], and Wortmannin as a negative control for PI3K activation [40,41]. The results indicated that Gefitinib significantly inhibits the PI3K/PIP3/AKT axis (Figure 4A) over the MAPK/ERK axis (Figure 4B) under the conditions used in this study. Clearly, although Wortmannin antagonizes PI3K (Figure 4C) and, as expected, impairs insulin-mediated AKT activation when given in co-treatment (Figure 4C, INS + WOR), it does not promote MBP expression, unlike Gefitinib (Figure 4D, respective sample). Gefitinib, as expected, inhibits insulin-mediated AKT phosphorylation and conversely insulin completely abrogates MBP expression under Gefitinib treatment by bypassing Gefitinib-mediated PI3K inactivation. Together these data show that MBP expression under Gefitinib treatment does not depend only on PI3K/PIP3/AKT signaling inhibition but that PI3K activation can turn off Gefitinib-mediated MBP expression, supporting the multi-receptor nature of Gefitinib-dependent MBP expression.

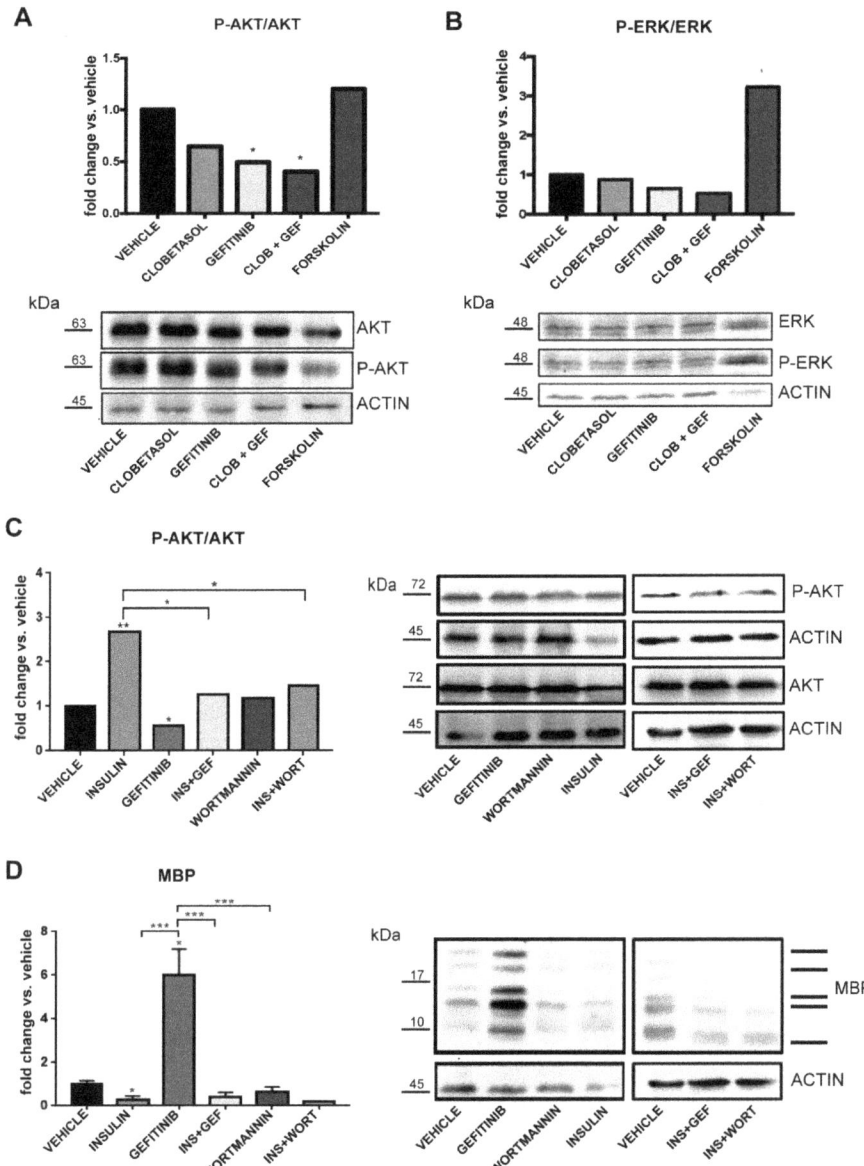

Figure 4. Analysis of the signaling pathways activated by Gefitinib treatment in Oli-neuM cells. (**A**,**B**) Immunoblot analysis Oli-neuM cell extracts after treatment with 1 μM Gefitinib, 5 μM Clobetasol, 5 μM Forskolin (as control treatment), or vehicle (DM + 0.5% DMSO). Quantitative analysis of protein levels: (**A**) top panel: anti-AKT (AKT) or phospho-AKT (P-AKT) antibody. Anti-actin antibody was used to normalize sample loading. (n = 3). Signal intensity was estimated on bands using ImageJ software tools, and data were plotted using GraphPad Prism as the fold change of P-AKT/AKT. A 2-fold change threshold versus vehicle was applied (indicated with *). Lower panel: representative image of immunoblots used for quantitative analysis. (**B**) Top panel: anti-ERK (ERK) or anti-phospho-ERK (P-ERK) antibody. Data and statistical analyses (n = 3) were performed as in (**A**). Lower panel: representative image of immunoblots used for quantitative analysis. (**C**,**D**) Immunoblot analysis of

Oli-neuM cell extracts after treatment with insulin (5 µg/mL), Gefitinib (1 µM), Wortmannin (1 µM), insulin+Gefitinib (INS + GEF), Wortmannin+Gefitinib (WORT+GEF), or vehicle (DM + 0.5% DMSO). (**C**) Left panel: quantitative analyses of the bands obtained after immunoblotting using an anti-AKT (AKT) or phospho-AKT (P-AKT) antibody (n = 3). An anti-actin antibody was used to normalize sample loading (n = 3). Signal intensity was estimated using ImageJ software, and data were plotted using GraphPad Prism as the fold change versus vehicle, arbitrarily set to 1. Statistical significance: two-tailed Student's t test was used for treatment versus vehicle, ANOVA one-way with Tukey's multiple comparison test was used to determine significance among different treatments. * $p < 0.05$, ** $p < 0.01$, *** $p < 0.001$, **** $p < 0.0001$. Right panel: representative immunoblot image of treatments. (**D**) Left panel: quantitative analysis of bands visualized by immunoblotting using an anti-MBP antibody. Data and statistical analyses were performed as in (**C**). Right panel: representative immunoblot images.

We reasoned that the Gefitinib treatment, by inhibiting the EGFR/PI3K/PIP3 pathway, might favor PIP2 re-localization at membranes and, thereby, PIP2 and MBP complex formation. As previously mentioned, the formation of the PIP2 and MBP complexes at the peak of MBP expression, by causing the release of the F-actin depolymerization proteins cofilin and gelsolin, promotes OL membrane enlargement [22,24,60]. To determine the existence of PIP2/MBP complexes in Clobetasol and Gefitinib co-treated Oli-neuM cells, we employed immunofluorescence confocal microscopy (see Materials and Methods) and anti-PIP2 and anti-MBP primary and the appropriate secondary antibodies. The PIP2/MBP complexes were visualized on acquired images by determining the Mean Pearson's correlation coefficient (PCC) and the mean Mander's overlap coefficient (MOC) of PIP2-(FITC) and MBP-(TRITC) signals in samples of treated compared to controls (Figure 5A; Figure S2). The resulting scatterplot of pixel intensity of co-localizing spots showed a clear correlation between PIP2 (green) and MBP (red) channels (n = 10). To visualize the structures to which these signals belong, a 3D surface reconstruction was performed using Imaris analysis tools (Figure 5B, blue box). This analysis showed vesicle-like carriers of about 600 nm containing PIP2 and MBP in the cytosol of Gefitinib and Clobetasol-treated Oli-neuM cells.

To establish if Oli-neuM cells treated with Clobetasol and Gefitinib had reached the final stage of differentiation that allows myelination of axons, we used cell culture chambers containing PS electrospun microfibers of 2–4 µm (PS chambers; Figure S3) suitable for microscopy inspection. This diameter of PS microfiber, by mimicking axons, allows primary OPCs to wrap along the fibers [25–28,46]. In our setup, Oli-neuM cells were seeded in the PS chamber 24 h prior to treatment (see Materials and Methods). Specifically, to establish the level of engagement of cells, we counted the proportion of cells with cytosol filled with MBP wrapped on the fibers (visualized in phase contrast) that also showed elongated nuclei (Hoechst; Figure 5C). Quantitative analysis of images showed that combined Clobetasol and Gefitinib treatment increases the number of Oli-neuM cells able to engage synthetic axons, compared to single or control treatments (Figure 5D). To determine the localization of PIP2 in Gefitinib and Clobetasol-treated cells during fiber engagement, we transfected Oli-neuM cells with plasmids carrying the pleckstrin homology (PH) domain of PLCδ1 fused to GFP (ΔPLCδ-pEGFP). The PLCδ1-PH domain is specifically recognized by PIP2 and thereby allows the visualization of PIP2 in fixed and living cells [43]. Clearly, PIP2-enriched membranes (Figure 6, green signals) wrap fibers over a long stretch in the Clobetasol and Gefitinib treated cells compared to vehicle control (Figure 6A–C), consistent with the role of Gefitinib and Clobetasol as remyelinating drugs.

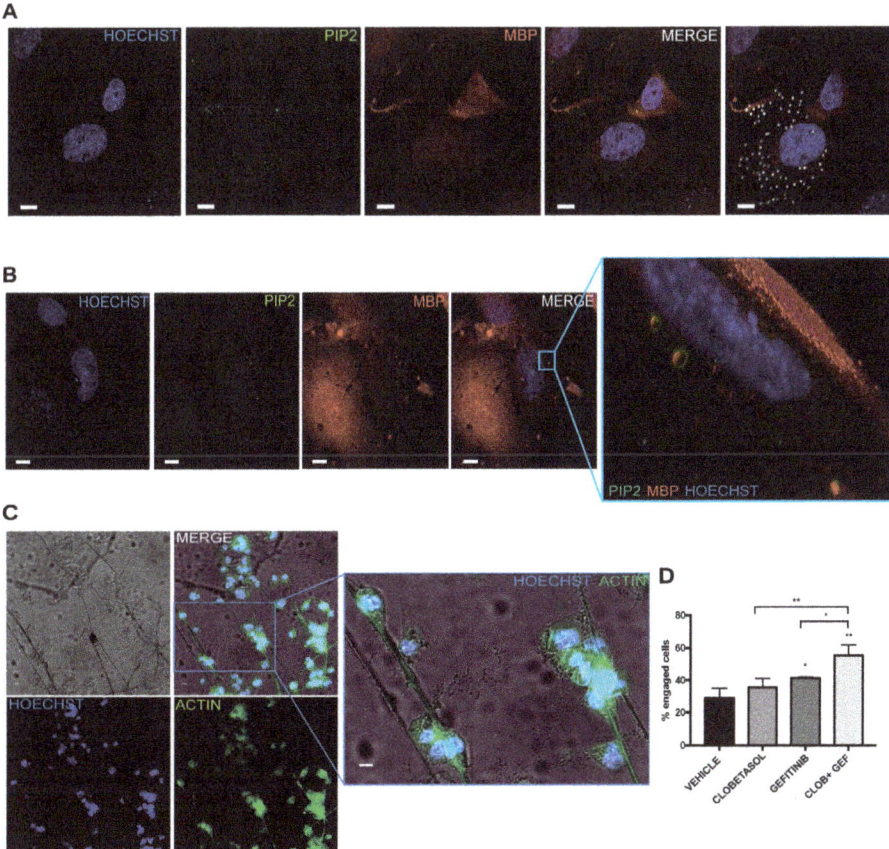

Figure 5. Clobetasol and Gefitinib co-treatment triggers MBP and PIP2 co-localization and enhances Oli-neuM engagement of polystyrene microfibers. (**A,B**) Confocal microscopy images of Oli-neuM cells treated with 5 µM Clobetasol and 1µM Gefitinib, stained with α-MBP (TRITC) and α-PIP2 (FITC). Nuclei (Hoechst). (**A**) Immunofluorescence images of cells showing PIP2 and MBP co-localization. Co-localization measurement details are shown in Figure S3. In the right-most panel, the co-localizing spots are highlighted by white dots. (**B**) Co-localization of MBP-PIP2. Colocalization analyses are in Figure S2. Confocal images of cells in which three-dimensional (3D) reconstruction has been performed. The blue boxed area in the MERGE panel indicates the region containing the co-localizing spots that is enlarged in the right panel. Blue boxed right panel: 3D volume reconstruction was performed using Imaris 6.21 suite on cropped images (Z-stack = 0.3 µm step size). Scale bar = 10 µm. (**C**) Epifluorescence IF microscopy images of Oli-neuM cells grown on PS microfiber chambers. Representative IF images of Oli-neuM cells treated for 72 h with 5 µM Clobetasol and 1 µM Gefitinib (CLOB GEF) cultured on supports containing electrospun PS microfibers (2–4 µm). Blue box shows an enlarged view of the region containing engaged cells. Cells were fixed and processed for IF microscopy as indicated in Materials and Methods. Fibers were visualized using phase contrast. Anti-actin (FITC), nuclei (HOECHST). Image acquisition was performed using a 20× objective, as indicated in Materials and Methods. Scale bar: 10 µm. (**D**) Engagement quantification after treatments. Image quantification was performed by analyzing 75 images/sample for each treatment (n = 3). Specifically, the percentage of engaged cells was estimated by counting nuclei located on fibers or within a range of 86 µm from the fiber. Data were plotted in the graph (n = 3, mean ± SEM) using GraphPad Prism as indicated in the text. Two-tailed paired Student's *t* test was used for statistical significance versus vehicle (NT), one-way ANOVA with Tukey's multiple comparison test was used to analyze statistical significance among different treatments. * $p < 0.05$, ** $p < 0.01$.

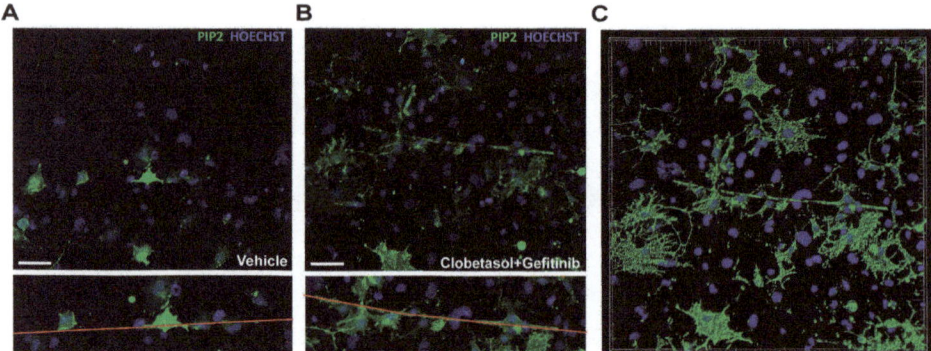

Figure 6. Clobetasol and Gefitinib promote lateral lengthening onto PS microfibers compared to vehicle-treated cells. Confocal microscopy images of PH-PLCδ-pEGFP-transfected Oli-neuM cells grown for 48 h in PS microfiber-containing growth chambers treated with (**A**) Vehicle (DM+ DMSO) or (**B**) 5 µM Clobetasol and 1 µM Gefitinib. Top (**A,B**) panels: confocal images, PIP2 (Green), Nuclei (Blue) Scale bar = 70µm. Lower (**A,B**) panels: detail of top images with enlargement of the cells engaging the PS microfiber. PS Microfibers are highlighted in red. Scale bar = 30 µm. (**C**) Volume reconstruction of image in panel (**B**), performed with Imaris software as described in Materials and Methods. Green = PIP2-containing membranes, blue = nuclei.

4. Discussion

The current study shows that EGFR inhibition per se favors MBP expression in pre-myelinating OLs and Gefitinib, by inhibiting EGFR as well as other EGFR/ErbB family members, is a potent promyelinating agent. Clobetasol and Gefitinib co-treatment, by co-regulating at least three of the receptors involved in OPC differentiation, namely Smo, GR (activation) and EGFR/ErbB (inhibition), mimic the natural signals promoting OPC differentiation until axon engagement. We show that Clobetasol and Gefitinib co-treatment maximizes MBP expression and PIP2 co-localization at endosome-like structures with consequent membrane expansion allowing synthetic axon engagement.

This work initiated with the in silico analysis of the chemical-protein network of drug targets that emerged from the study of Porcu et al. [8]. This analysis indicated the existence of a cross-talking network of receptors involved in Oli-neuM differentiation. We hypothesized that if appropriately stimulated/inhibited by the promyelinating drug, each receptor would promote signaling pathways leading to OPC differentiation. Based on these hypotheses, we began by studying the effects of EGFR/ErbB receptor(s) regulation by Gefitinib or EGFR gene silencing.

Using Gefitinib, we have clarified that EGFR/ErbB receptor(s) inhibition has two main effects: on the one hand, it contributes to upregulating MBP, RXRγ and Gli2 gene expression, while on the other hand, by downregulating the PI3K/PIP3/AKT signaling cascade at the peak of MBP expression, it enhances PIP2 and MBP interaction and thereby membrane expansion. We observed that while Gefitinib upregulates RXRγ and Gli2 gene transcription it has little effect on the expression of NR3C1 and Gli1. By comparing EGFR gene silencing with Gefitinib treatment we found that EGFR silencing contributes to upregulating MBP gene expression, as does chemical inhibition, but less effectively enhances RXRγ gene transcription and poorly affect Gli2 gene expression. Thus, EGFR genetic inhibition does not completely overlap Gefitinib action on OPC differentiation. We concluded that Gefitinib acts through EGFR inhibition but also through other pathways in promoting OPC differentiation.

Using RXRγ gene silencing, we showed that RXRγ is necessary to maximize MBP expression under Gefitinib or Clobetasol treatment. However, RXRγ silencing does not abolish either Gefitinib- or Clobetasol-mediated MBP expression. Thus, both drugs act on MBP expression via multiple pathways, one of which requires RXRγ.

How Gefitinib or Clobetasol treatment leads to RXRγ upregulation remains to be determined in our or in other systems [54]. The fact that the combined treatment with Clobetasol and siRXRγ returns Gli2 expression to basal levels shows that RXRγ acts before Gli2 in Clobetasol-mediated signaling to MBP and confirms that Clobetasol acts not only by GR mediated phosphorylation on MBP expression [9], but also via a RXRγ/Gli2/MBP pathway as we previously suggested [8].

A correlation between RXRγ upregulation and Gefitinib treatment has been previously indicated by the cooperative antitumor activity of the RXRγ-selective agonist Bexarotene and Gefitinib in preclinical models of non-small cell lung cancer [61]. PI3K inactivation by Gefitinib treatment can promote Retinoic Acid Receptor (RAR) gamma 2 transcriptional activity in cancer cells [62]. Thus, Gefitinib treatment might indirectly contribute to RXRγ upregulation by stimulating RXRγ dimerization with other nuclear factors, among which RARγ [55]. Moreover, RARβ, the vitamin D receptor (VDR), and the peroxisome proliferator activated receptor (gamma PPARγ) have been co-immunoprecipitated with RXRγ in cell lysates from OPC or OL primary cells, indicating that they might also be the active heterodimers during the OPC to OL differentiation [63]. In addition, other nuclear receptors regulating lipid homeostasis in myelinating OLs, such as Liver X Receptor (LXR), orphan Nur77 and Nurr1, and Farnesoid X receptor (FXR), can form dimers with RXRγ [55]. Thus, RXRγ upregulation by Gefitinib or Clobetasol treatment might contribute to coordinating lipid metabolism with MBP expression under EGFR and Smo signaling in myelinating OLs.

Several members of EGFR/ErbB have been previously shown to be involved in PNS and/or CNS myelination [34–36,64] and the role of EGF in promoting oligodendrogenesis till OPC differentiation has been recently established [36], but the signal that promotes EGFR/ErbB inhibition during OPC differentiation remains unclear [34,35,64–67]. Unfortunately, ErbB2, ErbB3, or ErbB4 mouse knock out models have not allowed to clarify the role of each receptor in brain development: they are either embryonic lethal or show postnatal death with neurodevelopmental and cardiac defects [64]. This work adds EGFR to the list of EGFR/ErbB family members potentially regulating MBP expression in differentiating OPC, by placing EGFR functional inhibition as required after Myrf expression to enhance MBP expression and to promote its interaction with PIP2. Further study will clarify the role of EGFR, if any, in OL engagement.

Clearly, Gefitinib, which inhibits multiple members of the EGFR/ErbB family [33], might act on RXRγ and Gli2 gene expression via regulation of one of the other of the EGFR/ErbB family members. Among the EGFR/ErbB family members that might participate in OPC differentiation, the ErbB2 receptor could be a potential partner of EGFR. ErbB2 is an orphan receptor regulated by heterodimerization with other ErbB family receptors, and is known to interact with the negative regulator of myelination, LINGO 1 [63]. It will be interesting to study EGFR and ErbB2 co-regulation during OPC differentiation. Moreover, it cannot be excluded that the role of EGFR in OPC differentiation is metabolic. In fact, it has been shown that the EGFR/src signaling pathway regulates volume-sensitive organic osmolyte efflux pathways in astrocytes and EGFR or PI3K inhibition by AG1478 or Wortmannin, respectively, results in reduced efflux of Taurine [68]. Taurine recently emerged from a metabolomics screening study as a compound able to promote OPC differentiation alone or in combination with Benztropine [69].

Consistent with the hypothesis that PI3K downregulation by Gefitinib does not promote MBP expression per se, Wortmannin, which specifically inhibits PI3K, does not have any effect on MBP expression. Furthermore, insulin, which stimulates the PI3K/PIP3/AKT axis [70], completely abrogates Gefitinib-mediated MBP expression in Oli-neuM. By downregulating EGFR/PI3K/PIP3/AKT signaling Gefitinib promotes PIP2 re-localization leading to a further increase of MBP expression compared to EGFR inhibition alone.

Using 3D reconstruction studies, we were able to visualize endosomal-like structures containing both PIP2 and MBP in Gefitinib and Clobetasol co-treated Oli-neuM cells. We observed that PIP2 accumulates at the tips of processes in 2D culture and is enriched at the sites of fiber engagement when cells are grown in 3D supports. Given the role of PIP2 in the re-localization of receptors, including

Smo, and cytoskeleton proteins to lipid rafts [71], it is tempting to speculate that the PIP2 enrichment at engaging membranes is the starting signal promoting wrapping during myelination.

In summary, our data support the view that Gefitinib, by inhibiting EGFR, promotes MBP expression and PIP2-mediated membrane enlargement, while other pathways regulate RXRγ gene expression under Clobetasol and Gefitinib treatment. Gefitinib, via PI3K/AKT pathway inhibition, could cause PIP2 re-localization thereby initiating the events leading, at the peak of MBP expression, to membrane expansion. Importantly, our combined genetic and chemical studies on the role of EGFR in OPC differentiation led to the observation that Gefitinib and Clobetasol combinatorial treatment potently increases MBP expression and OL engagement over single compound activity. This observation opens the way to study this drug combination in RRMS or other demyelination animal models and to their test in combinatorial therapies for their combinatorial remyelination properties.

Supplementary Materials: The following are available online at http://www.mdpi.com/2073-4409/8/8/844/s1.

Author Contributions: Conceptualization, Supervision, validation: A.R.-W. and A.R. Funding acquisition; Project Administration: E.T., A.R., A.R.-W. and M.T. (Marcella Trombetta); Methodology, validation, Investigation: A.R.-W., E.N., L.B., A.D.G., D.F., F.B., M.T. (Marta Tiberi), C.S. and E.R.; Formal Analyses; E.N., A.R., A.D.G., M.T.B., C.S. and E.R.; Data Curation: A.R.W., E.N., A.D.G.: A.R.-W., E.N., L.B. and A.D.G.; Writing–Original Draft; A.R.-W., E.N., A.D.G., L.B. and E.R.: Visualization. A.D.G., A.R., E.N., A.R.-W., E.R.

Funding: E.N. and A.D.G. received a Ph.D. fellowship from the Cell and Molecular biology PhD program, University of Rome "Tor Vergata". This project was supported by University of Rome Tor Vergata, "Mission: Sustainability" grant 2017 "Tissue engineering to study myelination processes". A.R. acknowledges support from Università Campus Bio-Medico di Roma ("INTESE" project, co-funded by Regione Lazio, grant# FILAS-RU-2014-1193).

Acknowledgments: We are deeply indebted to Cathal Wilson (Tigem, Naples) for critical discussion and manuscript English correction.

Conflicts of Interest: The authors declare no conflict of interest.

References

1. Plemel, J.R.; Liu, W.Q.; Yong, V.W. Remyelination Therapies: A New Direction and Challenge in Multiple Sclerosis. *Nat. Rev. Drug Discov.* **2017**, *16*, 617–634. [CrossRef]
2. Chamberlain, K.A.; Nanescu, S.E.; Psachoulia, K.; Huang, J.K. Oligodendrocyte Regeneration: Its Significance in Myelin Replacement and Neuroprotection in Multiple Sclerosis. *Neuropharmacology* **2016**, *110*, 633–643. [CrossRef]
3. Lopez Juarez, A.; He, D.; Richard Lu, Q. Oligodendrocyte Progenitor Programming and Reprogramming: Toward Myelin Regeneration. *Brain Res.* **2016**, *1638*, 209–220. [CrossRef]
4. Villoslada, P. Neuroprotective Therapies for Multiple Sclerosis and Other Demyelinating Diseases. *Mult. Scler. Demyelinating Disord.* **2016**, *1*, 1. [CrossRef]
5. Deshmukh, V.A.; Tardif, V.; Lyssiotis, C.A.; Green, C.C.; Kerman, B.; Kim, H.J.; Padmanabhan, K.; Swoboda, J.G.; Ahmad, I.; Kondo, T.; et al. A Regenerative Approach to the Treatment of Multiple Sclerosis. *Nature* **2013**, *502*, 327–332. [CrossRef]
6. Lariosa-Willingham, K.D.; Rosler, E.S.; Tung, J.S.; Dugas, J.C.; Collins, T.L.; Leonoudakis, D. A High Throughput Drug Screening Assay to Identify Compounds That Promote Oligodendrocyte Differentiation Using Acutely Dissociated and Purified Oligodendrocyte Precursor Cells. *BMC Res. Notes* **2016**, *9*. [CrossRef]
7. Mei, F.; Fancy, S.P.J.; Shen, Y.A.A.; Niu, J.; Zhao, C.; Presley, B.; Miao, E.; Lee, S.; Mayoral, S.R.; Redmond, S.A.; et al. Micropillar Arrays as a High-Throughput Screening Platform for Therapeutics in Multiple Sclerosis. *Nat. Med.* **2014**, *20*, 954–960. [CrossRef]
8. Porcu, G.; Serone, E.; De Nardis, V.; Di Giandomenico, D.; Lucisano, G.; Scardapane, M.; Poma, A.; Ragnini-Wilson, A. Clobetasol and Halcinonide Act as Smoothened Agonists to Promote Myelin Gene Expression and RxRγ Receptor Activation. *PLoS ONE* **2015**, *10*. [CrossRef]
9. Najm, F.J.; Madhavan, M.; Zaremba, A.; Shick, E.; Karl, R.T.; Factor, D.C.; Miller, T.E.; Nevin, Z.S.; Kantor, C.; Sargent, A.; et al. Drug-Based Modulation of Endogenous Stem Cells Promotes Functional Remyelination in Vivo. *Nature* **2015**, *522*, 216–220. [CrossRef]

10. Patel, S.S.; Tomar, S.; Sharma, D.; Mahindroo, N.; Udayabanu, M. Targeting Sonic Hedgehog Signaling in Neurological Disorders. *Neurosci. Biobehav. Rev.* **2017**, *74*, 76–97. [CrossRef]
11. Zuccaro, E.; Arlotta, P. The Quest for Myelin in the Adult Brain. *Nat. Cell Biol.* **2013**, *15*, 572–575. [CrossRef]
12. Ferent, J.; Zimmer, C.; Durbec, P.; Ruat, M.; Traiffort, E. Sonic Hedgehog Signaling Is a Positive Oligodendrocyte Regulator during Demyelination. *J. Neurosci.* **2013**, *33*, 1759–1772. [CrossRef]
13. Ferent, J.; Cochard, L.; Faure, H.; Taddei, M.; Hahn, H.; Ruat, M.; Traiffort, E. Genetic Activation of Hedgehog Signaling Unbalances the Rate of Neural Stem Cell Renewal by Increasing Symmetric Divisions. *Stem Cell Rep.* **2014**, *3*, 312–323. [CrossRef]
14. Samanta, J.; Salzer, J.L. Myelination: Actin Disassembly Leads the Way. *Dev. Cell* **2015**, *34*, 129–130. [CrossRef]
15. Del Giovane, A.; Ragnini-Wilson, A. Targeting Smoothened as a New Frontier in the Functional Recovery of Central Nervous System Demyelinating Pathologies. *Int. J. Mol. Sci.* **2018**, *19*, 3677. [CrossRef]
16. Infante, P.; Mori, M.; Alfonsi, R.; Ghirga, F.; Aiello, F.; Toscano, S.; Ingallina, C.; Siler, M.; Cucchi, D.; Po, A.; et al. Gli1/DNA Interaction Is a Druggable Target for Hedgehog-dependent Tumors. *EMBO J.* **2015**, *34*, 200–217. [CrossRef]
17. Samanta, J.; Grund, E.M.; Silva, H.M.; Lafaille, J.J.; Fishell, G.; Salzer, J.L. Inhibition of Gli1 Mobilizes Endogenous Neural Stem Cells for Remyelination. *Nature* **2015**, *526*, 448–452. [CrossRef]
18. Wang, L.C.; Almazan, G. Cdon, a Cell Surface Protein, Mediates Oligodendrocyte Differentiation and Myelination. *Glia* **2016**, *64*, 1021–1033. [CrossRef]
19. Emery, B.; Agalliu, D.; Cahoy, J.D.; Watkins, T.A.; Dugas, J.C.; Mulinyawe, S.B.; Ibrahim, A.; Ligon, K.L.; Rowitch, D.H.; Barres, B.A. Myelin Gene Regulatory Factor Is a Critical Transcriptional Regulator Required for CNS Myelination. *Cell* **2009**, *138*, 172–185. [CrossRef]
20. McKenzie, I.A.; Ohayon, D.; Li, H.; de Faria, J.P.; Emery, B.; Tohyama, K.; Richardson, W.D. Motor Skill Learning Requires Active Central Myelination. *Science* **2014**, *346*, 318–322. [CrossRef]
21. Duncan, G.J.; Plemel, J.R.; Assinck, P.; Manesh, S.B.; Muir, F.G.W.; Hirata, R.; Berson, M.; Liu, J.; Wegner, M.; Emery, B.; et al. Myelin Regulatory Factor Drives Remyelination in Multiple Sclerosis. *Acta Neuropathol.* **2017**, *134*, 403–422. [CrossRef] [PubMed]
22. Nawaz, S.; Kippert, A.; Saab, A.S.; Werner, H.B.; Lang, T.; Nave, K.-A.; Simons, M. Phosphatidylinositol 4,5-Bisphosphate-Dependent Interaction of Myelin Basic Protein with the Plasma Membrane in Oligodendroglial Cells and Its Rapid Perturbation by Elevated Calcium. *J. Neurosci.* **2009**, *29*, 4794–4807. [CrossRef] [PubMed]
23. Nawaz, S.; Sánchez, P.; Schmitt, S.; Snaidero, N.; Mitkovski, M.; Velte, C.; Bruckner, B.R.; Alexopoulos, I.; Czopka, T.; Rhee, J.S.; et al. Actin filament turnover drives leading edge growth during myelin sheath formation in the central nervous system. *Dev. Cell* **2015**, *34*, 139–151. [CrossRef] [PubMed]
24. Zuchero, J.B.; Fu, M.; Sloan, S.A.; Ibrahim, A.; Olson, A.; Zaremba, A.; Dugas, J.C.; Wienbar, S.; Caprariello, A.V.; Kantor, C.; et al. CNS Myelin Wrapping Is Driven by Actin Disassembly. *Dev. Cell* **2015**, *34*, 152–167. [CrossRef] [PubMed]
25. Bechler, M.E.; Byrne, L.; ffrench-Constant, C. CNS Myelin Sheath Lengths Are an Intrinsic Property of Oligodendrocytes. *Curr. Biol.* **2015**, *25*, 2411–2416. [CrossRef] [PubMed]
26. Espinosa-Hoyos, D.; Jagielska, A.; Homan, K.A.; Du, H.; Busbee, T.; Anderson, D.G.; Fang, N.X.; Lewis, J.A.; Vliet, K.J.V. Engineered 3D-Printed Artificial Axons. *Sci. Rep.* **2018**, *8*, 478. [CrossRef] [PubMed]
27. Káradóttir, R.T.; Stockley, J.H. Deconstructing Myelination: It All Comes down to Size. *Nat. Methods* **2012**, *9*, 883–884. [CrossRef]
28. Lee, Y.; Morrison, B.M.; Li, Y.; Lengacher, S.; Farah, M.H.; Hoffman, P.N.; Liu, Y.; Tsingalia, A.; Jin, L.; Zhang, P.-W.; et al. Oligodendroglia Metabolically Support Axons and Contribute to Neurodegeneration. *Nature* **2012**, *487*, 443–448. [CrossRef]
29. Urbanski, M.M.; Melendez-Vasquez, C.V. Preparation of Matrices of Variable Stiffness for the Study of Mechanotransduction in Schwann Cell Development. *Methods Mol. Biol.* **2018**, *1739*, 281–297. [CrossRef]
30. Chang, K.-J.; Redmond, S.A.; Chan, J.R. Remodeling Myelination: Implications for Mechanisms of Neural Plasticity. *Nat. Neurosci.* **2016**, *19*, 190–197. [CrossRef]
31. Yao, X.; Su, T.; Verkman, A.S. Clobetasol Promotes Remyelination in a Mouse Model of Neuromyelitis Optica. *Acta Neuropathol. Commun.* **2016**, *4*, 42. [CrossRef] [PubMed]

32. Wang, J.; Lu, J.; Bond, M.C.; Chen, M.; Ren, X.-R.; Lyerly, H.K.; Barak, L.S.; Chen, W. Identification of Select Glucocorticoids as Smoothened Agonists: Potential Utility for Regenerative Medicine. *Proc. Natl. Acad. Sci. USA* **2010**, *107*, 9323–9328. [CrossRef] [PubMed]
33. Verma, N.; Rai, A.K.; Kaushik, V.; Brünnert, D.; Chahar, K.R.; Pandey, J.; Goyal, P. Identification of Gefitinib Off-Targets Using a Structure-Based Systems Biology Approach; Their Validation with Reverse Docking and Retrospective Data Mining. *Sci. Rep.* **2016**, *6*, 33949. [CrossRef] [PubMed]
34. Joubert, L.; Foucault, I.; Sagot, Y.; Bernasconi, L.; Duval, F.; Alliod, C.; Frossard, M.-J.; Gobert, R.P.; Curchod, M.-L.; Salvat, C.; et al. Chemical Inducers and Transcriptional Markers of Oligodendrocyte Differentiation. *J. Neurosci. Res.* **2010**, *88*, 2546–2557. [CrossRef] [PubMed]
35. Koprivica, V.; Cho, K.-S.; Park, J.B.; Yiu, G.; Atwal, J.; Gore, B.; Kim, J.A.; Lin, E.; Tessier-Lavigne, M.; Chen, D.F.; et al. EGFR Activation Mediates Inhibition of Axon Regeneration by Myelin and Chondroitin Sulfate Proteoglycans. *Science* **2005**, *310*, 106–110. [CrossRef] [PubMed]
36. Starossom, S.C.; Campo Garcia, J.; Woelfle, T.; Romero-Suarez, S.; Olah, M.; Watanabe, F.; Cao, L.; Yeste, A.; Tukker, J.J.; Quintana, F.J.; et al. Chi3l3 Induces Oligodendrogenesis in an Experimental Model of Autoimmune Neuroinflammation. *Nat. Commun.* **2019**, *10*, 217. [CrossRef]
37. Amir-Levy, Y.; Mausner-Fainberg, K.; Karni, A. Treatment with Anti-EGF Ab Ameliorates Experimental Autoimmune Encephalomyelitis via Induction of Neurogenesis and Oligodendrogenesis. *Mult. Scler. Int.* **2014**, *2014*. [CrossRef]
38. Gonzalez-Perez, O.; Quiñones-Hinojosa, A. Dose-Dependent Effect of EGF on Migration and Differentiation of Adult Subventricular Zone Astrocytes. *Glia* **2010**, *58*, 975–983. [CrossRef]
39. Gonzalez-Perez, O.; Alvarez-Buylla, A. Oligodendrogenesis in the Subventricular Zone and the Role of Epidermal Growth Factor. *Brain Res. Rev.* **2011**, *67*, 147–156. [CrossRef]
40. Abliz, A.; Deng, W.; Sun, R.; Guo, W.; Zhao, L.; Wang, W. Wortmannin, PI3K/AKT signaling pathway inhibitor, attenuates thyroid injury associated with severe acute pancreatitis in rats. *Int. J. Clin. Exp. Pathol.* **2015**, *8*, 13821–13833.
41. Cantrell, W.; Huang, Y.; Menchaca, A.A.; Kulik, G.; Welker, M.E. Synthesis of PI3 Kinase Inhibition activity of a Wortmannin-Leucine Derivative. *Molecules* **2018**, *23*, 1792. [CrossRef]
42. Shin, M.; Yang, E.G.; Song, H.K.; Jeon, H. Insulin activates EGFR by stimulating its interaction with IGF-1R in low-EGFR-expressing TNBC cells. *Sci. Technol.* **2006**, *48*, 136–791. [CrossRef] [PubMed]
43. Szentpetery, Z.; Balla, A.; Kim, Y.J.; Lemmon, M.A.; Balla, T. Live cell imaging with protein domains capable of recognizing phosphatidylinositol 4,5-bisphosphate; a comparative study. *BMC Cell Biol.* **2009**, *10*, 67. [CrossRef] [PubMed]
44. Porcu, G.; Parsons, A.B.; Di Giandomenico, D.; Lucisano, G.; Mosca, M.G.; Boone, C.; Ragnini-Wilson, A. Combined P21-Activated Kinase and Farnesyltransferase Inhibitor Treatment Exhibits Enhanced Anti-Proliferative Activity on Melanoma, Colon and Lung Cancer Cell Lines. *Mol. Cancer* **2013**, *12*, 88. [CrossRef] [PubMed]
45. Sacco, F.; Gherardini, P.F.; Paoluzi, S.; Saez-Rodriguez, J.; Helmer-Citterich, M.; Ragnini-Wilson, A.; Castagnoli, L.; Cesareni, G. Mapping the Human Phosphatome on Growth Pathways. *Mol. Syst. Biol.* **2012**, *8*, 603. [CrossRef] [PubMed]
46. Hubler, Z.; Allimuthu, D.; Bederman, I.; Elitt, M.S.; Madhavan, M.; Allan, K.C.; Shick, H.E.; Garrison, E.; Karl, M.T.; Factor, D.C.; et al. Accumulation of 8,9-Unsaturated Sterols Drives Oligodendrocyte Formation and Remyelination. *Nature* **2018**, *560*, 372. [CrossRef] [PubMed]
47. Elbaz, B.; Popko, B. Molecular Control of Oligodendrocyte Development. *Trends Neurosci.* **2019**. [CrossRef]
48. Della Corte, C.M.; Bellevicine, C.; Vicidomini, G.; Vitagliano, D.; Malapelle, U.; Accardo, M.; Fabozzi, A.; Fiorelli, A.; Fasano, M.; Papaccio, F.; et al. SMO Gene Amplification and Activation of the Hedgehog Pathway as Novel Mechanisms of Resistance to Anti-Epidermal Growth Factor Receptor Drugs in Human Lung Cancer. *Clin. Cancer Res.* **2015**, *21*, 4686–4697. [CrossRef]
49. Rhen, T.; Cidlowski, J.A. Anti-inflammatory action of glucocorticoids—New mechanisms for old drugs. *N. Engl. J. Med.* **2005**, *353*, 1711–1723. [CrossRef]
50. White, R.; Gonsior, C.; Krämer-Albers, E.-M.; Stöhr, N.; Hüttelmaier, S.; Trotter, J. Activation of Oligodendroglial Fyn Kinase Enhances Translation of MRNAs Transported in HnRNP A2–Dependent RNA Granules. *J. Cell Biol.* **2008**, *181*, 579–586. [CrossRef]

51. White, R.; Krämer-Albers, E.-M. Axon-Glia Interaction and Membrane Traffic in Myelin Formation. *Front. Cell Neurosci.* **2014**, *7*. [CrossRef] [PubMed]
52. Emery, B.; Lu, Q.R. Transcriptional and epigenetic regulation of oligodendrocyte development and myelination in the central nervous system. *Cold Spring Harb. Perspect. Biol.* **2015**, *7*, a020461. [CrossRef] [PubMed]
53. Kim, S.; Kelland, E.E.; hong Kim, J.; Lund, B.T.; Chang, X.; Wang, K.; Weiner, L.P. The influence of retinoic acid on the human oligodendrocyte precursor cells by RNA-sequencing. *Biochem. Biophys. Rep.* **2017**, *9*, 166–172. [CrossRef] [PubMed]
54. Huang, J.K.; Jarjour, A.A.; Nait Oumesmar, B.; Kerninon, C.; Williams, A.; Krezel, W.; Kagechika, H.; Bauer, J.; Zhao, C.; Baron-Van Evercooren, A.; et al. Retinoid X Receptor Gamma Signaling Accelerates CNS Remyelination. *Nat. Neurosci.* **2011**, *14*, 45–53. [CrossRef] [PubMed]
55. Giner, X.C.; Cotnoir-White, D.; Mader, S.; Lévesque, D. Selective Ligand Activity at Nur/Retinoid X Receptor Complexes Revealed by Dimer-Specific Bioluminescence Resonance Energy Transfer-Based Sensors. *FASEB J.* **2015**, *29*, 4256–4267. [CrossRef] [PubMed]
56. Rimkus, T.K.; Carpenter, R.L.; Qasem, S.; Chan, M.; Lo, H.-W. Targeting the Sonic Hedgehog Signaling Pathway: Review of Smoothened and GLI Inhibitors. *Cancers (Basel)* **2016**, *8*, 22. [CrossRef] [PubMed]
57. Mangelberger, D.; Kern, D.; Loipetzberger, A.; Eberl, M.; Aberger, F. Cooperative Hedgehog-EGFR Signaling. *Front. Biosci. (Landmark Ed)* **2012**, *17*, 90–99. [CrossRef]
58. Riobo, N.A.; Saucy, B.; DiLizio, C.; Manning, D.R. Activation of Heterotrimeric G Proteins by Smoothened. *Proc. Natl. Acad. Sci. USA* **2006**, *103*, 12607–12612. [CrossRef]
59. Illiano, M.; Sapio, L.; Salzillo, A.; Capasso, L.; Caiafa, I.; Chiosi, E.; Spina, A.; Naviglio, S. Forskolin Improves Sensitivity to Doxorubicin of Triple Negative Breast Cancer Cells via Protein Kinase A-Mediated ERK1/2 Inhibition. *Biochem. Pharmacol.* **2018**, *152*, 104–113. [CrossRef]
60. Michailidis, I.E.; Rusinova, R.; Georgakopoulos, A.; Chen, Y.; Iyengar, R.; Robakis, N.K.; Logothetis, D.E.; Baki, L. Phosphatidylinositol-4,5-Bisphosphate Regulates Epidermal Growth Factor Receptor Activation. *Pflug. Arch. Eur. J. Physiol.* **2011**, *461*, 387–397. [CrossRef]
61. Bissonnette, R.P.; Fan, B.; Roegner, K.; Ng, S.; Corpuz, M.; Prudente, R. Cooperative antitumor activity between the retinoid X receptor (RXR)-selective agonist bexarotene and EGFR-tyrosine kinase inhibitors in preclinical models of NSCLC. *Int. J. Clin. Oncol.* **2006**, *18*, 17073.
62. Gianni, M.; Kopf, E.; Bastien, J.; Oulad-Abdelghani, M.; Garattini, E.; Chambon, P.; Rochette-Egly, C. Down-Regulation of the Phosphatidylinositol 3-Kinase/Akt Pathway Is Involved in Retinoic Acid-Induced Phosphorylation, Degradation, and Transcriptional Activity of Retinoic Acid Receptor Gamma 2. *J. Biol. Chem.* **2002**, *277*, 24859–24862. [CrossRef] [PubMed]
63. de la Fuente, A.G.; Errea, O.; van Wijngaarden, P.; Gonzalez, G.A.; Kerninon, C.; Jarjour, A.A.; Lewis, J.L.; Jones, C.A.; Nait-Oumesmar, B.; Zhao, C.; et al. Vitamin D receptor–retinoid X receptor heterodimer signaling regulates oligodendrocyte progenitor cell differentiation. *J. Cell Biol.* **2015**, *211*, 975–985. [CrossRef] [PubMed]
64. Birchmeier, C. ErbB receptors and the development of the nervous system. *Exp. Cell Res.* **2009**, *315*, 611–618. [CrossRef] [PubMed]
65. Lemmon, M.A.; Schlessinger, J.; Ferguson, K.M. The EGFR family: Not so prototypical receptor tyrosine kinases. *Cold Spring Harb. Perspect. Biol.* **2014**, *6*, a020768. [CrossRef] [PubMed]
66. Wilson, K.J.; Gilmore, J.L.; Foley, J.; Lemmon, M.A.; Riese, D.J., II. Functional selectivity of EGF family peptide growth factors: Implications for cancer. *Pharmacol. Ther.* **2009**, *122*, 1–8. [CrossRef] [PubMed]
67. Rico, B.; Marín, O. Neuregulin signaling, cortical circuitry development and schizophrenia. *Curr. Opin. Genet. Dev.* **2011**, *21*, 262–270. [CrossRef]
68. Cruz-Rangel, S.; Hernández-Benítez, R.; Vázquez-Juárez, E.; López-Dominguez, A.; Pasantes-Morales, H. Potentiation by Thrombin of Hyposmotic Glutamate and Taurine Efflux from Cultured Astrocytes: Signalling Chains. *Neurochem. Res.* **2008**, *33*, 1518–1524. [CrossRef]
69. Beyer, B.A.; Fang, M.; Sadrian, B.; Montenegro-Burke, J.R.; Plaisted, W.C.; Kok, B.P.C.; Saez, E.; Kondo, T.; Siuzdak, G.; Lairson, L.L. Metabolomics-based discovery of a metabolite that enhances oligodendrocyte maturation. *Nat. Chem. Biol.* **2018**, *14*, 22–28. [CrossRef]

70. Fidler, M.J.; Basu, S.; Buckingham, L.; Walters, K.; McCormack, S.; Batus, M.; Coon, J.; Bonomi, P. Utility of Insulin-like Growth Factor Receptor-1 Expression in Gefitinib-Treated Patients with Non-Small Cell Lung Cancer. *Anticancer Res.* **2012**, *32*, 1705–1710.
71. Shi, D.; Lv, X.; Zhang, Z.; Yang, X.; Zhou, Z.; Zhang, L.; Zhao, Y. Smoothened oligomerization/higher order clustering in lipid rafts is essential for high Hedgehog activity transduction. *J. Biol. Chem.* **2013**, *288*, 12605–12614. [CrossRef] [PubMed]

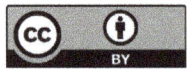

© 2019 by the authors. Licensee MDPI, Basel, Switzerland. This article is an open access article distributed under the terms and conditions of the Creative Commons Attribution (CC BY) license (http://creativecommons.org/licenses/by/4.0/).

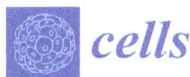

Article

Stereological Investigation of Regional Brain Volumes after Acute and Chronic Cuprizone-Induced Demyelination

Tanja Hochstrasser [1,2,*], Sebastian Rühling [1,2], Kerstin Hecher [1,2], Kai H. Fabisch [1,2], Uta Chrzanowski [1,2], Matthias Brendel [3], Florian Eckenweber [3], Christian Sacher [3], Christoph Schmitz [1] and Markus Kipp [2,*]

1. Department of Anatomy II, Ludwig-Maximilians-University of Munich, 80336 Munich, Germany
2. Institute of Anatomy, Rostock University Medical Center, 18057 Rostock, Germany
3. Department of Nuclear Medicine, University Hospital, Ludwig-Maximilians-University of Munich, 81377 Munich, Germany
* Correspondence: tanja.hochstrasser@med.uni-muenchen.de (T.H.); markus.kipp@med.uni-rostock.de (M.K.); Tel.: +49-89-2180-72705 (T.H.); Fax: +49-89-2180-72683 (T.H.)

Received: 16 July 2019; Accepted: 30 August 2019; Published: 3 September 2019

Abstract: Brain volume measurement is one of the most frequently used biomarkers to establish neuroprotective effects during pre-clinical multiple sclerosis (MS) studies. Furthermore, whole-brain atrophy estimates in MS correlate more robustly with clinical disability than traditional, lesion-based metrics. However, the underlying mechanisms leading to brain atrophy are poorly understood, partly due to the lack of appropriate animal models to study this aspect of the disease. The purpose of this study was to assess brain volumes and neuro-axonal degeneration after acute and chronic cuprizone-induced demyelination. C57BL/6 male mice were intoxicated with cuprizone for up to 12 weeks. Brain volume, as well as total numbers and densities of neurons, were determined using design-based stereology. After five weeks of cuprizone intoxication, despite severe demyelination, brain volumes were not altered at this time point. After 12 weeks of cuprizone intoxication, a significant volume reduction was found in the corpus callosum and diverse subcortical areas, particularly the internal capsule and the thalamus. Thalamic volume loss was accompanied by glucose hypermetabolism, analyzed by [^{18}F]-fluoro-2-deoxy-D-glucose (18F-FDG) positron-emission tomography. This study demonstrates region-specific brain atrophy of different subcortical brain regions after chronic cuprizone-induced demyelination. The chronic cuprizone demyelination model in male mice is, thus, a useful tool to study the underlying mechanisms of subcortical brain atrophy and to investigate the effectiveness of therapeutic interventions.

Keywords: multiple sclerosis; cuprizone; atrophy; design-based stereology; 18F-FDG

1. Introduction

Multiple sclerosis (MS) is a chronic, inflammatory demyelinating disease of the central nervous system. The majority of MS patients experience two clinical phases reflecting distinct but inter-related pathologies. The first phase is characterized by recurrent episodes of immune-driven inflammation and demyelination, from which the patients can recover completely (relapsing–remitting (RR) MS). In the second phase, a continuous progression of clinical, permanent disability can be observed, while the relapse frequency decreases [1,2]. This secondary disease phase is called secondary progressive MS (SPMS), and the findings of several imaging and pathological studies suggest that neuro-axonal damage plays a central role for the observed clinical disease progression [3–5]. Current therapeutic strategies for MS are beneficial during RRMS by modulating or suppressing immune function [6].

However, such therapies have no or just a moderate impact on the progressive phase, and therapeutic options effective in SPMS are still unsatisfactory [7].

Much of the research in MS focused on the inflammatory aspects of the disease. As a consequence, the inflammatory component of MS animal models, such as peripheral immune cell recruitment or T-cell-mediated oligodendrocyte pathology, was studied in detail [8–10]. In contrast, the neurodegenerative aspect of the disease is by far less frequently addressed and, if so, these studies merely focused on axonal degeneration [11,12]. In particular, brain atrophy, which is a key outcome measure during clinical studies [5,13,14], is almost never evaluated in MS animal models, although magnetic resonance imaging (MRI)-based protocols were published [15,16]. In MS patients, MRI measurements revealed white-matter lesions, as well as gray-matter atrophy of specific brain areas including cortical and subcortical gray matter [17–19]. The extent of atrophy was found to be more severe in the subcortex compared to the superficial cortex, and was found to correlate with cognitive performance and clinical disability in MS patients [19,20]. Thus, establishing the histological correlate of volumetric changes in the brain is of significant importance [21,22].

The cuprizone model is a well-established mouse model of MS. Following oral administration of the copper-chelating agent cuprizone, the mouse brain exhibits a variety of pathological alterations including demyelination of the white and gray matter, gliosis, and axonal damage [23,24]. While acute demyelination is usually induced by five weeks of cuprizone feeding, sustained (chronic) demyelination can be achieved by feeding mice with cuprizone for 12 weeks. Although axonal damage is found after acute and chronic demyelination in this model [11,12,25], there is little data available on neuronal loss and volumetric changes in the different vulnerable brain regions. Previous imaging studies revealed volumetric changes in the corpus callosum and the cortex after cuprizone intoxication [26–28]. Furthermore, histopathological studies showed neuronal pathologies, including loss of neurons in the hilus of the dentate gyrus, as well as loss of parvalbumin inhibitory interneurons in the hippocampus CA1 subregion of chronically demyelinated mice [29,30]. However, the extent of cortical and subcortical atrophy determined by standardized histological techniques (i.e., design-based stereology [31]) is still unexplored; therefore, the significance of this model to study the underlying mechanisms of brain atrophy in MS is unknown.

Thus, in the present study, we used design-based stereology to analyze callosal, cortical, and subcortical volumes, as well as neuron numbers and densities after acute and chronic cuprizone-induced demyelination.

2. Materials and Methods

2.1. Animals

Male C57BL/6J mice were purchased from Janvier (Le Genest-Saint-Isle, France), and were housed in a temperature-controlled environment (21–24 °C) with humidity levels between 55% and 65% on a 12-h light/dark cycle. Chow and water were provided ad libitum. All experiments were performed according to the Federation of European Laboratory Animal Science Association recommendations and were approved by the Review Board for the Care of Animal Subjects of the district government of Upper Bavaria (55.2-1-54-2532-73-15).

2.2. Cuprizone Intoxication and Tissue Processing

To induce acute or chronic demyelination, male mice (19–21g) were intoxicated with 0.25% cuprizone (bis(cyclohexanone)oxaldihydrazone, Sigma-Aldrich, St. Louis, MO, USA) mixed into ground standard rodent chow (Ssniff, Soest, Germany) for five or 12 weeks, respectively. Control groups were fed with cuprizone-free standard rodent chow. Detailed numbers of animals used for the different experiments are provided in the figure legends. After five or 12 weeks, the animals were perfused with ice-cold phosphate-buffered saline (PBS) followed by a 3.7% formaldehyde solution (pH 7.4). After overnight post-fixation in the same fixative, brains were carefully removed from the skull and processed for paraffin embedding or cryoprotection following established protocols [12,32]. For the preparation of paraffin sections, the brains were dehydrated, cleared with xylene, embedded in paraffin, and cut into 5-μm-thick coronal sections using a sliding microtome (Type SM 2000R; Leica Microsystems, Wetzlar, Germany). To prepare cryo-sections, post-fixed brains were rinsed in PBS and cryoprotected in sucrose solutions (10%, 20%, and finally 30% sucrose (w/v) in PBS) at 4 °C for 24 h in each solution. Thereafter, brains were frozen in isopentane (−70 °C, 1 min) on dry ice, cut into 40-μm-thick coronal serial sections on a cryostat (Type CM 1950; Leica Microsystems), and stored at −20 °C in a cryoprotective solution (30% ethylene glycol, 30% glycerol in PBS) until further processing.

For immunohistochemical analyses of paraffin sections, two consecutive sections (level R265 according to Reference [33]) were processed as previously described [34]. In brief, sections were deparaffinized, rehydrated, heat-unmasked by Tris–ethylene diamine tetraacetic acid (EDTA) (pH 9.0) and blocked in 5% normal goat serum or a mixture of 2% normal goat serum, 0.1% cold water fish skin gelatin, 1% bovine serum albumin, and 0.05% Tween-20. Sections were incubated with the following primary antibodies overnight at 4 °C: myelin proteolipid protein (PLP), 1:5000, RRID:AB_2237198, Bio-Rad, Hercules, CA, USA; ionized calcium-binding adapter molecule 1 (IBA1), 1:5000, RRID:AB_2665520, Wako, Neuss, Germany; amyloid precursor protein (APP), 1:5000, RRID:AB_94882, Merck-Millipore, Burlington, VT, USA. On the next day, sections were treated with 0.3% hydrogen peroxide in PBS, and the biotinylated secondary antibodies (goat anti-mouse immunoglobulin G (IgG), goat anti-rabbit IgG, 1:200; Vector labs, Burlingame, CA, USA) were applied for 1 h. Thereafter, sections were incubated in peroxidase-coupled avidin–biotin reagent (ABC kit, Vector labs) and the antigen–antibody complexes were finally visualized by 3,3'-diaminobenzidine (Dako, Hamburg, Germany). Sections were counterstained with standard hematoxylin to visualize cell nuclei if appropriate.

For stereological analyses of cryostat sections, every third section between levels R265 and R305 (according to Reference [33]; Figure 1) was selected with a random start (first series). In these regions, demyelination can be induced in a highly reproducible manner in the corpus callosum [35,36]. Demyelination is not only restricted to this white-matter tract but also involves other brain areas including the cerebral cortex, basal ganglia, and thalamus [23,37,38]. Sections were mounted on gelatinized glass slides, dried, and stained with cresyl violet (Nissl staining) [39]. For a second series of sections (every sixth section), free-floating immunofluorescence staining was performed. Sections were blocked in blocking solution (10% normal donkey serum/0.5% Triton X-100/PBS) and incubated with the primary antibodies (NeuN, 1:2000, RRID:AB_2298772, Merck-Millipore) for 48 h at 4 °C. Thereafter, sections were incubated with the secondary antibodies (donkey anti-mouse Alexa Fluor 488, 1:500; Life Technologies, Carlsbad, CA, USA) for 6 h. Cell nuclei were counterstained using DAPI (4,6-diamidino-2-phenyl-indole; Life Technologies), and sections were mounted on gelatinized glass slides and coverslipped using FluorPreserve reagent (Merck-Millipore).

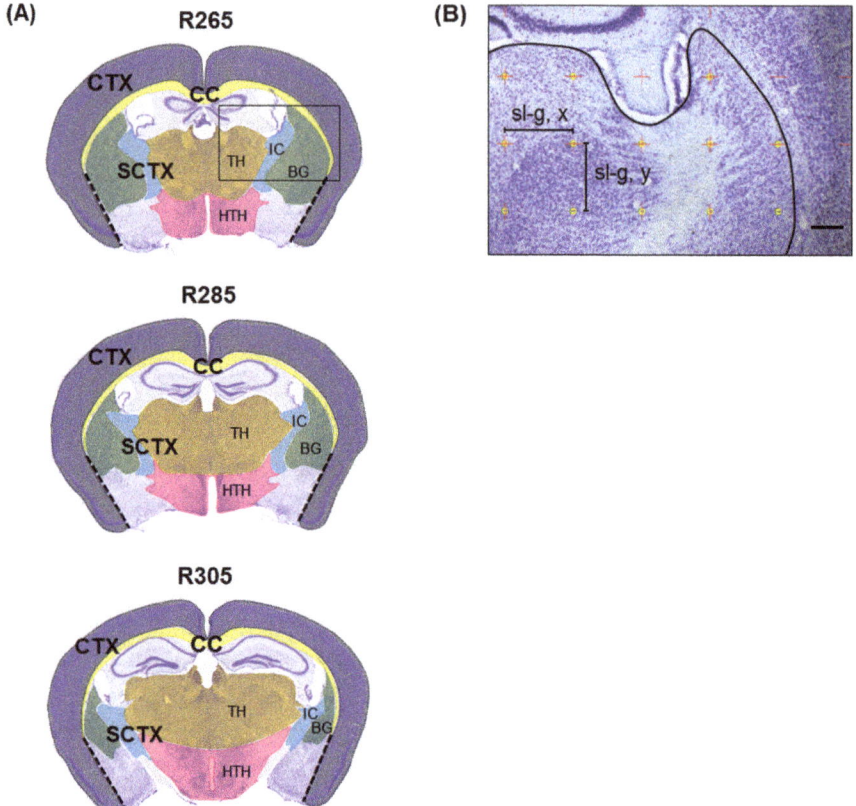

Figure 1. (**A**) Representative coronal sections of a mouse brain at levels R265, R285, and R305 (according to Reference [33]) showing regions investigated in the present study (corpus callosum (CC, yellow); cerebral cortex (CTX, gray); thalamus (TH, brown); hypothalamus (HTH, pink); internal capsule (IC, blue); basal ganglia (BG, green)). (**B**) Representative photomicrograph of a Nissl-stained coronal section (enlarged view of black square in (**A**)). The slide is superimposed with a rectangular grid (intersections are represented by red crosses; sl-g = side length in x- and y-directions of the grid) to estimate the volume of the designated areas. Grid intersections within the subcortical area are highlighted as yellow dots. Scale bar in (**B**) = 1 mm (**A**) and 200 µm (**B**).

2.3. Evaluation of Histological Parameters and Stereological Analysis

To validate demyelination and microgliosis in the cuprizone model, two consecutive (PLP- and IBA1-stained) sections per mouse were evaluated by densitometry of the staining intensity, and the results were averaged. Staining intensity of the region of interest (ROI) was quantified using ImageJ (NIH, version 1.47v, Bethesda, MD, USA) and is given as percentage myelination or percentage area of the entire ROI. For quantification of axonal damage, APP$^+$ spheroids were counted as previously described [23]. In general, densities are given in spheroids or cells per square millimeter (mm^2).

Stereological analyses were performed with the stereology software (Stereo Investigator, version 11.07; MBF Bioscience, Williston, ND, USA) and either a light microscope (Olympus BX51WI; Olympus, Tokyo, Japan) equipped with a motorized specimen stage (MBF Bioscience), UPlanApo objective (4×, numerical aperture (N.A.) = 0.16; Olympus), and a charge-coupled device (CCD) color video camera (U-CMAD-2; Olympus) or a modified fluorescence microscope (Olympus BX51; Olympus) equipped with a motorized specimen stage (MBF Bioscience), a customized spinning disk unit (DSU;

Olympus), UPlanSApo objective (20×, N.A. = 0.75; Olympus), Alexa Fluor 488 filter (excitation: 498 nm, emission: 520 nm; Chroma, Bellows Falls, VT, USA), and a Retiga 2000R CCD camera (Q-Imaging, Surrey, BC, Canada).

The first series of sections was stained with cresyl violet to analyze the volumes of the selected brain regions. The volumes of the distinct brain regions (cerebral cortex, subcortical area, corpus callosum, internal capsule, hypothalamus, thalamus, and basal ganglia (globus pallidus and caudoputamen)) were calculated using Cavalieri's principle [40]. Areas of brain regions were determined by tracing their boundaries on each section using the stereology software. Medial boundaries of the cortex (CTX) were defined by the corpus callosum and a line drawn between the basal tip of the corpus callosum and the basal end of the piriform area (shown in Figure 1A as dashed line). The thalamus, hypothalamus, basal ganglia, and internal capsule were summed up as the subcortical area (SCTX). To estimate the volume of the distinct brain regions, the slides were superimposed by a rectangular grid (Figure 1B, Table 1). Then, the volumes of brain regions were calculated by summing the counted points (grid intersections) from all sections (Table 1) and multiplying this value with the area associated with each point, the section interval, and the average cut section thickness.

Table 1. Details of the stereological estimation procedure.

	CC	CTX	SCTX	TH	HTH	BG	IC
sl-g (µm)	220	500	500	120	120	120	120
$\sum$points$_{area}$	337	669	985	5693	3192	2205	1943
sl-uvf (µm)	-	35	35	-	-	-	-
B (µm^2)	-	1225	1225	-	-	-	-
H (µm)	-	15	15	-	-	-	-
D (µm)	-	1100	1100	-	-	-	-
$\sum$UVCS	-	155	185	-	-	-	-
$\sum$neurons	-	653	555	-	-	-	-
sl-g (µm)	-	-	400	-	-	-	-
$\sum$points$_{perikarya}$	-	-	305	-	-	-	-
$\sum$points$_{neuropil}$	-	-	526	-	-	-	-

Details for stereological analysis of the corpus callosum (CC), cerebral cortex (CTX), subcortical area (SCTX), thalamus (TH), hypothalamus (HTH), basal ganglia (BG), and internal capsule (IC): sl-g = side length in x- and y-directions of the grids used to determine the volume; $\sum$points = mean number of counted points per animal; sl-uvf = side length in x- and y-directions of unbiased counting frames; B and H = base and height of the unbiased virtual counting spaces; D = distances between the unbiased virtual counting spaces in x- and y-directions; $\sum$UVCS = mean number of unbiased virtual counting spaces per animal; $\sum$neurons = mean number of counted neurons per animal.

The second series of sections was stained with anti-NeuN antibodies to analyze total neuronal numbers and densities within the distinct brain regions using the optical fractionator method [40,41]. The base of the unbiased virtual counting spaces (UVCS) was 1225 µm^2, the height was 15 µm, and the upper guard zone was 4 µm. The distance between the UVCS in x- and y-directions was 1100 µm and 1100 µm, respectively (Table 1). All neurons whose nucleus top came into focus within the UVCS were counted. Then, total neuronal numbers were calculated from the numbers of marked neurons (Table 1) and the corresponding sampling probability. Neuronal densities were calculated as the ratio of total numbers of neurons and the volume (measured section thickness × sum of all cross-sectional areas) of the region. The fractional volumes occupied by NeuN immunoreactive perikarya or the neuropil in the SCTX were estimated by counting randomly positioned test points (grid intersections) falling on nerve cell perikarya or the neuropil according to Cavalieri's principle.

2.4. [^{18}F]-Fluoro-2-deoxy-D-glucose Positron-Emission Tomography (FDG PET) Imaging

Chronic cuprizone-intoxicated mice (12 weeks of cuprizone) and controls were imaged with [^{18}F]-FDG-PET on the last day of treatment. Then, µPET imaging followed a standardized protocol [42]. In brief, 12.4 ± 2.1 MBq [^{18}F]-FDG was injected into the tail vein after a fasting period >3 h. Emission was acquired from 30 to 60 min post injection followed by a 15-min transmission scan. All images were co-registered to a [^{18}F]-FDG-PET mouse template and normalized to standardized uptake values (SUV). Predefined brain regions of the Mirrione mouse atlas implemented in PMOD v3.5 (PMOD technologies, Basel, Switzerland) were applied to extract individual regional glucose metabolism of all studied mice. Averaged SUV images of chronic cuprizone-intoxicated mice and control mice were used to calculate voxel-based percentage changes between both groups.

2.5. Statistical Analyses

For each group of animals, data are presented as individual values and means per group. Data were firstly analyzed using the Kolmogorov–Smirnov test for normality. Differences between groups were then analyzed using Student's *t*-test or the Mann–Whitney U test, as appropriate. Data were not corrected for multiple comparisons. The *p*-values and the applied statistical procedures are given in the respective figure legends. A *p*-value <0.05 was considered to be statistically significant. Calculations were performed using GraphPad Prism (GraphPad Software Inc., version 5.04; San Diego, CA, USA).

3. Results

3.1. Acute Demyelination Does Not Lead to Brain Volume Loss

We firstly investigated the severity of acute cuprizone-induced injury (i.e., demyelination, microglia activation, and axonal damage) in the different brain regions. To this end, animals were intoxicated with cuprizone for five weeks, and myelination (anti-PLP), microgliosis (anti-IBA1), and acute axonal damage (anti-APP) were compared to controls which were fed normal chow during the experimental period. In line with previous findings [23,34,36,43,44], immunohistochemical analyses revealed extensive demyelination of the medial corpus callosum, the cerebral cortex, and the subcortical area after five weeks of cuprizone intoxication (Figure 2A). Demyelination was most severe in the corpus callosum, followed by the cerebral cortex and the subcortical area. In the corpus callosum and the subcortical area, acute demyelination was paralleled by increased microglia densities (Figure 2B), in line with previous results from our group [23,36]. In the cerebral cortex, microglia activation was less severe, but IBA1$^+$ cells clearly showed an activated phenotype (swollen cell bodies and retracted processes; see Figure 2B). To examine the extent of acute axonal damage, we quantified APP$^+$ spheroids, a marker of acute axonal injury. As shown in Figure 2C, numerous APP$^+$-spheroids were found in the corpus callosum, the cerebral cortex, and the subcortical area of cuprizone-intoxicated animals. Such spheroids were not observed in control animals.

Furthermore, we investigated whether acute cuprizone-induced injury results in overall brain volume changes in the analyzed region (R265–R305). Mean overall volume was not altered in cuprizone-intoxicated versus control mice (control (Co): 63.68 mm^3 ± 1.15 mm^3; cuprizone (Cup): 64.34 mm^3 ± 0.89 mm^3; $p = 0.076$). Furthermore, we measured the volume of the corpus callosum, the cerebral cortex, and the subcortical area by stereological analysis. Despite extensive demyelination and axonal damage, individual brain volumes for the corpus callosum, cortex, and subcortical area were comparable in control and five weeks of cuprizone-intoxicated mouse brains (Figure 2D).

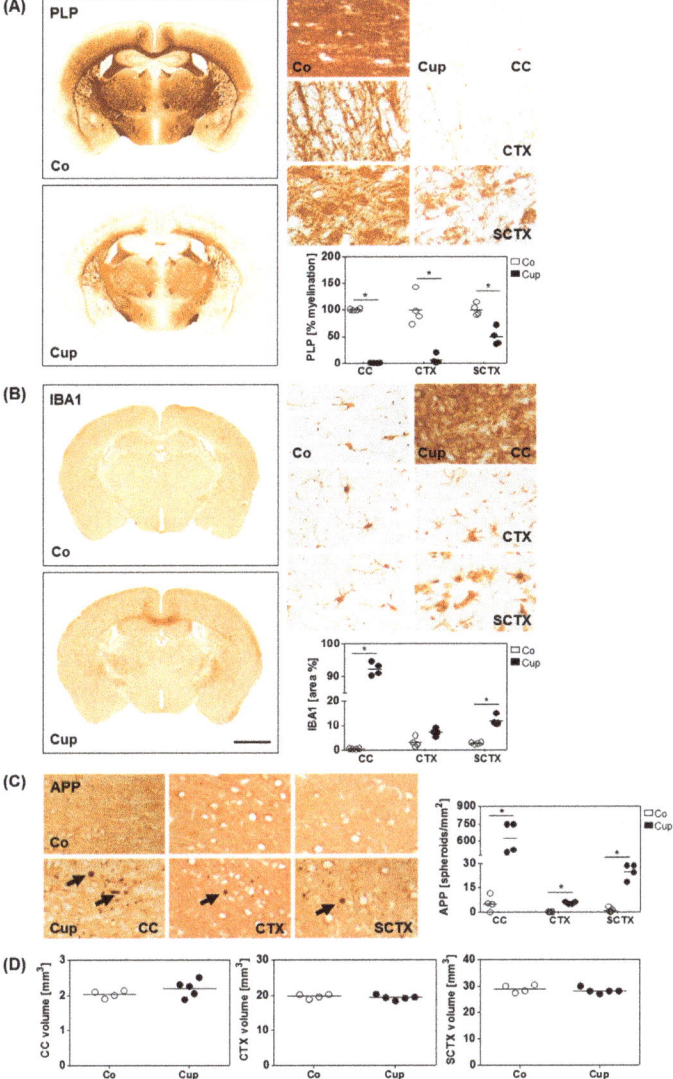

Figure 2. Acute demyelination does not lead to volumetric changes. (**A**) Quantification of myelination (anti-myelin proteolipid protein (PLP)) and (**B**) microgliosis (anti-ionized calcium-binding adapter molecule 1 (IBA1)) from controls (Co) ($n = 4$) and five weeks of cuprizone-intoxicated (Cup) mice ($n = 4$). Individual brain regions are shown in higher magnification: medial corpus callosum (CC), cortex (CTX), and subcortical area (SCTX). (**C**) Quantification of axonal damage (anti-amyloid precursor protein (APP)) with representative pictures of the medial CC, CTX, and SCTX from Co and Cup mice. Arrows indicate APP$^+$ spheroids. (**D**) Volumes of the CC, CTX, and the SCTX of Co ($n = 4$) and Cup mice ($n = 5$), analyzed with design-based stereology. Data are shown as individual values and means per group (lines). Statistical analysis revealed significant differences between Co and Cup in (**A**) (CC, $p = 0.03$, CTX, $p = 0.03$, SCTX, $p = 0.03$), (**B**) (CC, $p = 0.03$; SCTX, $p = 0.03$), and (**C**) (CC, $p = 0.02$, CTX, $p = 0.02$, SCTX, $p = 0.02$); *$p < 0.05$. Scale bar in (**B**) = 2 mm (**A**,**B**) and 17 µm (enlarged views (**A**,**B**)) and (**C**).

3.2. Chronic Demyelination Results in Regional Brain Volume Loss

In a next step, we investigated histopathological changes after chronic cuprizone intoxication. Therefore, mice were fed with cuprizone for 12 weeks, and myelination and microglia activation were evaluated. As shown in Figure 3A, severe loss of anti-PLP staining intensity was evident in several brain regions, including the corpus callosum and cerebral cortex of animals intoxicated for 12 weeks. Moreover, moderate but consistent demyelination was observed in the subcortical area. Of note, chronic demyelination was paralleled by increased microglia densities (Figure 3B). To analyze volumetric changes after chronic demyelination, we analyzed the overall brain volume (R265–R305). The overall volume of cuprizone-intoxicated mice was significantly smaller compared to control mice (Co: 67.16 mm^3 ± 0.66 mm^3; Cup: 65.28 mm^3 ± 0.38 mm^3; $p = 0.045$). Next, we measured the individual brain volumes after chronic cuprizone-induced demyelination. Mean volumes of the corpus callosum and the subcortical area were significantly smaller in cuprizone-intoxicated versus control mice. In particular, the volume of the corpus callosum was 1.96 mm^3 ± 0.10 mm^3 in control, and 1.59 mm^3 ± 0.09 mm^3 in cuprizone-intoxicated mice ($p = 0.02$), whereas the volume of the subcortical area was 30.96 mm^3 ± 0.34 mm^3 in control, and 29.11 mm^3 ± 0.14 mm^3 in cuprizone-intoxicated mice ($p = 0.0012$). No volume loss was observed in the cortex (Figure 3C).

As demonstrated above, a volume reduction after chronic cuprizone-induced demyelination was found in the subcortical area, which consists of distinct white- and gray-matter areas including different functional nuclei. Next, we were interested which subcortical region is most vulnerable in the cuprizone model. Thus, we decided to separately evaluate the volumes of the thalamus, hypothalamus, basal ganglia, and the internal capsule, and contrast atrophy with the extent of demyelination. As demonstrated in Figure 3D, anti-PLP staining intensities were clearly reduced in the thalamus, hypothalamus, and basal ganglia, yet demyelination was incomplete. In contrast, loss of anti-PLP staining intensity was moderate in the internal capsule (Figure 3D). Volumetric measurements revealed that the mean volumes of the internal capsule and the thalamus were significantly lower in cuprizone-intoxicated versus control mice. In particular, the volume of the internal capsule was 3.60 mm^3 ± 0.14 mm^3 in control, and 3.08 mm^3 ± 0.14 mm^3 in cuprizone-intoxicated mice ($p = 0.04$), whereas the volume of the thalamus was 10.18 mm^3 ± 0.24 mm^3 in control, and 9.45 mm^3 ± 0.20 mm^3 in cuprizone-intoxicated mice ($p = 0.02$). In contrast, the mean hypothalamus and basal ganglia volumes were not found to be reduced after chronic demyelination (Figure 3E).

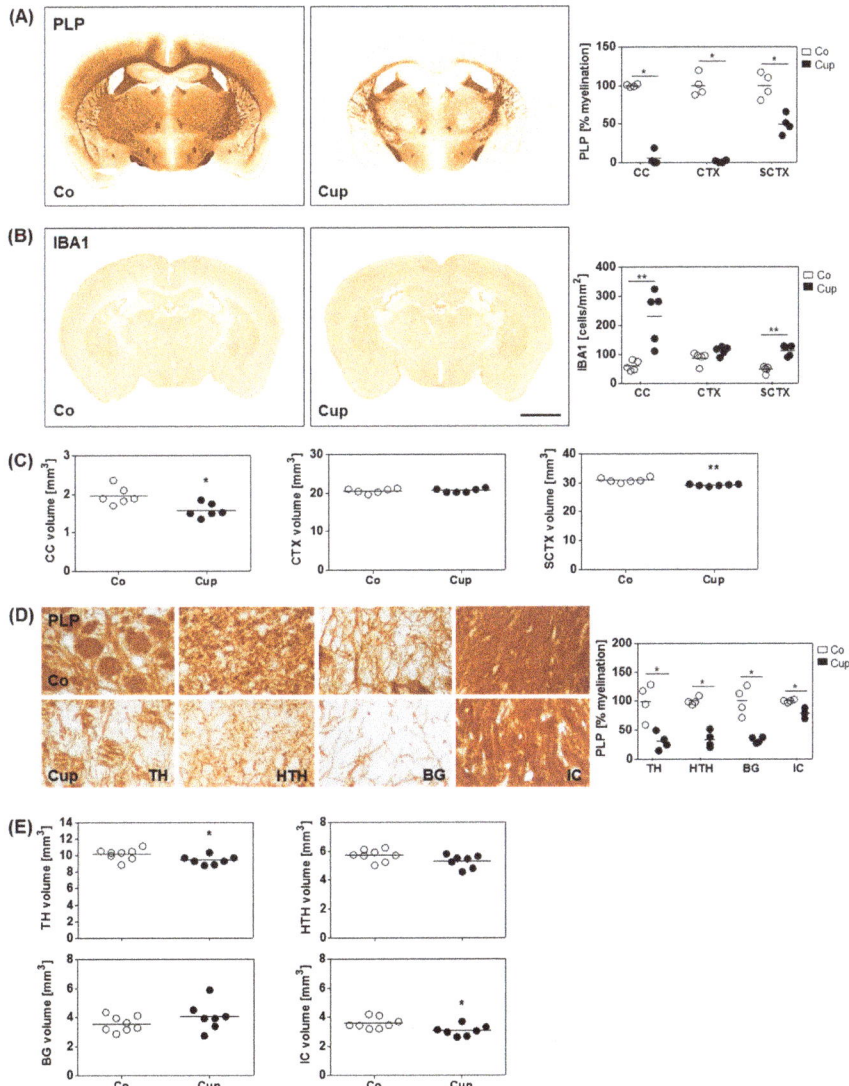

Figure 3. Chronic demyelination leads to subcortical volumetric reduction. (**A**) Quantification of myelination (anti-PLP) and (**B**) microgliosis (anti-IBA1) in the medial corpus callosum (CC), cortex (CTX), and subcortical area (SCTX) from controls (Co) ($n = 4$) and five weeks of cuprizone-intoxicated (Cup) mice ($n = 5$). (**C**) Volumes of the CC, CTX, and the SCTX of Co ($n = 6$) and Cup mice ($n = 6$) analyzed with design-based stereology. (**D**) Quantification of myelination with representative pictures of individual subcortical regions (thalamus (TH), hypothalamus (HTH), basal ganglia (BG), internal capsule (IC)) from Co ($n = 4$) and Cup mice ($n = 4$). (**E**) Volumes of the TH, HTH, STR, and IC of Co ($n = 8$) and Cup mice ($n = 7$). Data are shown as individual values and means per group (lines). Statistical analysis revealed significant differences between Co and Cup in (**A**) (CC, $p = 0.03$, CTX, $p = 0.03$, SCTX, $p = 0.03$), (**B**) (CC, $p = 0.008$; SCTX, $p = 0.008$), (**C**) (CC, $p = 0.02$; SCTX, $p = 0.0012$), (**D**) (TH, $p = 0.03$; HTH, $p = 0.03$; BG, $p = 0.03$; IC, $p = 0.03$), and **E** (TH, $p = 0.04$; IC, $p = 0.02$); *$p < 0.05$, **$p < 0.01$. Scale bar in (**B**) = 2 mm (**A**,**B**) and 17 μm (**D**).

3.3. Axonal Damage Rather Than Neuronal Loss Contributes to Brain Volume Loss

To investigate whether the observed subcortical volume reduction results from (i) neuronal cell body loss and/or (ii) acute axonal damage, we firstly quantified the mean numbers of neurons and mean densities of neurons in the cerebral cortex and the entire subcortical area using design-based stereology. In the cerebral cortex, no alterations in mean neuronal numbers and mean neuronal densities were detected in 12 weeks of cuprizone-intoxicated mice (Figure 4A,B). Of note, also in the subcortical area, the mean numbers and densities of neurons were comparable in 12 weeks of cuprizone-intoxicated mice as compared to age-matched controls (Figure 4A,B). Furthermore, in the entire subcortical area, the space occupied by perikarya and the neuropil was not significantly different in cuprizone-intoxicated versus control mice (Figure 4C).

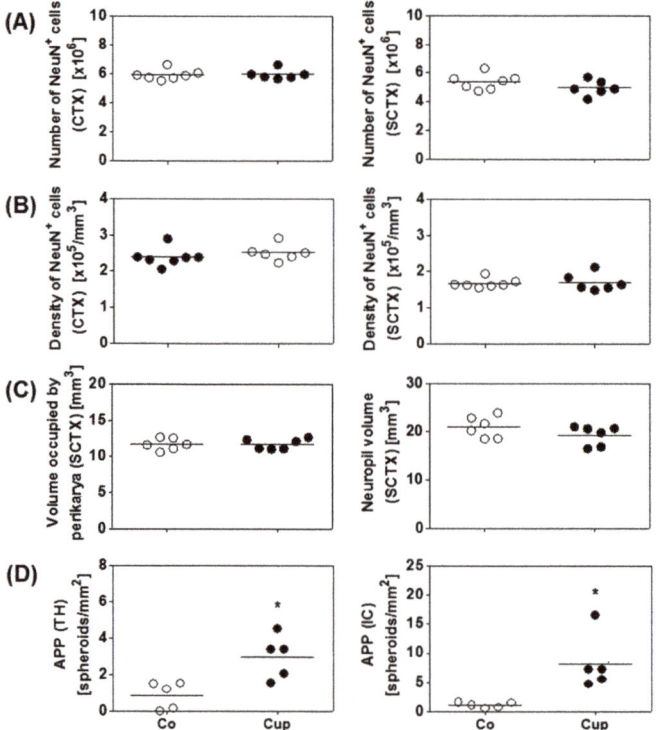

Figure 4. Effects of chronic demyelination on the neuro-axonal/-dendritic compartment. (**A**) Numbers and (**B**) densities of neurons in the cerebral cortex (CTX) and the subcortical area (SCTX) of control (Co) ($n = 6$) and 12 weeks of cuprizone-intoxicated (Cup) mice ($n = 6$) analyzed with design-based stereology. (**C**) Neuropil volumes and volumes occupied by nerve cell perikarya in the SCTX of Co ($n = 6$) and 12-week Cup mice ($n = 6$). (**D**) Quantification of amyloid precursor protein (APP)-positive spheroids in the thalamus (TH) and internal capsule (IC) of chronically demyelinated mice ($n = 5$). Data are shown as individual values and means per group (lines). Statistical analysis revealed significant differences between Co and Cup in (**D**) (TH, $p = 0.02$; IC, $p = 0.02$); *$p < 0.05$.

Secondly, we investigated the densities of APP$^+$ spheroids. We focused in this part of the study on the thalamus and the internal capsule because volume loss was found to be most severe in these two subcortical brain areas. As shown in Figure 4D, numerous APP$^+$ spheroids were found in the thalamus and the internal capsule of 12 weeks of cuprizone-intoxicated mice. Such spheroids were not observed in control animals (Figure 4D).

3.4. Mice with Chronic Demyelination Show Higher Uptake of [^{18}F]-FDG in the Thalamus

Neuroimaging is a central part of the diagnostic work-up of patients with suspected neurodegenerative disease, including MS. [^{18}F]-FDG PET is an attractive tool to study neurodegeneration on the metabolic level. Therefore, we were interested whether we could detect metabolic alterations after chronic demyelination. To this end, glucose metabolism in the mouse brain was analyzed using [^{18}F]-FDG μPET. Interestingly, we found a region-dependent increase of [^{18}F]-FDG uptake in cuprizone-treated mice. A visual interpretation of the [^{18}F]-FDG μPET scans indicated increased [^{18}F]-FDG μPET signal, particularly in the subcortical area (Figure 5A,B). A statistical comparison between predefined brain regions in the control and cuprizone-intoxicated mice showed significantly higher [^{18}F]-FDG uptake in the thalamus of 12 weeks of cuprizone-intoxicated mice (increase of 22%). There were no significant differences in [^{18}F]-FDG uptake in the cortex, hypothalamus, and basal ganglia in 12 weeks of cuprizone-intoxicated mice compared to age-matched controls (Figure 5C).

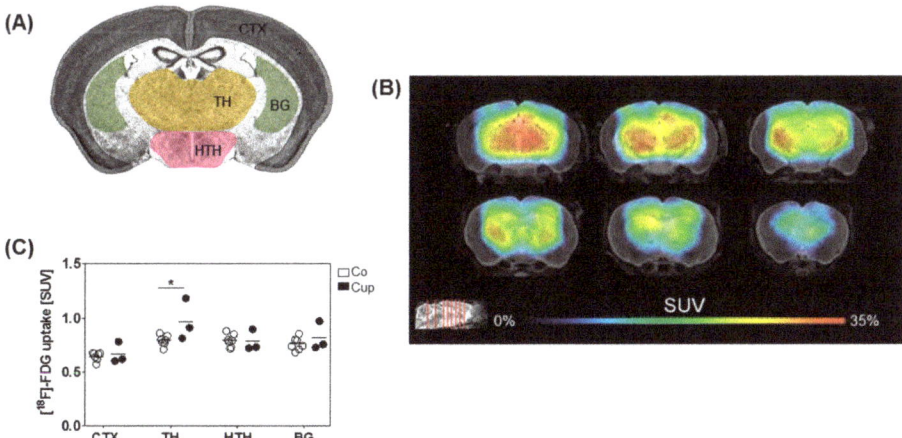

Figure 5. Altered [^{18}F]-fluoro-2-deoxy-D-glucose ([^{18}F]-FDG) ligand uptake after chronic cuprizone intoxication. (**A**) Schematic illustration of the different brain regions (cortex (CTX), thalamus (TH), hypothalamus (HTH), and basal ganglia (BG)), evaluated for [^{18}F]-FDG ligand uptake. (**B**) Cumulative heat map illustrating percentage increases of standardized uptake values (SUV) in cuprizone-treated mice relative to controls. (**C**) Quantification of the normalized [^{18}F]-FDG uptake in Co ($n = 7$) and 12-week Cup mice ($n = 3$). Data are shown as individual values and means per group (lines). Statistical analysis revealed significant differences between Co and Cup in (**C**) (TH, $p = 0.03$); *$p < 0.05$.

4. Discussion

This is the first study focusing on volume, neuronal densities, and total neuronal numbers in the cerebral cortex and subcortical area after acute and chronic cuprizone-induced demyelination. We could show that specific subregions display volume loss after chronic cuprizone-induced demyelination, particularly the corpus callosum, internal capsule, and the thalamus. Of note, volumetric changes were not paralleled by loss of NeuN$^+$ neuronal cell numbers or shrinkage of their perikarya, but by ongoing degeneration of axons, as demonstrated by the ongoing axonal transport deficit of APP.

Of note is the specific volume loss of the subcortex, whereas no significant volumetric changes were observed in the cerebral cortex. It is well known that, in addition to the corpus callosum, the cortex is a vulnerable brain region in the cuprizone model, demonstrating severe and almost complete demyelination after a five-week cuprizone intoxication period [37,45]. It was, therefore, somewhat surprising that we did not detect cortical atrophy in the cortex even after chronic cuprizone exposure. Since we only evaluated the entire cortex, we cannot rule out that specific cortical subregions, such as the somatosensory and somatomotor cortex, which are particularly vulnerable in the cuprizone model, show reduced volumes [24]. While axonal damage/injury was observed by many groups in the cuprizone model [11,12,30], a decrease in neuronal densities or neuronal cell numbers is less well appreciated. While Tiwari-Woodruff's lab demonstrated a loss of parvalbumin-expressing interneurons in the hippocampal CA1 region [29], Löscher's lab showed a loss of neurons in the hilus of the dentate gyrus [30]. While neuronal cell loss in the MS brain clearly exists [46], it is unclear which mechanisms trigger neurodegeneration. In the cuprizone model, demyelination alone seems not to be sufficient to trigger neuronal cell loss, at least in the investigated brain areas. Interestingly, recent post-mortem studies did not reveal any association between the extent of demyelination and the density of neurons in the MS neocortex [47,48]. We speculate that, in addition to metabolic stressors, auto-immune driven inflammatory mediators are necessary to induce neuronal cell loss in the neocortex and, consequently, cortical brain atrophy. A recently described novel MS animal model principally allows studying the interplay of innate and adaptive immunity [49–51], and we are currently investigating in ongoing studies the extent to which the liaison of metabolic and inflammatory brain injury triggers neuronal degeneration.

We are well aware that the underlying mechanisms of MS and cuprizone-induced injury are most likely not the same. Nevertheless, several important aspects of the MS pathology are nicely recapitulated by the cuprizone model. For example, mitochondrial density is increased within demyelinated axons in active MS [52] and cuprizone-induced lesions [53]. Furthermore, splitting of the inner myelin lamella, referred as dying-back oligodendrogliopathy, was reported in MS [54] and cuprizone-induced demyelination [55]. Finally, the presence of apoptotic oligodendrocytes, which express active caspase-3 during lesion formation, was described in MS [56] and the cuprizone model [57]. Thus, understanding mechanisms operant during cuprizone-induced demyelination might help to understand disease mechanisms in MS.

As pointed out above, significant brain volume loss was found in subcortical regions among the thalamus (see Figure 3E). The thalamus forms the largest part of the diencephalon and is eponymous for other diencephalic components such as the epithalamus and hypothalamus. This diencephalic brain region is highly interconnected with various cortical and subcortical areas. We speculate that the thalamus with its multiple reciprocal connections is sensitive to pathological processes occurring in different brain regions, thus acting as a "barometer" for diffuse brain parenchymal damage in MS [58]. Our findings are in line with a specific subcortical gray-matter atrophy found in MS patients [19,20,59,60]. In these MRI studies, subcortical gray-matter atrophy was most prominent in the thalamus, showing a volume reduction of 12–25%. From a functional point of view, it is interesting to note that the thalamus volume loss strongly correlated to patients' declining cognitive functions and physical disability [19,20,61,62], highlighting the thalamus as a central structure in the context of MS-related disability and disease progression.

Thalamic volume loss was found to be related to neuro-axonal pathology. Cifelli et al. found a reduction in both neuronal densities and N-acetylaspartate (NAA) concentration in the thalamus of MS patients [60]. In the present study, cuprizone-induced demyelination neither affected NeuN$^+$ neuronal numbers and densities nor the space occupied by perikarya. Noteworthy, our [^{18}F]-FDG-PET measurements indicated a significant hypermetabolism in the thalamus of cuprizone-intoxicated mice when compared to controls, fitting to preserved neuronal numbers in this brain region, as the vast majority of the [^{18}F]-FDG-PET signal is supposed to be related to neuronal energy metabolism [63]. Thus, it seems likely that equal neuronal numbers, together with increased glial activity after chronic cuprizone intoxication, will result in higher net energy consumption when compared to controls. Of note, there is still no evidence how much glial cells contribute to the cerebral energy consumption, although it is assumed that glucose metabolism decreases when microglia are dysfunctional [64].

Surprisingly, we did not find callosal volume loss after acute cuprizone-induced demyelination, despite significant axonal injury. This could have happened for a number of reasons. Firstly, in our study, we did not measure irreversible axonal degeneration or axonal loss, but rather a deficit of the anterograde axonal transport machinery. The gold-standard method to detect axonal loss is electron microscopy or thin plastic sections. Most previous studies which analyzed acute axonal injury in the cuprizone model visualized either axonal transport deficits or the expression changes of neurofilament proteins [11,65], which does not necessarily represent the true extent of irreversible axonal degeneration [66]. Secondly, due to the severe astrocytosis and microgliosis accompanying the cuprizone-induced demyelination, callosal volume loss might be "masked" despite axonal loss (if present). Thirdly, cuprizone intoxication results in spongy degeneration of the white matter [67], another pathological feature which might mask callosal volume loss. In MS, it was suggested that untreated inflammation and edema might increase the brain volume, leading to an underestimation of true tissue loss. Interestingly, anti-inflammatory therapies were associated with acceleration of brain volume loss, referred to as pseudoatrophy [68]. This is likely caused by the resolution of inflammation and edema rather than true brain atrophy. In our study, chronic cuprizone-induced demyelination did lead to a brain volume reduction despite ongoing microgliosis, suggesting true tissue loss. Furthermore, it was suggested that pseudoatrophy effects are greater in white-matter structures due to larger glial infiltration and activation compared to gray-matter structures. Thus, volume measurement of gray-matter structures might be more reliable to distinguish irreversible changes due to tissue loss from the reversible changes due to pseudoatrophy. The pathological substrate of subcortical volume loss in the cuprizone model is currently unknown. In principle, volume loss might be due to loss of the myelin sheath (i.e., demyelination), glia degeneration, neuronal cell loss, axonal degeneration, or synaptic pathology. Of note, in a post mortem analysis, widespread loss of dendritic spines was found in the cortex of MS patients. Dendritic spine loss occurred in demyelinated and non-demyelinated cortex regions, and preceded loss of cortical axons [69]. In this study, we could show that subcortical volume loss is not paralleled by a reduction of total neuronal cell numbers. However, subcortical neuropil volumes tended to decrease, suggesting degeneration in the axonal and/or dendritic compartment. Of note, in this study, we did not quantify the loss of cell types other than neurons, such as astrocytes or oligodendrocytes, by means of design-based stereology. It, thus, might well be that the observed atrophy in the thalamus, for example, is due to oligodendrocyte or astrocyte degeneration. In a recent study, we were able to show that astrocytes express the stress-associated transcription factor DNA damage-inducible transcript 3 after acute cuprizone-induced demyelination [32]. Further studies are needed to investigate this aspect in more detail.

As already pointed out above, the thalamus shares broad reciprocal connections with other brain regions, such as the cerebral cortex. These connections run within the internal capsule. In the present study, we observed volume reduction and axonal damage of the internal capsule, despite moderate demyelination. Thus, volume loss of the internal capsule might be due to the degeneration of efferent thalamic fiber tracts. This is consistent with findings demonstrating reduced NAA levels in normal-appearing white matter of the internal capsule in MS patients [70].

In summary, this study pointed out that the chronic, but not the acute cuprizone model may serve as a valuable tool to study subcortical brain volume loss. Further studies are now warranted to investigate which mechanisms are operant and how this brain volume loss can be ameliorated by pharmacological intervention.

Author Contributions: Conceptualization, T.H. and M.K.; formal analysis, T.H., S.R., K.H., and K.H.F.; investigation, T.H., S.R., K.H., K.H.F., U.C., F.E., and C.S. (Christian Sacher); methodology, T.H., M.B., C.S. (Christoph Schmitz), and M.K.; supervision, M.K.; visualization, T.H.; writing—original draft, T.H. and S.R.; writing—review and editing, M.B., C.S. (Christoph Schmitz), and M.K.

Acknowledgments: The authors thank Sarah Wübbel, Beate Aschauer, Astrid Baltruschat, and Barbara Mosler for their excellent and valuable technical assistance. The authors gratefully acknowledge Maren Kiessling for her valuable input regarding the stereological evaluation.

Conflicts of Interest: The authors declare no conflicts of interest.

References

1. Trapp, B.D.; Nave, K.A. Multiple sclerosis: An immune or neurodegenerative disorder? *Annu. Rev. Neurosci.* **2008**, *31*, 247–269. [CrossRef] [PubMed]
2. Rovaris, M.; Confavreux, C.; Furlan, R.; Kappos, L.; Comi, G.; Filippi, M. Secondary progressive multiple sclerosis: Current knowledge and future challenges. *Lancet Neurol.* **2006**, *5*, 343–354. [CrossRef]
3. Rudick, R.; Bö, L.; Trapp, B.D.; Peterson, J.; Ransohoff, R.M.; Mörk, S. Axonal Transection in the Lesions of Multiple Sclerosis. *New Engl. J. Med.* **1998**, *338*, 278–285.
4. Grimaud, J.; Barker, G.J.; Wang, L.; Lai, M.; MacManus, D.G.; Webb, S.L.; Thompson, A.J.; McDonald, W.I.; Tofts, P.S.; Miller, D.H. Correlation of magnetic resonance imaging parameters with clinical disability in multiple sclerosis: A preliminary study. *J. Neurol.* **1999**, *246*, 961–967. [CrossRef] [PubMed]
5. Calabrese, M.; Romualdi, C.; Poretto, V.; Favaretto, A.; Morra, A.; Rinaldi, F.; Perini, P.; Gallo, P. The changing clinical course of multiple sclerosis: A matter of gray matter. *Ann. Neurol.* **2013**, *74*, 76–83. [CrossRef] [PubMed]
6. Oh, J.; O'Connor, P.W. Established disease-modifying treatments in relapsing-remitting multiple sclerosis. *Curr. Opin. Neurol.* **2015**, *28*, 220–229. [CrossRef] [PubMed]
7. Wingerchuk, D.M.; Carter, J.L. Multiple Sclerosis: Current and Emerging Disease-Modifying Therapies and Treatment Strategies. *Mayo Clin. Proc.* **2014**, *89*, 225–240. [CrossRef]
8. Simmons, S.B.; Pierson, E.R.; Lee, S.Y.; Goverman, J.M. Modeling the Heterogeneity of Multiple Sclerosis in Animals. *Trends Immunol.* **2013**, *34*, 410–422. [CrossRef]
9. Patel, J.; Balabanov, R. Molecular Mechanisms of Oligodendrocyte Injury in Multiple Sclerosis and Experimental Autoimmune Encephalomyelitis. *Int. J. Mol. Sci.* **2012**, *13*, 10647–10659. [CrossRef]
10. Rossi, B.; Constantin, G. Live Imaging of Immune Responses in Experimental Models of Multiple Sclerosis. *Front. Immunol.* **2016**, *7*. [CrossRef]
11. Hoflich, K.M.; Beyer, C.; Clarner, T.; Schmitz, C.; Nyamoya, S.; Kipp, M.; Hochstrasser, T. Acute axonal damage in three different murine models of multiple sclerosis: A comparative approach. *Brain Res.* **2016**, *1650*, 125–133. [CrossRef] [PubMed]
12. Ruhling, S.; Kramer, F.; Schmutz, S.; Amor, S.; Jiangshan, Z.; Schmitz, C.; Kipp, M.; Hochstrasser, T. Visualization of the Breakdown of the Axonal Transport. Machinery: A Comparative Ultrastructural and Immunohistochemical Approach. *Mol. Neurobiol.* **2019**, *56*, 3984–3998. [CrossRef] [PubMed]
13. Derakhshan, M.; Caramanos, Z.; Giacomini, P.S.; Narayanan, S.; Maranzano, J.; Francis, S.J.; Arnold, D.L.; Collins, D.L. Evaluation of automated techniques for the quantification of grey matter atrophy in patients with multiple sclerosis. *Neuroimage* **2010**, *52*, 1261–1267. [CrossRef] [PubMed]
14. Fisher, E.; Lee, J.C.; Nakamura, K.; Rudick, R.A. Gray matter atrophy in multiple sclerosis: A longitudinal study. *Ann. Neurol.* **2008**, *64*, 255–265. [CrossRef] [PubMed]
15. MacKenzie-Graham, A.; Rinek, G.A.; Avedisian, A.; Gold, S.M.; Frew, A.J.; Aguilar, C.; Lin, D.R.; Umeda, E.; Voskuhl, R.R.; Alger, J.R. Cortical atrophy in experimental autoimmune encephalomyelitis: In vivo imaging. *Neuroimage* **2012**, *60*, 95–104. [CrossRef] [PubMed]
16. Wood, T.C.; Simmons, C.; Hurley, S.A.; Vernon, A.C.; Torres, J.; Dell'Acqua, F.; Williams, S.C.; Cash, D. Whole-brain ex-vivo quantitative MRI of the cuprizone mouse model. *PeerJ* **2016**, *4*. [CrossRef]
17. Bergsland, N.; Horakova, D.; Dwyer, M.G.; Dolezal, O.; Seidl, Z.K.; Vaneckova, M.; Krasensky, J.; Havrdova, E.; Zivadinov, R. Subcortical and cortical gray matter atrophy in a large sample of patients with clinically isolated syndrome and early relapsing-remitting multiple sclerosis. *AJNR Am. J. Neuroradiol.* **2012**, *33*, 1573–1578. [CrossRef] [PubMed]
18. De Stefano, N.; Matthews, P.M.; Filippi, M.; Agosta, F.; De Luca, M.; Bartolozzi, M.L.; Guidi, L.; Ghezzi, A.; Montanari, E.; Cifelli, A.; et al. Evidence of early cortical atrophy in MS: Relevance to white matter changes and disability. *Neurology* **2003**, *60*, 1157–1162. [CrossRef]
19. Batista, S.; Zivadinov, R.; Hoogs, M.; Bergsland, N.; Heininen-Brown, M.; Dwyer, M.G.; Weinstock-Guttman, B.; Benedict, R.H. Basal ganglia, thalamus and neocortical atrophy predicting slowed cognitive processing in multiple sclerosis. *J. Neurol.* **2012**, *259*, 139–146. [CrossRef]
20. Houtchens, M.K.; Benedict, R.H.; Killiany, R.; Sharma, J.; Jaisani, Z.; Singh, B.; Weinstock-Guttman, B.; Guttmann, C.R.; Bakshi, R. Thalamic atrophy and cognition in multiple sclerosis. *Neurology* **2007**, *69*, 1213–1223. [CrossRef]

21. Barkhof, F.; Calabresi, P.A.; Miller, D.H.; Reingold, S.C. Imaging outcomes for neuroprotection and repair in multiple sclerosis trials. *Nat. Rev. Neurol.* **2009**, *5*, 256–266. [CrossRef] [PubMed]
22. Sormani, M.P.; Arnold, D.L.; De Stefano, N. Treatment effect on brain atrophy correlates with treatment effect on disability in multiple sclerosis. *Ann. Neurol.* **2014**, *75*, 43–49. [CrossRef] [PubMed]
23. Wagenknecht, N.; Becker, B.; Scheld, M.; Beyer, C.; Clarner, T.; Hochstrasser, T.; Kipp, M. Thalamus Degeneration and Inflammation in Two Distinct Multiple Sclerosis Animal Models. *J. Mol. Neurosci.* **2016**, *60*, 102–114. [CrossRef] [PubMed]
24. Clarner, T.; Diederichs, F.; Berger, K.; Denecke, B.; Gan, L.; van der Valk, P.; Beyer, C.; Amor, S.; Kipp, M. Myelin debris regulates inflammatory responses in an experimental demyelination animal model and multiple sclerosis lesions. *Glia* **2012**, *60*, 1468–1480. [CrossRef] [PubMed]
25. Lindner, M.; Fokuhl, J.; Linsmeier, F.; Trebst, C.; Stangel, M. Chronic toxic demyelination in the central nervous system leads to axonal damage despite remyelination. *Neurosci. Lett.* **2009**, *453*, 120–125. [CrossRef]
26. Guglielmetti, C.; Veraart, J.; Roelant, E.; Mai, Z.; Daans, J.; Van Audekerke, J.; Naeyaert, M.; Vanhoutte, G.; Delgado, Y.P.R.; Praet, J.; et al. Diffusion kurtosis imaging probes cortical alterations and white matter pathology following cuprizone induced demyelination and spontaneous remyelination. *Neuroimage* **2016**, *125*, 363–377. [CrossRef]
27. Thiessen, J.D.; Zhang, Y.; Zhang, H.; Wang, L.; Buist, R.; Del Bigio, M.R.; Kong, J.; Li, X.M.; Martin, M. Quantitative MRI and ultrastructural examination of the cuprizone mouse model of demyelination. *NMR Biomed.* **2013**, *26*, 1562–1581. [CrossRef]
28. Wu, Q.Z.; Yang, Q.; Cate, H.S.; Kemper, D.; Binder, M.; Wang, H.X.; Fang, K.; Quick, M.J.; Marriott, M.; Kilpatrick, T.J.; et al. MRI identification of the rostral-caudal pattern of pathology within the corpus callosum in the cuprizone mouse model. *J. Magn Reson. Med.* **2008**, *27*, 446–453. [CrossRef]
29. Lapato, A.S.; Szu, J.I.; Hasselmann, J.P.C.; Khalaj, A.J.; Binder, D.K.; Tiwari-Woodruff, S.K. Chronic demyelination-induced seizures. *Neuroscience* **2017**, *346*, 409–422. [CrossRef]
30. Hoffmann, K.; Lindner, M.; Groticke, I.; Stangel, M.; Loscher, W. Epileptic seizures and hippocampal damage after cuprizone-induced demyelination in C57BL/6 mice. *Exp. Neurol.* **2008**, *210*, 308–321. [CrossRef]
31. Kipp, M.; Kiessling, M.C.; Hochstrasser, T.; Roggenkamp, C.; Schmitz, C. Design-Based Stereology for Evaluation of Histological Parameters. *J. Mol. Neurosci.* **2017**, *61*, 325–342. [CrossRef] [PubMed]
32. Fischbach, F.; Nedelcu, J.; Leopold, P.; Zhan, J.; Clarner, T.; Nellessen, L.; Beissel, C.; van Heuvel, Y.; Goswami, A.; Weis, J.; et al. Cuprizone-induced graded oligodendrocyte vulnerability is regulated by the transcription factor DNA damage-inducible transcript 3. *Glia* **2019**, *67*, 263–276. [CrossRef] [PubMed]
33. Sidman, R.L.; Angevine, J.B.; Pierce, E.T. *Atlas of the Mouse Brain and Spinal Cord*; Harvard University Press: Cambridge, UK, 1971; p. 261.
34. Hochstrasser, T.; Exner, G.L.; Nyamoya, S.; Schmitz, C.; Kipp, M. Cuprizone-Containing Pellets Are Less Potent to Induce Consistent Demyelination in the Corpus Callosum of C57BL/6 Mice. *J. Mol. Neurosci.* **2017**, *61*, 617–624. [CrossRef] [PubMed]
35. Chrzanowski, U.; Schmitz, C.; Horn-Bochtler, A.; Nack, A.; Kipp, M. Evaluation strategy to determine reliable demyelination in the cuprizone model. *Metab. Brain Dis.* **2019**, *34*, 681–685. [CrossRef] [PubMed]
36. Goldberg, J.; Clarner, T.; Beyer, C.; Kipp, M. Anatomical Distribution of Cuprizone-Induced Lesions in C57BL6 Mice. *J. Mol. Neurosci.* **2015**, *57*, 166–175. [CrossRef]
37. Skripuletz, T.; Lindner, M.; Kotsiari, A.; Garde, N.; Fokuhl, J.; Linsmeier, F.; Trebst, C.; Stangel, M. Cortical demyelination is prominent in the murine cuprizone model and is strain-dependent. *Am. J. Pathol.* **2008**, *172*, 1053–1061. [CrossRef] [PubMed]
38. Pott, F.; Gingele, S.; Clarner, T.; Dang, J.; Baumgartner, W.; Beyer, C.; Kipp, M. Cuprizone effect on myelination, astrogliosis and microglia attraction in the mouse basal ganglia. *Brain Res.* **2009**, *1305*, 137–149. [CrossRef]
39. Schmitz, C.; Bultmann, E.; Gube, M.; Korr, H. Neuron loss in the mouse hippocampus following prenatal injection of tritiated thymidine or saline. *Int. J. Dev. Neurosci.* **1999**, *17*, 185–190. [CrossRef]
40. Schmitz, C.; Hof, P. Design-based stereology in neuroscience. *Neurosci.* **2005**, *130*, 813–831. [CrossRef]
41. Schmitz, C.; Hof, P.R. Recommendations for straightforward and rigorous methods of counting neurons based on a computer simulation approach. *J. Chem. Neuroanat.* **2000**, *20*, 93–114. [CrossRef]
42. Brendel, M.; Probst, F.; Jaworska, A.; Overhoff, F.; Korzhova, V.; Albert, N.L.; Beck, R.; Lindner, S.; Gildehaus, F.J.; Baumann, K.; et al. Glial Activation and Glucose Metabolism in a Transgenic Amyloid Mouse Model.: A Triple-Tracer PET Study. *J. Nucl. Med.* **2016**, *57*, 954–960. [CrossRef] [PubMed]

43. Leopold, P.; Schmitz, C.; Kipp, M. Animal Weight Is an Important Variable for Reliable Cuprizone-Induced Demyelination. *J. Mol. Neurosci.* **2019**, *68*, 522–528. [CrossRef] [PubMed]
44. Esser, S.; Gopfrich, L.; Bihler, K.; Kress, E.; Nyamoya, S.; Tauber, S.C.; Clarner, T.; Stope, M.B.; Pufe, T.; Kipp, M.; et al. Toll-Like Receptor 2-Mediated Glial Cell Activation in a Mouse Model. of Cuprizone-Induced Demyelination. *Mol. Neurobiol.* **2018**, *55*, 6237–6249. [CrossRef] [PubMed]
45. Cerina, M.; Narayanan, V.; Gobel, K.; Bittner, S.; Ruck, T.; Meuth, P.; Herrmann, A.M.; Stangel, M.; Gudi, V.; Skripuletz, T.; et al. The quality of cortical network function recovery depends on localization and degree of axonal demyelination. *Brain Behav. Immun.* **2017**, *59*, 103–117. [CrossRef] [PubMed]
46. Peterson, J.W.; Bo, L.; Mork, S.; Chang, A.; Trapp, B.D. Transected neurites, apoptotic neurons, and reduced inflammation in cortical multiple sclerosis lesions. *Ann. Neurol.* **2001**, *50*, 389–400. [CrossRef] [PubMed]
47. Klaver, R.; Popescu, V.; Voorn, P.; Galis-de Graaf, Y.; van der Valk, P.; de Vries, H.E.; Schenk, G.J.; Geurts, J.J. Neuronal and axonal loss in normal-appearing gray matter and subpial lesions in multiple sclerosis. *J. Neuropathol. Exp. Neurol.* **2015**, *74*, 453–458. [CrossRef]
48. Carassiti, D.; Altmann, D.R.; Petrova, N.; Pakkenberg, B.; Scaravilli, F.; Schmierer, K. Neuronal loss, demyelination and volume change in the multiple sclerosis neocortex. *Neuropathol. Appl. Neurobiol.* **2018**, *44*, 377–390. [CrossRef]
49. Chrzanowski, U.; Bhattarai, S.; Scheld, M.; Clarner, T.; Fallier-Becker, P.; Beyer, C.; Rohr, S.O.; Schmitz, C.; Hochstrasser, T.; Schweiger, F.; et al. Oligodendrocyte degeneration and concomitant microglia activation directs peripheral immune cells into the forebrain. *Neurochem. Int.* **2019**, *126*, 139–153. [CrossRef]
50. Ruther, B.J.; Scheld, M.; Dreymueller, D.; Clarner, T.; Kress, E.; Brandenburg, L.O.; Swartenbroekx, T.; Hoornaert, C.; Ponsaerts, P.; Fallier-Becker, P.; et al. Combination of cuprizone and experimental autoimmune encephalomyelitis to study inflammatory brain lesion formation and progression. *Glia* **2017**, *65*, 1900–1913. [CrossRef]
51. Scheld, M.; Ruther, B.J.; Grosse-Veldmann, R.; Ohl, K.; Tenbrock, K.; Dreymuller, D.; Fallier-Becker, P.; Zendedel, A.; Beyer, C.; Clarner, T.; et al. Neurodegeneration Triggers Peripheral Immune Cell Recruitment into the Forebrain. *J. Neurosci.* **2016**, *36*, 1410–1415. [CrossRef]
52. Witte, M.E.; Bo, L.; Rodenburg, R.J.; Belien, J.A.; Musters, R.; Hazes, T.; Wintjes, L.T.; Smeitink, J.A.; Geurts, J.J.; De Vries, H.E.; et al. Enhanced number and activity of mitochondria in multiple sclerosis lesions. *J. Pathol.* **2009**, *219*, 193–204. [CrossRef] [PubMed]
53. Ohno, N.; Chiang, H.; Mahad, D.J.; Kidd, G.J.; Liu, L.; Ransohoff, R.M.; Sheng, Z.H.; Komuro, H.; Trapp, B.D. Mitochondrial immobilization mediated by syntaphilin facilitates survival of demyelinated axons. *Proc. Natl. Acad. Sci. USA* **2014**, *111*, 9953–9958. [CrossRef] [PubMed]
54. Rodriguez, M.; Scheithauer, B. Ultrastructure of Multiple Sclerosis. *Ultrastruct. Pathol.* **1994**, *18*, 3–13. [CrossRef] [PubMed]
55. Ludwin, S.K.; Johnson, E.S. Evidence for a "dying-back" gliopathy in demyelinating disease. *Ann. Neurol.* **1981**, *9*, 301–305. [PubMed]
56. Prineas, J.W.; Parratt, J.D. Oligodendrocytes and the early multiple sclerosis lesion. *Ann. Neurol.* **2012**, *72*, 18–31. [CrossRef]
57. Buschmann, J.P.; Berger, K.; Awad, H.; Clarner, T.; Beyer, C.; Kipp, M. Inflammatory response and chemokine expression in the white matter corpus callosum and gray matter cortex region during cuprizone-induced demyelination. *J. Mol. Neurosci.* **2012**, *48*, 66–76. [CrossRef] [PubMed]
58. Kipp, M.; Wagenknecht, N.; Beyer, C.; Samer, S.; Wuerfel, J.; Nikoubashman, O. Thalamus pathology in multiple sclerosis: From biology to clinical application. *Cell. Mol. Life Sci.* **2015**, *72*, 1127–1147. [CrossRef] [PubMed]
59. Wylezinska, M.; Cifelli, A.; Jezzard, P.; Palace, J.; Alecci, M.; Matthews, P.M. Thalamic neurodegeneration in relapsing-remitting multiple sclerosis. *Neurology* **2003**, *60*, 1949–1954. [CrossRef]
60. Cifelli, A.; Arridge, M.; Jezzard, P.; Esiri, M.M.; Palace, J.; Matthews, P.M. Thalamic neurodegeneration in multiple sclerosis. *Ann. Neurol.* **2002**, *52*, 650–653. [CrossRef]
61. Schoonheim, M.M.; Popescu, V.; Rueda Lopes, F.C.; Wiebenga, O.T.; Vrenken, H.; Douw, L.; Polman, C.H.; Geurts, J.J.; Barkhof, F. Subcortical atrophy and cognition: Sex effects in multiple sclerosis. *Neurology* **2012**, *79*, 1754–1761. [CrossRef]

62. Magon, S.; Chakravarty, M.M.; Amann, M.; Weier, K.; Naegelin, Y.; Andelova, M.; Radue, E.W.; Stippich, C.; Lerch, J.P.; Kappos, L.; et al. Label-fusion-segmentation and deformation-based shape analysis of deep gray matter in multiple sclerosis: The impact of thalamic subnuclei on disability. *Hum. Brain Mapp.* **2014**, *35*, 4193–4203. [CrossRef] [PubMed]
63. Herholz, K. Perfusion SPECT and FDG-PET. *Int. Psychogeriatr.* **2011**, *23*, S25–S31. [CrossRef] [PubMed]
64. Kleinberger, G.; Brendel, M.; Mracsko, E.; Wefers, B.; Groeneweg, L.; Xiang, X.; Focke, C.; Deussing, M.; Suarez-Calvet, M.; Mazaheri, F.; et al. The FTD-like syndrome causing TREM2 T66M mutation impairs microglia function, brain perfusion, and glucose metabolism. *EMBO J.* **2017**, *36*, 1837–1853. [CrossRef] [PubMed]
65. Irvine, K.A.; Blakemore, W.F. Age increases axon loss associated with primary demyelination in cuprizone-induced demyelination in C57BL/6 mice. *J. Neuroimmunol.* **2006**, *175*, 69–76. [CrossRef] [PubMed]
66. Nikic, I.; Merkler, D.; Sorbara, C.; Brinkoetter, M.; Kreutzfeldt, M.; Bareyre, F.M.; Bruck, W.; Bishop, D.; Misgeld, T.; Kerschensteiner, M. A reversible form of axon damage in experimental autoimmune encephalomyelitis and multiple sclerosis. *Nat. Med.* **2011**, *17*, 495–499. [CrossRef] [PubMed]
67. Carlton, W.W. Spongiform encephalopathy induced in rats and guinea pigs by cuprizone. *Exp. Mol. Pathol.* **1969**, *10*, 274–287. [CrossRef]
68. De Stefano, N.; Airas, L.; Grigoriadis, N.; Mattle, H.P.; O'Riordan, J.; Oreja-Guevara, C.; Sellebjerg, F.; Stankoff, B.; Walczak, A.; Wiendl, H.; et al. Clinical relevance of brain volume measures in multiple sclerosis. *CNS Drugs* **2014**, *28*, 147–156. [CrossRef] [PubMed]
69. Jurgens, T.; Jafari, M.; Kreutzfeldt, M.; Bahn, E.; Bruck, W.; Kerschensteiner, M.; Merkler, D. Reconstruction of single cortical projection neurons reveals primary spine loss in multiple sclerosis. *Brain* **2016**, *139*, 39–46. [CrossRef] [PubMed]
70. Lee, M.A.; Blamire, A.M.; Pendlebury, S.; Ho, K.H.; Mills, K.R.; Styles, P.; Palace, J.; Matthews, P.M. Axonal injury or loss in the internal capsule and motor impairment in multiple sclerosis. *Arch. Neurol.* **2000**, *57*, 65–70. [CrossRef] [PubMed]

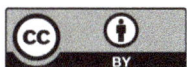

© 2019 by the authors. Licensee MDPI, Basel, Switzerland. This article is an open access article distributed under the terms and conditions of the Creative Commons Attribution (CC BY) license (http://creativecommons.org/licenses/by/4.0/).

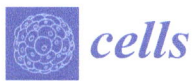

Article

Quantitative Imaging of White and Gray Matter Remyelination in the Cuprizone Demyelination Model Using the Macromolecular Proton Fraction

Marina Khodanovich [1,*], Anna Pishchelko [1], Valentina Glazacheva [1], Edgar Pan [1], Andrey Akulov [2], Mikhail Svetlik [1], Yana Tyumentseva [1], Tatyana Anan'ina [1] and Vasily Yarnykh [1,3]

1. Laboratory of Neurobiology, Research Institute of Biology and Biophysics, Tomsk State University, Tomsk 634050, Russia
2. Institute of Cytology and Genetics, Siberian Branch of the Russian Academy of Sciences, Novosibirsk 630090, Russia
3. Department of Radiology, University of Washington, Seattle, WA 98109, USA
* Correspondence: khodanovich@mail.tsu.ru; Tel.: +7-3822-529-600

Received: 13 September 2019; Accepted: 1 October 2019; Published: 5 October 2019

Abstract: Macromolecular proton fraction (MPF) has been established as a quantitative clinically-targeted MRI myelin biomarker based on recent demyelination studies. This study aimed to assess the capability of MPF to quantify remyelination using the murine cuprizone-induced reversible demyelination model. MPF was measured in vivo using the fast single-point method in three animal groups (control, cuprizone-induced demyelination, and remyelination after cuprizone withdrawal) and compared to quantitative immunohistochemistry for myelin basic protein (MBP), myelinating oligodendrocytes (CNP-positive cells), and oligodendrocyte precursor cells (OPC, NG2-positive cells) in the corpus callosum, caudate putamen, hippocampus, and cortex. In the demyelination group, MPF, MBP-stained area, and oligodendrocyte count were significantly reduced, while OPC count was significantly increased as compared to both control and remyelination groups in all anatomic structures ($p < 0.05$). All variables were similar in the control and remyelination groups. MPF and MBP-stained area strongly correlated in each anatomic structure (Pearson's correlation coefficients, $r = 0.80$–0.90, $p < 0.001$). MPF and MBP correlated positively with oligodendrocyte count ($r = 0.70$–0.84, $p < 0.01$ for MPF; $r = 0.81$–0.92, $p < 0.001$ for MBP) and negatively with OPC count ($r = -0.69$–-0.77, $p < 0.01$ for MPF; $r = -0.72$–-0.89, $p < 0.01$ for MBP). This study provides immunohistological validation of fast MPF mapping as a non-invasive tool for quantitative assessment of de- and remyelination in white and gray matter and indicates the feasibility of using MPF as a surrogate marker of reparative processes in demyelinating diseases.

Keywords: macromolecular proton fraction; MPF; myelin; magnetic resonance imaging; cuprizone model; demyelination; remyelination; oligodendrocyte precursors; oligodendrocytes; immunohistochemistry

1. Introduction

New therapies enabling regeneration of damaged myelin may offer potential for restoring neurological function in multiple sclerosis (MS) and other demyelinating diseases [1–3]. Quantitative imaging biomarkers of remyelination are of critical importance for the development and clinical testing of myelin repair therapies [4,5]. Partial remyelination associated with the recruitment and proliferation of oligodendrocyte precursor cells (OPC) is a known phenomenon in MS lesions, which, however, usually fails to completely restore damaged brain tissue [1,6,7]. Although significant efforts were focused on identifying magnetic resonance imaging (MRI) signatures of remyelination in MS lesions [4,8,9], no existing technique provides sufficient sensitivity and specificity to myelin to be used as a routine clinical tool for remyelination monitoring [4]. Furthermore, the lesions detectable by MRI are known to represent only a small part of MS pathology, which is characterized by widespread microscopic demyelination of white and gray matter [10–12]. Assessment of remyelination in normal-appearing brain tissues remains unachievable by using any clinical imaging method to date.

A new MRI method, fast macromolecular proton fraction (MPF) mapping [12–20], has demonstrated promise as a reliable clinical and preclinical tool for quantitative imaging of demyelination [12,14–18] and myelin development [19,20]. This method is based on the magnetization transfer (MT) effect and enables quantification of the number of macromolecular protons that are involved into cross-relaxations with water protons [13]. In recent clinical studies, MPF mapping provided the capability to quantify microscopic demyelination in both white and gray matter caused by MS [12,15] and mild traumatic brain injury [16]. MPF mapping has been extensively validated by histology in animal models including the normal brain and C6 glioma in rats [21], cuprizone-induced demyelination in mice [17], and ischemic stroke in rats [18], where it demonstrated strong correlations with the myelin content across white and gray matter anatomic structures and lesions. However, to the best of our knowledge, this method has not been tested in the setting of remyelination.

Cuprizone-induced toxic demyelination in mice is a common animal model of MS [22–26], which is frequently used in preclinical studies of remyelination therapies [5,23–25]. In this model, demyelination is induced by the administration of the copper chelator cuprizone, causing selective oligodendrocyte apoptosis followed by extensive demyelination of both white and gray matter [22–26]. If cuprizone treatment is discontinued within a certain timeframe, spontaneous remyelination and functional recovery (complete or incomplete depending on treatment regimen) typically occur [22–26]. Although cuprizone intoxication is considered a reductionist model of MS devoid of the autoimmune inflammatory component, it reproduces certain pathological features of human disease including diffuse demyelination of white and gray matter, microglial activation, astrogliosis, axonal damage, and remyelination associated with OPC proliferation and oligodendrocyte repopulation [22–26]. The cuprizone model also offers substantial convenience for the evaluation of quantitative imaging methods targeted at the assessment of normal-appearing brain tissues, because cuprizone induces demyelination that affects the whole brain at the microscopic level without the formation of focal lesions, and appears to a variable extent across anatomic structures [17,24–26].

The primary objective of this study was to assess the capability of fast MPF mapping to quantify remyelination in white and gray matter using the cuprizone model. Additionally, we sought to investigate a relationship between MPF and markers of oligodendrogenesis, such as the number of oligodendrocytes and OPC, which are frequently used as outcome measures in preclinical studies of myelin repair therapies.

2. Materials and Methods

2.1. Animals and Experimental Design

All animal experiments were performed in accordance with the rules adopted by the European Convention for the Protection of Vertebrate Animals used for Experimental and Other Scientific Purposes. The experimental protocol was approved by the Bioethical Committee of the Institute of Cytology and Genetics of the Siberian Branch of the Russian Academy of Sciences (Protocol number 25) and the Bioethical Committee of the Biological Institute at Tomsk State University (Protocol number 3, Registration No. 8). Eight-week-old CD1 male mice were obtained from the vivarium of the E.D. Goldberg Institute of Pharmacology and Regenerative Medicine of the Siberian Branch of the Russian Academy of Sciences (Tomsk, Russian Federation). Animals were housed with a 12-h dark-light cycle at a temperature of 21 ± 2 °C, and humidity of 40 ± 2%. Food and water were provided ad libitum.

After 10 days of quarantine, the animals were divided into three groups: the control group (n = 4), the demyelination group (n = 4), and the remyelination group (n = 5). Mice in the demyelination group received 0.5% cuprizone (Bis(cyclohexanone)oxaldihydrazone, Sigma-Aldrich, St. Louis, MO, USA) with standard chow for 10 weeks. The remyelination group returned to a normal diet after 5 weeks of cuprizone treatment. The controls received standard chow for 10 weeks. After 10 weeks of cuprizone treatment, the mice were MRI-scanned with an MPF mapping protocol. Imaging was performed under isoflurane anesthesia (1.5–2% in oxygen) with respiratory monitoring during the scan. The mice were then transcardially perfused with 4% paraformaldehyde (PFA) under ether anesthesia. Brains were removed and fixed overnight in PFA at 4 °C. The brains were then cryoprotected in a graded concentration of sucrose in phosphate buffer (24 h at 10% and 24 h at 20%) at 4 °C, frozen in liquid nitrogen, and stored at −80 °C prior to immunohistochemical staining.

2.2. MRI Acquisition and Processing

The mice were imaged on an 11.7 Tesla horizontal-bore animal MRI scanner (BioSpec 117/16 USR; Bruker BioSpin, Ettlingen, Germany) with the manufacturer's four-channel mouse brain surface coil. A fast high-resolution single-point 3D MPF mapping protocol was implemented as described previously [17]. The protocol included the following sequences applied in the coronal plane with a 3D field-of-view of 20 × 20 × 24 mm:

(1) MT-weighted spoiled gradient echo (GRE): repetition time (TR) = 22 ms, echo time (TE) = 2.5 ms, flip angle (FA) = 9°, spectral bandwidth (BW) = 125 kHz, off-resonance saturation by the Gaussian pulse with an offset frequency of 4500 kHz, effective FA = 900°, a duration of 10 ms, 3D matrix 200 × 200 × 48, spatial resolution 100 × 100 × 500 μm^3, four signal acquisitions, and a scan time of 10 min 34 s;

(2) T_1-weighted spoiled GRE: TR = 16 ms, TE = 2.5 ms, FA = 16°, BW = 125 kHz, 3D matrix 200 × 200 × 48, spatial resolution 100 × 100 × 500 μm^3, four signal acquisitions, and a scan time of 7 min 41 s;

(3) Proton-density (PD)-weighted spoiled GRE: TR = 16 ms, TE = 2.5 ms, FA = 3°, BW = 125 kHz, 3D matrix 200 × 200 × 48, spatial resolution 100 × 100 × 500 μm^3, four signal acquisitions, and a scan time of 7 min 41 s;

(4) B_0 mapping using the dual-TE phase-difference method: TR = 20 ms, TE1 = 2.4 ms, TE2 = 4.1 ms, FA = 8°, BW = 200 kHz, 3D matrix 100 × 100 × 48, spatial resolution 200 × 200 × 500 μm^3, one signal acquisition, and a scan time of 1 min 36 s;

(5) B_1 mapping using the dual-TR actual flip-angle imaging (AFI) method: TR1 = 13 ms, TR2 = 65 ms, TE = 3.7 ms, FA = 60°, BW = 59.5 kHz, 3D matrix 100 × 100 × 48, spatial resolution 200 × 200 × 500 μm^3, one signal acquisition, and a scan time of 4 min 45 s.

The GRE and AFI sequences were implemented with optimal radiofrequency and gradient spoiling based on the excitation pulse phase increments of 169° for GRE and 39° for AFI [27]. In all sequences, linear phase-encoding order with fractional (75%) k-space acquisition in the slab selection direction was used. The total scan time was about 35 min.

Reconstruction of MPF maps was carried out using custom-written C-language software based on the single-point algorithm with synthetic reference image normalization and correction of B_0 and B_1 field non-uniformities, as detailed elsewhere [13,14,17].

2.3. Immunohistochemistry

Coronal brain sections with 10 μm thickness were prepared using an HM525 cryostat (Thermo Fisher Scientific, Walldorf, Germany). Sections were obtained at two brain locations: −1.58 mm and +0.74 mm from bregma according to the mouse brain atlas [28].

Sections were stained using immunohistochemistry for myelin basic protein (MBP, the marker of myelin), 2′,3′-cyclic-nucleotide 3′-phosphodiesterase (CNP, the marker of myelinating oligodendrocytes), and neuro-glial antigen 2 (NG2, the marker of oligodendrocyte precursors). The primary antibodies were: goat polyclonal anti-MBP, (sc-13914, Santa Cruz Biotechnology, Dallas, TX, USA); mouse monoclonal anti-CNPase (Cat#MAB326, Merck Millipore, Burlington, MA, USA), rabbit polyclonal anti-NG2 (H-300), (sc-20162, Santa Cruz Biotechnology, USA), and goat polyclonal anti-DCX (C-18), (sc-8066, Santa Cruz Biotechnology, USA). The secondary antibody was donkey anti-goat AlexaFluor® 488 (green color, code 705-545-147, Jackson ImmunoResearch, West Grove, PA, USA) or donkey anti-rabbit AlexaFluor® 488 (green color, code 711-545-152, Jackson ImmunoResearch).

Slides were covered with mounting medium with DAPI (4′,6-diamidino-2-phenylindole, blue color, nuclear counter stain). Photography was performed using an Axio Imager Z2 microscope (Carl Zeiss, Oberkochen, Germany) and AxioVision 4.8 (Carl Zeiss) software with a MozaiX module, which enables reconstruction of the whole brain images by stitching a series of mosaic images. Additionally, 2′,3′-cyclic-nucleotide 3′-phosphodiesterase (CNP), neural/glial antigen 2 (NG2) stained sections were photographed using a confocal laser microscope LSM 780 NLO (Carl Zeiss).

2.4. Image Analysis

MPF maps and microphotographs of MBP-, CNP-, and NG2-stained brain sections were analyzed using freely available ImageJ software (National Institutes of Health, Bethesda, MD, USA). Two brain locations (−1.58 mm and +0.74 mm from bregma) defined according to the mouse brain atlas [28] were chosen for quantitative analysis. Quantitative imaging variables were assessed in the regions-of-interest (ROIs) of standard sizes placed within the following anatomic structures: the central and distal parts of the corpus callosum, center of the caudate putamen, cortex, and hippocampus. The scheme of image analysis is presented in Figure 1. MPF values were quantified as previously described [17]. Myelin density on the MBP microphotographs was quantified in the above structures by the Otsu thresholding method [29] implemented as a plugin for ImageJ software [30]. A percentage of the total area of detected objects in the binarized images (Figure 1) was used as a surrogate measure of MBP density [31]. Myelinating oligodendrocytes (CNP-positive cells) and OPC (NG2-positive cells) were counted manually in the similarly positioned ROIs.

2.5. Statistical Analysis

All statistical analyses were carried out using Statistica 10.0 for Windows (StatSoft Inc, Tulsa, OK, USA). Mean values and standard errors of the mean were calculated for each variable in each anatomical structure. Normality of the data within animal groups and residuals in regression analyses was assessed using the Shapiro-Wilk's test. No significant deviations from the normal distribution were found, and therefore, parametric analyses were used. MPF values and quantitative histology data were compared between the control, demyelination, and remyelination groups using a two-way repeated measures analysis of variance (ANOVA) followed by post hoc least significant difference (LSD) tests for individual anatomical structures.

The effects of demyelination and remyelination on MPF and histological variables in each anatomic structure were characterized by the effect sizes (Cohen's d) calculated as the ratios of the mean differences to the pooled standard deviation. The d values for demyelination were calculated from the differences between the control and demyelination groups. The d values for remyelination were calculated from the differences between the demyelination and remyelination groups. Pearson's correlation coefficient (r) and linear regression analysis were used to determine associations between variables across anatomical structures and animals. Statistical significance was defined as a p value less than 0.05.

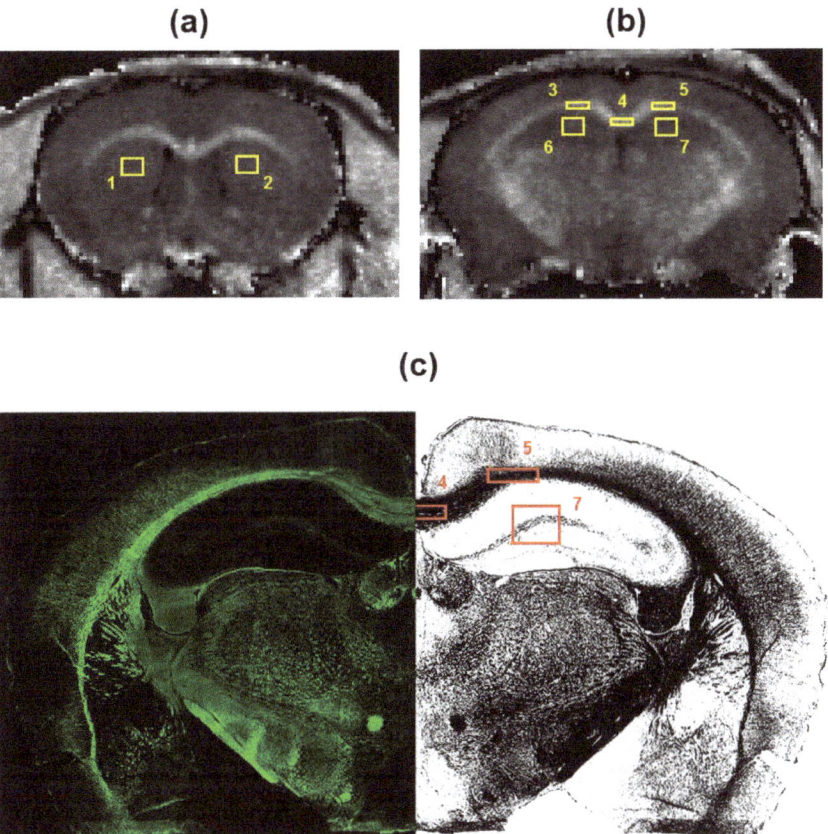

Figure 1. The scheme of image processing for macromolecular proton fraction (MPF) maps (**a,b**) and myelin basic protein (MBP)-stained images (**c**). Cross-sections of a 3D MPF map of a control mouse taken at the locations of +0.74 mm (a) and −1.58 mm (b) from bregma and superimposed with regions-of-interest (ROIs) corresponding to the following brain structures: 1, 2—caudate putamen; 3, 4, 5—corpus callosum; 6, 7—hippocampus, 8, 9, 10, 11—cortex. MBP-stained image at the location of −1.58 mm from bregma (c) is presented in the native (left) and binarized (right) forms with ROIs corresponding to the corpus callosum (5,6), hippocampus (7), and cortex (10,11).

3. Results

3.1. Effects of Demyelination and Remyelination on MPF, MBP Density, and the Counts of Myelinating Oligodendrocytes and OPC

Example MPF maps of the murine brain from the control, demyelination, and remyelination groups at the two brain locations are demonstrated in Figure 2. Representative microphotographs corresponding to the investigated brain structures in the three animal groups taken from MBP-, CNP-, and NG2-stained sections are shown in Figures 3–5, respectively. Summary statistics and group comparisons for MPF measurements and quantitative histological variables are presented in Figure 6. Cuprizone-treated mice demonstrated reduced contrast between white and gray matter on MPF maps as compared to control mice, particularly in the corpus callosum, whereas the maps from animals in the remyelination group showed visually normal tissue contrast (Figure 2). MPF values in both the corpus callosum and gray matter structures (caudate putamen, cortex, and hippocampus) were significantly smaller in the demyelination group as compared to the control and remyelination groups (Figure 6a). The control and remyelination groups did not show significant differences in MPF (Figure 6a). MBP immunostaining showed visible loss of myelin in all structures in the demyelination group and restoration of myelination patterns in the remyelination group (Figure 3). MBP quantitation by the percentage of the stained area showed a significant decrease in myelin density in all structures in the demyelination group relative to both control and remyelination groups and the absence of significant differences between the control and remyelination groups (Figure 6b). The count of myelinating oligodendrocytes showed a similar trend and was significantly reduced in the demyelination group as compared to the control and remyelination groups (Figure 4, Figure 6c). In the remyelination group, the CNP-positive cell count in the corpus callosum was significantly lower than that in controls, while no significant differences were found for other structures (Figure 6c). The amount of OPC showed an opposite trend, with a significant increase in the demyelination group relative to both control and demyelination groups in all brain structures (Figure 6d). There were no significant differences in the NG2-positive cell count between the control and remyelination groups. Another interesting observation is substantial changes in OPC morphology in the demyelination group, where these cells exhibited shorter and fewer processes or bipolar or star-like structures reflecting variable stages of immaturity. Notably, OPC in remyelinated animals showed highly branched morphology, similar to the control animals (Figure 5b).

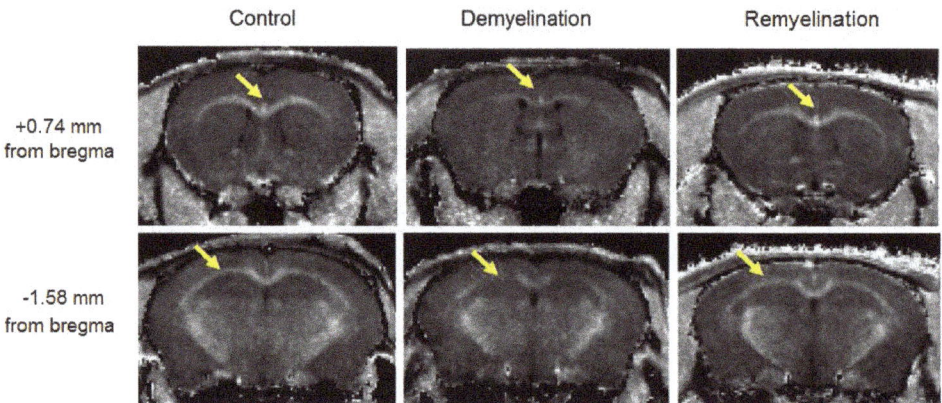

Figure 2. Example MPF maps of the mice from the control (left), demyelination (center), and remyelination (right) groups. Cross-sections of 3D MPF maps were taken through the caudate putamen (+0.74 mm from bregma, top) and hippocampus (−1.58 mm from bregma, bottom). Arrows show a visible reduction in MPF in the corpus callosum. MPF maps are presented with the grayscale range corresponding to 2–16% and window centered at 9%.

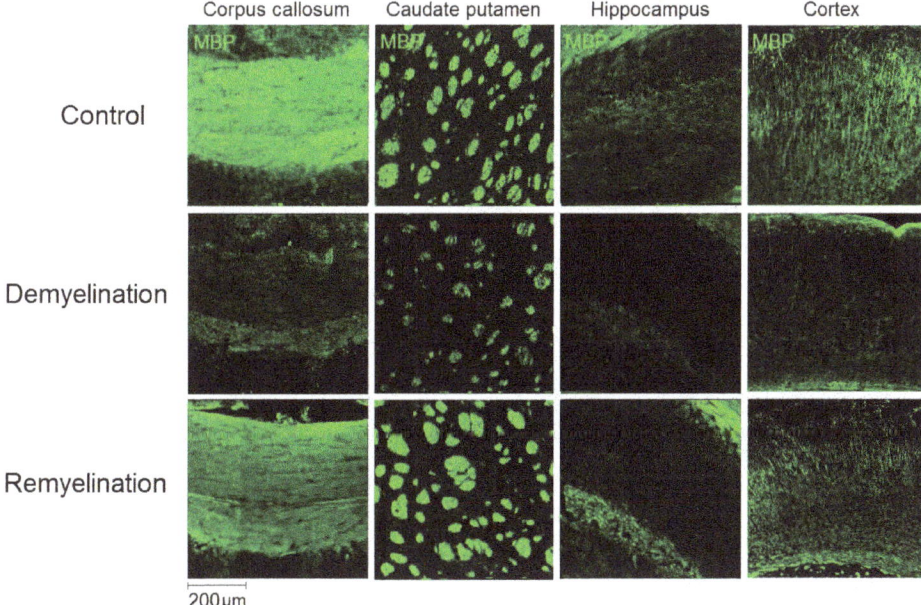

Figure 3. Effect of cuprizone-induced demyelination and remyelination after cuprizone discontinuation on MBP immunostaining. Example microphotographs of MBP-stained sections are presented for the corpus callosum, caudate putamen, cortex, and hippocampus with magnification of ×100.

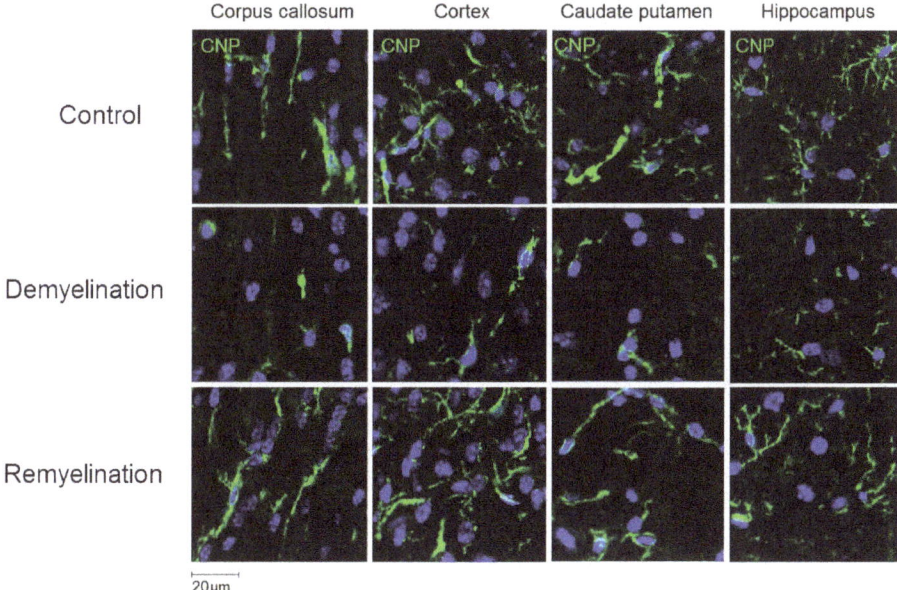

Figure 4. Effect of cuprizone-induced demyelination and remyelination after cuprizone discontinuation on the number of myelinating oligodendrocytes (CNP-positive cells). Example microphotographs of CNP-stained sections are presented for the corpus callosum, caudate putamen, cortex, and hippocampus with magnification of ×200.

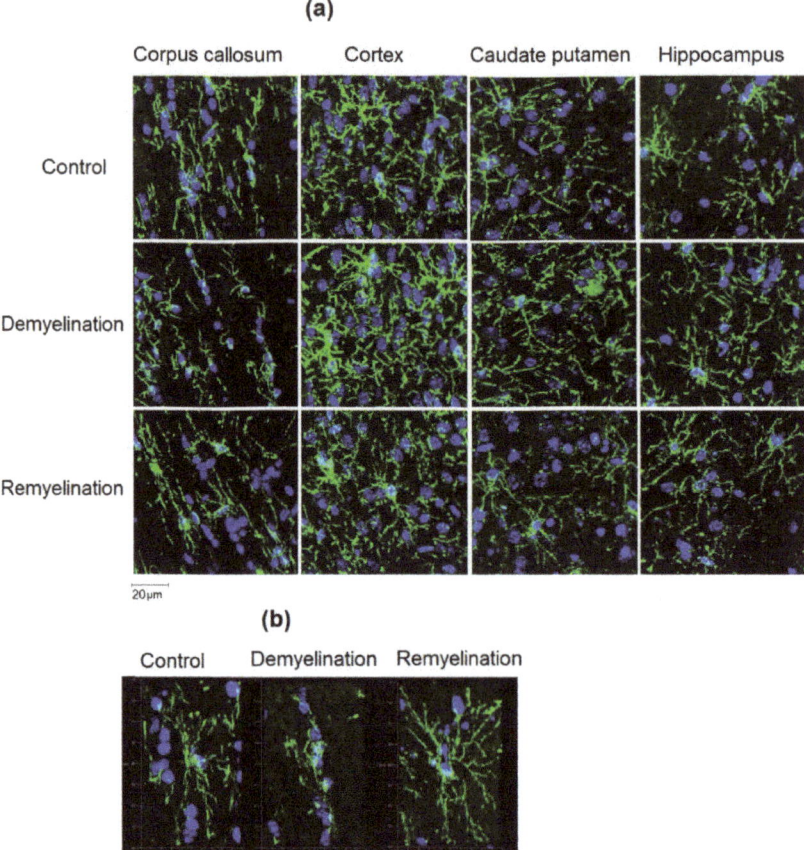

Figure 5. Effect of cuprizone-induced demyelination and remyelination after cuprizone discontinuation on the amount of OPC (NG2-positive cells). (**a**) Example microphotographs of NG2-stained sections corresponding to the corpus callosum, caudate putamen, cortex, and hippocampus with magnification of ×200. (**b**) 3D reconstructions of separate NG2-positive cells in the corpus callosum illustrating distinctions in OPC morphology. Magnification: ×200.

Effect sizes characterizing de- and remyelination across the studied brain regions in a uniform dimensionless scale are summarized in Table 1. For all variables and anatomic regions, the effect sizes appeared very large (d > 1.3) according to the commonly used classification [32]. The d values tended to be larger in the absolute scale for MBP staining and CNP-positive cell count and comparable for MPF and NG2-positive cell count. For all variables except for the NG2-positive cell count, the effect sizes were fairly homogenous across the anatomic regions (Table 1).

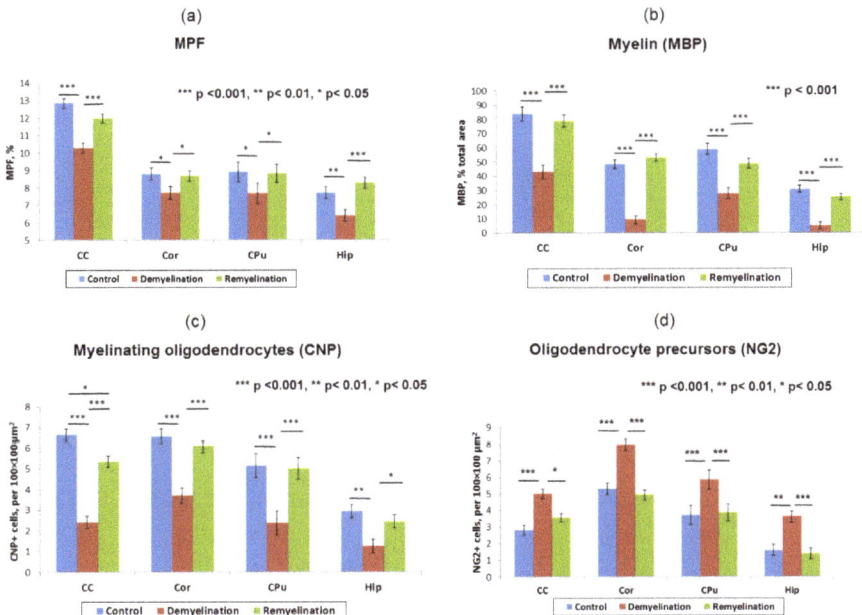

Figure 6. Summary statistics of MPF measurements and quantitative histological variables in the brain anatomic structures across the control, demyelination, and remyelination animal groups: MPF values (**a**), myelin content according to the percentage of MBP staining area (**b**), the count of myelinating oligodendrocytes (CNP-positive cells) (**c**), and OPC count (NG2-positive cells) (**d**). Anatomic structures are abbreviated as follows: CC—corpus callosum, Cor—cortex, CPu—caudate putamen, and Hip—hippocampus. Significant differences between the groups according to the LSD test are marked by asterisks: * – $p < 0.05$, ** – $p < 0.01$, and *** – $p < 0.001$. Error bars represent standard errors of the mean.

Table 1. Effect sizes (Cohen's d) with 95% confidence intervals (CI) corresponding to the demyelination and remyelination states in the corpus callosum, caudate putamen, cortex, and hippocampus based on MPF and quantitative histology variables.

Variable	Control-Demyelination: d [−CI, +CI]				Demyelination-Remyelination: d [−CI, +CI]			
	CC	CPu	Cor	Hip	CC	CPu	Cor	Hip
MPF	2.7 [0.8, 4.6]	2.3 [0.5, 4.5]	2.2 [0.5, 4.0]	2.2 [0.5, 4.0]	−2.3 [−4.0, −0.6]	−2.1 [−3.7, −0.5]	−1.8 [−3.4, −0.3]	−2.8 [−4.7, −1.0]
MBP area percentage	3.9 [1.6, 6.3]	3.8 [1.5, 6.1]	5.6 [2.2, 8.0]	4.6 [1.9, 7.2]	−3.1 [−5.1, −1.2]	−2.8 [−4.6, −0.9]	−4.4 [−6.8, −2.0]	−4.0 [−6.3, −1.7]
CNP-positive cell count	5.7 [2.6, 8.8]	3.8 [1.5, 6.1]	2.9 [0.9, 4.9]	3.0 [1.9, 7.2]	−5.4 [−8.2, −2.6]	−4.3 [−6.6, −1.9]	−3.5 [−5.6, −1.4]	−2.4 [−4.2, −0.7]
NG2-positive cell count	−4.4 [−7.0, −1.8]	−1.7 [−7.0, −1.8]	−3.5 [−7.0, −1.8]	−2.6 [−7.0, −1.8]	2.7 [0.9, 4.6]	1.6 [0.1, 3.2]	4.0 [1.7, 6.2]	3.0 [1.1, 4.9]

3.2. Correlations between MPF and Quantitative Histology Variables

The results of linear regression analyses for MPF values as a function of the myelin content, the number of myelinating oligodendrocytes and OPC are presented in Figure 7. The summary of regression analyses for all variables is provided in Table 2.

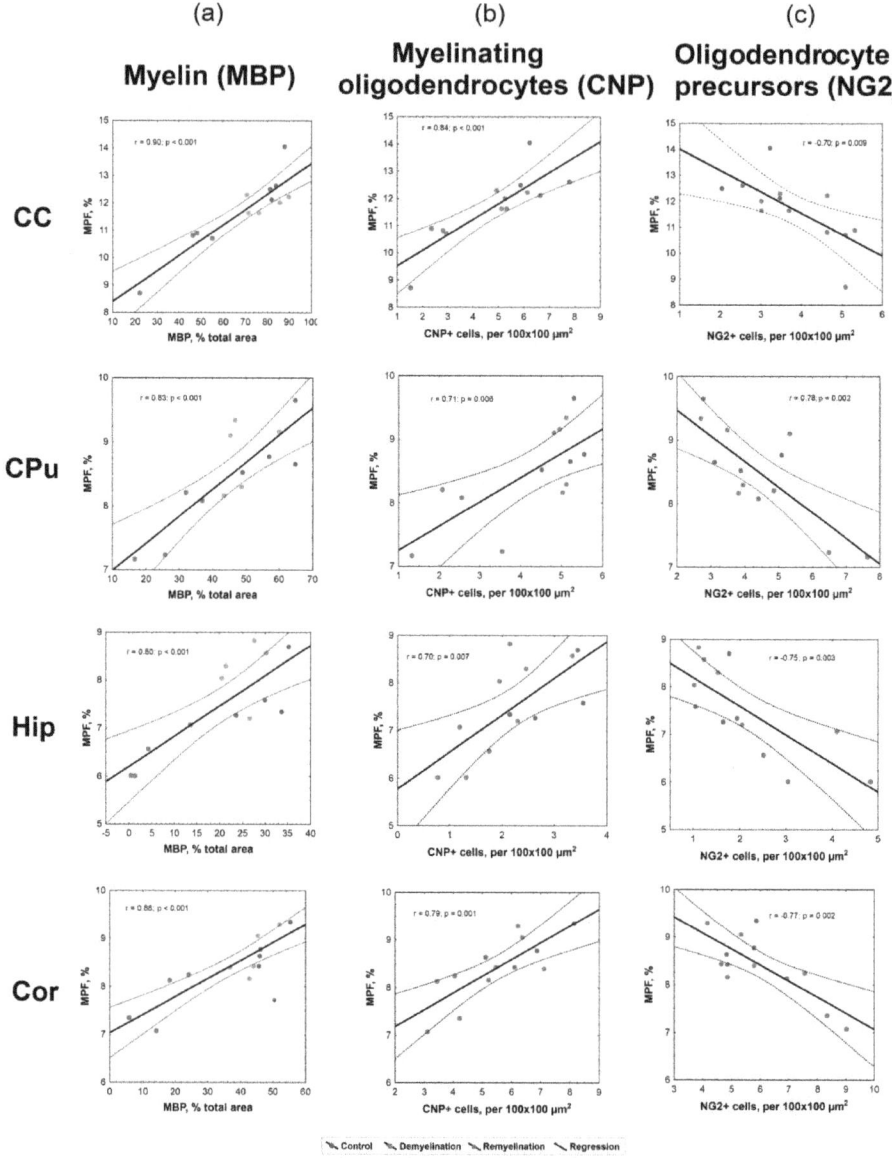

Figure 7. Linear regression analysis of MPF values vs. myelin content according to MBP staining (**a**), the number of myelinating oligodendrocytes according to CNP staining (**b**), and the number of OPC according to NG2 staining (**c**) in the corpus callosum, caudate putamen, hippocampus, and cortex. Blue, red and green dots correspond to the control, demyelination, and remyelination groups, respectively. Black lines depict the plots of the regression equations for the pooled datasets including all groups. Dotted lines represent confidence intervals of the regression lines.

Table 2. Linear regression analysis of associations between MPF, MBP-stained percentage of the total area, CNP-positive cell count, and NG2-positive cell count in the corpus callosum, caudate putamen, hippocampus, and cortex.

Parameters	Brain Structure	r	r²	p	Slope (95% CI), p	Intercept (95% CI), p
MPF vs. MBP % total area	CC	0.90	0.82	<0.001	0.06 (0.04, 0.07), <0.001	7.84 (6.57, 9.12), <0.001
	CPu	0.83	0.69	<0.001	0.04 (0.02, 0.06), <0.001	6.57 (5.68, 7.46), <0.001
	Hip	0.80	0.64	<0.001	0.06 (0.03, 0.09), 0.001	6.20 (5.46, 6.95), <0.001
	Cor	0.88	0.78	<0.001	0.04 (0.02, 0.05), <0.001	7.04 (6.52, 7.56), <0.001
MPF vs CNP + cells	CC	0.84	0.71	<0.001	0.57 (0.33, 0.81), <0.001	8.96 (7.70, 10.21), <0.001
	CPu	0.71	0.51	0.006	0.38 (0.13, 0.63), 0.006	6.87 (5.76, 7.98), <0.001
	Hip	0.70	0.50	0.007	0.77 (0.26, 1.29), 0.007	5.78 (4.54, 7.01), <0.001
	Cor	0.79	0.63	0.001	0.35 (0.17, 0.53), 0.001	6.49 (5.46, 7.51), <0.001
MPF vs NG2 + cells	CC	−0.69	0.47	0.009	−0.82 (−1.40, −0.25), 0.009	14.83 (12.57, 17.10), <0.001
	CPu	−0.76	0.58	0.006	−0.67 (−1.04, −0.29), 0.002	14.67 (12.94, 16.41), <0.001
	Hip	−0.75	0.57	0.003	−0.60 (−0.95, −0.25), 0.003	8.79 (7.95, 9.63), <0.001
	Cor	−0.77	0.59	0.002	−0.34 (−0.52, −0.15), 0.002	10.43 (9.28, 11.59), <0.001
MBP % total area vs CNP + cells	CC	0.92	0.85	<0.001	10.13 (7.36, 12.87), <0.001	20.32 (6.02, 34.61), 0.01
	CPu	0.85	0.72	<0.001	8.49 (4.46, 12.52), <0.001	7.47 (−9.04, 23.98), 0.34
	Hip	0.82	0.67	<0.001	11.43 (6.11, 16.74), <0.001	−4.90 (−17.57, 7.77), 0.41
	Cor	0.81	0.66	<0.001	8.49 (4.46, 12.52), <0.001	−10.05 (−32.95, 12.86), 0.36
MBP % total area vs NG2 + cells	CC	−0.72	0.62	0.005	−13.87 (−22.78, −4.96), 0.005	121.88 (86.93, 156.82), <0.001
	CPu	−0.81	0.65	<0.001	−8.21 (−12.18, −4.25), <0.001	81.81 (63.41, 100.20), <0.001
	Hip	−0.74	0.54	0.004	−7.45 (−11.98, −2.91), 0.004	36.59 (25.57, 47.62), <0.001
	Cor	−0.89	0.78	<0.001	−9.14 (−12.32, −5.96), <0.001	91.48 (71.83, 111.13), <0.001
CNP + cells vs NG2 + cells	CC	−0.79	0.62	0.001	−1.39 (−2.11, −0.67), 0.001	10.10 (7.28, 12.93), <0.001
	CPu	−0.68	0.47	0.01	−0.66 (−1.12, −0.19), 0.01	7.14 (4.99, 9.31), <0.001
	Hip	−0.79	0.62	0.001	−0.57 (−0.87, −0.27), 0.001	3.45 (2.73, 4.17), <0.001
	Cor	−0.63	0.39	0.02	−0.62 (−1.13, −0.11), 0.02	9.22 (6.07, 12.38), <0.001

Abbreviation: CI, confidence interval; CC, corpus callosum; CPu, caudate putamen; Hip, hippocampus; Cor, cortex.

Correlations between all variables appeared statistically significant for each investigated brain anatomic structure (corpus callosum, caudate putamen, hippocampus, and cortex). MPF values strongly correlated with MBP-stained percentage of the total area (r = 0.80–0.90, $p < 0.001$), as seen in Figure 6a. Both MPF and MBP staining demonstrated strong positive correlations with the count of CNP-positive myelinating oligodendrocytes (Figure 6b, Table 2), although correlations for MPF (r = 0.70–0.84, $p < 0.01$) were slightly weaker than those for MBP (r = 0.81–0.92, $p < 0.001$). MPF and MBP also showed strong negative correlations with the amount of NG2-positive OPC (r = −0.69−−0.77, $p < 0.01$ for MPF; r = −0.72−−0.89, $p < 0.01$ for MBP), while the counts of CNP-positive and NG2-positive cells were negatively correlated in all anatomic structures (Figure 6c, Table 2).

4. Discussion

The results of this study demonstrate the capability of fast MPF mapping to accurately and reliably quantify remyelination in both white and gray matter. MPF showed very similar patterns of changes as compared to the immunohistochemical myelin marker MBP including a significant decrease caused by the cuprizone treatment and restoration to the nearly normal level after treatment discontinuation. These findings are further supported by strong correlations between MPF and MBP immunofluorescence in all investigated white and gray matter anatomic structures including the corpus callosum, caudate putamen, hippocampus, and cortex. It is important to emphasize that correlations between MPF and MBP in this study were assessed separately for each structure and, therefore, could not be driven by intrinsic distinctions in the myelin content between white and gray matter.

In the aspect of demyelination, our results confirm the conclusions of the previous study [17], which demonstrated close agreement between MPF and quantitative myelin histology in the assessment of cuprizone-induced myelin loss in white and gray matter across a series of anatomic structures. It should be pointed out that the earlier results [17] were achieved with luxol fast blue histological staining, whereas this study utilized immunohistochemistry with MBP. Similar findings obtained with different myelin markers provide extra confidence to the interpretation of MPF measurements in terms of the myelin content.

Cuprizone-induced demyelination has been extensively studied by various MRI methods as overviewed earlier [17]. At the same time, fewer MRI studies investigated remyelination in this model [33–43]. The majority of these publications [33–40] were limited to analyzing the behavior of imaging variables in the corpus callosum, which is known as the most susceptible to cuprizone-induced demyelination anatomic structure [22–26]. Several quantitative and non-quantitative imaging techniques, such as conventional T_1- and T_2-weighted imaging [34,43], T_2 mapping [38,43], diffusion tensor imaging (DTI) [33,36,38,40,42,43], diffusion kurtosis imaging (DKI) [38,42], and magnetization transfer imaging in the traditional semi-quantitative [34,35,38,39,41] and quantitative [37] variants demonstrated significant trends in the corresponding imaging parameters consistent with de- and remyelination in the corpus callosum. Among the above studies, significant correlations of variable strength (absolute values of correlation coefficients in a range of 0.6–0.9) between myelin histology [35,37,39–41] or electron microscopy [34,38] and imaging variables in the corpus callosum were found for normalized T_1- and T_2-weighted signal intensities [34], T_2 values [38], DTI-related indexes (mean diffusivity, radial diffusivity, and fractional anisotropy) [38,40], MT ratio (MTR, conventional semi-quantitative MT imaging index) [34,35,39,41], and pool size ratio (PSR) derived from quantitative MT measurements [37]. To the best of our knowledge, only four studies [33,41–43] investigated changes in MRI parameters associated with both de- and remyelination in regions other than corpus callosum anatomic regions, including a series of white matter fiber tracts [33,43], cortical gray matter [41–43], and subcortical gray matter structures (caudate putamen [41,43] and thalamus [43]). In some white matter regions outside the corpus callosum, T_2 values showed significant differences associated with de- and remyelination [43], while the trends for diffusion tensor metrics were non-significant [33,43]. In the deep gray matter structures, the significant effects of de- and remyelination were found for T_2 in the caudate putamen and thalamus [43] and for MTR in the caudate putamen [41]. MTR was also weakly (r = 0.46) but significantly correlated with histologically measured myelin content in the caudate putamen [41]. In the cortex, quantitative changes in T_2 were significant for demyelination but failed to detect remyelination [43]. No significant effects of cortical demyelination or remyelination were identified for MTR [41]. DKI was the only quantitative MRI technique that was able to detect significant cortical changes consistent with cuprizone-induced demyelination and subsequent recovery [42]. However, DKI indexes in white and gray matter were reported to change in opposite directions [42], thus suggesting that the observed DKI parameter alterations were driven by factors other than myelination. None of earlier cuprizone model studies has reported quantitative correlations between histological myelin measures and imaging variables in the cortex and hippocampus. As evidenced by this and previous studies, only the fast MPF mapping method enables reliable in vivo quantitation of both demyelination and remyelination in a variety of white and gray matter structures, being in close agreement with histology.

Our observations in the investigated anatomic structures are in overall agreement with earlier immunopathological studies, which reported prominent cuprizone-induced myelin loss and oligodendrocyte depletion in the corpus callosum [22–26,40,44–48], cortex [45–48], caudate putamen [41,48,49], and hippocampus [45,48,50,51]. Similar to previous publications, we also observed remyelination accompanied with recovery of oligodendrocyte population in the corpus callosum [22–26,40,44–47], cortex [45–47], caudate putamen [41], and hippocampus [45] after cuprizone discontinuation. These processes were paralleled by an increased OPC count in all structures during the demyelination phase followed by its restoration to a nearly normal level during the remyelination phase. Similar patterns of OPC population changes were reported for the corpus callosum [40,44,45], cortex [45,47], and hippocampus [45], though some studies did not find significant OPC proliferation in the basal ganglia [49] and hippocampus [51]. These discrepancies may be explained by the use of different OPC markers and/or distinctions in the time frame of oligodendroglial response between white and gray matter structures [45,47]. The results of our study indicate close quantitative agreement between molecular and cellular components of myelin loss and repair in the cuprizone model including myelin content changes assessed by both MBP and MPF, and the number of myelinating oligodendrocytes and OPC in all anatomic structures. While this study was not focused on the elucidation of detailed temporal profiles of cellular responses during de- and remyelination, our data suggest a high degree of synchrony between underlying cellular events in both white and gray matter in agreement with earlier studies [44,46].

The presented results have several implications for the design of future preclinical studies of remyelinating therapies. First, based on very strong correlations between MPF and histological myelin content measures, this and previous [17–19] studies suggest that fast MPF mapping can be used interchangeably with myelin histology in animal studies, particularly if several time points are needed. Our results demonstrate that the effect sizes for MPF, while being slightly lower than those for histological variables, are still very large (>2 for all anatomic structures). Additional gain in statistical power can be achieved due to longitudinal measurements using MPF as opposed to the study designs based on histological endpoints only. Second, this study shows that both imaging and histological outcomes in the cuprizone model should be assessed not only for the corpus callosum but also for different gray matter structures (cortex, striatum, hippocampus), where the effects of both demyelination and remyelination are highly significant. Cortical demyelination is known to represent a separate and highly clinically relevant aspect of MS pathology [10–12], while cortical MS lesions have been shown to hold an extensive remyelination potential compared to white matter lesions [52,53]. Accordingly, the advent of an imaging method enabling reliable assessment of cortical remyelination may substantially impact future preclinical and clinical studies of myelin repair therapies. Third, our results may be helpful in the interpretation of the OPC count as an outcome measure in preclinical myelin repair studies. The dynamics of OPC population is known to demonstrate a biphasic behavior with an increase during cuprizone-induced demyelination followed by a decrease during recovery after cuprizone discontinuation [22–26]. However, the significance of OPC count as a biomarker in preclinical studies of remyelination therapies using the cuprizone model remains an open question due to a possible mismatch between temporal profiles of mature oligodendrocyte repopulation, remyelination, and OPC proliferation. Recent meta-analysis [5] showed that the histological or immunohistochemical myelin assessment and oligodendrocyte count provided consistent results as outcome measures for prospective remyelination therapies, while the performance of OPC count was rather controversial with a non-significant overall effect. Our results demonstrate strong negative correlations between the OPC count and both the population of myelinating oligodendrocytes and myelin content measures (MBP and MPF). These correlations indicate that OPC count may provide extra confidence in the assessment of therapeutic efficacy and suggest that its reduction towards the normal level should be viewed as a favorable treatment outcome in acute demyelination settings. At the same time, more research is needed to identify the utility of OPC assessment in the treatment of chronic demyelination where the OPC pool may be intrinsically depleted [54].

While this study provides a compelling evidence of the utility of fast MPF mapping as a means to quantify remyelination in the acute cuprizone intoxication model, some aspects of the application of this method to other animal models of MS need further research. Besides cuprizone, common MS models include inflammatory demyelination caused by immunization with myelin antigens (experimental autoimmune encephalomyelitis (EAE)) or infectious agents (Theiler's murine encephalomyelitis virus and murine hepatitis virus) and toxic demyelination induced by focal administration of lysolecithin or ethidium bromide [25,55]. Newer models involving different demyelination mechanisms, such as inducible conditional knock-out of the myelin regulatory factor (iCKO-Myrf) in mice [56] and feline irradiated diet-induced demyelination (FIDID) [57] were also described. All these models capture certain pathological features of MS, though there is no single model that could entirely mimic the human disease. In contrast to acute cuprizone intoxication where remyelination is typically rapid and complete [22–26], only partial remyelination occurs in some other models including prolonged cuprizone administration [22–26,54], EAE [25,55], FIDID [57], and iCKO-Myrf [56]. Arguably, these models may be more relevant to chronic MS lesions in humans, where complete remyelination usually does not happen [1,6,7]. Due to a reduced effect size associated with remyelination, such models may pose challenges in the application of MPF mapping or any other quantitative imaging approach for the assessment of remyelination in either spontaneous or treatment-related settings. Another potential challenge may be associated with edema, which is a common feature of the inflammatory models [58] and present to a lesser extent in the cuprizone model [59]. A recent study [18] demonstrated that MPF measurements in the acute ischemic stroke model may be confounded by edema, though myelin remains the main factor driving MPF changes in the ischemic lesion. More sophisticated MPF mapping techniques with a reduced sensitivity to tissue water content alterations [60,61] may be advantageous in the applications to inflammatory MS models as well as MS lesions in humans.

The key practical advantage of the fast MPF mapping method is the simplicity of clinical translation. This method has already been successfully applied in several clinical studies of MS [12,15] and traumatic brain injury [16] with the use of 3 Tesla research MRI equipment. In these studies [12,15,16], MPF mapping demonstrated the capability to quantify demyelination not only in white matter but also in cortical and subcortical gray matter. Recent studies [19,20,62] demonstrated the feasibility of MPF mapping using a routine 1.5 Tesla clinical MRI scanner in conjunction with the design of ultrafast protocols enabling collection of source images within a few minutes. Furthermore, due to the inherent insensitivity of MPF to magnetic field strength [63], the data obtained in humans on clinical scanners can be quantitatively compared to the values measured in animal models with the use of specialized high-field MRI equipment. An additional advantage of MPF mapping in both clinical and preclinical studies is its independence of changes in tissue relaxation times T_1 and T_2 caused by paramagnetic ions, particularly iron [15]. Abnormal iron deposition in the subcortical gray matter anatomic structures is a known pathological feature of MS [15,64,65]. A growing body of evidence suggests that an altered iron metabolism is closely associated with myelin pathology in both human MS disease and animal demyelination models [66–69]. Sensitivity to tissue relaxation properties is a known problem in alternative approaches for myelin imaging, such as multi-component relaxation methods [70–72] and MTR, while MPF mapping overcomes this limitation [12,15]. Taken together, the results of this and previous applications [12–21] suggest that the fast MPF mapping technology can provide a method of choice for preclinical and clinical studies of myelin repair therapies.

5. Conclusions

The results of this study provide comprehensive immunohistological validation of the fast MPF mapping method as a non-invasive quantitative tool for preclinical and clinical studies of de- and remyelination in both white and gray matter. Strong correlations between MPF and quantitative immunochemistry of the major protein component of myelin (MBP) support the use of MPF as a myelin biomarker in a variety of neurological conditions. Our results also demonstrate close quantitative agreement between oligodendroglial response and myelin content changes in the cuprizone model. Correlations of MPF with both myelin content and oligodendrogenesis indicate the feasibility of using this parameter as a uniform surrogate marker of reparative processes in demyelinating diseases.

Author Contributions: M.K. and V.Y. designed the study. V.G. and E.P. were responsible for the development of the animal model. A.A. and V.Y. performed MRI studies. A.P., V.G., T.A. and M.S. performed image analysis. Y.T., A.P., and T.A. performed tissue processing and immunohistochemical labeling. M.K. performed statistical analysis and wrote the manuscript. V.Y. developed an MRI protocol and image processing software and critically revised the manuscript. All authors reviewed and approved the final version of the manuscript.

Funding: The study was performed under support from the Ministry of Education and Science of the Russian Federation within State Assignment Project No. 18.2583.2017/4.6. Immunohistochemical studies were carried out with support from the Russian Science Foundation, project No. 18-15-00229.

Acknowledgments: The authors thank Ms. Svetlana Kildyaeva for proofreading the manuscript.

Conflicts of Interest: The authors declare no conflict of interest.

References

1. Franklin, R.J.; Ffrench-Constant, C. Remyelination in the CNS: from biology to therapy. *Nat. Rev. Neurosci.* **2008**, *9*, 839–855. [CrossRef] [PubMed]
2. Kremer, D.; Akkermann, R.; Küry, P.; Dutta, R. Current advancements in promoting remyelination in multiple sclerosis. *Mult. Scler.* **2019**, *25*, 7–14. [CrossRef] [PubMed]
3. Kipp, M. Remyelination strategies in multiple sclerosis: a critical reflection. *Expert. Rev. Neurother.* **2016**, *16*, 1–3. [CrossRef] [PubMed]
4. Mallik, S.; Samson, R.S.; Wheeler-Kingshott, C.A.; Miller, D.H. Imaging outcomes for trials of remyelination in multiple sclerosis. *J. Neurol. Neurosurg. Psychiatry* **2014**, *85*, 1396–1404. [CrossRef] [PubMed]
5. Hooijmans, C.R.; Hlavica, M.; Schuler, F.A.F.; Good, N.; Good, A.; Baumgartner, L.; Galeno, G.; Schneider, M.P.; Jung, T.; de Vries, R.; et al. Remyelination promoting therapies in multiple sclerosis animal models: a systematic review and meta-analysis. *Sci. Rep.* **2019**, *29*, 822. [CrossRef] [PubMed]
6. Chang, A.; Tourtellotte, W.W.; Rudick, R.; Trapp, B.D. Premyelinating oligodendrocytes in chronic lesions of multiple sclerosis. *N. Engl. J. Med.* **2002**, *17*, 165–173. [CrossRef]
7. Kipp, M.; Victor, M.; Martino, G.; Franklin, R.J. Endogeneous remyelination: Findings in human studies. *CNS Neurol. Disord. Drug Targets* **2012**, *11*, 598–609. [CrossRef]
8. Barkhof, F.; Bruck, W.; De Groot, C.J.; Bergers, E.; Hulshof, S.; Geurts, J.; Polman, C.H.; van der Valk, P. Remyelinated lesions in multiple sclerosis: magnetic resonance image appearance. *Arch. Neurol.* **2003**, *60*, 1073–1081. [CrossRef]
9. Van den Elskamp, I.J.; Knol, D.L.; Vrenken, H.; Karas, G.; Meijerman, A.; Filippi, M.; Kappos, L.; Fazekas, F.; Wagner, K.; Pohl, C.; et al. Lesional magnetization transfer ratio: a feasible outcome for remyelinating treatment trials in multiple sclerosis. *Mult. Scler.* **2010**, *16*, 660–669. [CrossRef]
10. Kutzelnigg, A.; Lucchinetti, C.F.; Stadelmann, C.; Brück, W.; Rauschka, H.; Bergmann, M.; Schmidbauer, M.; Parisi, J.E.; Lassmann, H. Cortical demyelination and diffuse white matter injury in multiple sclerosis. *Brain* **2005**, *128*, 2705–2712. [CrossRef]
11. Seewann, A.; Vrenken, H.; Kooi, E.J.; van der Valk, P.; Knol, D.L.; Polman, C.H.; Pouwels, P.J.; Barkhof, F.; Geurts, J.J. Imaging the tip of the iceberg: Visualization of cortical lesions in multiple sclerosis. *Mult. Scler.* **2011**, *17*, 1202–1210. [CrossRef] [PubMed]
12. Yarnykh, V.L.; Bowen, J.D.; Samsonov, A.; Repovic, P.; Mayadev, A.; Qian, P.; Gangadharan, B.; Keogh, B.P.; Maravilla, K.R.; Henson, L.K. Fast Whole-Brain Three-dimensional Macromolecular Proton Fraction Mapping in Multiple Sclerosis. *Radiology* **2015**, *274*, 210–220. [CrossRef] [PubMed]
13. Yarnykh, V.L. Fast macromolecular proton fraction mapping from a single off-resonance magnetization transfer measurement. *Magn. Reson. Med.* **2012**, *68*, 166–178. [CrossRef] [PubMed]
14. Yarnykh, V.L. Time-efficient, high-resolution, whole brain three-dimensional macromolecular proton fraction mapping. *Magn. Reson. Med.* **2016**, *75*, 100–2106. [CrossRef]
15. Yarnykh, V.L.; Krutenkova, E.P.; Aitmagambetova, G.; Repovic, P.; Mayadev, A.; Qian, P.; Jung Henson, L.K.; Gangadharan, B.; Bowen, J.D. Iron-Insensitive Quantitative Assessment of Subcortical Gray Matter Demyelination in Multiple Sclerosis Using the Macromolecular Proton Fraction. *Am. J. Neuroradiol.* **2018**, *39*, 618–625. [CrossRef]
16. Petrie, E.C.; Cross, D.J.; Yarnykh, V.L.; Richards, T.; Martin, N.M.; Pagulayan, K.; Hoff, D.; Hart, K.; Mayer, C.; Tarabochia, M.; et al. Neuroimaging, Behavioral, and Psychological Sequelae of Repetitive Combined Blast/Impact Mild Traumatic Brain Injury in Iraq and Afghanistan War Veterans. *J. Neurotrauma.* **2014**, *31*, 425–436. [CrossRef]
17. Khodanovich, M.Y.; Sorokina, I.V.; Glazacheva, V.Y.; Akulov, A.E.; Nemirovich-Danchenko, N.M.; Romashchenko, A.V.; Tolstikova, T.G.; Mustafina, L.R.; Yarnykh, V.L. Histological validation of fast macromolecular proton fraction mapping as a quantitative myelin imaging method in the cuprizone demyelination model. *Sci. Rep.* **2017**, *7*, 46686. [CrossRef]
18. Khodanovich, M.Y.; Kisel, A.A.; Akulov, A.E.; Atochin, D.N.; Kudabaeva, M.S.; Glazacheva, V.Y.; Svetlik, M.V.; Medvednikova, Y.A.; Mustafina, L.R.; Yarnykh, V.L. Quantitative assessment of demyelination in ischemic stroke in vivo using macromolecular proton fraction mapping. *J. Cereb. Blood Flow Metab.* **2018**, *38*, 919–931. [CrossRef]

19. Yarnykh, V.L.; Prihod'ko, I.Y.; Savelov, A.A.; Korostyshevskaya, A.M. Quantitative Assessment of Normal Fetal Brain Myelination Using Fast Macromolecular Proton Fraction Mapping. *Am. J. Neuroradiol.* **2018**, *39*, 341–1348. [CrossRef]
20. Korostyshevskaya, A.M.; Prihod'ko, I.Y.; Savelov, A.A.; Yarnykh, V.L. Direct comparison between apparent diffusion coefficient and macromolecular proton fraction as quantitative biomarkers of the human fetal brain maturation. *J. Magn. Reson. Imag.* **2019**, *50*, 52–61. [CrossRef]
21. Underhill, H.R.; Rostomily, R.C.; Mikheev, A.M.; Yuan, C.; Yarnykh, V.L. Fast bound pool fraction imaging of the in vivo rat brain: Association with myelin content and validation in the C6 glioma model. *Neuroimage* **2011**, *54*, 2052–2065. [CrossRef] [PubMed]
22. Matsushima, G.K.; Morell, P. The neurotoxicant, cuprizone, as a model to study demyelination and remyelination in the central nervous system. *Brain Pathol.* **2001**, *11*, 107–116. [CrossRef] [PubMed]
23. Kipp, M.; Clarner, T.; Dang, J.; Copray, S.; Beyer, C. The cuprizone animal model: new insights into an old story. *Acta Neuropathol.* **2009**, *118*, 723–736. [CrossRef] [PubMed]
24. Skripuletz, T.; Gudi, V.; Hackstette, D.; Stangel, M. De- and remyelination in the CNS white and grey matter induced by cuprizone: The old, the new, and the unexpected. *Histol. Histopathol.* **2011**, *26*, 1585–1597. [CrossRef]
25. Kipp, M.; Nyamoya, S.; Hochstrasser, T.; Amor, S. Multiple sclerosis animal models: a clinical and histopathological perspective. *Brain Pathol.* **2017**, *27*, 123–137. [CrossRef]
26. Gudi, V.; Gingele, S.; Skripuletz, T.; Stangel, M. Glial response during cuprizone-induced de-and remyelination in the CNS: lessons learned. *Front. Cell Neurosci.* **2014**, *8*, 73. [CrossRef]
27. Yarnykh, V.L. Optimal radiofrequency and gradient spoiling for improved accuracy of T1 and B1 measurements using fast steady-state techniques. *Magn. Reson. Med.* **2010**, *63*, 1610–1626. [CrossRef]
28. Paxinos, G.; Franklin, K. *The Mouse Brain in Stereotaxic Coordinates*, 2nd ed.; Academic Press: London, UK, 2001.
29. Otsu, N. A Threshold Selection Method from Gray-Level Histograms. *IEEE Trans. Syst. Man. Cybern.* **1979**, *9*, 62–66. [CrossRef]
30. Otsu Thresholding. Available online: https://imagej.nih.gov/ij/plugins/otsu-thresholding.html (accessed on 10 August 2019).
31. Ercan, E.; Han, J.M.; Di Nardo, A.; Winden, K.; Han, M.J.; Hoyo, L.; Saffari, A.; Leask, A.; Geschwind, D.H.; Sahin, M. Neuronal CTGF/CCN2 negatively regulates myelination in a mouse model of tuberous sclerosis complex. *J. Exp. Med.* **2017**, *214*, 681–697. [CrossRef]
32. Sullivan, G.M.; Feinn, R. Using Effect Size–or Why the P Value Is Not Enough. *J. Grad. Med. Educ.* **2012**, *4*, 279–282. [CrossRef]
33. Song, S.K.; Yoshino, J.; Le, T.Q.; Lin, S.J.; Sun, S.W.; Cross, A.H.; Armstrong, R.C. Demyelination increases radial diffusivity in corpus callosum of mouse brain. *Neuroimage* **2005**, *26*, 132–140. [CrossRef] [PubMed]
34. Merkler, D.; Boretius, S.; Stadelmann, C.; Ernsting, T.; Michaelis, T.; Frahm, J.; Brück, W. Multicontrast MRI of remyelination in the central nervous system. *NMR Biomed.* **2005**, *18*, 395–403. [CrossRef] [PubMed]
35. Zaaraoui, W.; Deloire, M.; Merle, M.; Girard, C.; Raffard, G.; Biran, M.; Inglese, M.; Petry, K.G.; Gonen, O.; Brochet, B.; et al. Monitoring demyelination and remyelination by magnetization transfer imaging in the mouse brain at 9.4 T. *MAGMA* **2008**, *21*, 357–362. [CrossRef] [PubMed]
36. Harsan, L.A.; Steibel, J.; Zaremba, A.; Agin, A.; Sapin, R.; Poulet, P.; Guignard, B.; Parizel, N.; Grucker, D.; Boehm, N.; et al. Recovery from chronic demyelination by thyroid hormone therapy: myelinogenesis induction and assessment by diffusion tensor magnetic resonance imaging. *J. Neurosci.* **2008**, *28*, 14189–14201. [CrossRef] [PubMed]
37. Turati, L.; Moscatelli, M.; Mastropietro, A.; Dowell, N.G.; Zucca, I.; Erbetta, A.; Cordiglieri, C.; Brenna, G.; Bianchi, B.; Mantegazza, R.; et al. In vivo quantitative magnetization transfer imaging correlates with histology during de- and remyelination in cuprizone-treated mice. *NMR Biomed.* **2015**, *28*, 327–337. [CrossRef] [PubMed]
38. Jelescu, I.O.; Zurek, M.; Winters, K.V.; Veraart, J.; Rajaratnam, A.; Kim, N.S.; Babb, J.S.; Shepherd, T.M.; Novikov, D.S.; Kim, S.G.; et al. In vivo quantification of demyelination and recovery using compartment-specific diffusion MRI metrics validated by electron microscopy. *Neuroimage* **2016**, *132*, 104–114. [CrossRef]

39. Tagge, I.; O'Connor, A.; Chaudhary, P.; Pollaro, J.; Berlow, Y.; Chalupsky, M.; Bourdette, D.; Woltjer, R.; Johnson, M.; Rooney, W. Spatio-Temporal Patterns of Demyelination and Remyelination in the Cuprizone Mouse Model. *PLoS ONE* **2016**, *11*, e0152480. [CrossRef]
40. Yano, R.; Hata, J.; Abe, Y.; Seki, F.; Yoshida, K.; Komaki, Y.; Okano, H.; Tanaka, K.F. Quantitative temporal changes in DTI values coupled with histological properties in cuprizone-induced demyelination and remyelination. *Neurochem. Int.* **2018**, *119*, 151–158. [CrossRef]
41. Fjær, S.; Bø, L.; Lundervold, A.; Myhr, K.M.; Pavlin, T.; Torkildsen, O.; Wergeland, S. Deep gray matter demyelination detected by magnetization transfer ratio in the cuprizone model. *PLoS ONE* **2013**, *8*, e84162. [CrossRef]
42. Guglielmetti, C.; Veraart, J.; Roelant, E.; Mai, Z.; Daans, J.; Van Audekerke, J.; Naeyaert, M.; Vanhoutte, G.; Delgado Y Palacios, R.; Praet, J.; et al. Diffusion kurtosis imaging probes cortical alterations and white matter pathology following cuprizone induced demyelination and spontaneous remyelination. *Neuroimage* **2016**, *125*, 363–377. [CrossRef]
43. Petiet, A.; Aigrot, M.S.; Stankoff, B. Gray and White Matter Demyelination and Remyelination Detected with Multimodal Quantitative MRI Analysis at 11.7T in a Chronic Mouse Model of Multiple Sclerosis. *Front. Neurosci.* **2016**, *10*, 491. [CrossRef] [PubMed]
44. Mason, J.L.; Jones, J.J.; Taniike, M.; Morell, P.; Suzuki, K.; Matsushima, G.K. Mature oligodendrocyte apoptosis precedes IGF-1 production and oligodendrocyte progenitor accumulation and differentiation during demyelination/remyelination. *J. Neurosci Res.* **2000**, *61*, 251–262. [CrossRef]
45. Baxi, E.G.; DeBruin, J.; Jin, J.; Strasburger, H.J.; Smith, M.D.; Orthmann-Murphy, J.L.; Schott, J.T.; Fairchild, A.N.; Bergles, D.E.; Calabresi, P.A. Lineage tracing reveals dynamic changes in oligodendrocyte precursor cells following cuprizone-induced demyelination. *Glia* **2017**, *65*, 2087–2098. [CrossRef] [PubMed]
46. Skripuletz, T.; Lindner, M.; Kotsiari, A.; Garde, N.; Fokuhl, J.; Linsmeier, F.; Trebst, C.; Stangel, M. Cortical Demyelination Is Prominent in the Murine Cuprizone Model and Is Strain-Dependent. *Am. J. Pathol.* **2008**, *172*, 1053–1061. [CrossRef] [PubMed]
47. Gudi, V.; Moharregh-Khiabani, D.; Skripuletz, T.; Koutsoudaki, P.N.; Kotsiari, A.; Skuljec, J.; Trebst, C.; Stangel, M. Regional differences between grey and white matter in cuprizone induced demyelination. *Brain Res.* **2009**, *1283*, 127–138. [CrossRef] [PubMed]
48. Yang, H.J.; Wang, H.; Zhang, Y.; Xiao, L.; Clough, R.W.; Browning, R.; Li, X.M.; Xu, H. Region-specific susceptibilities to cuprizone-induced lesions in the mouse forebrain: Implications for the pathophysiology of schizophrenia. *Brain Res.* **2009**, *1270*, 121–130. [CrossRef] [PubMed]
49. Pott, F.; Gingele, S.; Clarner, T.; Dang, J.; Baumgartner, W.; Beyer, C.; Kipp, M. Cuprizone effect on myelination, astrogliosis and microglia attraction in the mouse basal ganglia. *Brain Res.* **2009**, *1305*, 137–149. [CrossRef]
50. Norkute, A.; Hieble, A.; Braun, A.; Johann, S.; Clarner, T.; Baumgartner, W.; Beyer, C.; Kipp, M. Cuprizone treatment induces demyelination and astrocytosis in the mouse hippocampus. *J. Neurosci. Res.* **2009**, *87*, 1343–1355. [CrossRef]
51. Koutsoudaki, P.N.; Skripuletz, T.; Gudi, V.; Moharregh-Khiabani, D.; Hildebrandt, H.; Trebst, C.; Stangel, M. Demyelination of the hippocampus is prominent in the cuprizone model. *Neurosci. Lett.* **2009**, *451*, 83–88. [CrossRef]
52. Chang, A.; Staugaitis, S.M.; Dutta, R.; Batt, C.E.; Easley, K.E.; Chomyk, A.M.; Yong, V.W.; Fox, R.J.; Kidd, G.J.; Trapp, B.D. Cortical remyelination: a new target for repair therapies in multiple sclerosis. *Ann. Neurol.* **2012**, *72*, 918–926. [CrossRef]
53. Albert, M.; Antel, J.; Brück, W.; Stadelmann, C. Extensive cortical remyelination in patients with chronic multiple sclerosis. *Brain Pathol.* **2007**, *17*, 129–138. [CrossRef] [PubMed]
54. Mason, J.L.; Toews, A.; Hostettler, J.D.; Morell, P.; Suzuki, K.; Goldman, J.E.; Matsushima, G.K. Oligodendrocytes and progenitors become progressively depleted within chronically demyelinated lesions. *Am. J. Pathol.* **2004**, *164*, 1673–1682. [CrossRef]
55. Lassmann, H.; Bradl, M. Multiple sclerosis: experimental models and reality. *Acta Neuropathol.* **2017**, *133*, 223–244. [CrossRef] [PubMed]
56. Hartley, M.D.; Banerji, T.; Tagge, I.J.; Kirkemo, L.L.; Chaudhary, P.; Calkins, E.; Scanlan, T.S. Myelin repair stimulated by CNS-selective thyroid hormone action. *JCI Insight* **2019**, *4*, 126329. [CrossRef] [PubMed]

57. Field, A.S.; Samsonov, A.; Alexander, A.L.; Mossahebi, P.; Duncan, I.D. Conventional and quantitative MRI in a novel feline model of demyelination and endogenous remyelination. *J. Magn. Reson. Imag.* **2019**, *49*, 1304–1311. [CrossRef]
58. Nathoo, N.; Yong, V.W.; Dunn, J.F. Understanding disease processes in multiple sclerosis through magnetic resonance imaging studies in animal models. *Neuroimage Clin.* **2014**, *4*, 743–756. [CrossRef]
59. Berghoff, S.A.; Düking, T.; Spieth, L.; Winchenbach, J.; Stumpf, S.K.; Gerndt, N.; Kusch, K.; Ruhwedel, T.; Möbius, W.; Saher, G. Blood-brain barrier hyperpermeability precedes demyelination in the cuprizone model. *Acta Neuropathol. Commun.* **2017**, *5*, 94. [CrossRef]
60. Mossahebi, P.; Yarnykh, V.L.; Samsonov, A. Analysis and correction of biases in cross-relaxation MRI due to biexponential longitudinal relaxation. *Magn. Reson. Med.* **2014**, *71*, 830–838. [CrossRef]
61. Mossahebi, P.; Alexander, A.L.; Field, A.S.; Samsonov, A.A. Removal of cerebrospinal fluid partial volume effects in quantitative magnetization transfer imaging using a three-pool model with nonexchanging water component. *Magn. Reson. Med.* **2015**, *74*, 1317–1326. [CrossRef]
62. Korostyshevskaya, A.M.; Savelov, A.A.; Papusha, L.I.; Druy, A.E.; Yarnykh, V.L. Congenital medulloblastoma: Fetal and postnatal longitudinal observation with quantitative MRI. *Clin. Imag.* **2018**, *52*, 172–176. [CrossRef]
63. Naumova, A.V.; Akulov, A.E.; Khodanovich, M.Y.; Yarnykh, V.L. High-resolution three-dimensional macromolecular proton fraction mapping for quantitative neuroanatomical imaging of the rodent brain in ultra-high magnetic fields. *Neuroimage* **2017**, *147*, 985–993. [CrossRef] [PubMed]
64. Haider, L.; Simeonidou, C.; Steinberger, G.; Hametner, S.; Grigoriadis, N.; Deretzi, G.; Kovacs, G.G.; Kutzelnigg, A.; Lassmann, H.; Frischer, J.M. Multiple sclerosis deep grey matter: the relation between demyelination, neurodegeneration, inflammation and iron. *J. Neurol. Neurosurg. Psychiatry* **2014**, *85*, 1386–1395. [CrossRef] [PubMed]
65. Stephenson, E.; Nathoo, N.; Mahjoub, Y.; Dunn, J.F.; Yong, V.W. Iron in multiple sclerosis: Roles in neurodegeneration and repair. *Nat. Rev. Neurol* **2014**, *10*, 459–468. [CrossRef] [PubMed]
66. Varga, E.; Pandur, E.; Abrahám, H.; Horváth, A.; Ács, P.; Komoly, S.; Miseta, A.; Sipos, K. Cuprizone Administration Alters the Iron Metabolism in the Mouse Model of Multiple Sclerosis. *Cell Mol. Neurobiol.* **2018**, *38*, 1081–1097. [CrossRef] [PubMed]
67. Pandur, E.; Pap, R.; Varga, E.; Jánosa, G.; Komoly, S.; Fórizs, J.; Sipos, K. Relationship of Iron Metabolism and Short-Term Cuprizone Treatment of C57BL/6 Mice. *Int. J. Mol. Sci.* **2019**, *20*, 2257. [CrossRef] [PubMed]
68. Lee, N.J.; Ha, S.-K.; Sati, P.; Absinta, M.; Nair, G.; Luciano, N.J.; Leibovitch, E.C.; Yen, C.C.; Rouault, T.A.; Silva, A.C.; et al. Potential role of iron in repair of inflammatory demyelinating lesions. *J. Clin. Invest.* **2019**. [CrossRef]
69. Nathoo, N.; Agrawal, S.; Wu, Y.; Haylock-Jacobs, S.; Yong, V.W.; Foniok, T.; Barnes, S.; Obenaus, A.; Dunn, J.F. Susceptibility-weighted imaging in the experimental autoimmune encephalomyelitis model of multiple sclerosis indicates elevated deoxyhemoglobin, iron deposition and demyelination. *Mult. Scler.* **2013**, *19*, 721–731. [CrossRef] [PubMed]
70. MacKay, A.; Whittall, K.; Adler, J.; Li, D.; Paty, D.; Graeb, D. In vivo visualization of myelin water in brain by magnetic resonance. *Magn. Reson. Med.* **1994**, *31*, 673–677. [CrossRef]
71. Deoni, S.C.; Rutt, B.K.; Arun, T.; Pierpaoli, C.; Jones, D.K. Gleaning multicomponent T1 and T2 information from steady-state imaging data. *Magn. Reson. Med.* **2008**, *60*, 1372–1387. [CrossRef]
72. Hwang, D.; Kim, D.-H.; Du, Y.P. In vivo multi-slice mapping of myelin water content using T2* decay. *Neuroimage* **2010**, *52*, 198–204. [CrossRef]

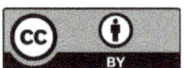 © 2019 by the authors. Licensee MDPI, Basel, Switzerland. This article is an open access article distributed under the terms and conditions of the Creative Commons Attribution (CC BY) license (http://creativecommons.org/licenses/by/4.0/).

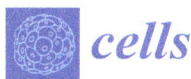

Review

From OPC to Oligodendrocyte: An Epigenetic Journey

Assia Tiane [1,3], Melissa Schepers [1,3], Ben Rombaut [1,3], Raymond Hupperts [2,3], Jos Prickaerts [3], Niels Hellings [1], Daniel van den Hove [3,4] and Tim Vanmierlo [1,3,*]

1. Department of Immunology, Biomedical Research Institute, Hasselt University, Hasselt 3500, Belgium; assia.tiane@uhasselt.be (A.T.); melissa.schepers@uhasselt.be (M.S.); ben.rombaut@uhasselt.be (B.R.); niels.hellings@uhasselt.be (N.H.)
2. Department of Neurology, Zuyderland Medical Center, Sittard-Geleen 6130 MB, The Netherlands; r.hupperts@zuyderland.nl
3. Department Psychiatry and Neuropsychology, European Graduate School of Neuroscience, School for Mental Health and Neuroscience, Maastricht University, Maastricht 6200 MD, The Netherlands; jos.prickaerts@maastrichtuniversity.nl (J.P.); d.vandenhove@maastrichtuniversity.nl (D.v.d.H.)
4. Department of Psychiatry, Psychosomatics and Psychotherapy, University of Wuerzburg, Wuerzburg 97080, Germany
* Correspondence: tim.vanmierlo@uhasselt.be

Received: 20 September 2019; Accepted: 10 October 2019; Published: 11 October 2019

Abstract: Oligodendrocytes provide metabolic and functional support to neuronal cells, rendering them key players in the functioning of the central nervous system. Oligodendrocytes need to be newly formed from a pool of oligodendrocyte precursor cells (OPCs). The differentiation of OPCs into mature and myelinating cells is a multistep process, tightly controlled by spatiotemporal activation and repression of specific growth and transcription factors. While oligodendrocyte turnover is rather slow under physiological conditions, a disruption in this balanced differentiation process, for example in case of a differentiation block, could have devastating consequences during ageing and in pathological conditions, such as multiple sclerosis. Over the recent years, increasing evidence has shown that epigenetic mechanisms, such as DNA methylation, histone modifications, and microRNAs, are major contributors to OPC differentiation. In this review, we discuss how these epigenetic mechanisms orchestrate and influence oligodendrocyte maturation. These insights are a crucial starting point for studies that aim to identify the contribution of epigenetics in demyelinating diseases and may thus provide new therapeutic targets to induce myelin repair in the long run.

Keywords: oligodendrocyte; epigenetics; myelination

---

1. Introduction

Oligodendrocytes (OLs) are myelinating glial cells within the central nervous system (CNS) that insulate neuronal axons to provide them with trophic, metabolic and functional support. OLs are generated from oligodendrocyte precursor cells (OPCs) via a consecutive process of cell cycle exit, maturation, and differentiation [1]. OPCs arise during early development, persist throughout a lifetime and occupy around 5%–10% of the total number of cells in the brain [2,3]. In response to both intrinsic molecular cues and extracellular signals, OPCs are able to withdraw from their proliferative stage and differentiate into myelin-producing OLs [4]. Consequently, alterations in these extrinsic stimuli, such as an increase in inhibitory ECM molecules (LINGO, glycosaminoglycans, fibronectin) or secreted factors (BMP, FGF), hamper differentiation, possibly via an upstream effect on transcriptional and epigenetic processes that regulate OL differentiation [5]. Indeed, current evidence indicates that epigenetic mechanisms, comprising DNA methylation, histone modifications and microRNAs (miRNAs), play an essential role in the regulation of OL lineage development. As such, epigenetic signatures translate extracellular signals into functional cellular changes and coordinate the transcriptional machinery that is responsible for the differentiation process [6,7]. This review provides an overview of the current understanding of the physiological process of OL lineage development and how the different epigenetic mechanisms are involved in the regulation of this process (Figure 1). Furthermore, we discuss how this epigenetic fingerprinting is altered during ageing and in neurological conditions.

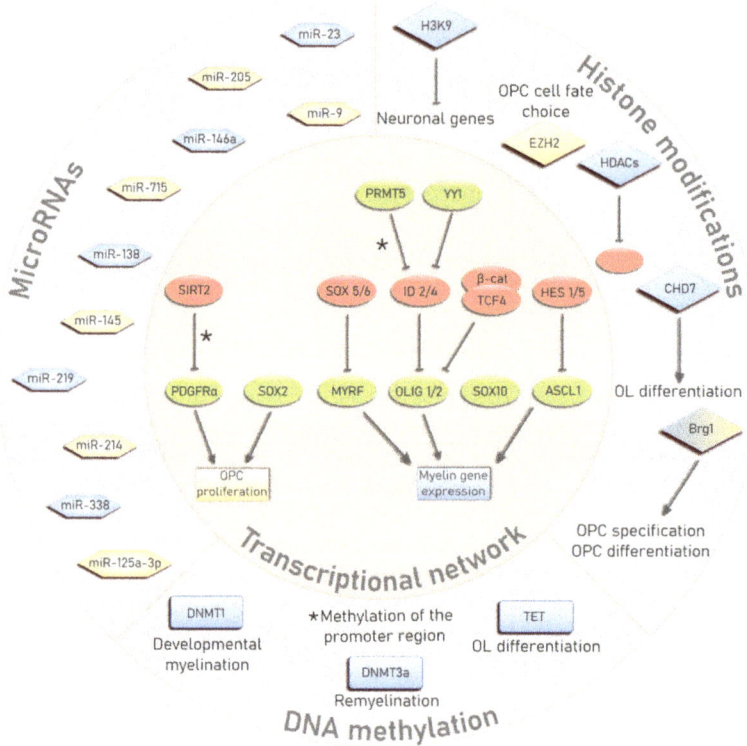

Figure 1. An overview of the transcriptional and epigenetic regulation of oligodendrocyte precursor cell (OPC) proliferation and oligodendrocyte (OL) development. Transcription factors that exert a positive or negative effect on these processes are depicted in green and red, respectively. Pro-proliferative factors are visualized in yellow, whereas pro-differentiation factors are blue. * Methylation of the promoter region.

2. OL Differentiation and the Transcriptional Network

OPCs arise from the ventricular zone during early development, proliferate and migrate their way into the different developing areas of the brain, where they differentiate into myelin-forming OLs [8]. Unlike most progenitor cells, OPCs persist throughout life as adult, self-renewing OPCs that can differentiate into newly formed myelinating OLs to maintain myelin plasticity or in response to damaging signals [9]. The differentiation of OPC into mature and myelin-producing OLs is a gradual and well-defined process that can be divided into four successive stages: proliferative OPCs, pre-OLs, differentiated OLs and myelinating OLs [10]. This process of OL differentiation, both during early development and in adult stages, is controlled by the combination of OL-specific transcription factors, extracellular signals, epigenetic modifications and signaling pathways. It is necessary to maintain a homeostatic balance between these molecular cues to allow for proper differentiation.

The regulatory network of transcription factors that controls OL lineage development has been extensively studied over the past decades [9,11,12]. These transcription factors regulate OPC proliferation, migration and differentiation and at the same time serve as stage-specific cell identity markers of the OL lineage [11]. In general, a distinction can be made between positive regulators, which boost and stimulate OL differentiation, and negative regulators, which function as inhibitory transcription factors for myelin genes and keep OPCs in a proliferative and non-differentiated state.

The main transcription factors that regulate OL lineage progression belong to the helix-loop-helix (HLH) family, such as the oligodendrocyte transcription factors (OLIG), hairy and enhancer-of-split homologs (HES) and inhibitor or differentiation (ID) proteins. OLIG2 is considered as one of the major and indispensable transcription factors during different stages of OL development. It is an essential factor during OPC specification, enhances OPC migration during early development, but also functions as a promoting factor of OL differentiation and regeneration in the adult life [13–15]. In contrast to OLIG2, the closely related OLIG1 is not directly involved during early brain development, but rather promotes OL differentiation and myelination after injury [16,17]. The achaete-scute homolog 1 (ASCL1 or MASH1) is another member of the HLH family that promotes early OPC specification and OL development [18]. Although it was considered to be mainly involved in early oligodendrogenesis, ASCL1 is also shown to be important during adult OL regeneration and remyelination [19]. In contrast, HES proteins, such as HES1 and HES5, function as differentiation inhibitors either by recruiting other repressor proteins to myelin gene promoters, or by inhibiting ASCL1 [12]. Similarly, the ID HLH transcription factors ID2 and ID4 inhibit OPC differentiation by binding to other members of the HLH family (OLIG1/2, ASCL1) and preventing their translocation from the cytoplasm to the nucleus [20,21].

Another family of transcriptional regulators are HMG-domain transcription factors, that are classified as the sex determining region Y-box (SOX) family, of which SOX10 is a well-established regulator involved in terminal OL differentiation and myelination, through its direct binding to the promoter region of myelin genes to enhance their [22,23]. Interestingly, SOX10 is expressed in all stages of the OL lineage and can thus serve as a general marker for OPCs/OLs [24]. In contrast, SOX5 and SOX6 inhibit OL differentiation by competing with SOX10 binding sites, thereby antagonizing its function [25]. SOX2 on the other hand, maintains OPCs in a proliferative and undifferentiated stage, but is indispensable for OPC expansion and OL regeneration during CNS remyelination [26,27]. Transcription factor 4 (TCF4, also known as TCFL2) is another important HMG-domain transcription factor and is a downstream effector of the Wnt signaling pathway. Through its binding to β-catenin, TCF4 acts as an inhibitor of myelin gene expression and impairs (re)myelination [28].

An additional class of OL-related transcription factors are zinc finger proteins (ZFP). Yin Yang 1 (YY1) stimulates OL differentiation by silencing inhibitor proteins, such as ID4 and TCF4 [29]. Other ZFPs that enhance OL maturation and differentiation are ZFP191, ZFP488 and the Smad interacting protein 1 (SIP1) [30–33]. Myelin regulatory factor (MYRF) was only recently discovered as a crucial regulator of CNS myelination [34]. MYRF is exclusively expressed in post-mitotic cells of the OL lineage, which signifies its essential role during terminal differentiation. The synergistic effect of MYRF and SOX10 leads to myelin gene activation and drives CNS myelination [23,34].

All the transcriptional regulators influence OL differentiation mainly by controlling the expression of genes that encode for the essential myelin-associated proteins, such as the myelin basic protein (MBP), proteolipid protein (PLP) and myelin-associated glycoprotein (MAG) [35,36]. The transcription factors either enhance or inhibit the expression of these myelin genes by directly binding to their promoter region, which eventually results in a spatiotemporal expression of myelin genes during the process of OL lineage development [37].

3. The Epigenetic Triumvirate in OL Development

OL lineage development and the regulation of the associated transcriptional program is highly influenced by various epigenetic processes. Epigenetic mechanisms are defined as modifications that affect gene expression without altering the DNA sequence itself and are heritable from mother to daughter cell [38,39]. Epigenetic control of gene expression is sustained via DNA methylation, modifications at histone tails of chromatin, and miRNAs. The interplay between these different modifications changes the physiological form of the DNA, thereby influencing the accessibility of specific transcription factors to their target regions in the genome [39,40]. In the following part of this review, we discuss how the different levels of epigenetic regulation influence OL differentiation and CNS myelination.

3.1. DNA Methylation

DNA methylation, in particular CG methylation, is one of the most studied and long-lasting epigenetic modifications. CG methylation involves the addition of a methyl-group (–CH3) to a cytosine base followed by a guanine nucleotide, referred to as 5'cytosine–guanine–3' dinucleotide (CpG) site. Although various definitions exist, so-called 'CpG islands' cover regions of more than 300 bp with a C/G-content of 50% at minimum and are mostly found within the promoters of protein coding genes [41]. Methylation of these CpG islands is generally associated with gene silencing due to the inability of transcription factors to bind to the methylated promoter region or via an additional recruitment of other repressor proteins [42,43]. DNA methylation is established by DNA methyltransferases (DNMTs) that add a methyl-group to cytosine (5mC). There are two distinct forms of DNMTs, DNMT1 and DNMT3a/b, which either maintain DNA methylation during replication or induce de novo methylation, respectively [44,45]. Contrarily, DNA methylation can be removed via gradual degradation of 5mC by the ten-eleven translocation (TET) enzymes [46,47], although DNMTs may serve the same purpose under certain conditions [48,49]. Hydroxylation of 5mC into hydroxy-methylated cytosine (5hmC) is the first step of the demethylation process. Interestingly, 5hmC patterns have shown to be abundantly present in the CNS of mammals [47,50]. 5hmC was first identified as an intermediate epigenetic mark during active DNA demethylation but has also been shown to represent a potentially independent and functionally distinct epigenetic marker in the brain [51,52].

One of the first studies that linked DNA methylation to OL development showed that neonatal rats treated with the DNMT-inhibitor 5-azacytidine (5-aza), displayed disrupted gliogenesis, concomitant with hypomyelination of the 11-day-old optic nerve. Postnatal inhibition of DNA methylation resulted in a reduced number of oligodendrocytes, whilst the number of astrocytes was less affected, indicating a higher vulnerability of OPCs to changes in DNA methylation [53]. Likewise, ablation of the *Dnmt1* gene in embryonic progenitor cells led to OPC growth arrest and resulted in severe hypomyelination. Moreover, this loss of *Dnmt1* seemed to alter splicing events, such as exon skipping and intron retention, in genes related to myelination, lipid metabolism and the cell cycle, indicating a crucial role of DNA methylation in relation to alternative splicing during neonatal OL development [54]. Although DNMT1 seemed to be an important regulator during developmental myelination, it seems to play a less prominent role during remyelination of the adult CNS [55]. After lysolecithin-induced demyelination of adult murine spinal cord white matter, higher levels of DNA methylation in differentiating OLs are accompanied by an increased expression of DNMT3a. Transgenic mice that lack *Dnmt3a* showed impaired OL differentiation and a reduced ability to remyelinate affected axons after injury [55]. Together, these studies suggest that maintenance of DNA methylation is important to ensure proper gliogenesis during developmental myelination, whilst de novo methylation is needed for the differentiation of adult OPCs into remyelinating OLs. On the opposite side of the methylation spectrum, TET enzymes also strongly influence OL differentiation [56]. Even though the three TET enzymes show different subcellular localization and unique expression patterns, they all seem to be equally important during OL development. Interestingly, knock-down of the *Tet* mRNA levels was associated with increased expression of HLH inhibitory transcription factors, such as ID2 and HES5, leading to suppression of myelin gene expression [56]. It however remains unclear whether TET enzymes directly inhibit the expression of these genes or whether the observed transcriptional change is mediated in an indirect manner. In general, epigenome-wide studies of stage-specific cells are still needed to unravel how and which exact CpG sites or islands change in their methylation status during OL lineage progression.

In relation to the transcriptional regulatory network of OL development, it has been shown that DNA methylation can regulate the temporal expression of these transcription factors. In a study of Huang et al., PRMT5 was identified as a pro-differentiation factor that binds to CpG-rich islands within the ID2 and ID4 genes. Subsequent DNA methylation of these regions led to silencing of the transcriptional inhibitors and resulted in OL differentiation [57]. In a similar fashion, SIRT2 was shown to translocate to the nucleus, inducing DNA methylation in the platelet-derived growth factor receptor α (PDGFRα) promoter region and initiating glial differentiation [58]. Interestingly, both PRMT5 and SIRT2 are classified as histone-modification enzymes, yet they are also known to induce epigenetic changes at the level of DNA methylation, thereby emphasizing the intricate relationship between different epigenetic mechanisms.

3.2. Histone Modifications

Histone modifications encompass a wide range of post-translational changes on histone tails, such as histone (de)acetylation, methylation, ubiquitination, and phosphorylation. These modifications can act separately or together to orchestrate chromatin dynamics and structure. Depending on the obtained histone code, DNA accessibility for polymerases and transcription factors can be either promoted or hampered [59].

The most prevalent type of histone modifications is (de)acetylation of the lysine (K) residues. Acetylation is established by histone acetyltransferases (HATs), whilst removal of the acetyl groups is maintained by histone deacetylases (HDACs). Histone acetylation neutralizes the positive charge of the lysine residues, resulting in a weaker interaction between the histone proteins and the DNA, eventually leading to an 'open' chromatin structure. Consequently, HDACs function to make the chromatin more compact, thereby preventing transcriptional processes from occurring [59,60]. Whereas not that many studies have directly assessed the role of HATs in OL development, HDACs have been shown to be heavily involved in different aspects of this process. In general, pharmacological inhibition of HDACs is associated with a decrease in OL maturation and differentiation, suggesting a crucial role of HDACs during OL development [61–64]. Treatment of OL in vitro cultures with the HDAC inhibitor trichostatin A (TSA), prevented the suppression of inhibitory transcription factors, such as ID2 and SOX11, in rats [63], and ID4, SOX2, and TCF4 in humans [64]. These data indicate that HDAC-mediated repression of genes that keep OPCs in a proliferative and undifferentiated state is necessary for the early onset of OL lineage progression. Indeed, it has been shown that HDAC functionality is restricted to a specific temporal window, as HDAC inhibitors seem to only suppress myelination during the early phase of OPC differentiation, but not after onset of myelination [62]. These observations are in line with recent findings, which show that HDACs are predominantly expressed in early OPC stages, compared to other stages of OL differentiation [65].

Interestingly, HDACs can also regulate and promote OL development in a (partly) histone-independent manner, as interaction of HDACs with other transcriptional regulators can result in repressive complexes that counteract the expression of OPC differentiation inhibitors. For instance, studies conducted on murine OPCs have shown that the pro-differentiation factor YY1 is recruited via HDAC1 to the promoter region of *Id2*, *Id4* and *Hes5*, where it can block the expression of these genes [66]. Protein deacetylation of OLIG1 by HDACs prevents its physical interaction with the inhibitory ID2 protein, stimulates its nuclear transportation and promotes OPC differentiation [67]. Furthermore, HDAC1/2 interact with TCF4 and antagonize its binding to β-catenin, thereby preventing its downstream function as an inhibitor of myelin gene expression [28].

Another type of histone modification that has been associated with OL development is histone methylation. Histone methylation can occur either on lysine or arginine side chains and is associated with both activation and repression of transcription, depending on the site of methylation [60]. During OL differentiation, the activity of the Histone H3 Lysine 9 (H3K9) methylation enzyme increases. This is accompanied by an increase of the associated repressive H3K9me3 mark at genes that regulate neuronal lineage development [68]. Furthermore, the catalytic subunit (EZH2) of the polycomb repressive complex (PRC) that is responsible for trimethylation of histone 3 (H3K27me3), promotes OPC cell fate choice from progenitor cells and stimulates OPC proliferation [69,70]. A decrease in histone H4R5 methylation via pharmacological inhibition or genetic ablation of PRMT5 results in poor OL differentiation and hypomyelination [71]. Likewise, deletion of PRMT1 leads to severe hypomyelination due to impaired OL maturation and disturbed myelin gene expression in OLIG2-positive cells [72].

Next to the abovementioned histone-modifying enzymes, ATP-dependent chromatin remodeling complexes have also been recently shown to influence and orchestrate OPC differentiation. These complexes make use of ATP as an energy source to reposition nucleosomes, thereby altering histone accessibility and gene transcription [73]. The helicase component of the SWI/SNF-related chromatin remodeling complex brahma-related 1 (Brg1, also known as Smarca4) is highly expressed in OPCs and is an essential factor during OPC specification and at the onset of OL differentiation. BRG1 interacts with the *Olig2* promoter in order to regulate its expression during early development [74]. As a positive feedback loop, BRG1 is consequently recruited by OLIG2 to enhance the expression of OL-associated genes [75]. One of these targets of BRG1 and OLIG2 is *Cdh7*, an ATP-dependent chromatin remodeler of the chromodomain helicase DNA-binding (CHD) family. CHD7 is highly expressed in differentiating OLs, and functions synergistically with SOX10 to enhance myelin-associated gene expression. Furthermore, CHD7 promotes the expression of other positive transcription factors during OL maturations, such as *Myrf* and *Olig1* [76]. Interestingly, deletion of either ATP-dependent remodeler (BRG1 or CHD7) resulted in a dysmyelinating phenotype in mice, suggesting that even though they have different targets and influence OL development at distinct stages, both BRG1 and CHD7 are indispensable factors during OL development and myelination [75,76].

3.3. MicroRNAs

Small non-coding RNAs (ncRNAs) are powerful endogenous regulators of gene expression. Many ncRNAs have been comprehensively described, such as Piwi-interacting RNAs (piRNAs), small interfering RNAs (siRNAs) and miRNAs, with these latter being the most widespread and abundant ncRNAs [77]. MiRNAs are small ncRNA molecules with an average length of 21–25 nucleotides and are most often transcribed from non-coding and coding protein introns [78]. By means of base-pair complementarity, a mature miRNA binds the seed-sequence at the 3′ untranslated region (3′UTR) of the target mRNA and subsequently negatively regulates its translation by repressing or degrading the mRNA [79–81]. Nevertheless, base-pair complementarity between miRNA and target RNA can sometimes be incomplete so that a single miRNA can target multiple 3′ UTR sequencing, leading to a cumulative reduction of gene expression that may orchestrate a common molecular pathway such as cell proliferation, development and differentiation [82].

During OL development, a coordinated interplay between multiple miRNAs determines OPC cell fate by downregulating intrinsic and extrinsic transcription factor expression [83,84]. The importance of miRNA-mediated gene repression in OPC differentiation is highlighted in animals lacking the DICER1 enzyme, which is an essential enzyme responsible for processing pre-microRNA (pre-miRNA) thereby forming mature miRNA. DICER1 mutant mice display a lack of mature miRNAs which is featured by a disrupted CNS myelination pattern due to the lack of differentiated OPCs [85,86]. MicroRNAome studies revealed a 10–100-fold induction of miR-219, miR-338 and miR-138 during OL differentiation [85,86]. Since direct targets of miR-219 include genes essential for maintaining OPC proliferation (e.g., *Sox6*, *Hes5* and *Pdgfra*), its increase stimulates OPCs to exit from the proliferative cycle and enter differentiation [85]. By suppressing *Hes5* and *Sox6*, miR-219 indirectly elevates the expression of monocarboxylate transporters, leading to increased OL numbers and enhanced protein levels of MBP and CNP, which subsequently attenuates cuprizone-induced demyelination [87]. MiR-219 is additionally important for metabolic regulation of lipid formation and maintenance during OL maturation, rendering miR-219 essential in both early and late stages of OL differentiation [86]. MiR-219 cooperates synergistically with miRNA-138, which is essential for reaching the immature phase of OL differentiation, to regulate CNS myelination. Boosting the expression of solely these two miRNAs is sufficient to induce OL differentiation in vitro [88,89]. Furthermore, differentiation of human endometrial-derived stromal cells towards OLs is stimulated when miR-338 is overexpressed, emphasizing the importance of this miRNA in the regulation of OPC differentiation [90,91].

In contrast to the induction of several miRNAs, miR-9 is downregulated during OL differentiation [92,93]. In line with this, depleting miR-9 in OPCs stimulates OL differentiation, presumably through an increase in peripheral myelin protein 22 (PMP22) and serum response factor (srf) transcripts [92,94]. During OL differentiation, a comparable expression pattern of the developmentally regulated miR-125a-3p is observed. Oligodendroglial differentiation and maturation is impaired upon miR-125a-3p overexpression, which can be attributed to a decreased expression of genes involved in the differentiation process (e.g., GTPase RhoA, Neuregulin and p38) [95–98]. On the contrary, antago-miR treatment that inhibits miR-125-3p expression and subsequently stimulates OL differentiation, indicates the importance of miR-125a-3p suppression during oligodendroglial maturation [95].

Many other miRNAs have been described to be either positively or negatively involved in OL differentiation processes. In vivo studies have shown an increased generation of myelin proteins upon miR-146a overexpression in primary OPCs following demyelinating injuries, thereby highlighting the positive relationship between miR-146a and OL differentiation [99,100]. Similarly, miR 23 promotes CNS myelination via the suppression of lamin B1, which is a negative regulator of OL differentiation [101]. On the other hand, many miRNAs inhibit OL differentiation and therefore need to be downregulated during the transition of OPCs to OLs. The translation of essential proteins of the CNS myelin, such as myelin-associated oligodendrocyte basic protein (MOBP), claudin11/O4 and MBP, is suppressed by miR-214 [102,103], miR-205 [102] and miR-715 [97], respectively. Moreover, miR-145 has been shown to pair to its seeding sequence located in the 3′UTR of the gene coding for Myrf and consequently inhibits OPC differentiation [103,104]. Therefore, downregulating miR-214, miR-205, miR-715 and miR-145 is sufficient for the differentiation of OPCs into mature OLs. In contrast to regulating OL differentiation, at least one miRNA cluster, miR-17-92, has been shown to be involved in OPC expansion by targeting, among others, PTEN, and therefore regulating OL numbers both in vitro and in vivo [89,105]. Taken together, miRNAs have been shown to be critically involved in different steps of the process of OL development. Data have demonstrated that miRNA expression is dynamically and precisely regulated to control cellular differentiation, which offers new avenues for further therapeutic target identification for myelin-related pathologies.

4. Implications in Ageing and CNS Myelin Disorders

Current knowledge about the strong involvement of epigenetic mechanisms in OL development has led to new perspectives on OL- and myelin-related pathologies. Over the past years, a considerable amount of research has been conducted with regard to aberrant epigenetic regulation and its impact on OL regeneration and myelin repair. Hence, in this part of the review, we focus on what is known about epigenetic malfunctioning during OL regeneration and remyelination, both in the context of ageing and myelin-related pathologies.

4.1. Ageing

It is generally known that regenerative processes become less efficient with increasing age. A classic example is age-related deficits in remyelination, a process which is entirely dependent on OL regeneration to restore the myelin sheath [106–108]. The age-associated decrease in remyelination efficiency is attributed to a reduced level of OPC recruitment. Moreover, recruited OPCs show an impaired ability to differentiate into remyelinating OLs [107]. The relationship between ageing and epigenetic alterations has already been proposed before [109–111] and provides an incentive to link age-associated remyelination failure to changes in the epigenome of aged OPCs or OLs.

Up to now, only one study has connected changes in methylation in OPCs/OLs to cellular ageing [112]. Rat OPCs from the spinal cord showed an age-dependent decrease in methylation levels. Interestingly, no changes regarding TET activity or expression were observed. The global hypomethylation in aged

OPCs rather correlated with a reduced expression and activity of DNMTs, and in particular DNMT1 [112]. Regarding histone modifications, mature OLs from the corpus callosum of older animals show increased levels of histone acetylation and a decreased rate of histone methylation, compared to younger mice. These histone changes were correlated with re-expression of inhibitory HLH-transcription factors, such as HES5 and ID4 [113]. As mentioned before, HDAC recruitment to these promoter regions is crucial for OPC differentiation and myelin formation. OPCs in demyelinated regions of older mice, however, fail in the recruitment of HDACs, resulting in the accumulation of transcriptional inhibitors and poor remyelination [114].

In a study conducted by Pusic et al., aged rats were exposed to a youthful environment in a Marlau-style enrichment cage to assess the effect on remyelination capacity [115,116]. Environmental enrichment promoted remyelination in aged rats, to a level comparable to younger animals. Interestingly, they found that serum-derived exosomes from both young and environmentally enriched stimulated rats displayed increased levels of miR-219, which is known to inhibit the expression of inhibitory myelin gene regulators and therefore promotes OL differentiation [115]. Exosomal delivery of such miRNAs could therefore be regarded as a potential therapeutic strategy to boost remyelination both in young and aged individuals.

4.2. Multiple Sclerosis

Multiple sclerosis (MS) is a multi-faceted immune-driven demyelinating disease of the CNS. MS is characterized by inflammation-induced demyelination during the early stages, which eventually results in gradual neurological disability as the disease progresses [117,118]. The concordance rate of identical twins to develop MS averages between 6%–30%, suggesting that the disease is only partially driven by genetic polymorphisms, but is largely attributed to environmental stimuli [119]. An increasing body of evidence suggests a role of epigenetically regulated mechanisms in the pathophysiology of MS. Numerous links have been made between environmental risk factors for MS and epigenetic changes [120–122]. Yet, most studies concerning epigenetics in MS are focused on the early, inflammatory stage of the disease [123–125]. Another important aspect of the disease is the subsequent endogenous repair process underlying remyelination of axons in order to cope with inflammatory damage. In the chronic stages of MS, however, these repair processes are hampered due to a differentiation block in OPCs [126,127]. New regenerative therapies, such as Opicinimab (anti-LINGO), are currently tested for their potential to boost remyelination in lesions that still contain undifferentiated OPCs [128]. Interestingly, even though the influence of epigenetics in progressive MS pathology is not clear yet, emerging data suggest an existing role in OL differentiation and maturation.

Analysis of MS postmortem samples revealed increased levels of MBP citrullination, a post-translational modification which renders the MBP protein less stable, leads to the degradation of myelin and can eventually result in the development of an auto-immune response against myelin [129,130]. MBP citrullination is carried out by the peptidyl arginine deiminase type-2 (PAD2) enzyme. Interestingly, the promoter region of the *PAD2* gene is hypomethylated in normal appearing white matter (NAWM) of MS patients, compared to control samples [130]. This implies that *PAD2* hypomethylation leads to a higher expression of the enzyme, which finally results in the destabilization and degradation of the myelin sheath in MS white matter. *PAD2* hypomethylation is, surprisingly, not brain-specific but can also be observed in peripheral blood mononuclear cells (PBMCs) of MS patients [131]. In a similar fashion, cell-free DNA (cfDNA) in peripheral blood samples of MS patients with an active disease course showed hypomethylated patterns of the *MOG* gene, which is associated with OL cell death and demyelinating events in the brain [132]. The correlation of methylation patterns between the brain and blood has gained interest over the past years for its potential application as a biomarker for neurodegenerative diseases [133–135], and could therefore also be used to monitor disease progression in MS.

An epigenome-wide DNA methylation study (EWAS) was conducted on MS NAWM postmortem samples. Genes responsible for OL survival (*BCL2L2*, *NDRG1*) and myelination (*MBP*, *SOX8*) were hypermethylated and decreased in expression in MS-affected tissue, compared to controls [136]. While representing a valuable study, it is important to note that no distinction has been made between regular cytosine methylation and 5-hydroxymethylation (5hmC). Considering the functional consequences of 5hmC, but also to prevent underrepresentation of methylated cytosine values, 5hmC analysis should be taken along in CNS EWAS studies.

Another study that analyzed postmortem brain tissue of MS patients showed higher levels of histone acetylation in oligodendrocytes within chronic MS lesions, compared to non-neurological controls. These changes are associated with elevated HAT transcript levels and higher expression of inhibitory regulators (*TCF7L2*, *ID2*, *SOX2*). In contrast, OLs present in early MS lesions show the presence of deacetylated histones [137]. Since histone acetylation impairs OL differentiation and remyelination, these data could partially explain the poor remyelination capacity associated with progressive MS patients.

MiRNA analysis of brain samples of progressive MS patients showed upregulated levels of different miRNAs (miR-155, miR-338, miR-491), which target enzymes that are involved in the production of neurosteroids [138]. Opposing results were obtained from another study, in which they show that these miRNAs are downregulated in chronic, inactive MS lesions, compared to control white matter samples [139]. The discrepancy between these studies could be attributed to differences in the analyzed tissue, their control sample selection or the method of miRNA analysis, which makes it difficult to directly compare them to each other. Interestingly, the most significant downregulated hit from the latter study is miR-219, which, together with miR-338, is essential for OPC cell cycle exit and differentiation into myelin-producing OLs [85,88,91]. The absence of these miRNAs could thus underlie the differentiation block of OPCs in chronic demyelinated lesion of progressive MS patients. Moreover, miR-219 expression is also decreased in the cerebrospinal fluid (CSF) of MS patients, rendering it a possible biomarker for MS diagnosis [140].

It is however noteworthy that most of the abovementioned studies have been conducted on bulk tissue, leading to a possible noise introduced by the cellular heterogeneity. Since the observed epigenetic changes could be strongly influenced by cellular variation or cell numbers, cell type-specific validation is recommended to circumvent such bias [141,142].

4.3. Other Diseases with Myelopathy

Even though MS is regarded as the most common myelopathy of the CNS, many other neurological diseases are characterized by oligodendroglial injury and myelin disruption. Here, we briefly discuss how epigenetic changes impact OL regeneration and remyelination in relation to these other demyelinating diseases.

Ischemic stroke, caused by a cerebral artery occlusion, is an important cause of death worldwide and the majority of survivors often struggle from severe neurological disabilities throughout the lifespan. Molecularly, ischemic stroke can be characterized by a disrupted architecture of neuronal synapses, neuronal loss and loss of glial cells, including oligodendrocytes, leading to prominent white matter demyelination [143]. During stroke recovery, endogenous repair processes are initiated and include axonal growth, synaptic plasticity, angiogenesis, neurogenesis, and oligodendrogenesis. Interestingly, during early brain recovery following ischemic stroke, HDAC1 and HDAC2 levels were shown to be increased in white matter OPCs at the peri-infarct region [144,145]. Mature OLs showed a retained increase of HDAC2 following stroke, while HDAC1 levels were decreased, indicating that individual HDACs family members play distinct roles during recovery after stroke [144]. In line, pan-HDAC inhibitors have repeatedly shown to protect OLs from ischemia-induced cell death and subsequently increase oligodendrogenesis [146–148]. However, contradictory results have been observed for the pan HDAC inhibitor suberoylanilide hydroxamic acid (SAHA) as its treatment suppressed OPC survival, leading to detrimental effects for the myelinating brain during stroke recovery [149]. Interestingly, not only HDAC modifications have shown their importance during oligodendrogenesis following stroke, but also miRNAs have been widely investigated for their therapeutic and diagnostic properties [150]. In ischemic white matter regions, miR-9 and miR-200b levels were decreased, concomitant with an increased differentiation state of OL lineage cells [94,151]. However, the majority of the investigated miRNAs showed an increased expression pattern following stroke. For example, rodent models for ischemic stroke showed a high presence of miR-146a, miR-138, miR-338, miR-423-5p, miR-200b, miR-298, miR-205, miR-107 and miR-145 [99,152–154], all of which have a negative impact on OPC proliferation, which is actually necessary in the early phase after stroke injury to replenish the pool of lost OPCs. Interestingly, circulating miRNA levels have been measured in stroke patients to provide new therapeutic and minimally invasive diagnostic insights. Measuring miR-146a levels, for example, can segregate the acute phase from the subacute phase during ischemic stroke, thereby highlighting the usefulness of miRNAs for future stroke research [155].

X-linked adrenoleukodystrophy (X-ALD) is a genetic disorder caused by a mutation in the *ABCD1* gene and characterized by progressive demyelination of the CNS [156]. An important aspect of this disease is the absence of remyelination capacities, even after successful hematopoietic stem cell transplantation [157]. X-ALD patients endure progressive impairment of cognition, vision, hearing and motoric function, eventually leading to total disability [158]. An EWAS, conducted on white matter samples of the prefrontal cortex of X-ALD patients, revealed differential DNA methylation in genes involved in OL differentiation. Myelin genes, such as *MBP*, *PLP1*, *MOG* and *CNP* were hypermethylated in X-ALD patients compared to age-matched controls. Furthermore, transcriptional inhibitors (*ID4* and *SOX2*) displayed an increased expression in these patients, suggesting a disturbed HDAC activity [157]. In line with this, treatment with SAHA prevented OL cell loss both in vitro and in vivo by counteracting the very long chain fatty acid (VLCFA) derangement associated with X-ALD pathology [159]. Another type of leukodystrophy, adult-onset autosomal dominant leukodystrophy (ADLD) is characterized by duplication of the gene that codes for lamin B1 (*LMNB1*), which leads to overexpression of LMNB1 and causes severe myelin loss [160]. Interestingly, miR-23 has been identified as a negative regulator of lamin B by targeting its transcript levels and could therefore be considered as a therapeutic strategy for ADLD [161].

Schizophrenia has also been associated with OL dysfunction. Interestingly, the CpG island within the promoter region of *SOX10* is hypermethylated in brains of patients with schizophrenia, which is directly associated with a decreased expression of *SOX10* and other OL-related genes [162].

5. Therapeutic Perspectives: From Pharmaceuticals to (epi) Gene Therapy to IPSCs

It is clear that epigenetic modifications strongly influence OL development and functional remyelination in a wide variety of diseases. Targeting these epigenetic alterations could therefore be considered as a new therapeutic strategy to overcome remyelination failure. Most attempts to pharmacologically manipulate epigenetic modulations are based on the use of inhibitors of epigenetic enzymes, such as 5-aza, TSA and valproic acid (VPA) [163,164]. However, such pan-epigenetic inhibitors are non-specific due to their pleiotropic impact at a genome-wide level. Furthermore, these compounds are known to have low chemical stability and are cytotoxic at higher doses, which limits their potency to be used in a cellular microenvironment [165,166]. Recent improvements in the field of epigenetic editing have disclosed the use of DNA-binding proteins, such as zinc-finger proteins (ZFPs), transcription activator-like effectors (TALEs) and type II clustered regularly interspaced short palindromic repeat (CRISPR)/Cas9, as new synthetic epigenomic engineering tools [167–170]. These DNA-binding proteins are linked to epigenetic modifiers and serve to guide them to a specific region in the genome, thereby altering the epigenome at specific loci. Even though many advances have been made regarding these new epigenetic editing techniques, their applicability in the clinic may require, next to ethical considerations, additional research as their safety and efficacy remain to be disclosed. In particular, the off-target effects and undesired genomic binding of these DNA-binding proteins are still considered as one of the major hurdles for their therapeutic application [171].

Autologous cell-based therapies have emerged as a promising technique to restore OL dysfunction. Mature and fully differentiated OLs derived from induced pluripotent stem cells (iPSCs) have shown to successfully remyelinate axons in rodents [172]. Interestingly, human iPSC-derived OPCs show the same epigenetic signature during their differentiation process into mature OLs as seen in normal OL development [173]. Furthermore, generation of oligodendrocytes from progressive MS patient-derived iPSCs results in functional and myelinating cells, in contrast to the resident non-myelinating OPCs in the CNS [174]. Since the epigenetic signature of OPCs/OLs can be disturbed in a pathological context, reprogramming patient-derived iPSCs into OLs and repopulating lesion sites with these cells could be considered as a promising remyelinating strategy.

6. Concluding Remarks

In this review, we have discussed how different epigenetic modifications influence OL development and lineage progression and how this is dysregulated in demyelinating conditions. Epigenetic mechanisms function as a precise gateway control system that governs the transcriptional machinery in a spatiotemporal manner. In CNS demyelinating diseases, these epigenetic mechanisms are found to be altered, concomitant with increased levels of transcriptional inhibitors and resulting in a differentiation block of OPCs. Targeting these epigenetic processes, either by pan-inhibitors or via CRISPR/Cas9-mediated epigenetic editing, could therefore be a potential strategy to boost OL differentiation and (re)myelination. Taken together, epigenetic research has earned its place within the universe of OL development and further studies will contribute to the complete understanding of CNS myelin disorders.

Funding: This work was funded by the Research Foundation of Flanders (FWO Vlaanderen, 1S25119N) and the Charcot Foundation.

Conflicts of Interest: The authors declare no conflict of interest.

References

1. Bradl, M.; Lassmann, H. Oligodendrocytes: Biology and pathology. *Acta. Neuropathol.* **2010**, *119*, 37–53. [CrossRef] [PubMed]
2. Dawson, M.R.; Polito, A.; Levine, J.M.; Reynolds, R. NG2-expressing glial progenitor cells: An abundant and widespread population of cycling cells in the adult rat CNS. *Mol. Cell. Neurosci.* **2003**, *24*, 476–488. [CrossRef]
3. Fernandez, C.A.; Gaultier, A. Adult oligodendrocyte progenitor cells—Multifaceted regulators of the CNS in health and disease. *Brain Behav. Immun.* **2016**, *57*, 1–7. [CrossRef] [PubMed]
4. Bergles, D.E.; Richardson, W.D. Oligodendrocyte Development and Plasticity. *Cold Spring Harb. Perspect. Biol.* **2015**, *8*, 020453. [CrossRef] [PubMed]
5. Wheeler, N.A.; Fuss, B. Extracellular cues influencing oligodendrocyte differentiation and (re)myelination. *Exp. Neurol.* **2016**, *283*, 512–530. [CrossRef] [PubMed]
6. Koch, M.W.; Metz, L.M.; Kovalchuk, O. Epigenetic changes in patients with multiple sclerosis. *Nat. Rev. Neurol.* **2013**, *9*, 35–43. [CrossRef] [PubMed]
7. Liu, J.; Moyon, S.; Hernandez, M.; Casaccia, P. Epigenetic control of oligodendrocyte development: Adding new players to old keepers. *Curr. Opin. Neurobiol.* **2016**, *39*, 133–138. [CrossRef] [PubMed]
8. Gonzalez-Perez, O.; Alvarez-Buylla, A. Oligodendrogenesis in the subventricular zone and the role of epidermal growth factor. *Brain Res. Rev.* **2011**, *67*, 147–156. [CrossRef] [PubMed]
9. Elbaz, B.; Popko, B. Molecular Control of Oligodendrocyte Development. *Trends Neurosci.* **2019**, *42*, 263–277. [CrossRef] [PubMed]
10. Armada-Moreira, A.; Ribeiro, F.F.; Sebastião, A.M.; Xapelli, S. Neuroinflammatory modulators of oligodendrogenesis. *Neuroimmunol. Neuroinflammation* **2015**, *2*, 263–273.
11. Sock, E.; Wegner, M. Transcriptional control of myelination and remyelination. *Trends cell boil.* **2011**, *21*, 585–593. [CrossRef] [PubMed]
12. Li, H.; He, Y.; Richardson, W.D.; Casaccia, P. Two-tier transcriptional control of oligodendrocyte differentiation. *Curr. Opin. Neurobiol.* **2009**, *19*, 479–485. [CrossRef]
13. Zhu, X.; Zuo, H.; Maher, B.J.; Serwanski, D.R.; LoTurco, J.J.; Lu, Q.R.; Nishiyama, A. Olig2-dependent developmental fate switch of NG2 cells. *Dev. Camb. Engl.* **2012**, *139*, 2299–2307. [CrossRef] [PubMed]

14. Wegener, A.; Deboux, C.; Bachelin, C.; Frah, M.; Kerninon, C.; Seilhean, D.; Weider, M.; Wegner, M.; Nait-Oumesmar, B. Gain of Olig2 function in oligodendrocyte progenitors promotes remyelination. *Brain A J. Neurol.* **2015**, *138*, 120–135. [CrossRef] [PubMed]
15. Maire, C.L.; Wegener, A.; Kerninon, C.; Nait Oumesmar, B. Gain-of-Function of Olig Transcription Factors Enhances Oligodendrogenesis and Myelination. *Stem Cells* **2010**, *28*, 1611–1622. [CrossRef]
16. Arnett, H.A.; Fancy, S.P.; Alberta, J.A.; Zhao, C.; Plant, S.R.; Kaing, S.; Raine, C.S.; Rowitch, D.H.; Franklin, R.J.; Stiles, C.D. bHLH transcription factor Olig1 is required to repair demyelinated lesions in the CNS. *Science* **2004**, *306*, 2111–2115. [CrossRef] [PubMed]
17. Dai, J.; Bercury, K.K.; Ahrendsen, J.T.; Macklin, W.B. Olig1 function is required for oligodendrocyte differentiation in the mouse brain. *J. Neurosci.* **2015**, *35*, 4386–4402. [CrossRef]
18. Sugimori, M.; Nagao, M.; Parras, C.M.; Nakatani, H.; Lebel, M.; Guillemot, F.; Nakafuku, M. Ascl1 is required for oligodendrocyte development in the spinal cord. *Dev. Camb. Engl.* **2008**, *135*, 1271–1281. [CrossRef]
19. Nakatani, H.; Martin, E.; Hassani, H.; Clavairoly, A.; Maire, C.L.; Viadieu, A.; Kerninon, C.; Delmasure, A.; Frah, M.; Weber, M.; et al. Ascl1/Mash1 Promotes Brain Oligodendrogenesis during Myelination and Remyelination. *J. Neurosci.* **2013**, *33*, 9752–9768. [CrossRef]
20. Samanta, J.; Kessler, J.A. Interactions between ID and OLIG proteins mediate the inhibitory effects of BMP4 on oligodendroglial differentiation. *Dev. Camb. Engl.* **2004**, *131*, 4131–4142. [CrossRef]
21. Wang, S.; Sdrulla, A.; Johnson, J.E.; Yokota, Y.; Barres, B.A. A role for the helix-loop-helix protein Id2 in the control of oligodendrocyte development. *Neuron* **2001**, *29*, 603–614. [CrossRef]
22. Turnescu, T.; Arter, J.; Reiprich, S.; Tamm, E.R.; Waisman, A.; Wegner, M. Sox8 and Sox10 jointly maintain myelin gene expression in oligodendrocytes. *Glia* **2018**, *66*, 279–294. [CrossRef] [PubMed]
23. Hornig, J.; Frob, F.; Vogl, M.R.; Hermans-Borgmeyer, I.; Tamm, E.R.; Wegner, M. The transcription factors Sox10 and Myrf define an essential regulatory network module in differentiating oligodendrocytes. *PLoS Genet.* **2013**, *9*, 1003907. [CrossRef] [PubMed]
24. Stolt, C.C.; Rehberg, S.; Ader, M.; Lommes, P.; Riethmacher, D.; Schachner, M.; Bartsch, U.; Wegner, M. Terminal differentiation of myelin-forming oligodendrocytes depends on the transcription factor Sox10. *Genes Dev.* **2002**, *16*, 165–170. [CrossRef] [PubMed]
25. Stolt, C.C.; Schlierf, A.; Lommes, P.; Hillgartner, S.; Werner, T.; Kosian, T.; Sock, E.; Kessaris, N.; Richardson, W.D.; Lefebvre, V.; et al. SoxD proteins influence multiple stages of oligodendrocyte development and modulate SoxE protein function. *Dev. Cell* **2006**, *11*, 697–709. [CrossRef] [PubMed]
26. Zhao, C.; Ma, D.; Zawadzka, M.; Fancy, S.P.; Elis-Williams, L.; Bouvier, G.; Stockley, J.H.; de Castro, G.M.; Wang, B.; Jacobs, S.; et al. Sox2 Sustains Recruitment of Oligodendrocyte Progenitor Cells following CNS Demyelination and Primes Them for Differentiation during Remyelination. *J. Neurosci. Neurosci.* **2015**, *35*, 11482–11499. [CrossRef] [PubMed]
27. Zhang, S.; Zhu, X.; Gui, X.; Croteau, C.; Song, L.; Xu, J.; Wang, A.; Bannerman, P.; Guo, F. Sox2 Is Essential for Oligodendroglial Proliferation and Differentiation during Postnatal Brain Myelination and CNS Remyelination. *J. Neurosci.* **2018**, *38*, 1802–1820. [CrossRef] [PubMed]
28. Ye, F.; Chen, Y.; Hoang, T.; Montgomery, R.L.; Zhao, X.H.; Bu, H.; Hu, T.; Taketo, M.M.; van Es, J.H.; Clevers, H.; et al. HDAC1 and HDAC2 regulate oligodendrocyte differentiation by disrupting the beta-catenin-TCF interaction. *Nat. Neurosci.* **2009**, *12*, 829–838. [CrossRef] [PubMed]
29. He, Y.; Dupree, J.; Wang, J.; Sandoval, J.; Li, J.; Liu, H.; Shi, Y.; Nave, K.A.; Casaccia-Bonnefil, P. The transcription factor Yin Yang 1 is essential for oligodendrocyte progenitor differentiation. *Neuron* **2007**, *55*, 217–230. [CrossRef]
30. Howng, S.Y.; Avila, R.L.; Emery, B.; Traka, M.; Lin, W.; Watkins, T.; Cook, S.; Bronson, R.; Davisson, M.; Barres, B.A.; et al. ZFP191 is required by oligodendrocytes for CNS myelination. *Genes Dev.* **2010**, *24*, 301–311. [CrossRef]
31. Biswas, S.; Chung, S.H.; Jiang, P.; Dehghan, S.; Deng, W. Development of glial restricted human neural stem cells for oligodendrocyte differentiation in vitro and in vivo. *Sci. Rep.* **2019**, *9*, 9013. [CrossRef] [PubMed]
32. Soundarapandian, M.M.; Selvaraj, V.; Lo, U.G.; Golub, M.S.; Feldman, D.H.; Pleasure, D.E.; Deng, W. Zfp488 promotes oligodendrocyte differentiation of neural progenitor cells in adult mice after demyelination. *Sci. Rep.* **2011**, *1*, 2. [CrossRef] [PubMed]

33. Weng, Q.; Chen, Y.; Wang, H.; Xu, X.; Yang, B.; He, Q.; Shou, W.; Chen, Y.; Higashi, Y.; van den Berghe, V.; et al. Dual-mode modulation of Smad signaling by Smad-interacting protein Sip1 is required for myelination in the central nervous system. *Neuron* **2012**, *73*, 713–728. [CrossRef] [PubMed]
34. Emery, B.; Agalliu, D.; Cahoy, J.D.; Watkins, T.A.; Dugas, J.C.; Mulinyawe, S.B.; Ibrahim, A.; Ligon, K.L.; Rowitch, D.H.; Barres, B.A. Myelin gene regulatory factor is a critical transcriptional regulator required for CNS myelination. *Cell* **2009**, *138*, 172–185. [CrossRef]
35. Fulton, D.; Paez, P.M.; Campagnoni, A.T. The Multiple Roles of Myelin Protein Genes During the Development of the Oligodendrocyte. *Asn. Neuro.* **2010**, *2*, AN20090051. [CrossRef]
36. Aggarwal, S.; Yurlova, L.; Simons, M. Central nervous system myelin: Structure, synthesis and assembly. *Trends Cell Biol.* **2011**, *21*, 585–593. [CrossRef]
37. Emery, B.; Lu, Q.R. Transcriptional and Epigenetic Regulation of Oligodendrocyte Development and Myelination in the Central Nervous System. *Cold Spring Harb. Perspect. Biol.* **2015**, *7*, a020461. [CrossRef]
38. Dulac, C. Brain function and chromatin plasticity. *Nature* **2010**, *465*, 728–735. [CrossRef]
39. Allis, C.D.; Jenuwein, T. The molecular hallmarks of epigenetic control. *Nat. Rev. Genet.* **2016**, *17*, 487. [CrossRef]
40. Copray, S.; Huynh, J.L.; Sher, F.; Casaccia-Bonnefil, P.; Boddeke, E. Epigenetic mechanisms facilitating oligodendrocyte development, maturation and aging. *Glia* **2009**, *57*, 1579–1587. [CrossRef]
41. Illingworth, R.S.; Gruenewald-Schneider, U.; Webb, S.; Kerr, A.R.W.; James, K.D.; Turner, D.J.; Smith, C.; Harrison, D.J.; Andrews, R.; Bird, A.P. Orphan CpG Islands Identify Numerous Conserved Promoters in the Mammalian Genome. *PLoS Genet.* **2010**, *6*, e1001134. [CrossRef] [PubMed]
42. Jones, P.L.; Veenstra, G.J.; Wade, P.A.; Vermaak, D.; Kass, S.U.; Landsberger, N.; Strouboulis, J.; Wolffe, A.P. Methylated DNA and MeCP2 recruit histone deacetylase to repress transcription. *Nat. Genet.* **1998**, *19*, 187–191. [CrossRef] [PubMed]
43. Fuks, F.; Hurd, P.J.; Wolf, D.; Nan, X.; Bird, A.P.; Kouzarides, T. The methyl-CpG-binding protein MeCP2 links DNA methylation to histone methylation. *J. Biol. Chem.* **2003**, *278*, 4035–4040. [CrossRef] [PubMed]
44. Day, J.J.; Kennedy, A.J.; Sweatt, J.D. DNA Methylation and Its Implications and Accessibility for Neuropsychiatric Therapeutics. *Annu. Rev. Pharmacol. Toxicol.* **2015**, *55*, 591–611. [CrossRef] [PubMed]
45. Chen, Z.X.; Riggs, A.D. DNA methylation and demethylation in mammals. *J. Biol. Chem.* **2011**, *286*, 18347–18353. [CrossRef] [PubMed]
46. Hu, L.; Lu, J.; Cheng, J.; Rao, Q.; Li, Z.; Hou, H.; Lou, Z.; Zhang, L.; Li, W.; Gong, W.; et al. Structural insight into substrate preference for TET-mediated oxidation. *Nature* **2015**, *527*, 118–122. [CrossRef] [PubMed]
47. Kriaucionis, S.; Heintz, N. The nuclear DNA base 5-hydroxymethylcytosine is present in Purkinje neurons and the brain. *Science* **2009**, *324*, 929–930. [CrossRef] [PubMed]
48. Chen, C.-C.; Wang, K.-Y.; Shen, C.-K.J. The mammalian de novo DNA methyltransferases DNMT3A and DNMT3B are also DNA 5-hydroxymethylcytosine dehydroxymethylases. *J. Biol. Chem.* **2012**, *287*, 33116–33121. [CrossRef]
49. Chen, C.C.; Wang, K.Y.; Shen, C.K. DNA 5-methylcytosine demethylation activities of the mammalian DNA methyltransferases. *J. Biol. Chem.* **2013**, *288*, 9084–9091. [CrossRef] [PubMed]
50. Globisch, D.; Munzel, M.; Muller, M.; Michalakis, S.; Wagner, M.; Koch, S.; Bruckl, T.; Biel, M.; Carell, T. Tissue distribution of 5-hydroxymethylcytosine and search for active demethylation intermediates. *PLoS ONE* **2010**, *5*, 15367. [CrossRef]
51. Roubroeks, J.A.Y.; Smith, R.G.; van den Hove, D.L.A.; Lunnon, K. Epigenetics and DNA methylomic profiling in Alzheimer's disease and other neurodegenerative diseases. *J. Neurochem.* **2017**, *143*, 158–170. [CrossRef]
52. van den Hove, D.L.; Chouliaras, L.; Rutten, B.P. The role of 5-hydroxymethylcytosine in aging and Alzheimer's disease: Current status and prospects for future studies. *Curr. Alzheimer Res.* **2012**, *9*, 545–549. [CrossRef] [PubMed]
53. Ransom, B.R.; Yamate, C.L.; Black, J.A.; Waxman, S.G. Rat optic nerve: Disruption of gliogenesis with 5-azacytidine during early postnatal development. *Brain Res.* **1985**, *337*, 41–49. [CrossRef]
54. Moyon, S.; Huynh, J.L.; Dutta, D.; Zhang, F.; Ma, D.; Yoo, S.; Lawrence, R.; Wegner, M.; John, G.R.; Emery, B.; et al. Functional Characterization of DNA Methylation in the Oligodendrocyte Lineage. *Cell Rep.* **2016**, *15*, 748–760. [CrossRef]
55. Moyon, S.; Ma, D.; Huynh, J.L.; Coutts, D.J.C.; Zhao, C.; Casaccia, P.; Franklin, R.J.M. Efficient Remyelination Requires DNA Methylation. *eNeuro* **2017**, *4*, ENEURO.0336–0316.2017. [CrossRef] [PubMed]

56. Zhao, X.; Dai, J.; Ma, Y.; Mi, Y.; Cui, D.; Ju, G.; Macklin, W.B.; Jin, W. Dynamics of ten-eleven translocation hydroxylase family proteins and 5-hydroxymethylcytosine in oligodendrocyte differentiation. *Glia* **2014**, *62*, 914–926. [CrossRef] [PubMed]
57. Huang, J.; Vogel, G.; Yu, Z.; Almazan, G.; Richard, S. Type II arginine methyltransferase PRMT5 regulates gene expression of inhibitors of differentiation/DNA binding Id2 and Id4 during glial cell differentiation. *J. Biol. Chem.* **2011**, *286*, 44424–44432. [CrossRef] [PubMed]
58. Fang, N.; Cheng, J.; Zhang, C.; Chen, K.; Zhang, C.; Hu, Z.; Bi, R.; Furber, K.L.; Thangaraj, M.; Nazarali, A.J.; et al. Sirt2 epigenetically down-regulates PDGFRalpha expression and promotes CG4 cell differentiation. *Cell Cycle* **2019**, *18*, 1095–1109. [CrossRef]
59. Bannister, A.J.; Kouzarides, T. Regulation of chromatin by histone modifications. *Cell Res.* **2011**, *21*, 381. [CrossRef]
60. He, H.; Hu, Z.; Xiao, H.; Zhou, F.; Yang, B. The tale of histone modifications and its role in multiple sclerosis. *Hum. Genom.* **2018**, *12*, 31. [CrossRef]
61. Marin-Husstege, M.; Muggironi, M.; Liu, A.; Casaccia-Bonnefil, P. Histone deacetylase activity is necessary for oligodendrocyte lineage progression. *J. Neurosci.* **2002**, *22*, 10333–10345. [CrossRef] [PubMed]
62. Shen, S.; Li, J.; Casaccia-Bonnefil, P. Histone modifications affect timing of oligodendrocyte progenitor differentiation in the developing rat brain. *J. Cell Biol.* **2005**, *169*, 577–589. [CrossRef] [PubMed]
63. Swiss, V.A.; Nguyen, T.; Dugas, J.; Ibrahim, A.; Barres, B.; Androulakis, I.P.; Casaccia, P. Identification of a gene regulatory network necessary for the initiation of oligodendrocyte differentiation. *PLoS ONE* **2011**, *6*, e18088. [CrossRef] [PubMed]
64. Conway, G.D.; O'Bara, M.A.; Vedia, B.H.; Pol, S.U.; Sim, F.J. Histone deacetylase activity is required for human oligodendrocyte progenitor differentiation. *Glia* **2012**, *60*, 1944–1953. [CrossRef] [PubMed]
65. Egawa, N.; Shindo, A.; Hikawa, R.; Kinoshita, H.; Liang, A.C.; Itoh, K.; Lok, J.; Maki, T.; Takahashi, R.; Lo, E.H.; et al. Differential roles of epigenetic regulators in the survival and differentiation of oligodendrocyte precursor cells. *Glia* **2019**, *67*, 718–728. [CrossRef] [PubMed]
66. He, Y.; Sandoval, J.; Casaccia-Bonnefil, P. Events at the transition between cell cycle exit and oligodendrocyte progenitor differentiation: The role of HDAC and YY1. *Neuron Glia Biol.* **2007**, *3*, 221–231. [CrossRef] [PubMed]
67. Dai, J.; Bercury, K.K.; Jin, W.; Macklin, W.B. Olig1 Acetylation and Nuclear Export Mediate Oligodendrocyte Development. *J. Neurosci.* **2015**, *35*, 15875–15893. [CrossRef] [PubMed]
68. Liu, J.; Magri, L.; Zhang, F.; Marsh, N.O.; Albrecht, S.; Huynh, J.L.; Kaur, J.; Kuhlmann, T.; Zhang, W.; Slesinger, P.A.; et al. Chromatin landscape defined by repressive histone methylation during oligodendrocyte differentiation. *J. Neurosci.* **2015**, *35*, 352–365. [CrossRef]
69. Sher, F.; Rößler, R.; Brouwer, N.; Balasubramaniyan, V.; Boddeke, E.; Copray, S. Differentiation of Neural Stem Cells into Oligodendrocytes: Involvement of the Polycomb Group Protein Ezh2. *Stem Cells* **2008**, *26*, 2875–2883. [CrossRef]
70. Koreman, E.; Sun, X.; Lu, Q.R. Chromatin remodeling and epigenetic regulation of oligodendrocyte myelination and myelin repair. *Mol. Cell. Neurosci.* **2018**, *87*, 18–26. [CrossRef]
71. Scaglione, A.; Patzig, J.; Liang, J.; Frawley, R.; Bok, J.; Mela, A.; Yattah, C.; Zhang, J.; Teo, S.X.; Zhou, T.; et al. PRMT5-mediated regulation of developmental myelination. *Nat. Commun.* **2018**, *9*, 2840. [CrossRef] [PubMed]
72. Hashimoto, M.; Murata, K.; Ishida, J.; Kanou, A.; Kasuya, Y.; Fukamizu, A. Severe Hypomyelination and Developmental Defects Are Caused in Mice Lacking Protein Arginine Methyltransferase 1 (PRMT1) in the Central Nervous System. *J. Biol. Chem.* **2016**, *291*, 2237–2245. [CrossRef] [PubMed]
73. Gregath, A.; Lu, Q.R. Epigenetic modifications-insight into oligodendrocyte lineage progression, regeneration, and disease. *FEBS Lett.* **2018**, *592*, 1063–1078. [CrossRef] [PubMed]
74. Matsumoto, S.; Banine, F.; Feistel, K.; Foster, S.; Xing, R.; Struve, J.; Sherman, L.S. Brg1 directly regulates Olig2 transcription and is required for oligodendrocyte progenitor cell specification. *Dev. Biol.* **2016**, *413*, 173–187. [CrossRef] [PubMed]
75. Yu, Y.; Chen, Y.; Kim, B.; Wang, H.; Zhao, C.; He, X.; Liu, L.; Liu, W.; Wu, L.M.; Mao, M.; et al. Olig2 targets chromatin remodelers to enhancers to initiate oligodendrocyte differentiation. *Cell* **2013**, *152*, 248–261. [CrossRef] [PubMed]

76. He, D.; Marie, C.; Zhao, C.; Kim, B.; Wang, J.; Deng, Y.; Clavairoly, A.; Frah, M.; Wang, H.; He, X.; et al. Chd7 cooperates with Sox10 and regulates the onset of CNS myelination and remyelination. *Nat. Neurosci* **2016**, *19*, 678–689. [CrossRef] [PubMed]
77. Fabian, M.R.; Sundermeier, T.R.; Sonenberg, N. Understanding how miRNAs post-transcriptionally regulate gene expression. *Prog. Mol. Subcell. Biol.* **2010**, *50*, 1–20.
78. Rodriguez, A.; Griffiths-Jones, S.; Ashurst, J.L.; Bradley, A. Identification of mammalian microRNA host genes and transcription units. *Genome Res.* **2004**, *14*, 1902–1910. [CrossRef]
79. Lewis, B.P.; Shih, I.H.; Jones-Rhoades, M.W.; Bartel, D.P.; Burge, C.B. Prediction of mammalian microRNA targets. *Cell* **2003**, *115*, 787–798. [CrossRef]
80. He, L.; Hannon, G.J. MicroRNAs: Small RNAs with a big role in gene regulation. *Nat. Rev. Genet.* **2004**, *5*, 522–531. [CrossRef]
81. Eulalio, A.; Huntzinger, E.; Nishihara, T.; Rehwinkel, J.; Fauser, M.; Izaurralde, E. Deadenylation is a widespread effect of miRNA regulation. *RNA* **2009**, *15*, 21–32. [CrossRef] [PubMed]
82. Sayed, D.; Abdellatif, M. MicroRNAs in development and disease. *Physiol. Rev.* **2011**, *91*, 827–887. [CrossRef] [PubMed]
83. Barca-Mayo, O.; Lu, Q.R. Fine-Tuning Oligodendrocyte Development by microRNAs. *Front. Neurosci.* **2012**, *6*, 13. [CrossRef] [PubMed]
84. Fitzpatrick, J.M.; Anderson, R.C.; McDermott, K.W. MicroRNA: Key regulators of oligodendrocyte development and pathobiology. *Int. J. Biochem. Cell Biol.* **2015**, *65*, 134–138. [CrossRef] [PubMed]
85. Dugas, J.C.; Cuellar, T.L.; Scholze, A.; Ason, B.; Ibrahim, A.; Emery, B.; Zamanian, J.L.; Foo, L.C.; McManus, M.T.; Barres, B.A. Dicer1 and miR-219 Are required for normal oligodendrocyte differentiation and myelination. *Neuron* **2010**, *65*, 597–611. [CrossRef] [PubMed]
86. Shin, D.; Shin, J.Y.; McManus, M.T.; Ptacek, L.J.; Fu, Y.H. Dicer ablation in oligodendrocytes provokes neuronal impairment in mice. *Ann. Neurol.* **2009**, *66*, 843–857. [CrossRef] [PubMed]
87. Liu, S.; Ren, C.; Qu, X.; Wu, X.; Dong, F.; Chand, Y.K.; Fan, H.; Yao, R.; Geng, D. miR-219 attenuates demyelination in cuprizone-induced demyelinated mice by regulating monocarboxylate transporter 1. *Eur. J. Neurosci.* **2017**, *45*, 249–259. [CrossRef] [PubMed]
88. Wang, H.; Moyano, A.L.; Ma, Z.; Deng, Y.; Lin, Y.; Zhao, C.; Zhang, L.; Jiang, M.; He, X.; Ma, Z.; et al. miR-219 Cooperates with miR-338 in Myelination and Promotes Myelin Repair in the CNS. *Dev. Cell* **2017**, *40*, 566–582. [CrossRef] [PubMed]
89. Dugas, J.C.; Notterpek, L. MicroRNAs in oligodendrocyte and Schwann cell differentiation. *Dev. Neurosci.* **2011**, *33*, 14–20. [CrossRef] [PubMed]
90. Zhao, X.; He, X.; Han, X.; Yu, Y.; Ye, F.; Chen, Y.; Hoang, T.; Xu, X.; Mi, Q.S.; Xin, M.; et al. MicroRNA-mediated control of oligodendrocyte differentiation. *Neuron* **2010**, *65*, 612–626. [CrossRef] [PubMed]
91. Ebrahimi-Barough, S.; Massumi, M.; Kouchesfahani, H.M.; Ai, J. Derivation of pre-oligodendrocytes from human endometrial stromal cells by using overexpression of microRNA 338. *J. Mol. Neurosci. Mn* **2013**, *51*, 337–343. [CrossRef]
92. Smirnova, L.; Grafe, A.; Seiler, A.; Schumacher, S.; Nitsch, R.; Wulczyn, F.G. Regulation of miRNA expression during neural cell specification. *Eur. J. Neurosci.* **2005**, *21*, 1469–1477. [CrossRef]
93. Lau, P.; Verrier, J.D.; Nielsen, J.A.; Johnson, K.R.; Notterpek, L.; Hudson, L.D. Identification of dynamically regulated microRNA and mRNA networks in developing oligodendrocytes. *J. Neurosci.* **2008**, *28*, 11720–11730. [CrossRef]
94. Buller, B.; Chopp, M.; Ueno, Y.; Zhang, L.; Zhang, R.L.; Morris, D.; Zhang, Y.; Zhang, Z.G. Regulation of serum response factor by miRNA-200 and miRNA-9 modulates oligodendrocyte progenitor cell differentiation. *Glia* **2012**, *60*, 1906–1914. [CrossRef]
95. Lecca, D.; Marangon, D.; Coppolino, G.T.; Mendez, A.M.; Finardi, A.; Costa, G.D.; Martinelli, V.; Furlan, R.; Abbracchio, M.P. MiR-125a-3p timely inhibits oligodendroglial maturation and is pathologically up-regulated in human multiple sclerosis. *Sci. Rep.* **2016**, *6*, 34503. [CrossRef]
96. Huang, B.; Luo, W.; Sun, L.; Zhang, Q.; Jiang, L.; Chang, J.; Qiu, X.; Wang, E. MiRNA-125a-3p is a negative regulator of the RhoA-actomyosin pathway in A549 cells. *Int. J. Oncol.* **2013**, *42*, 1734–1742. [CrossRef]
97. Dong, Y.; Li, P.; Ni, Y.; Zhao, J.; Liu, Z. Decreased microRNA-125a-3p contributes to upregulation of p38 MAPK in rat trigeminal ganglions with orofacial inflammatory pain. *PLoS ONe* **2014**, *9*, e111594. [CrossRef]

98. Yin, F.; Zhang, J.N.; Wang, S.W.; Zhou, C.H.; Zhao, M.M.; Fan, W.H.; Fan, M.; Liu, S. MiR-125a-3p regulates glioma apoptosis and invasion by regulating Nrg1. *PLoS ONE* **2015**, *10*, e0116759. [CrossRef]
99. Liu, X.S.; Chopp, M.; Pan, W.L.; Wang, X.L.; Fan, B.Y.; Zhang, Y.; Kassis, H.; Zhang, R.L.; Zhang, X.M.; Zhang, Z.G. MicroRNA-146a Promotes Oligodendrogenesis in Stroke. *Mol. Neurobiol.* **2017**, *54*, 227–237. [CrossRef]
100. Zhang, J.; Zhang, Z.G.; Lu, M.; Wang, X.; Shang, X.; Elias, S.B.; Chopp, M. MiR-146a promotes remyelination in a cuprizone model of demyelinating injury. *Neuroscience* **2017**, *348*, 252–263. [CrossRef]
101. Lin, S.T.; Huang, Y.; Zhang, L.; Heng, M.Y.; Ptacek, L.J.; Fu, Y.H. MicroRNA-23a promotes myelination in the central nervous system. *Proc. Natl. Acad Sci. USA* **2013**, *110*, 17468–17473. [CrossRef]
102. Bronstein, J.M.; Tiwari-Woodruff, S.; Buznikov, A.G.; Stevens, D.B. Involvement of OSP/claudin-11 in oligodendrocyte membrane interactions: Role in biology and disease. *J. Neurosci. Res.* **2000**, *59*, 706–711. [CrossRef]
103. Letzen, B.S.; Liu, C.; Thakor, N.V.; Gearhart, J.D.; All, A.H.; Kerr, C.L. MicroRNA expression profiling of oligodendrocyte differentiation from human embryonic stem cells. *PLoS ONE* **2010**, *5*, e10480. [CrossRef]
104. Hoffmann, S.A.; Hos, D.; Kuspert, M.; Lang, R.A.; Lovell-Badge, R.; Wegner, M.; Reiprich, S. Stem cell factor Sox2 and its close relative Sox3 have differentiation functions in oligodendrocytes. *Dev. Camb. Engl.* **2014**, *141*, 39–50. [CrossRef]
105. Budde, H.; Schmitt, S.; Fitzner, D.; Opitz, L.; Salinas-Riester, G.; Simons, M. Control of oligodendroglial cell number by the miR-17-92 cluster. *Dev. Camb. Engl.* **2010**, *137*, 2127–2132. [CrossRef]
106. Shields, S.A.; Gilson, J.M.; Blakemore, W.F.; Franklin, R.J. Remyelination occurs as extensively but more slowly in old rats compared to young rats following gliotoxin-induced CNS demyelination. *Glia* **1999**, *28*, 77–83. [CrossRef]
107. Sim, F.J.; Zhao, C.; Penderis, J.; Franklin, R.J. The age-related decrease in CNS remyelination efficiency is attributable to an impairment of both oligodendrocyte progenitor recruitment and differentiation. *J. Neurosci.* **2002**, *22*, 2451–2459. [CrossRef]
108. Nicaise, A.M.; Wagstaff, L.J.; Willis, C.M.; Paisie, C.; Chandok, H.; Robson, P.; Fossati, V.; Williams, A.; Crocker, S.J. Cellular senescence in progenitor cells contributes to diminished remyelination potential in progressive multiple sclerosis. *Proc. Natl. Acad. Sci. USA* **2019**, *116*, 9030–9039. [CrossRef]
109. Ryan, J.M.; Cristofalo, V.J. Histone acetylation during aging of human cells in culture. *Biochem. Biophys. Res. Commun.* **1972**, *48*, 735–742. [CrossRef]
110. Chouliaras, L.; Lardenoije, R.; Kenis, G.; Mastroeni, D.; Hof, P.R.; van Os, J.; Steinbusch, H.W.M.; van Leeuwen, F.W.; Rutten, B.P.F.; van den Hove, D.L.A. Age-related Disturbances in DNA (hydroxy)methylation in APP/PS1 Mice. *Transl. Neurosci.* **2018**, *9*, 190–202. [CrossRef]
111. Calvanese, V.; Lara, E.; Kahn, A.; Fraga, M.F. The role of epigenetics in aging and age-related diseases. *Ageing Res. Rev.* **2009**, *8*, 268–276. [CrossRef]
112. Zhou, J.; Wu, Y.C.; Xiao, B.J.; Guo, X.D.; Zheng, Q.X.; Wu, B. Age-related Changes in the Global DNA Methylation Profile of Oligodendrocyte Progenitor Cells Derived from Rat Spinal Cords. *Curr. Med Sci.* **2019**, *39*, 67–74. [CrossRef]
113. Shen, S.; Liu, A.; Li, J.; Wolubah, C.; Casaccia-Bonnefil, P. Epigenetic memory loss in aging oligodendrocytes in the corpus callosum. *Neurobiol. Aging* **2008**, *29*, 452–463. [CrossRef]
114. Shen, S.; Sandoval, J.; Swiss, V.A.; Li, J.; Dupree, J.; Franklin, R.J.; Casaccia-Bonnefil, P. Age-dependent epigenetic control of differentiation inhibitors is critical for remyelination efficiency. *Nat. Neurosci* **2008**, *11*, 1024–1034. [CrossRef]
115. Pusic, A.D.; Kraig, R.P. Youth and environmental enrichment generate serum exosomes containing miR-219 that promote CNS myelination. *Glia* **2014**, *62*, 284–299. [CrossRef]
116. Fares, R.P.; Belmeguenai, A.; Sanchez, P.E.; Kouchi, H.Y.; Bodennec, J.; Morales, A.; Georges, B.; Bonnet, C.; Bouvard, S.; Sloviter, R.S.; et al. Standardized environmental enrichment supports enhanced brain plasticity in healthy rats and prevents cognitive impairment in epileptic rats. *PLoS ONE* **2013**, *8*, e53888. [CrossRef]
117. Loma, I.; Heyman, R. Multiple Sclerosis: Pathogenesis and Treatment. *Curr. Neuropharmacol.* **2011**, *9*, 409–416. [CrossRef]
118. Zurawski, J.; Stankiewicz, J. Multiple Sclerosis Re-Examined: Essential and Emerging Clinical Concepts. *Am. J. Med.* **2017**, *10*, 1016.

119. Ebers, G.C.; Bulman, D.E.; Sadovnick, A.D.; Paty, D.W.; Warren, S.; Hader, W.; Murray, T.J.; Seland, T.P.; Duquette, P.; Grey, T.; et al. A population-based study of multiple sclerosis in twins. *New Engl. J. Med.* **1986**, *315*, 1638–1642. [CrossRef]
120. Ascherio, A.; Munger, K.L.; Lennette, E.T.; Spiegelman, D.; Hernan, M.A.; Olek, M.J.; Hankinson, S.E.; Hunter, D.J. Epstein-Barr virus antibodies and risk of multiple sclerosis: A prospective study. *JAMA* **2001**, *286*, 3083–3088. [CrossRef]
121. Tsai, C.N.; Tsai, C.L.; Tse, K.P.; Chang, H.Y.; Chang, Y.S. The Epstein-Barr virus oncogene product, latent membrane protein 1, induces the downregulation of E-cadherin gene expression via activation of DNA methyltransferases. *Proc. Natl. Acad Sci. USA* **2002**, *99*, 10084–10089. [CrossRef]
122. Baranzini, S.E.; Mudge, J.; van Velkinburgh, J.C.; Khankhanian, P.; Khrebtukova, I.; Miller, N.A.; Zhang, L.; Farmer, A.D.; Bell, C.J.; Kim, R.W.; et al. Genome, epigenome and RNA sequences of monozygotic twins discordant for multiple sclerosis. *Nature* **2010**, *464*, 1351–1356. [CrossRef]
123. Graves, M.C.; Benton, M.; Lea, R.A.; Boyle, M.; Tajouri, L.; Macartney-Coxson, D.; Scott, R.J.; Lechner-Scott, J. Methylation differences at the HLA-DRB1 locus in CD4+ T-Cells are associated with multiple sclerosis. *Mult. Scler. J.* **2013**, *20*, 1033–1041. [CrossRef]
124. Liggett, T.; Melnikov, A.; Tilwalli, S.; Yi, Q.; Chen, H.; Replogle, C.; Feng, X.; Reder, A.; Stefoski, D.; Balabanov, R.; et al. Methylation patterns of cell-free plasma DNA in relapsing-remitting multiple sclerosis. *J. Neurol. Sci.* **2010**, *290*, 16. [CrossRef]
125. Guan, H.; Nagarkatti, P.S.; Nagarkatti, M. CD44 Reciprocally Regulates the Differentiation of Encephalitogenic Th1/Th17 and Th2/Regulatory T Cells through Epigenetic Modulation Involving DNA Methylation of Cytokine Gene Promoters, Thereby Controlling the Development of Experimental Autoimmune Encephalomyelitis. *J. Immunol.* **2011**, *186*, 6955–6964.
126. Franklin, R.J.; Ffrench-Constant, C. Remyelination in the CNS: From biology to therapy. *Nat. Rev. Neurosci.* **2008**, *9*, 839–855. [CrossRef]
127. Kuhlmann, T.; Miron, V.; Cui, Q.; Wegner, C.; Antel, J.; Bruck, W. Differentiation block of oligodendroglial progenitor cells as a cause for remyelination failure in chronic multiple sclerosis. *Brain: J. Neurol.* **2008**, *131*, 1749–1758. [CrossRef]
128. Cadavid, D.; Mellion, M.; Hupperts, R.; Edwards, K.R.; Calabresi, P.A.; Drulović, J.; Giovannoni, G.; Hartung, H.-P.; Arnold, D.L.; Fisher, E.; et al. Safety and efficacy of opicinumab in patients with relapsing multiple sclerosis (SYNERGY): A randomised, placebo-controlled, phase 2 trial. *Lancet Neurol.* **2019**, *18*, 845–856. [CrossRef]
129. Moscarello, M.A.; Wood, D.D.; Ackerley, C.; Boulias, C. Myelin in multiple sclerosis is developmentally immature. *J. Clin. Investig.* **1994**, *94*, 146–154. [CrossRef]
130. Mastronardi, F.G.; Noor, A.; Wood, D.D.; Paton, T.; Moscarello, M.A. Peptidyl argininedeiminase 2 CpG island in multiple sclerosis white matter is hypomethylated. *J. Neurosci. Res.* **2007**, *85*, 2006–2016. [CrossRef]
131. Calabrese, R.; Zampieri, M.; Mechelli, R.; Annibali, V.; Guastafierro, T.; Ciccarone, F.; Coarelli, G.; Umeton, R.; Salvetti, M.; Caiafa, P. Methylation-dependent PAD2 upregulation in multiple sclerosis peripheral blood. *Mult. Scler.* **2012**, *18*, 299–304. [CrossRef]
132. Olsen, J.A.; Kenna, L.A.; Tipon, R.C.; Spelios, M.G.; Stecker, M.M.; Akirav, E.M. A Minimally-invasive Blood-derived Biomarker of Oligodendrocyte Cell-loss in Multiple Sclerosis. *EBioMedicine* **2016**, *10*, 227–235. [CrossRef]
133. Al-Mahdawi, S.; Anjomani Virmouni, S.; Pook, M.A. DNA Methylation in Neurodegenerative Diseases A2. In *Epigenetic Biomarkers and Diagnostics*; Giménez, G., Luis, J., Eds.; Academic Press: Boston, ME, USA, 2016; pp. 401–415.
134. Jakubowski, J.L.; Labrie, V. Epigenetic Biomarkers for Parkinson's Disease: From Diagnostics to Therapeutics. *J. Parkinson's Dis.* **2016**, *7*, 1–12. [CrossRef]
135. Pihlstrom, L.; Berge, V.; Rengmark, A.; Toft, M. Parkinson's disease correlates with promoter methylation in the alpha-synuclein gene. *Mov. Disord.* **2015**, *30*, 577–580. [CrossRef]
136. Huynh, J.L.; Garg, P.; Thin, T.H.; Yoo, S.; Dutta, R.; Trapp, B.D.; Haroutunian, V.; Zhu, J.; Donovan, M.J.; Sharp, A.J.; et al. Epigenome-wide differences in pathology-free regions of multiple sclerosis-affected brains. *Nat. Neurosci* **2014**, *17*, 121–130. [CrossRef]

137. Pedre, X.; Mastronardi, F.; Bruck, W.; Lopez-Rodas, G.; Kuhlmann, T.; Casaccia, P. Changed histone acetylation patterns in normal-appearing white matter and early multiple sclerosis lesions. *J. Neurosci.* **2011**, *31*, 3435–3445. [CrossRef]
138. Noorbakhsh, F.; Ellestad, K.K.; Maingat, F.; Warren, K.G.; Han, M.H.; Steinman, L.; Baker, G.B.; Power, C. Impaired neurosteroid synthesis in multiple sclerosis. *Brain J. Neurol.* **2011**, *134*, 2703–2721. [CrossRef]
139. Junker, A.; Krumbholz, M.; Eisele, S.; Mohan, H.; Augstein, F.; Bittner, R.; Lassmann, H.; Wekerle, H.; Hohlfeld, R.; Meinl, E. MicroRNA profiling of multiple sclerosis lesions identifies modulators of the regulatory protein CD47. *Brain J. Neurol.* **2009**, *132*, 3342–3352. [CrossRef]
140. Bruinsma, I.B.; van Dijk, M.; Bridel, C.; van de Lisdonk, T.; Haverkort, S.Q.; Runia, T.F.; Steinman, L.; Hintzen, R.Q.; Killestein, J.; Verbeek, M.M.; et al. Regulator of oligodendrocyte maturation, miR-219, a potential biomarker for MS. *J. Neuroinflamm.* **2017**, *14*, 235. [CrossRef]
141. Mendizabal, I.; Berto, S.; Usui, N.; Toriumi, K.; Chatterjee, P.; Douglas, C.; Huh, I.; Jeong, H.; Layman, T.; Tamminga, C.A.; et al. Cell type-specific epigenetic links to schizophrenia risk in the brain. *Genome Biol.* **2019**, *20*, 135. [CrossRef]
142. Kozlenkov, A.; Roussos, P.; Timashpolsky, A.; Barbu, M.; Rudchenko, S.; Bibikova, M.; Klotzle, B.; Byne, W.; Lyddon, R.; Di Narzo, A.F.; et al. Differences in DNA methylation between human neuronal and glial cells are concentrated in enhancers and non-CpG sites. *Nucleic Acids Res.* **2014**, *42*, 109–127. [CrossRef] [PubMed]
143. Hao, L.; Zou, Z.; Tian, H.; Zhang, Y.; Zhou, H.; Liu, L. Stem Cell-Based Therapies for Ischemic Stroke. *Biomed Res. Int.* **2014**, *2014*, 17. [CrossRef] [PubMed]
144. Kassis, H.; Chopp, M.; Liu, X.S.; Shehadah, A.; Roberts, C.; Zhang, Z.G. Histone deacetylase expression in white matter oligodendrocytes after stroke. *Neurochem. Int.* **2014**, *77*, 17–23. [CrossRef] [PubMed]
145. Felling, R.J.; Song, H. Epigenetic mechanisms of neuroplasticity and the implications for stroke recovery. *Exp. Neurol.* **2015**, *268*, 37–45. [CrossRef] [PubMed]
146. Liu, X.S.; Chopp, M.; Kassis, H.; Jia, L.F.; Hozeska-Solgot, A.; Zhang, R.L.; Chen, C.; Cui, Y.S.; Zhang, Z.G. Valproic acid increases white matter repair and neurogenesis after stroke. *Neuroscience* **2012**, *220*, 313–321. [CrossRef] [PubMed]
147. Kim, H.J.; Chuang, D.M. HDAC inhibitors mitigate ischemia-induced oligodendrocyte damage: Potential roles of oligodendrogenesis, VEGF, and anti-inflammation. *Am. J. Transl. Res.* **2014**, *6*, 206–223. [PubMed]
148. Ziemka-Nalecz, M.; Jaworska, J.; Sypecka, J.; Polowy, R.; Filipkowski, R.K.; Zalewska, T. Sodium Butyrate, a Histone Deacetylase Inhibitor, Exhibits Neuroprotective/Neurogenic Effects in a Rat Model of Neonatal Hypoxia-Ischemia. *Mol. Neurobiol.* **2017**, *54*, 5300–5318. [CrossRef] [PubMed]
149. Dincman, T.A.; Beare, J.E.; Ohri, S.S.; Gallo, V.; Hetman, M.; Whittemore, S.R. Histone deacetylase inhibition is cytotoxic to oligodendrocyte precursor cells in vitro and in vivo. *Int. J. Dev. Neurosci.* **2016**, *54*, 53–61. [CrossRef]
150. Tan, K.S.; Armugam, A.; Sepramaniam, S.; Lim, K.Y.; Setyowati, K.D.; Wang, C.W.; Jeyaseelan, K. Expression profile of MicroRNAs in young stroke patients. *PLoS ONE* **2009**, *4*, 7689. [CrossRef]
151. Delaloy, C.; Liu, L.; Lee, J.A.; Su, H.; Shen, F.; Yang, G.Y.; Young, W.L.; Ivey, K.N.; Gao, F.B. MicroRNA-9 coordinates proliferation and migration of human embryonic stem cell-derived neural progenitors. *Cell Stem Cell* **2010**, *6*, 323–335. [CrossRef]
152. Birch, D.; Britt, B.C.; Dukes, S.C.; Kessler, J.A.; Dizon, M.L. MicroRNAs participate in the murine oligodendroglial response to perinatal hypoxia-ischemia. *Pediatric Res.* **2014**, *76*, 334–340. [CrossRef] [PubMed]
153. Li, J.S.; Yao, Z.X. MicroRNA patents in demyelinating diseases: A new diagnostic and therapeutic perspective. *Recent Pat. Dna Gene Seq.* **2012**, *6*, 47–55. [CrossRef] [PubMed]
154. Dharap, A.; Vemuganti, R. Ischemic pre-conditioning alters cerebral microRNAs that are upstream to neuroprotective signaling pathways. *J. Neurochem.* **2010**, *113*, 1685–1691. [CrossRef] [PubMed]
155. Li, S.H.; Su, S.Y.; Liu, J.L. Differential Regulation of microRNAs in Patients with Ischemic Stroke. *Curr. Neurovascular Res.* **2015**, *12*, 214–221. [CrossRef]
156. Engelen, M.; Kemp, S.; Poll-The, B.T. X-linked adrenoleukodystrophy: Pathogenesis and treatment. *Curr. Neurol. Neurosci. Rep.* **2014**, *14*, 486. [CrossRef] [PubMed]
157. Schluter, A.; Sandoval, J.; Fourcade, S.; Diaz-Lagares, A.; Ruiz, M.; Casaccia, P.; Esteller, M.; Pujol, A. Epigenomic signature of adrenoleukodystrophy predicts compromised oligodendrocyte differentiation. *Brain Pathol.* **2018**, *10*, 12595. [CrossRef] [PubMed]

158. Engelen, M.; Kemp, S.; de Visser, M.; van Geel, B.M.; Wanders, R.J.A.; Aubourg, P.; Poll-The, B.T. X-linked adrenoleukodystrophy (X-ALD): Clinical presentation and guidelines for diagnosis, follow-up and management. *Orphanet J. Rare Dis.* **2012**, *7*, 51. [CrossRef] [PubMed]
159. Singh, J.; Khan, M.; Pujol, A.; Baarine, M.; Singh, I. Histone deacetylase inhibitor upregulates peroxisomal fatty acid oxidation and inhibits apoptotic cell death in abcd1-deficient glial cells. *PLoS ONE* **2013**, *8*, e70712. [CrossRef]
160. Lin, S.-T.; Ptácek, L.J.; Fu, Y.-H. Adult-onset autosomal dominant leukodystrophy: Linking nuclear envelope to myelin. *J. Neurosci.* **2011**, *31*, 1163–1166. [CrossRef]
161. Lin, S.T.; Fu, Y.H. miR-23 regulation of lamin B1 is crucial for oligodendrocyte development and myelination. *Dis. Models Mech.* **2009**, *2*, 178–188. [CrossRef]
162. Iwamoto, K.; Bundo, M.; Yamada, K.; Takao, H.; Iwayama-Shigeno, Y.; Yoshikawa, T.; Kato, T. DNA methylation status of SOX10 correlates with its downregulation and oligodendrocyte dysfunction in schizophrenia. *J. Neurosci.* **2005**, *25*, 5376–5381. [CrossRef] [PubMed]
163. Fabianowska-Majewska, K.; Wyczechowska, D.; Czyz, M. Inhibition of dna methylation by 5-aza-2′-deoxycytidine correlates with induction of K562 cells differentiation. *Adv. Exp. Med. Biol.* **2000**, *486*, 343–347. [PubMed]
164. Raj, K.; Mufti, G.J. Azacytidine (Vidaza®) in the treatment of myelodysplastic syndromes. *Ther. Clin. Risk Manag.* **2006**, *2*, 377–388. [CrossRef] [PubMed]
165. Gnyszka, A.; Jastrzebski, Z.; Flis, S. DNA methyltransferase inhibitors and their emerging role in epigenetic therapy of cancer. *Anticancer Res.* **2013**, *33*, 2989–2996. [PubMed]
166. Stresemann, C.; Lyko, F. Modes of action of the DNA methyltransferase inhibitors azacytidine and decitabine. *Int. J. Cancer* **2008**, *123*, 8–13. [CrossRef]
167. Waryah, C.B.; Moses, C.; Arooj, M.; Blancafort, P. Zinc Fingers, TALEs, and CRISPR Systems: A Comparison of Tools for Epigenome Editing. *Methods Mol. Biol.* **2018**, *1767*, 19–63.
168. Thakore, P.I.; Black, J.B.; Hilton, I.B.; Gersbach, C.A. Editing the Epigenome: Technologies for Programmable Transcriptional Modulation and Epigenetic Regulation. *Nat. Methods* **2016**, *13*, 127–137. [CrossRef]
169. Laity, J.H.; Lee, B.M.; Wright, P.E. Zinc finger proteins: New insights into structural and functional diversity. *Curr. Opin. Struct. Biol.* **2001**, *11*, 39–46. [CrossRef]
170. Rots, M.G.; Jeltsch, A. Editing the Epigenome: Overview, Open Questions, and Directions of Future Development. *Methods Mol. Biol.* **2018**, *1767*, 3–18.
171. Dai, W.J.; Zhu, L.Y.; Yan, Z.Y.; Xu, Y.; Wang, Q.L.; Lu, X.J. CRISPR-Cas9 for in vivo Gene Therapy: Promise and Hurdles. *Mol. Ther. Nucleic Acids* **2016**, *5*, 349. [CrossRef]
172. Wang, S.; Bates, J.; Li, X.; Schanz, S.; Chandler-Militello, D.; Levine, C.; Maherali, N.; Studer, L.; Hochedlinger, K.; Windrem, M.; et al. Human iPSC-derived oligodendrocyte progenitor cells can myelinate and rescue a mouse model of congenital hypomyelination. *Cell Stem Cell* **2013**, *12*, 252–264. [CrossRef] [PubMed]
173. Douvaras, P.; Rusielewicz, T.; Kim, K.H.; Haines, J.D.; Casaccia, P.; Fossati, V. Epigenetic Modulation of Human Induced Pluripotent Stem Cell Differentiation to Oligodendrocytes. *Int. J. Mol. Sci.* **2016**, *17*, 614. [CrossRef] [PubMed]
174. Douvaras, P.; Wang, J.; Zimmer, M.; Hanchuk, S.; O'Bara, M.A.; Sadiq, S.; Sim, F.J.; Goldman, J.; Fossati, V. Efficient Generation of Myelinating Oligodendrocytes from Primary Progressive Multiple Sclerosis Patients by Induced Pluripotent Stem Cells. *Stem Cell Rep.* **2014**, *3*, 250–259. [CrossRef] [PubMed]

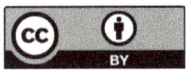

© 2019 by the authors. Licensee MDPI, Basel, Switzerland. This article is an open access article distributed under the terms and conditions of the Creative Commons Attribution (CC BY) license (http://creativecommons.org/licenses/by/4.0/).

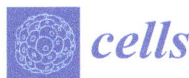

Article

Laquinimod Supports Remyelination in Non-Supportive Environments

Stella Nyamoya [1,2,†], Julia Steinle [2,†], Uta Chrzanowski [3], Joel Kaye [4], Christoph Schmitz [3], Cordian Beyer [2] and Markus Kipp [2,5,*]

1. Institute of Anatomy, Rostock University Medical Center, 18057 Rostock, Germany; Stella.Nyamoya@rwth-aachen.de
2. Institute of Neuroanatomy and JARA-BRAIN, Faculty of Medicine, RWTH Aachen University, 52074 Aachen, Germany; Julia.Steinle@rwth-aachen.de (J.S.); CBeyer@ukaachen.de (C.B.)
3. Department of Anatomy II, Ludwig-Maximilians-University of Munich, 80336 Munich, Germany; Uta.Chrzanowski@med.uni-muenchen.de (U.C.); Christoph_Schmitz@med.uni-muenchen.de (C.S.)
4. AyalaPharma, VP Research & Nonclinical Development, Rehovot 7670104, Israel; joel.k@ayalapharma.com
5. Centre for Transdisciplinary Neurosciences, Rostock University Medical Center, 18057 Rostock, Germany
* Correspondence: Markus.Kipp@med.uni-rostock.de; Tel.: +49-(0)-381-494-8401
† These authors contributed equally to this work.

Academic Editor: Sassan Hafizi
Received: 10 October 2019; Accepted: 22 October 2019; Published: 31 October 2019

Abstract: Inflammatory demyelination, which is a characteristic of multiple sclerosis lesions, leads to acute functional deficits and, in the long term, to progressive axonal degeneration. While remyelination is believed to protect axons, the endogenous-regenerative processes are often incomplete or even completely fail in many multiple sclerosis patients. Although it is currently unknown why remyelination fails, recurrent demyelination of previously demyelinated white matter areas is one contributing factor. In this study, we investigated whether laquinimod, which has demonstrated protective effects in active multiple sclerosis patients, protects against recurrent demyelination. To address this, male mice were intoxicated with cuprizone for up to eight weeks and treated with either a vehicle solution or laquinimod at the beginning of week 5, where remyelination was ongoing. The brains were harvested and analyzed by immunohistochemistry. At the time-point of laquinimod treatment initiation, oligodendrocyte progenitor cells proliferated and matured despite ongoing demyelination activity. In the following weeks, myelination recovered in the laquinimod- but not vehicle-treated mice, despite continued cuprizone intoxication. Myelin recovery was paralleled by less severe microgliosis and acute axonal injury. In this study, we were able to demonstrate that laquinimod, which has previously been shown to protect against cuprizone-induced oligodendrocyte degeneration, exerts protective effects during oligodendrocyte progenitor differentiation as well. By this mechanism, laquinimod allows remyelination in non-supportive environments. These results should encourage further clinical studies in progressive multiple sclerosis patients.

Keywords: multiple sclerosis; remyelination; cuprizone; neurodegeneration; laquinimod

---

1. Introduction

Multiple sclerosis (MS) has a complex pathomechanism, leading to the formation of inflammatory demyelinating lesions within the central nervous system (CNS). Such lesions, which can be found in white and grey matter, are characterized by the loss of oligodendrocytes to a variable extent, focal and diffuse myelin pathology, and astrocyte and microglia activation, as well as damage to nerve cells [1-6]. On the clinical level, distinct disease courses can be distinguished: At the beginning of the disease most patients suffer from the sudden occurrence of new neurological symptoms, which usually disappear after several weeks [7]. This initial disease course is called relapsing-remitting MS (RRMS), which means that symptoms appear (i.e., a relapse) and then fade away, either partially or completely (i.e., remitting). By definition, during the RRMS disease phase, the level of clinical disability remains stable in between two relapses. After several years (10–15 years), the frequency of relapses decreases, and patients clinically deteriorate independent of the relapses. This so-called secondary-progressive MS (SPMS) course is characterized by chronically progressive clinical worsening over time, with or without superimposed relapses. In about 15% of patients, the disease is characterized by neurologic worsening (accumulation of disability) from the onset of symptoms, without early relapses or remissions. Here, this is called primary-progressive MS (PPMS). Depending on the location of the demyelinated lesions within the CNS, clinical symptoms can vary substantially between different patients [8,9]. While inflammation is believed to be the pathological correlate of relapses during RRMS, neurodegeneration, especially axonal damage, is thought to be the underlying substratum of irreversible clinical disability accumulating during the progressive stage of the disease [10,11].

The mechanisms underlying the progressive neurodegeneration in MS are currently unknown, but the failure of remyelination appears to play a significant role. Remyelination is a very complex biological process and can be classified, on the cellular level, as four consecutive steps: (i) Proliferation of oligodendrocyte progenitor cells (OPCs); (ii) OPC migration towards the demyelinated axons; (iii) OPC differentiation; and finally, (iv) interaction of the premature oligodendrocyte with the axon (i.e., axon wrapping) [12]. It has been accepted since early neuropathological studies that in MS, demyelinated lesions can remyelinate, although there are extremely limited data on the quantitative extent and natural history of this repair process [13–15]. The existence of so called 'shadow plaques', representing remyelinated lesions, clearly demonstrates that the complete repair of MS plaques is principally possible, although it is more common to observe only limited repair at the edge of lesions [16,17]. It is not clear why in some patients remyelination is widespread while in others it is sparse. Clearly, remyelination is neuroprotective, and if remyelination fails, different biochemical mechanisms can trigger delayed axonal degeneration, along with an increased energy demand of impulse conduction along excitable demyelinated axons [18], a lack of axonal trophic support provided by oligodendrocytes [19], a lethal rise in intra-axonal calcium levels [20], or the higher vulnerability of demyelinated axons against cytotoxic substances. Of note, several reports suggest that the recurrent demyelination of demyelinated white matter areas is one of the factors underlying remyelination failure in MS [21–23]. For example, in a detailed histopathological study, around 15% of remyelinated shadow plaques showed evidence of a superimposed, new demyelinating activity [21]. In another study, serial magnetization transfer imaging in RRMS and SPMS patients showed that in both patient cohorts new lesions form in previously lesional tissue that appears to be experiencing a second round of inflammatory demyelination (i.e., repeat lesions) [23]. In line with these findings, several pre-clinical studies have shown that recurrent episodes of demyelination occur at sites of previous demyelination [24–26]. Indeed, demyelinated foci can be a potent trigger for peripheral immune cell recruitment [27–29]. An increased understanding of how inflammation alters cell intrinsic and extrinsic factors to, in turn, influence OPC proliferation, recruitment, differentiation, and, ultimately, remyelination, is crucial for the development of novel therapies that target disease progression. Moreover, a need exists to elucidate the factors that contribute to successful remyelination as well as those that result from its failure.

One of the models which allows such questions to be addressed is the cuprizone model. In this model, oral intoxication with copper-chelator cuprizone induces, oligodendrocyte apoptosis within days, which is closely followed by the activation of the innate immune cells of the brain, i.e., astrocytes and microglia, finally leading to the demyelination of distinct white and grey matter brain areas. Although OPCs are activated during the course of cuprizone intoxication [30], remyelination fails due to an ongoing cuprizone-induced mature oligodendrocyte injury. In this study, we tested the hypothesis that laquinimod, which has been shown to ameliorate cuprizone-induced demyelination [31,32], supports remyelination in non-supportive environments. To this end, mice were intoxicated with cuprizone for up to 8 weeks and treated with laquinimod, starting at the beginning of week 5, when the endogenous remyelination pathways are activated in this model. We can show that daily laquinimod treatment induces myelin recovery, which is paralleled by an amelioration of axonal degeneration.

2. Material and Methods

2.1. Animals and Experimental Setup

C57BL/6 mice were purchased either from Janvier Labs, Le Genest-Saint-Isle, France or provided by TEVA. All experimental procedures were approved by the Review Board for the Care of Animal Subjects of the district government (Regierung Oberbayern; reference number 55.2-154-2532-73-15; Germany) and the local ethics committee of Teva Pharmaceutical Industries Ltd. The animals were randomly allocated to the different experimental groups and were kept under standard laboratory conditions with access to food and water ad libitum. Demyelination was induced by intoxicating mice with a diet containing 0.3% cuprizone (bis(cyclohexanone)oxaldihydrazone) mixed into pellets and or standard pelleted rodent chow for the indicated treatment period. The control mice (5 animals per group) were fed standard pelleted rodent chow for the entire duration of the study. The following treatment groups were included in the study: Control animals (CO), 4-weeks CPZ (cuprizone), where the animals were intoxicated with cuprizone for 4 weeks; 6-week CPZ and vehicle, where the animals were intoxicated with cuprizone for 6 weeks. With this group, at the beginning of week 5, the animals were subjected daily to an oral gavage with the vehicle solution (100 µL); 6-week CPZ and laquinimod (LAQ), where the animals were intoxicated with cuprizone for 6 weeks. With the group, at the beginning of week 5, the animals were subjected daily to an oral gavage with the laquinimod solution (100 µL); 8-week CPZ and vehicle, where the animals were intoxicated with cuprizone for 8 weeks. With this group, at the beginning of week 5, the animals were subjected daily to an oral gavage with the vehicle solution (100 µL); 8-week CPZ and LAQ, where the animals were intoxicated with cuprizone for 8 weeks. With this group, at the beginning of week 5, the animals were subjected daily to an oral gavage with the laquinimod solution (100 µL). See Figure 1A for a schematic illustration of the experiment setup. An additional cohort of C57BL/6 mice was intoxicated with 0.25% cuprizone mixed in the ground rodent chow for the duration of 1 (5 animals), 3 (4 animals), or 5 weeks (5 animals) to study OPC responses.

2.2. Tissue Preparation

For the histological and immunohistochemical studies, the preparation of tissue was performed as previously described [33,34]. In brief, mice were transcardially perfused with ice-cold PBS (Phosphate-buffered saline), followed by a 3.7% formalin solution (pH 7.4). After overnight post-fixation in the same fixative, the brains were dissected and embedded in paraffin, and coronal 5-µm-thick sections were prepared for immunohistochemistry. The coronal slices were analyzed at level 265 according to the mouse brain atlas published by Sidman et al. (http://www.hms.harvard.edu/research/brain/atlas.html).

2.3. Luxol Fast Blue (LFB) Periodic Acid–Schiff (PAS) Stain and Myelin Status Scoring

The intact and damaged myelin were both histochemically visualized using Luxol fast blue / periodic acid–Schiff (LFB/PAS) stains. To this end, the slides were deparaffinized in 4 × 5 min xylene, rinsed 3 × 3 min in 100% ethanol, followed by 2 × 5 min in 96% ethanol. The sections were then subsequently incubated in a LFB solution (0.1 g Luxol fast blue; 7709, Carl Roth, Karlsruhe, Germany) in 100 mL 96% ethanol plus 500 µL acetic acid (3738, Carl Roth, Germany), overnight at 60 °C. On the next day, the sections were dipped into 96% ethanol, followed by water, and processed in a lithium carbonate solution (0.05 g lithium carbonate [1.05680.0250, Merck, Darmstadt, Germany] in 100 mL aqua (dist.). The sections were further differentiated in 70% ethanol for a few seconds and rinsed in water. Afterwards, oxidation was performed in periodic acid (0.5 g periodic acid [1.00524.0025, Merck, Germany] in 100 mL aqua dist.). Sections were rinsed, followed by incubation in Schiff's reaction

(1.09033.0500, Merck, Germany) for 15 min, then rinsed in warm tap water for 5 min and counterstained with hematoxylin (1.04302.0025, Merck, Germany) for 1 min. The sections were dehydrated and subsequently mounted in DePeX (18243, Serva Electrophoresis GmbH, Heidelberg, Germany) for further analyses. Myelination in the corpus callosum was analyzed by scoring the LFB/PAS stained sections, ranging from 100% ("normal" myelination) to 0% (complete demyelination). Two evaluators blinded to the treatment groups performed the scoring, and the results were averaged.

2.4. Immunohistochemistry and Densitometric Analyses

For immunohistochemistry, sections were rehydrated and, if necessary, antigens were unmasked with heat in a Tris/EDTA (pH 9.0) or citrate (pH 6.0) buffer. After washing in PBS, sections were incubated overnight (4 °C) with the different primary antibody solutions (Table 1). The following primary antibody concentrations were applied: Anti-PLP 1:5000, anti-MAG 1:2500, anti-IBA1 1:10000, anti-APP 1:5000, anti-APC/CC1 1:250, and anti-OLIG2 1:2000. The next day, the slides were incubated in a biotinylated secondary antibody solution [(i) horse anti-mouse IgG, 1:50; (ii) goat anti-rabbit IgG, 1:50] for 1 h and then incubated in a peroxidase-coupled avidin–biotin complex solution (ABC-HRP kit; PK-6100, RRID AB 2336819, Vector Laboratories, USA). Finally, the slides were incubated in 3,3′-diaminobenzidine (K3468, DAKO, Germany) as a peroxidase substrate. A detailed list of applied antibodies is given in Tables 1 and 2.

Table 1. Primary antibodies used in this study.

Name	Host/Clone	Order Number	RRID	Supplier
MAG	Mouse monoclonal	ab89780	AB_2042411	Abcam
IBA1	Rabbit polyclonal	019-19741	AB_839504	WAKO
APP (A4)	Mouse monoclonal	MAB348	AB_94882	Millipore
APC (Ab-7)	Mouse monoclonal	OP80	AB_2057371	Millipore
PLP	Mouse monoclonal	MCA839G	AB_2237198	Biorad
OLIG2	Mouse monoclonal	MABN50	AB_10807410	Millipore
Ki67	Rabbit monoclonal	ab16667	AB_302459	Abcam

Table 2. Secondary antibodies used in this study.

Name	Host/Clone	Order Number	RRID	Supplier
Biotinylated Goat Anti-Rabbit IgG	Goat Polyclonal	BA-1000	AB_2313606	Vector Laboratories
Biotinylated Horse Anti-Mouse IgG	Horse Polyclonal	BA-2000	AB_2313581	Vector Laboratories
Donkey anti-Rabbit IgG (H+L) Highly Cross-Adsorbed Secondary Antibody, Alexa Fluor 488	Donkey Polyclonal	A21206	AB_2535792	Thermo Fisher Scientific
Goat anti-Mouse IgG2a Cross-Adsorbed Secondary Antibody, Alexa Fluor 546	Goat Polyclonal	A21133	AB_2535772	Thermo Fisher Scientific

The stained and processed sections were digitalized using a Nikon Eclipse 80i microscope (Nikon Instruments, Düsseldorf, Germany) equipped with a DS-2MV camera. The open source program ImageJ 1.48v (NIH, Bethesda, MD, USA) was used to evaluate the staining intensities using semi-automated densitometrical evaluation after a threshold setting. Relative staining intensities were then semi-quantified in binary converted images, and the results were presented as percentage areas. Cell and spheroid numbers were quantified after manually delineating the region of interest (ROI;

i.e., the midline of the corpus callosum). The ROI-area was quantified, and results were presented as cells or spheroids/mm^2. Additional slides were scanned using the Nikon Eclipse E200 microscope (Nikon Instruments, Germany) equipped with a Basler acA1920-40um camera (Basler AG, Ahrensburg, Germany) and manual scanning software (manualWSI software, Microvisioneer, München, Germany). Cell numbers were quantified after manually delineating the ROI using the program ViewPoint (PreciPoint GmbH, Freising, Germany). Two evaluators blinded to the treatment groups performed the scoring and the results were averaged.

2.5. Immunofluorescence Double Labelling

For the immunofluorescence double labeling experiments, the sections were rehydrated, the sites of antigens unmasked by heating in a Tris/EDTA (pH 9.0) or citrate (pH 6.0) buffer, blocked with PBS containing 2% heat-inactivated fetal calf serum ([FCS], A15-152, PAA, Germany) and 1% bovine serum albumin ([BSA], 0163, Carl Roth, Karlsruhe, Germany), and incubated overnight (4 °C) with the first primary mouse anti-OLIG2 antibody (1:1000) diluted in the blocking solution to visualize oligodendrocytes. After washing, the sections were incubated with the appropriate fluorescent secondary antibody (1:500, anti-mouse Alexa Fluor 546) diluted in the blocking solution for 1 h (room temperature). The sections were subsequently washed and incubated overnight (4 °C), with the second rabbit anti-Ki67 primary antibody (1:1500) diluted in the blocking solution to visualize proliferating cells. After washing, the sections were incubated with the second fluorescent secondary antibody (1:500, anti-rabbit Alexa Fluor 488) diluted in the blocking solution for 1 h. Subsequently, sections were incubated with a Hoechst 33342 solution (1:10000, H3570, Thermo Fisher Scientific, Waltham, MA, USA) diluted in PBS for the staining of cell nuclei. A detailed list of applied antibodies is given in Tables 1 and 2. The stained and processed sections were documented with the Leica microscope DMI6000B working station (Leica Microsystems, Wetzlar, Germany). Cell numbers were quantified after manually delineating the corpus callosum using the open source program ImageJ 1.48v (NIH, USA). Single and double positive cells were counted within the region of interest. Two evaluators (S.N. and J.S./U.C.) blinded to the treatment groups performed the scoring, and the results were averaged. To rule out unspecific binding of the fluorescent secondary antibodies to primary antibodies, appropriate negative controls were performed by first incubating sections with the primary antibodies and subsequently incubating these sections with the wrong fluorescent secondary antibody. Unspecific secondary antibody binding to the tissue itself was checked by performing negative controls by incubating sections with each of the fluorescent secondary antibodies alone (data not shown).

2.6. Statistical Analyses

The statistical analyses were performed using GraphPad Prism 5. The data are presented as arithmetic means ± SEM. Non-Gaussian distribution was assumed. The data were analyzed with either the Mann–Whitney or Kruskal–Wallis test, followed by Dunn's multiple comparison test. Here, results where $p < 0.05$ were considered statistically significant. The following symbols were used to indicate the level of significance: * $p < 0.05$, ** $p < 0.005$, and *** $p < 0.001$.

3. Results

To determine the potential effect of laquinimod (LAQ) on intrinsic remyelination capacity during continuous toxin-induced demyelination, mice were intoxicated with cuprizone (CPZ) for either 6 or 8 weeks. At the beginning of week 5, both cohorts were treated with either the vehicle or laquinimod solution until the end of the experiment (see Figure 1A for the detailed experimental setup).

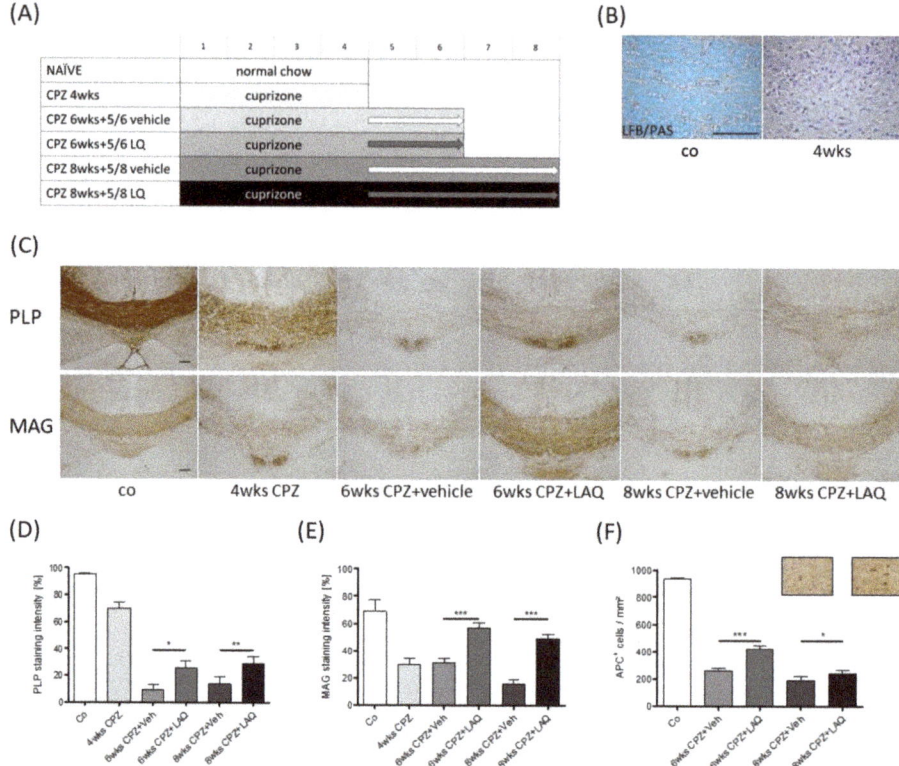

Figure 1. Influence of laquinimod on remyelination in the non-supportive environment. (**A**) Schematic depiction of the experimental setup. Numbers indicate the duration of the experiment in weeks. The control group is colored in white, cuprizone (CPZ) intoxication groups are colored in grayscale and black. The arrows indicate treatment with either the vehicle (Veh, light gray) or laquinimod (LAQ, dark gray) solutions. (**B**) Representative image of Luxol fast blue / periodic acid–Schiff (LFB/PAS) staining of a control animal and an animal intoxicated with cuprizone for 4 weeks. (**C**) Representative images of anti-PLP and anti-MAG stained sections of the midline corpus callosum. Densitometric analysis of (**D**) anti-PLP and (**E**) anti-MAG staining intensity (repetitive Mann–Whitney test, as indicated). (**F**) Quantification of APC$^+$ cell numbers (repetitive Mann Whitney test as indicated). Representative images of anti-APC immunohistochemical stained sections of the medial corpus callosum of 8 weeks cuprizone plus vehicle (left) or laquinimod (right) treatment groups. Scale bar: 100 μm. The following symbols were used to indicate the level of significance: * $p < 0.05$, ** $p < 0.005$, and *** $p < 0.001$.

To analyze the extent of de- and re-myelination, LFB/PAS, anti-PLP, and anti-MAG stains were performed, and the staining intensity was quantified in the midline of the corpus callosum (Figure 1D,E). At the end of week 4, myelin pathology was clearly evident in the LFB/PAS stained sections, indicated by a pronounced loss of LFB staining intensity (Figure 1B). Anti-PLP (co 95.1 ± 1.05%, 4 wks CPZ 69.9 ± 4.26%) and anti-MAG (co 68.9 ± 8.56%, 4 wks CPZ 30.0 ± 4.52%) staining intensity loss was less severe, yet clearly evident. To analyze, whether laquinimod protects new-born myelinating oligodendrocytes, and thus support endogenous remyelination in a non-supportive environment, another cohort of mice was treated daily with either the vehicle or laquinimod solution, starting at the beginning of week 5. To allow early remyelination, mice were sacrificed at week 6. As demonstrated in Figure 1, the anti-PLP and anti-MAG staining intensities were higher in the laquinimod-treated mice compared to the vehicle-treated mice. To verify these findings, a third cohort of mice was sacrificed at week 8 (i.e., after 4 weeks of laquinimod treatment), and the myelination status of the corpus callosum was analyzed. Comparable to what we found at week 6, the anti-PLP and anti-MAG staining intensities were higher in the laquinimod-treated mice compared to the vehicle-treated mice.

To analyze, whether higher myelination levels in laquinimod-treated groups are paralleled by higher densities of mature oligodendrocytes, we quantified the densities of anti-APC$^+$ cells in the different treatment groups (Figure 1F). A severe reduction of APC$^+$ cell densities was found in both vehicle treated groups (co 932.8 ± 8.04 cells/mm^2, 6 weeks CPZ and Veh 261.5 ± 15.34 cells/mm^2, 8 weeks CPZ and Veh 188.6 ± 31.41 cells/mm^2), whereas the number of APC$^+$ cells were significantly higher in the laquinimod-treated groups (6 weeks CPZ and LAQ 420.7 ± 21.78 cells/mm^2, 8 weeks CPZ and LAQ 240.9 ± 24.32 cells/mm^2).

To verify whether remyelination was ongoing at the time point when we started the laquinimod treatment (i.e., at the beginning of week 5), we analyzed the densities of proliferating OPC in OLIG2/Ki67-double stained sections during the course of cuprizone-induced demyelination. As demonstrated in Figure 2A, the number of OLIG2$^+$/Ki67$^+$ cells, resembling proliferating OPCs, were low in control animals and animals intoxicated for 1 week with cuprizone, but high (~70 cells/mm^2) at weeks 3 and 5. The percentage of Ki67$^+$ cells among all OLIG2$^+$ cells was highest at week 3 and decreased till week 5 (Figure 2B). Furthermore, the number of APC$^+$ cells was low at weeks 1 and 3 but recovered at week 5 (Figure 2D). These results implicate that remyelination was already ongoing at week 3 and entered the OPC differentiation stage at week 5. Taken together, these results suggest that while remyelination fails during a continuous cuprizone-intoxication protocol in vehicle-treated mice, myelin recovery occurs in laquinimod-treated mice.

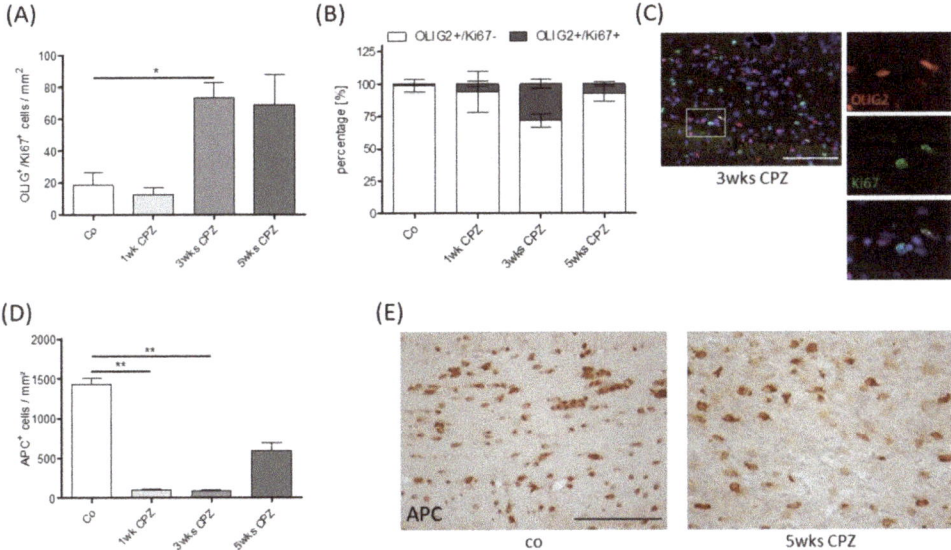

Figure 2. Oligodendrocyte pathology. (**A**) Quantity of OLIG2$^+$ and Ki67$^+$ single and double positive cells during the course of cuprizone-induced demyelination (Kruskal–Wallis test followed by Dunn's multiple comparison test). (**B**) Percentage of single and double positive cells in relation to the entire OLIG2$^+$ cell population. (**C**) Representative image of OLIG2$^+$ and Ki67$^+$ double positive cells. (**D**) Quantification of APC$^+$ cell numbers (Kruskal–Wallis test followed by Dunn's multiple comparison test). (**E**) Representative images of anti-APC stained sections in the medial corpus callosum. Scale bar: 100 μm. The following symbols were used to indicate the level of significance: * $p < 0.05$, ** $p < 0.005$.

The recent work of our lab suggests that the extent of microglia activation is an important determinant for acute axonal injury in this model [35]. To analyze whether the activation status of microglia cells was affected by the laquinimod treatment, anti-IBA1 stains were performed, and differences in staining intensities were assessed via densitometric analyses. As demonstrated in Figure 3A,C, microglia activation was clearly evident in both vehicle-treated groups. Of note, anti-IBA1 staining intensities were considerably less severe at week 6 (6 weeks CPZ and Veh 36.8 ± 3.41% versus 6 weeks CPZ and LAQ 23.0 ± 1.96%), and tended to be lower at week 8 (8 weeks CPZ and Veh 23.8 ± 2.35% versus 8 weeks CPZ and LAQ 18.0 ± 2.09%) in the laquinimod-treated groups compared to the vehicle-treated groups. To determine the extent of acute axonal injury, we quantified the accumulation of synaptic vesicles by anti-APP stains (Figure 3B,D). As expected, APP$^+$ spheroids were virtually absent in the control animals, whereas numerous could be found in the vehicle-treated mice. Here, the numbers were, by trend, lower in laquinimod-treated mice at week 8 (APP: CPZ and Veh 25.8 ± 5.79 spheroids/mm^2 versus CPZ and LAQ 10.3 ± 1.86 spheroids/mm^2).

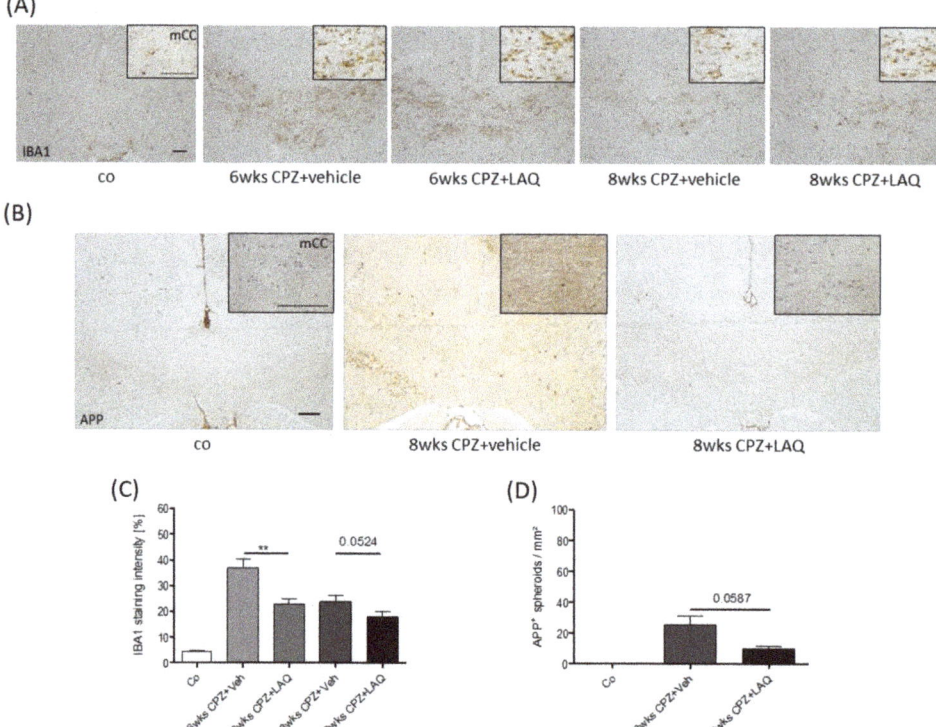

Figure 3. Microglia/monocyte accumulation and axonal damage. (**A**) Accumulation of microglia/monocytes visualized by anti-IBA1 immunohistochemistry. Inserts show the medial corpus callosum in higher magnification. (**B**) Axonal injury visualized by anti-APP immunohistochemistry. (**C**) Densitometric analysis of anti-IBA1 stains (Mann–Whitney test). (**D**) APP$^+$ spheroid density quantification (Mann–Whitney test). Scale bar: 100μm. The following symbols were used to indicate the level of significance: ** $p < 0.005$.

Finally, we were interested whether laquinimod modulates the proliferation of OPC. To this end, the proportion of proliferating (Ki67$^+$) oligodendrocytes (OLIG2$^+$) was quantified in the different treatment groups. Low numbers of proliferating OLIG2$^+$-cells were found in the control animals (~0.55%), whereas numerous were found after 6 weeks of cuprizone intoxication. However, no difference was observed between the vehicle- (~5.96%) versus laquinimod-treated (~5.91%) groups (see Supplementary Figure).

4. Discussion

In this study, we have applied the following characteristic of the cuprizone model: During continuous cuprizone intoxication, remyelination fails because differentiating oligodendrocytes become vulnerable to the cuprizone toxin during differentiation. The results of in vitro studies suggest that cuprizone is selectively toxic for mature oligodendrocytes, whereas OPCs are not affected [36]. Furthermore, microglia, astrocytes, and SH-SY5Y cells were resistant to cuprizone [36,37]. We assume that once OPCs reach a certain differentiation stage, they become vulnerable against cuprizone and die, which results in the failure of remyelination during a continuous intoxication period [38]. However, if cuprizone is removed from the diet, OPCs can fully differentiate and remyelinate the affected white and grey matter brain areas. In consistence with this idea, it has been demonstrated that cuprizone retards the differentiation of oligodendrocytes in vitro [39]. Cell counts have suggested that cuprizone inhibits the maturation of oligodendrocytes without diminishing the numbers of precursors. Although it remains unclear why mature oligodendrocytes are preferentially vulnerable to cuprizone, the recent results of our lab suggest that an impaired protein folding machinery, together with stress reactions within the endoplasmic reticulum, might play an important role [40]. Oligodendrocytes protrude processes, where at the end of which, sheet-like extensions are formed, namely, myelin membranes, which ensheath axons in a multilamellar fashion to provide proper saltatory nerve conduction as well as trophic and metabolic support. Myelin membranes are unique in that approximately 70% of their dry weight consists of lipids, in particular, cholesterol, and the galactolipids galactosylceramide and sulfatide. Furthermore, myelin also contains a specific repertoire of myelin proteins, among which PLP and myelin basic protein (MBP) are the most abundant ones. All elements of this myelination machinery require a careful mutual orchestration. For example, mitochondria and the endoplasmic reticulum are two major organelles implicated in the cholesterol biosynthesis machinery. Mitochondria, for example, provide acetyl-CoAs, which are needed for cholesterol biosynthesis. On the other hand, the endoplasmic reticulum plays major roles during the propagation of secretory and membrane proteins. Since both cellular compartments, namely, the mitochondria and the endoplasmic reticulum, are functionally disturbed in the cuprizone model [40–42], alterations in protein–lipid trafficking or misfolding in conformational changes of myelin proteins may cause mature oligodendrocyte degeneration.

To investigate, whether newly formed oligodendrocytes are protected by laquinimod, it was essential to initiate the treatment at a time point where OPC differentiation had already started in the experimental mice. As demonstrated in Figure 2, we found low numbers of proliferating OLIG2$^+$ cells in the control and 1 week cuprizone-intoxicated mice, whereas numerous were found at weeks 3 and 5. Furthermore, the quantification of APC/CC1$^+$ cell numbers revealed low numbers at weeks 1 and 3, but this rapidly rebounded by the fifth week of cuprizone treatment, despite continued intoxication [43]. These data suggest that the process of remyelination, i.e., OPC proliferation and maturation, is an ongoing process between weeks 3 and 5 in this model. In line with this assumption, a recent study of our group demonstrated the presence of stressed OLIG2$^+$ cells after week 5 [40], implicating that the OPCs had reached a differentiation level which had rendered them prone to the toxic effects of cuprizone. Furthermore, previous studies have indicated that the first OPCs begin to accumulate in the corpus callosum 2 weeks after initiating the cuprizone challenge, and peak between 2 to 3 weeks thereafter [30,44,45]. Thus, remyelination in the corpus callosum occurs even before demyelination is complete. Interestingly, a recent study revealed that densities of APC/CC1$^+$ oligodendrocytes at 6 weeks of recovery from a cuprizone intoxication protocol were greater than that of control mice, suggesting that cuprizone-induced injury leads to differentiation of more oligodendrocytes than would be expected without injury [43]. In support of this, the density of PDGFRα^+ OPCs at 4 weeks of cuprizone-treatment was approximately 2.5 times greater than the age-matched controls, indicating that there was a massive mobilization of progenitors after demyelination to differentiate and remyelinate the corpus callosum. To conclude, the results provided in this study and reports from others using the same model system strongly suggest that, in this study, laquinimod treatment was initiated at a time point when early remyelination cascades were already active.

Laquinimod is an immunomodulatory drug with potential anti-inflammatory and neuroprotective effects, and has been tested in MS animal models as well as in clinical studies [46,47]. Clinical trials have shown that the number of active lesions in RRMS patients are reduced and that brain volume reduction is ameliorated by laquinimod [48–50]. Pre-clinical studies have revealed that laquinimod has the capacity to reduce demyelination in the cuprizone model and in EAE (Experimental autoimmune encephalomyelitis) [31,32,47]. Furthermore, laquinimod prevents axonal damage, synaptic loss, and modulates immune response [31,32,51–53]. A number of studies suggest that laquinimod might as well be protective in other CNS pathologies than MS. For example, beneficial effects have been reported in models of Huntington's disease [54–56] or in a model of traumatic brain injury [57]. However, in other experimental neurodegeneration models, such as in a model of Alzheimer's disease, laquinimod did not show protective effects [58]. Two big clinical phase three trials were conducted to study the effectiveness of laquinimod in RRMS patients, the BRAVO (Benefit-Risk Assessment of Avonex and Laquinimod) trial [59] and ALLEGRO (Assessment of Oral Laquinimod in Preventing Progression in Multiple Sclerosis) trial [50]. In the BRAVO study, once-daily oral laquinimod resulted in statistically nonsignificant reductions in annualized relapse rate and disability progression, but significant reductions in brain atrophy versus a placebo. In the ALLEGRO trial, oral laquinimod administered once daily slowed the progression of disability and reduced the rate of relapse in patients with RRMS. Unfortunately, laquinimod failed to slow brain atrophy and disease progression in PPMS patients enrolled in the ARPEGGIO phase two clinical trial. Laquinimod was also evaluated as a potential therapy for Huntington's disease in the LEGATO-HD phase two clinical trial [60], however, it failed to meet its primary objective of improving motor function in Huntington's disease patients after 12 months of treatment. Most of the pre-clinical MS studies with laquinimod were performed using EAE, which recapitulates the autoimmune aspect of MS [61–64]. While auto-immune driven inflammatory demyelination is an important component of the RRMS disease stage, it is believed that autoimmunity plays a minor role in PPMS. This is best demonstrated by the finding that the classical immunomodulatory drugs [65,66] or immunosuppressive interventions [67] are largely ineffective in PPMS patients. Beyond that, histopathological studies have demonstrated that there is significantly more inflammation in SPMS (as judged by the frequency of perivascular cuffing and cellularity of the parenchyma) than in PPMS [68], and imaging studies have shown that PPMS patients have lower mean brain T2 and T1 hypointensity lesion loads than SPMS patients [69]. Why exactly the observed beneficial effects of laquinimod in pre-clinical studies did not translate into a positive impact in PPMS patients is currently unknown. On the one hand, the pathogenesis of PPMS is still largely unknown. Implicated mechanisms include the chronification of inflammation behind the relatively intact blood brain barrier, diffuse meningeal inflammation, reactive oxygen and nitrogen species produced by microglia, inducing mitochondrial dysfunction, neuronal Ca^{2+} overload, and others (see [70] for a recent review on that topic). On the other hand, classical pre-clinical animal models, especially EAE, poorly reflect the complex pathogenesis of PPMS.

In this study, we have applied a pre-clinical MS model which shares several characteristics of progressive MS, among innate driven myelin and axonal injury, functional activation of oxidative stress pathways [71], or the relative preservation of the blood-brain-barrier [72]. We were able to show that laquinimod supports remyelination in the non-supportive environment used in this model. While the results of most studies suggest that remyelination is neuroprotective [73–75], the results of Manrique-Hoyos and colleagues suggest that axonal degeneration continues to progress at a low level even if remyelination is complete. In their studies, animals showed an initial recovery of locomotor performance after acute cuprizone-induced demyelination. However, long after remyelination was completed (approximately 6 months after the last demyelinating episode), locomotor performance again declined in remyelinated animals as compared to the age-matched controls. This functional decline was accompanied by brain atrophy and callosal axonal loss [76]. It thus might be that laquinimod indeed restores myelin integrity in PPMS patients which does, however, not result in a superior clinical outcome or a preservation of brain atrophy. Clearly, a more complete understanding of the mechanisms involved in the pathogenesis of progressive MS phenotypes and animal models that incorporate these pathogenic characteristics is urgently needed. Comparably, further studies are needed to elucidate the underlying mechanisms of laquinimod's protective effects in this model. As demonstrated in Figure 3, laquinimod ameliorated microglia reactivity. Microglial activation is a common feature of diverse CNS diseases, and although in some instances this activation can be damaging, the protective and regenerative functions of microglia have been revealed [77]. In the context of myelination disorders, it has been demonstrated that microglia can support remyelination in the CNS after injury via the clearance of debris, secretion of growth factors and cytokines, and through modulation of the extracellular matrix [78–80]. Furthermore, microglia contribute to developmental myelinogenesis and to oligodendrocyte progenitor maintenance during adulthood [78,81,82]. Beyond that, astrocytes orchestrate myelin repair by modulating microglia activity [83]. Since laquinimod can regulate glial/macrophage cell function [57,63], it might well be that parts of the observed protective effects of laquinimod in this study are due to a direct interaction with astrocytes and/or microglia.

5. Conclusions

In this study we were able to demonstrate that laquinimod, which has previously been shown to protect against cuprizone-induced oligodendrocyte degeneration, exerts protective effects during OPC differentiation as well. By this mechanism, laquinimod allows remyelination in non-supportive environments. These results should encourage further clinical studies in SPMS patients. Of note, laquinimod could have a significant place in the therapy of more advanced stages of disease but careful clinical studies assessing properly this potential should be conducted.

Supplementary Materials: The following are available online at http://www.mdpi.com/2073-4409/8/11/1363/s1. Figure S1: Percentage of proliferating (Ki67$^+$) oligodendrocytes (OLIG2$^+$) of control, 4 weeks of cuprizone intoxication, 6 and 8 weeks of cuprizone intoxication and vehicle or laquinimod groups.

Author Contributions: Conceptualization, J.K. and M.K.; methodology, J.K. and M.K.; validation, S.N., J.S., U.C. and M.K.; formal analysis, S.N., J.S. and M.K.; investigation, S.N., J.S., U.C. and M.K.; resources, J.K., C.B., C.S. and M.K.; data curation, S.N., J.S., U.C. and M.K.; writing—original draft preparation, S.N., J.S. and M.K.; writing—review and editing, S.N., J.S., J.K. and M.K.; visualization, S.N., J.S. and M.K.; supervision, C.B., C.S. and M.K.; project administration, M.K., J.K.; funding acquisition, J.K. and M.K.

Funding: This study was supported by the Robert Pfleger Stiftung (M.K.) and the Deutsche Forschungsgemeinschaft (#398138584).

Acknowledgments: The technical support from A. Baltruschat, B. Aschauer, S. Wübbel, H. Helten, L. Litinetsky and P. Ibold is acknowledged. The study was financially supported by Teva Pharmaceutical Industries Ltd.

Conflicts of Interest: The authors declare no conflict of interest

References

1. Haider, L.; Simeonidou, C.; Steinberger, G.; Hametner, S.; Grigoriadis, N.; Deretzi, G.; Frischer, J.M. Multiple sclerosis deep grey matter: The relation between demyelination, neurodegeneration, inflammation and iron. *J. Neurol Neurosurg Psychiatry* **2014**, *85*, 1386–1395. [CrossRef] [PubMed]
2. Ferguson, B.; Matyszak, M.K.; Esiri, M.M.; Perry, V.H. Axonal damage in acute multiple sclerosis lesions. *Brain* **1997**, *120*, 393–399. [CrossRef]
3. Kuhlmann, T.; Lingfeld, G.; Bitsch, A.; Schuchardt, J.; Bruck, W. Acute axonal damage in multiple sclerosis is most extensive in early disease stages and decreases over time. *Brain* **2002**, *125*, 2202–2212. [CrossRef] [PubMed]
4. Bauer, J.; Rauschka, H.; Lassmann, H. Inflammation in the nervous system: The human perspective. *Glia* **2001**, *36*, 235–243. [CrossRef] [PubMed]
5. Barnett, M.H.; Prineas, J.W. Relapsing and remitting multiple sclerosis: Pathology of the newly forming lesion. *Ann. Neurol.* **2004**, *55*, 458–468. [CrossRef]

6. Lucchinetti, C.; Bruck, W.; Parisi, J.; Scheithauer, B.; Rodriguez, M.; Lassmann, H. Heterogeneity of multiple sclerosis lesions: for the pathogenesis of demyelination. *Ann. Neurol.* **2000**, *47*, 707–717. [CrossRef]
7. Naldi, P.; Collimedaglia, L.; Vecchio, D.; Rosso, M.G.; Perl, F.; Stecco, A.; Monaco, F.; Leone, M.A. Predictors of attack severity and duration in multiple sclerosis: prospective study. *Open Neurol. J.* **2011**, *5*, 75–82. [CrossRef]
8. Vidal-Jordana, A.; Montalban, X. Multiple Sclerosis: Epidemiologic, Clinical, and Therapeutic Aspects. *Neuroimaging Clin. N. Am.* **2017**, *27*, 195–204. [CrossRef]
9. Confavreux, C.; Vukusic, S. The clinical course of multiple sclerosis. *Handb. Clin. Neurol.* **2014**, *122*, 343–369.
10. Tartaglia, M.C.; Narayanan, S.; Francis, S.J.; Santos, A.C.; De Stefano, N.; Lapierre, Y.; Arnold, D.L. The relationship between diffuse axonal damage and fatigue in multiple sclerosis. *Arch. Neurol.* **2004**, *61*, 201–207. [CrossRef]
11. De Stefano, N.; Matthews, P.M.; Fu, L.; Narayanan, S.; Stanley, J.; Francis, G.S.; Antel, J.P.; Arnold, D.L. Axonal damage correlates with disability in patients with relapsing-remitting multiple sclerosis. Results of a longitudinal magnetic resonance spectroscopy study. *Brain* **1998**, *121*, 1469–1477. [CrossRef] [PubMed]
12. Kipp, M.; Amor, S. FTY720 on the way from the base camp to the summit of the mountain: Relevance for remyelination. *Mult. Scler.* **2012**, *18*, 258–263. [CrossRef] [PubMed]
13. Perier, O.; Gregoire, A. Electron microscopic features of multiple sclerosis lesions. *Brain* **1965**, *88*, 937–952. [CrossRef] [PubMed]
14. Rodriguez, M.; Scheithauer, B. Ultrastructure of multiple sclerosis. *Ultrastruct Pathol.* **1994**, *18*, 3–13. [CrossRef] [PubMed]
15. Prineas, J.W.; Kwon, E.E.; Cho, E.S.; Sharer, L.R. Continual breakdown and regeneration of myelin in progressive multiple sclerosis plaques. *Ann. N. Y. Acad. Sci.* **1984**, *436*, 11–32. [CrossRef] [PubMed]
16. Prineas, J.W.; Connell, F. Remyelination in multiple sclerosis. *Ann. Neurol.* **1979**, *5*, 22–31. [CrossRef] [PubMed]
17. Prineas, J.W.; Barnard, R.O.; Kwon, E.E.; Sharer, L.R.; Cho, E.S. Multiple sclerosis: Remyelination of nascent lesions. *Ann. Neurol.* **1993**, *33*, 137–151. [CrossRef]
18. Trapp, B.D.; Stys, P.K. Virtual hypoxia and chronic necrosis of demyelinated axons in multiple sclerosis. *Lancet Neurol.* **2009**, *8*, 280–291. [CrossRef]
19. Funfschilling, U.; Supplie, L.M.; Mahad, D.; Boretius, S.; Saab, A.S.; Edgar, J.; Brinkmann, B.G.; Kassmann, C.M.; Tzvetanova, I.D.; Mobius, W.; et al. Glycolytic oligodendrocytes maintain myelin and long-term axonal integrity. *Nature* **2012**, *485*, 517–521. [CrossRef]
20. Smith, K.J. Sodium channels and multiple sclerosis: Roles in symptom production, damage and therapy. *Brain Pathol.* **2007**, *17*, 230–242. [CrossRef]
21. Prineas, J.W.; Barnard, R.O.; Revesz, T.; Kwon, E.E.; Sharer, L.; Cho, E.S. Multiple sclerosis. Pathology of recurrent lesions. *Brain* **1993**, *116*, 681–693. [CrossRef] [PubMed]
22. Willoughby, E.W.; Grochowski, E.; Li, D.K.; Oger, J.; Kastrukoff, L.F.; Paty, D.W. Serial magnetic resonance scanning in multiple sclerosis: A second prospective study in relapsing patients. *Ann. Neurol.* **1989**, *25*, 43–49. [CrossRef] [PubMed]
23. Brown, R.A.; Narayanan, S.; Arnold, D.L. Imaging of repeated episodes of demyelination and remyelination in multiple sclerosis. *Neuroimage Clin.* **2014**, *6*, 20–25. [CrossRef] [PubMed]
24. Johnson, E.S.; Ludwin, S.K. The demonstration of recurrent demyelination and remyelination of axons in the central nervous system. *Acta Neuropathol.* **1981**, *53*, 93–98. [CrossRef]
25. Mason, J.L.; Langaman, C.; Morell, P.; Suzuki, K.; Matsushima, G.K. Episodic demyelination and subsequent remyelination within the murine central nervous system: Changes in axonal calibre. *Neuropathol. Appl. Neurobiol.* **2001**, *27*, 50–58. [CrossRef]
26. Penderis, J.; Shields, S.A.; Franklin, R.J. Impaired remyelination and depletion of oligodendrocyte progenitors does not occur following repeated episodes of focal demyelination in the rat central nervous system. *Brain* **2003**, *126*, 1382–1391. [CrossRef]
27. Ruther, B.J.; Scheld, M.; Dreymueller, D.; Clarner, T.; Kress, E.; Brandenburg, L.O.; Swartenbroekx, T.; Hoornaert, C.; Ponsaerts, P.; Fallier-Becker, P.; et al. Combination of cuprizone and experimental autoimmune encephalomyelitis to study inflammatory brain lesion formation and progression. *Glia* **2017**, *65*, 1900–1913. [CrossRef]

28. Scheld, M.; Ruther, B.J.; Grosse-Veldmann, R.; Ohl, K.; Tenbrock, K.; Dreymuller, D.; Fallier-Becker, P.; Zendedel, A.; Beyer, C.; Clarner, T.; et al. Neurodegeneration Triggers Peripheral Immune Cell Recruitment into the Forebrain. *J. Neurosci.* **2016**, *36*, 1410–1415. [CrossRef]
29. Baxi, E.G.; DeBruin, J.; Tosi, D.M.; Grishkan, I.V.; Smith, M.D.; Kirby, L.A.; Gocke, A.R. Transfer of myelin-reactive th17 cells impairs endogenous remyelination in the central nervous system of cuprizone-fed mice. *J. Neurosci* **2015**, *35*, 8626–8639. [CrossRef]
30. Nyamoya, S.; Leopold, P.; Becker, B.; Beyer, C.; Hustadt, F.; Schmitz, C.; Michel, A.; Kipp, M. G-Protein-Coupled Receptor Gpr17 Expression in Two Multiple Sclerosis Remyelination Models. *Mol. Neurobiol.* **2019**, *56*, 1109–1123. [CrossRef]
31. Kramann, N.; Menken, L.; Hayardeny, L.; Hanisch, U.K.; Bruck, W. Laquinimod prevents cuprizone-induced demyelination independent of Toll-like receptor signaling. *Neurol. Neuroimmunol. Neuroinflamm.* **2016**, *3*, e233. [CrossRef] [PubMed]
32. Brück, W.; Pförtner, R.; Pham, T.; Zhang, J.; Hayardeny, L.; Piryatinsky, V.; Hanisch, U.K.; Regen, T.; van Rossum, D.; Brakelmann, L.; et al. Reduced astrocytic NF-kappaB activation by laquinimod protects from cuprizone-induced demyelination. *Acta Neuropathol.* **2012**, *124*, 411–424.
33. Clarner, T.; Janssen, K.; Nellessen, L.; Stangel, M.; Skripuletz, T.; Krauspe, B.; Hess, F.M.; Denecke, B.; Beutner, C.; Linnartz-Gerlach, B.; et al. CXCL10 triggers early microglial activation in the cuprizone model. *J. Immunol.* **2015**, *194*, 3400–3413. [CrossRef] [PubMed]
34. Goldberg, J.; Clarner, T.; Beyer, C.; Kipp, M. Anatomical Distribution of Cuprizone-Induced Lesions in C57BL6 Mice. *J. Mol. Neurosci.* **2015**, *57*, 166–175. [CrossRef]
35. Hoflich, K.M.; Beyer, C.; Clarner, T.; Schmitz, C.; Nyamoya, S.; Kipp, M.; Hochstrasser, T. Acute axonal damage in three different murine models of multiple sclerosis: A comparative approach. *Brain Res.* **2016**, *1650*, 125–133. [CrossRef]
36. Benardais, K.; Kotsiari, A.; Skuljec, J.; Koutsoudaki, P.N.; Gudi, V.; Singh, V.; Vulinovic, F.; Skripuletz, T.; Stangel, M. Cuprizone [bis(cyclohexylidenehydrazide)] is selectively toxic for mature oligodendrocytes. *Neurotox Res.* **2013**, *24*, 244–250. [CrossRef]
37. Benetti, F.; Ventura, M.; Salmini, B.; Ceola, S.; Carbonera, D.; Mammi, S.; Zitolo, A.; D'Angelo, P.; Urso, E.; Maffia, M.; et al. Cuprizone neurotoxicity, copper deficiency and neurodegeneration. *Neurotoxicology* **2010**, *31*, 509–517. [CrossRef]
38. Slowik, A.; Schmidt, T.; Beyer, C.; Amor, S.; Clarner, T.; Kipp, M. The sphingosine 1-phosphate receptor agonist FTY720 is neuroprotective after cuprizone-induced CNS demyelination. *Br. J. Pharm.* **2015**, *172*, 80–92. [CrossRef]
39. Cammer, W. The neurotoxicant, cuprizone, retards the differentiation of oligodendrocytes in vitro. *J. Neurol. Sci.* **1999**, *168*, 116–120. [CrossRef]
40. Fischbach, F.; Nedelcu, J.; Leopold, P.; Zhan, J.; Clarner, T.; Nellessen, L.; Beissel, C.; van Heuvel, Y.; Goswami, A.; Weis, J.; et al. Cuprizone-induced graded oligodendrocyte vulnerability is regulated by the transcription factor DNA damage-inducible transcript 3. *Glia* **2019**, *67*, 263–276. [CrossRef]
41. Faizi, M.; Salimi, A.; Seydi, E.; Naserzadeh, P.; Kouhnavard, M.; Rahimi, A.; Pourahmad, J. Toxicity of cuprizone a Cu(2+) chelating agent on isolated mouse brain mitochondria: A justification for demyelination and subsequent behavioral dysfunction. *Toxicol. Mech. Methods* **2016**, *26*, 276–283. [CrossRef] [PubMed]
42. Hoppel, C.L.; Tandler, B. Biochemical effects of cuprizone on mouse liver and heart mitochondria. *Biochem. Pharm.* **1973**, *22*, 2311–2318. [CrossRef]
43. Baxi, E.G.; DeBruin, J.; Jin, J.; Strasburger, H.J.; Smith, M.D.; Orthmann-Murphy, J.L.; Schott, J.T.; Fairchild, A.N.; Bergles, D.E.; Calabresi, P.A. Lineage tracing reveals dynamic changes in oligodendrocyte precursor cells following cuprizone-induced demyelination. *Glia* **2017**, *65*, 2087–2098. [CrossRef] [PubMed]
44. Gudi, V.; Moharregh-Khiabani, D.; Skripuletz, T.; Koutsoudaki, P.N.; Kotsiari, A.; Skuljec, J.; Trebst, C.; Stangel, M. Regional differences between grey and white matter in cuprizone induced demyelination. *Brain Res.* **2009**, *1283*, 127–138. [CrossRef]
45. Xing, Y.L.; Roth, P.T.; Stratton, J.A.; Chuang, B.H.; Danne, J.; Ellis, S.L.; Ng, S.W.; Kilpatrick, T.J.; Merson, T.D. Adult neural precursor cells from the subventricular zone contribute significantly to oligodendrocyte regeneration and remyelination. *J. Neurosci.* **2014**, *34*, 14128–14146. [CrossRef]

46. Moore, S.; Khalaj, A.J.; Yoon, J.; Patel, R.; Hannsun, G.; Yoo, T.; Sasidhar, M.; Martinez-Torres, L.; Hayardeny, L.; Tiwari-Woodruff, S.K. Therapeutic laquinimod treatment decreases inflammation, initiates axon remyelination, and improves motor deficit in a mouse model of multiple sclerosis. *Brain Behav.* **2013**, *3*, 664–682. [CrossRef]
47. Wegner, C.; Stadelmann, C.; Pfortner, R.; Raymond, E.; Feigelson, S.; Alon, R.; Timan, B.; Hayardeny, L.; Bruck, W. Laquinimod interferes with migratory capacity of T cells and reduces IL-17 levels, inflammatory demyelination and acute axonal damage in mice with experimental autoimmune encephalomyelitis. *J. Neuroimmunol.* **2010**, *227*, 133–143. [CrossRef]
48. Comi, G.; Pulizzi, A.; Rovaris, M.; Abramsky, O.; Arbizu, T.; Boiko, A.; Gold, R.; Havrdova, E.; Komoly, S.; Selmaj, K.; et al. Effect of laquinimod on MRI-monitored disease activity in patients with relapsing-remitting multiple sclerosis: A multicentre, randomised, double-blind, placebo-controlled phase IIb study. *Lancet* **2008**, *371*, 2085–2092. [CrossRef]
49. Polman, C.; Barkhof, F.; Sandberg-Wollheim, M.; Linde, A.; Nordle, O.; Nederman, T. Treatment with laquinimod reduces development of active MRI lesions in relapsing MS. *Neurology* **2005**, *64*, 987–991. [CrossRef]
50. Comi, G.; Jeffery, D.; Kappos, L.; Montalban, X.; Boyko, A.; Rocca, M.A.; Filippi, M.; Group, A.S. Placebo-controlled trial of oral laquinimod for multiple sclerosis. *N. Engl. J. Med.* **2012**, *366*, 1000–1009. [CrossRef]
51. Schulze-Topphoff, U.; Shetty, A.; Varrin-Doyer, M.; Molnarfi, N.; Sagan, S.A.; Sobel, R.A. Laquinimod, a quinoline-3-carboxamide, induces type II myeloid cells that modulate central nervous system autoimmunity. *PLoS ONE* **2012**, *7*, e33797. [CrossRef] [PubMed]
52. Jolivel, V.; Luessi, F.; Masri, J.; Kraus, S.H.; Hubo, M.; Poisa-Beiro, L.; Furlan, R. Modulation of dendritic cell properties by laquinimod as a mechanism for modulating multiple sclerosis. *Brain* **2013**, *136*, 1048–1066. [CrossRef] [PubMed]
53. Ruffini, F.; Rossi, S.; Bergamaschi, A.; Brambilla, E.; Finardi, A.; Motta, C.; Comi, G. Laquinimod prevents inflammation-induced synaptic alterations occurring in experimental autoimmune encephalomyelitis. *Mult. Scler.* **2013**, *19*, 1084–1094. [CrossRef] [PubMed]
54. Ruffini, F.; Rossi, S.; Bergamaschi, A.; Brambilla, E.; Finardi, A.; Motta, C.; Comi, G. Laquinimod Treatment Improves Myelination Deficits at the Transcriptional and Ultrastructural Levels in the YAC128 Mouse Model. of Huntington Disease. *Mol. Neurobiol.* **2019**, *56*, 4464–4478.
55. Ellrichmann, G.; Blusch, A.; Fatoba, O.; Brunner, J.; Reick, C.; Hayardeny, L.; Gold, R. Laquinimod treatment in the R6/2 mouse model. *Sci Rep.* **2017**, *7*, 4947. [CrossRef]
56. Garcia-Miralles, M.; Hong, X.; Tan, L.J.; Caron, N.S.; Huang, Y.; To, X.V.; Lin, R.Y.; Franciosi, S.; Papapetropoulos, S.; Hayardeny, L.; et al. Laquinimod rescues striatal, cortical and white matter pathology and results in modest behavioural improvements in the YAC128 model of Huntington disease. *Sci. Rep.* **2016**, *6*, 31652. [CrossRef]
57. Katsumoto, A.; Miranda, A.S.; Butovsky, O.; Teixeira, A.L.; Ransohoff, R.M.; Lamb, B.T. Laquinimod attenuates inflammation by modulating macrophage functions in traumatic brain injury mouse model. *J. Neuroinflamm.* **2018**, *15*, 26. [CrossRef]
58. Hussain, R.Z.; Miller-Little, W.A.; Lambracht-Washington, D.; Jaramillo, T.C.; Takahashi, M.; Zhang, S.; Fu, M.; Cutter, G.R.; Hayardeny, L.; Powell, C.M.; et al. Laquinimod has no effects on brain volume or cellular CNS composition in the F1 3xTg-AD/C3H mouse model of Alzheimer's disease. *J. Neuroimmunol.* **2017**, *309*, 100–110. [CrossRef]
59. Vollmer, T.L.; Sorensen, P.S.; Selmaj, K.; Zipp, F.; Havrdova, E.; Cohen, J.A.; Sasson, N.; Gilgun-Sherki, Y.; Arnold, D.L.; Group, B.S. A randomized placebo-controlled phase III trial of oral laquinimod for multiple sclerosis. *J. Neurol.* **2014**, *261*, 773–783. [CrossRef]
60. Rodrigues, F.B.; Wild, E.J. Clinical Trials Corner: September 2017. *J. Huntingt. Dis.* **2017**, *6*, 255–263. [CrossRef]
61. Wilmes, A.T.; Reinehr, S.; Kuhn, S.; Pedreiturria, X.; Petrikowski, L.; Faissner, S.; Ayzenberg, I.; Stute, G.; Gold, R.; Dick, H.B.; et al. Laquinimod protects the optic nerve and retina in an experimental autoimmune encephalomyelitis model. *J. Neuroinflamm.* **2018**, *15*, 183. [CrossRef] [PubMed]

62. Luhder, F.; Kebir, H.; Odoardi, F.; Litke, T.; Sonneck, M.; Alvarez, J.I.; Winchenbach, J.; Eckert, N.; Hayardeny, L.; Sorani, E.; et al. Laquinimod enhances central nervous system barrier functions. *Neurobiol. Dis.* **2017**, *102*, 60–69. [CrossRef] [PubMed]
63. Gentile, A.; Musella, A.; De Vito, F.; Fresegna, D.; Bullitta, S.; Rizzo, F.R.; Centonze, D.; Mandolesi, G. Laquinimod ameliorates excitotoxic damage by regulating glutamate re-uptake. *J. Neuroinflamm.* **2018**, *15*, 5. [CrossRef] [PubMed]
64. Kaye, J.; Piryatinsky, V.; Birnberg, T.; Hingaly, T.; Raymond, E.; Kashi, R.; Amit-Romach, E.; Caballero, I.S.; Towfic, F.; Ator, M.A.; et al. Laquinimod arrests experimental autoimmune encephalomyelitis by activating the aryl hydrocarbon receptor. *Proc. Natl. Acad. Sci. USA* **2016**, *113*, E6145–E6152. [CrossRef] [PubMed]
65. Hawker, K.; O'Connor, P.; Freedman, M.S.; Calabresi, P.A.; Antel, J.; Simon, J.; Hauser, S.; Waubant, E.; Vollmer, T.; Panitch, H.; et al. Rituximab in patients with primary progressive multiple sclerosis: Results of a randomized double-blind placebo-controlled multicenter trial. *Ann. Neurol.* **2009**, *66*, 460–471. [CrossRef] [PubMed]
66. Lublin, F.; Miller, D.H.; Freedman, M.S.; Cree, B.A.C.; Wolinsky, J.S.; Weiner, H.; Lubetzki, C.; Hartung, H.P.; Montalban, X.; Uitdehaag, B.M.J.; et al. Oral fingolimod in primary progressive multiple sclerosis (INFORMS): A phase 3, randomised, double-blind, placebo-controlled trial. *Lancet* **2016**, *387*, 1075–1084. [CrossRef]
67. Rumbach, L.; Racadot, E.; Armspach, J.P.; Namer, I.J.; Bonneville, J.F.; Wijdenes, J.; Marescaux, C.; Herve, P.; Chambron, J. Biological assessment and MRI monitoring of the therapeutic efficacy of a monoclonal anti-T CD4 antibody in multiple sclerosis patients. *Mult. Scler.* **1996**, *1*, 207–212. [CrossRef]
68. Revesz, T.; Kidd, D.; Thompson, A.J.; Barnard, R.O.; McDonald, W.I. A comparison of the pathology of primary and secondary progressive multiple sclerosis. *Brain* **1994**, *117*, 759–765. [CrossRef]
69. Stevenson, V.L.; Miller, D.H.; Rovaris, M.; Barkhof, F.; Brochet, B.; Dousset, V.; Dousset, V.; Filippi, M.; Montalban, X.; Polman, C.H.; et al. Primary and transitional progressive MS: A clinical and MRI cross-sectional study. *Neurology* **1999**, *52*, 839–845. [CrossRef]
70. Correale, J.; Gaitan, M.I.; Ysrraelit, M.C.; Fiol, M.P. Progressive multiple sclerosis: From pathogenic mechanisms to treatment. *Brain* **2017**, *140*, 527–546. [CrossRef]
71. Draheim, T.; Liessem, A.; Scheld, M.; Wilms, F.; Weissflog, M.; Denecke, B.; Kensler, T.W.; Zendedel, A.; Beyer, C.; Kipp, M.; et al. Activation of the astrocytic Nrf2/ARE system ameliorates the formation of demyelinating lesions in a multiple sclerosis animal model. *Glia* **2016**, *64*, 2219–2230. [CrossRef] [PubMed]
72. McMahon, E.J.; Suzuki, K.; Matsushima, G.K. Peripheral macrophage recruitment in cuprizone-induced CNS demyelination despite an intact blood-brain barrier. *J. Neuroimmunol.* **2002**, *130*, 32–45. [CrossRef]
73. Verden, D.; Macklin, W.B. Neuroprotection by central nervous system remyelination: Molecular, cellular, and functional considerations. *J. Neurosci. Res.* **2016**, *94*, 1411–1420. [CrossRef] [PubMed]
74. Mayer, R.F. Conduction velocity in the central nervous system of the cat during experimental demyelination and remyelination. *Int. J. Neurosci.* **1971**, *1*, 287–308. [CrossRef] [PubMed]
75. Irvine, K.A.; Blakemore, W.F. Remyelination protects axons from demyelination-associated axon degeneration. *Brain* **2008**, *131*, 1464–1477. [CrossRef] [PubMed]
76. Manrique-Hoyos, N.; Jurgens, T.; Gronborg, M.; Kreutzfeldt, M.; Schedensack, M.; Kuhlmann, T.; Schrick, C.; Bruck, W.; Urlaub, H.; Simons, M.; et al. Late motor decline after accomplished remyelination: Impact for progressive multiple sclerosis. *Ann. Neurol.* **2012**, *71*, 227–244. [CrossRef] [PubMed]
77. Lloyd, A.F.; Miron, V.E. The pro-remyelination properties of microglia in the central nervous system. *Nat. Rev. Neurol.* **2019**, *15*, 447–458. [CrossRef]
78. Olah, M.; Amor, S.; Brouwer, N.; Vinet, J.; Eggen, B.; Biber, K.; Boddeke, H.W. Identification of a microglia phenotype supportive of remyelination. *Glia* **2012**, *60*, 306–321. [CrossRef]
79. Kotter, M.R.; Li, W.W.; Zhao, C.; Franklin, R.J. Myelin impairs CNS remyelination by inhibiting oligodendrocyte precursor cell differentiation. *J. Neurosci.* **2006**, *26*, 328–332. [CrossRef]
80. Lampron, A.; Larochelle, A.; Laflamme, N.; Prefontaine, P.; Plante, M.M.; Sanchez, M.G.; Yong, V.W.; Stys, P.K.; Tremblay, M.E.; Rivest, S. Inefficient clearance of myelin debris by microglia impairs remyelinating processes. *J. Exp. Med.* **2015**, *212*, 481–495. [CrossRef]
81. Hagemeyer, N.; Hanft, K.M.; Akriditou, M.A.; Unger, N.; Park, E.S.; Stanley, E.R.; Staszewski, O.; Dimou, L.; Prinz, M. Microglia contribute to normal myelinogenesis and to oligodendrocyte progenitor maintenance during adulthood. *Acta Neuropathol.* **2017**, *134*, 441–458. [CrossRef] [PubMed]

82. Wlodarczyk, A.; Holtman, I.R.; Krueger, M.; Yogev, N.; Bruttger, J.; Khorooshi, R.; Benmamar-Badel, A.; de Boer-Bergsma, J.J.; Martin, N.A.; Karram, K.; et al. A novel microglial subset plays a key role in myelinogenesis in developing brain. *Embo J.* **2017**, *36*, 3292–3308. [CrossRef] [PubMed]
83. Skripuletz, T.; Hackstette, D.; Bauer, K.; Gudi, V.; Pul, R.; Voss, E.; Berger, K.; Kipp, M.; Baumgartner, W.; Stangel, M. Astrocytes regulate myelin clearance through recruitment of microglia during cuprizone-induced demyelination. *Brain* **2013**, *136*, 147–167. [CrossRef] [PubMed]

Sample Availability: Samples of the brain sections are available from the authors.

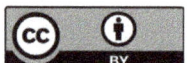

© 2019 by the authors. Licensee MDPI, Basel, Switzerland. This article is an open access article distributed under the terms and conditions of the Creative Commons Attribution (CC BY) license (http://creativecommons.org/licenses/by/4.0/).

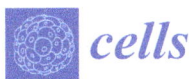

Article

Detrimental Impact of Energy Drink Compounds on Developing Oligodendrocytes and Neurons

Meray Serdar, Annika Mordelt, Katharina Müser, Karina Kempe, Ursula Felderhoff-Müser, Josephine Herz [†] and Ivo Bendix *,[†]

Department of Paediatrics I, Neonatology & Experimental perinatal Neurosciences, University Hospital Essen, University Duisburg-Essen, 45147 Essen, Germany; meray.serdar@uk-essen.de (M.S.); annika.mordelt@stud.uni-due.de (A.M.); katharina.mueser@freenet.de (K.M.); karina.kempe@uk-essen.de (K.K.); Ursula.Felderhoff@uk-essen.de (U.F.-M.); josephine.herz@uk-essen.de (J.H.)
* Correspondence: ivo.bendix@uk-essen.de; Tel.: +49-201-723-2114
[†] These authors contributed equally to this work.

Received: 26 September 2019; Accepted: 31 October 2019; Published: 3 November 2019

Abstract: The consumption of energy drinks is continuously rising, particularly in children and adolescents. While risks for adverse health effects, like arrhythmia, have been described, effects on neural cells remain elusive. Considering that neurodevelopmental processes like myelination and neuronal network formation peak in childhood and adolescence we hypothesized that developing oligodendrocytes and neurons are particularly vulnerable to main energy drink components. Immature oligodendrocytes and hippocampal neurons were isolated from P0-P1 Wistar rats and were incubated with 0.3 mg/mL caffeine and 4 mg/mL taurine alone or in combination for 24 h. Analysis was performed immediately after treatment or after additional three days under differentiating conditions for oligodendrocytes and standard culture for neurons. Oligodendrocyte degeneration, proliferation, and differentiation were assessed via immunocytochemistry and immunoblotting. Neuronal integrity was investigated following immunocytochemistry by analysis of dendrite outgrowth and axonal morphology. Caffeine and taurine induced an increased degeneration and inhibited proliferation of immature oligodendrocytes accompanied by a decreased differentiation capacity. Moreover, dendritic branching and axonal integrity of hippocampal neurons were negatively affected by caffeine and taurine treatment. The negative impact of caffeine and taurine on developing oligodendrocytes and disturbed neuronal morphology indicates a high risk for disturbed neurodevelopment in children and adolescents by excessive energy drink consumption.

Keywords: energy drinks; caffeine; taurine; neuron; oligodendrocytes

1. Introduction

The consumption of energy drinks has exponentially increased due to the expectation of increased mental and physical performance. This makes them particularly attractive for children, adolescents, and young adults at reproductive age, who are the main consumers of energy drinks, comprising 30 to 50% of all consumers [1,2]. A significant increase in adolescents who died after excessive consumption of energy drinks in combination with or without alcohol was noted in recent years [3]. Furthermore, several studies reported negative health effects of short- and long-term consumption of energy drinks, such as aggressive behaviour, arrhythmia, increased heart rate, and sleep disturbances [4–6]. These effects were mainly attributed to the high caffeine and sugar concentrations [3,7]. To date there are no studies analysing a potential risk of energy drink consumption on key neurodevelopmental processes of the central nervous system (CNS). Childhood and adolescence is a period of rapid body growth but also an important period of brain development. White matter volume, i.e., myelination increases linearly with increasing age, beginning at the end of the second trimester and continuing into the third decade of life [8–10]. Furthermore, grey matter volume and formation, reorganization of neuronal projections reach its maximum during childhood and adolescence [9].

Considering the continuously rising number of children and adolescents consuming energy drinks and the fact that brain development is in a crucial phase, neuronal and glial cell types of the still immature brain might be particularly vulnerable to high doses of energy drink compounds. Al Basher et al. and Reis et al. provided first indications for detrimental effects of energy drinks on the developing brain resulting in anxiety disorders in later life [4,11]. With regard to the molecular components of energy drinks, potentially harmful to neural cells, it was suggested that caffeine and taurine either alone or in combination might be involved [12]. However, these data were obtained in the human neuroblastoma cell line SH-SY5Y. Effects on primary developing CNS cell types remain unclear.

In the present study, we investigated the impact of caffeine and taurine alone or in combination on primary immature oligodendrocytes and hippocampal neurons, focusing on degeneration, proliferation, and differentiation capacity of immature oligodendrocytes as well as on dendritic branching and axonal morphology of hippocampal neurons.

2. Materials and Methods

2.1. Drugs

Caffeine and taurine were purchased from Sigma Aldrich (Taufkirchen, Germany). Both components were dissolved to a final concentration of 0.3 mg/mL caffeine and 4 mg/mL taurine in the appropriate medium of oligodendrocytes and neurons. The selected concentrations are based on a previous report in neuronal SH-SY5Y cells [12].

2.2. Primary Cell Culture

2.2.1. Oligodendrocytes

Neonatal rat mixed glia cells were isolated from P0–P1 old Wistar rats as previously described [13–16]. Cells were cultured in Dulbecco's modified Eagle's medium (DMEM, Gibco, Erlangen, Germany) supplemented with 20% foetal calf serum, 1% penicillin/streptomycin. After 10–12 days, immature oligodendrocytes, attached to the astrocyte layer of the mixed glia culture, were isolated by shaking overnight at 230 rpm. The collected cells were pre-plated for 30 min at 5% CO_2 and 37 °C to remove contaminating microglia and astrocytes. Floating cells were collected in proliferation medium (DMEM, 1×B27 (Gibco), 10 ng/mL plated derived growth factor (PDGF, PanBiotech, Aidenbach, Germany), 10 ng/mL basic fibroblast growth factor (bFGF, PanBiotech)) and plated on poly-dl-ornithine-coated (Sigma-Aldrich, Taufkirchen, Germany) cover slips or culture plates (100,000 cells/mL). At this stage the purity of culture was approximately around 95%, assessed by expression of the immature oligodendrocyte surface progenitor marker A2B5 [17]. Oligodendrocyte precursor cells were cultivated in proliferation medium for 3 days before treatment with 0.3 mg/mL caffeine, 4 mg/mL taurine, and the combination of both for 24 h at 5% CO_2 and 37 °C in humidified air. To quantify the effect of caffeine and taurine on myelination capacity of oligodendrocytes, cells were cultivated in differentiation medium (DMEM, 1× B27, 10 ng/mL ciliary neurotrophic factor (CNTF, PanBiotech), 15 µM triiodothyronine (T3, Sigma-Aldrich)) for another 3 days after treatment. Cells were lysed for western blot analysis or fixed with 2% paraformaldehyde (PFA) for analysis via immunocytochemistry (ICC).

2.2.2. Hippocampal Neurons

In the present study, neurons were isolated from the hippocampus, the main structure of learning and memory formation involving adult neurogenesis and synaptogenesis [18], which has been suggested to be impaired by energy drink components [19]. Hippocampal neurons were isolated from P0–P1 old Wistar rats according to described methods [20]. Briefly, hippocampi were carefully dissected from the cerebrum and enzymatically digested with trypsin (2.5%, Sigma-Aldrich) and deoxyribonuclease (DNase, 1%, Sigma-Aldrich). Subsequently the hippocampi were mechanically disrupted by a glass pipette followed by pre-plating of the cell suspension for 30 min to remove contaminating astrocytes. 80,000 cells/mL were seeded on double coated poly-L-lysine and laminin (Sigma-Aldrich) Falcondishes (Amsterdam, Netherlands) in neurobasal media (NB, Gibco) containing B27, 1% glutamine, and 1% penicillin/streptomycin for 24 h. Afterwards, neuron-enriched cultures were treated with 3 µM cytosine beta-D-arabinofuranosyl cytosine (AraC, Sigma-Aldrich) for 48 h to inhibit proliferation of contaminating astrocytes [20], resulting in a purity of approximately 80%. Neurons were treated as described for oligodendrocyte cultures. Appropriate controls were cultivated under standard culture conditions in NB medium. Both substances were dissolved in the NB medium. Cells were fixated with 2% PFA immediately after the treatment or after cultivation for another 3 days in NB medium.

2.3. Western-Blot Analysis

For immunoblot analysis oligodendrocytes were plated in 6-well plates. Cells of three wells for each condition were lysed in ice-cooled radioimmunoprecipitation assay (RIPA) buffer containing protease inhibitors. The homogenate was centrifuged at 14,000× g (4 °C) for 10 min. The protein concentration in the supernatant cytosolic extract was determined using the bicinchoninic acid assay (BCA assay; Thermo Fisher Scientific, Erlangen, Germany). Ten µg of protein were denatured in Laemmli sample buffer at 95 °C for 5 min. Proteins were separated by 15% sodium dodecyl sulphate polyacrylamide gel electrophoresis, and blotted onto nitrocellulose membranes (0.2 µm pore, Sigma-Aldrich). Equal loading and transfer of proteins was confirmed by staining with Ponceau S solution (Sigma-Aldrich). Five percent nonfat dry milk was used for blocking of nonspecific antibody binding in Tris buffered saline/0.1% Tween (TBST) at room temperature for 60 min. Membranes were incubated overnight (4 °C) with the primary monoclonal rabbit anti-cleaved Caspase-3 (cCaspase-3) antibody (1:1000, Cell Signaling Technology, Frankfurt am Main, Germany; molecular weight 19 kDa) or mouse anti-glyceraldehyde 3-phosphate dehydrogenase (GAPDH) antibody (1:50,000; Sigma-Aldrich; molecular weight 37 kDa) in 5% nonfat dry milk in TBST. Horseradish peroxidase-conjugated secondary antibodies (DAKO, Hamburg, Germany) were diluted 1:5000 (anti-mouse) or 1:2000 (anti-rabbit) in 5% non-fat dry milk in TBST. For visualization and densitometric analysis ChemiDoc XRS$^+$ imaging system and ImageLab software (6.0.1, Bio-Rad, Munich, Germany) was used. Density ratios between cCaspase-3 protein and the reference protein GAPDH were calculated for each (=1) sample per experiment. These ratios were normalized to control (i.e., without treatment) per experiment. The mean of four independent experiments was used for graphical presentation.

2.4. Immunocytochemistry

Following fixation, cells were incubated with blocking solution (5% normal goat serum in 0.1% Triton X-100 in phosphate-buffered-solution (PBS)) for 1 h at room temperature followed by incubation with primary antibodies in PBS with 5% goat serum at 4°C overnight. The following antibodies were used: anti-oligodendrocyte transcription factor 2 (polyclonal rabbit anti-Olig2, 1:500; monoclonal mouse anti-Olig2, 1:300, Millipore, Darmstadt, Germany), anti-A2B5 (monoclonal mouse anti-A2B5, 1:500, Millipore, Germany), anti-proliferating cell nuclear antigen (polyclonal rabbit anti-PCNA, 1:800, Cell Signaling Technology), anti-myelin basic protein (monoclonal mouse anti-MBP, 1:500, Covance, Munich, Germany), anti-microtubuli associated protein 2 (polyclonal mouse anti-Map2, 1:500, Sigma-Aldrich), and anti-TAU (polyclonal rabbit anti-TAU, 1:500, GeneTex, Germany). Specific antibody binding was visualized by incubation with the appropriate secondary antibodies (anti-mouse Alexa Fluor 555; anti-mouse Alexa Fluor 488; anti-rabbit Alexa Fluor 555; anti-rabbit Alexa Fluor 488; anti-rabbit Alexa Fluor 647, Invitrogen, Erlangen, Germany; all 1:1000) for 1 h at room temperature. Nuclei were counterstained with 4′,6-diamidino-2-phenylindole (DAPI, 1 µg/mL). Cover slips were mounted onto glass slides with DAKO Fluorescent Mounting Medium and kept in the dark at 4 °C. Cells were analysed via confocal microscopy (A1plus, Eclipse Ti, with NIS Elements AR software, Nikon, Düsseldorf, Germany).

2.5. Confocal Microscopy and Quantitative Analysis

Analysis was performed with confocal microscopy (A1plus, Eclipse Ti, with NIS Elements AR software, Nikon) using a 10× objective. Four laser lines (laser diode, 405 nm; Ar laser, 514 nm; G-HeNe-laser, 543 nm and Rh-laser 647 nm) and three different filters (450/50-405 LP, 515/20-540 LP, 585/65-640 LP) were used for image acquisition. Oligodendrocytes were analysed in a total of 15 random fields of view (each 1.6 mm^2) derived from three independent experiments (5 images per experiment and group). The number of total (Olig2) and proliferating (PCNA) oligodendrocytes as well as the area of A2B5 were analysed automatically using the NIS Elements AR software 4.0 (Nikon). Since reductions of total MBP-positive cells after initiation of differentiation might have resulted from a total reduction of immature A2B5-positive oligodendrocytes after acute treatment, i.e., before initiation of differentiation, the percentage of MBP-positive cells of total Olig2-positive cells was quantified. As, under differentiating conditions, immature oligodendrocytes do not proliferate and substances were not present during this culture period, percentage values of MBP+ cells provide information about the general capacity of all initially surviving oligodendrocytes independent of acute treatment effects on cell numbers. To investigate morphological changes of neurons, 8–10 random fields (each 0.395 mm^2) per experiment were analysed in Map2/TAU co-staining by using the 20× objective. The images were converted to Tiff-images using the NIS Elements AR software 4.0 (Nikon, Germany). Analysis of dendrite branches and length was performed with ImageJ (NIH, Java 1.8.0) using the NeuronJ plugin [21].

2.6. Statistical Analysis

Data are expressed as scatter plots with bars including mean values with standard deviation (SD). Data were analysed using GraphPad Prism 6 (Statcon, Witzenhausen, Germany). Differences between groups were determined by one-way analysis of variance (one-way ANOVA) followed by Bonferroni post hoc test for multiple comparison. p-values < 0.05 were considered as statistically significant. Detailed results of statistical analysis are provided in Supplementary Tables S1 and S2 in the Supplementary Material.

3. Results

3.1. The Main Compounds of Energy Drinks Caffeine and Taurine Induce Cell Degeneration and Inhibit Proliferation of Immature Oligodendrocytes

The selected treatment design with 0.3 mg/mL caffeine and 4 mg/mL taurine for 24 h is mainly based on a previous in vitro study on neural cells [12] and concentrations in commercially available energy drinks considering the increasing rise of high acute and high chronic consumers [22]. Immediately after treatment, oligodendrocytes were stained for the pan-oligodendrocyte marker Olig2 and the immature cell marker A2B5 (Figure 1A). We observed a significant reduction of immature oligodendrocytes by 40–50% in the presence of caffeine, taurine, and the combination of both (Olig2/mm^2: $F_{3,56}$ = 17.33; mean: control 314.2, caffeine 192.2, taurine 188.6, caffeine + taurine 188.1; A2B5 area/mm^2: $F_{3,56}$ = 18.43; mean: control 0.21, caffeine 0.14, taurine 0.11 and caffeine +taurine 0.11, Figure 1B,C).

Since reduced cell density may have been caused either by increased cell degeneration and/or reduced proliferation, we analysed proliferation of immature oligodendrocytes via immunocytochemistry for the marker PCNA (Figure 2A,B). These analyses demonstrated a significantly reduced proliferation of immature oligodendrocytes incubated with caffeine, taurine, and the combination of both (% PCNA-positive Olig2: $F_{3,56}$ = 40.10, mean: control 40.15, caffeine 8.67, taurine 19.71 and caffeine+ taurine 15.97, Figure 2B). Analysis of apoptosis by western blot for cleaved-Caspase-3 [23] revealed a significant three-fold increase in the combined treatment compared to control ($F_{3,12} = 6.886$; mean cCaspase-3/GAPDH ratio: caffeine + taurine 3.05 compared to control (=1); Figure 2C). Of note, single taurine treatment did not affect apoptotic cell death, resulting in a significant difference between taurine single and the combined treatment with caffeine (Figure 2C).

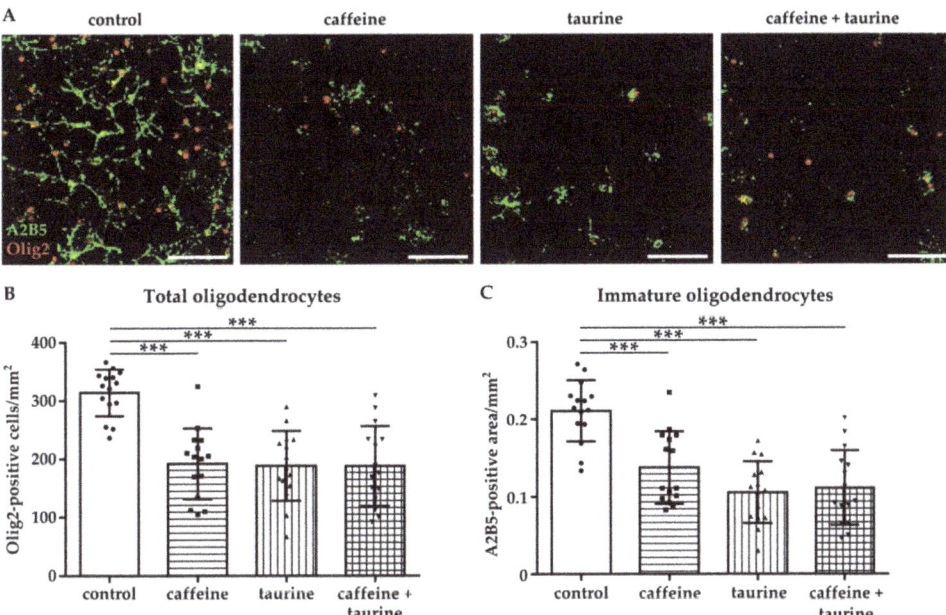

Figure 1. Caffeine and taurine alone or in combination induce immature oligodendrocyte cell loss. After three days under standard culture conditions primary immature oligodendrocytes were incubated with or without 0.3 mg/mL caffeine, 4 mg/mL taurine, and the combination of both for 24 h. (**A**) Representative images of immunofluorescence staining of immature oligodendrocytes (A2B5 green, Olig2 red). (**B**) Quantification of Olig2 positive cells. The density of immature oligodendrocytes was determined by measuring the A2B5 positive area (**C**). Data are derived from 15 images per group out of three independent experiments (depicted by circle = control, square = caffeine, triangle up = taurine, triangle down = caffeine + taurine). Scale bar 400 μm. *** $p < 0.001$, one-way ANOVA followed by Bonferroni post hoc test.

3.2. Differentiation Capacity of Oligodendrocytes is Reduced by Caffeine and Taurine

To investigate whether the treatment of the main energy drink ingredients caffeine and taurine influence differentiation capacity of oligodendrocytes, we analysed the expression of MBP three days after substance treatment and induction of differentiation (Figure 3A). In accordance with acute treatment effects the number of oligodendrocytes remained reduced under differentiating, i.e., non-proliferating conditions (Figure 3B). In addition to an acute decrease in immature A2B5-positive oligodendrocytes (Figure 1), differentiation capacity of surviving oligodendrocytes was significantly reduced to 85% by caffeine and taurine with the single as well as combined treatment ($F_{3,56} = 17.43$; mean % MBP of total Olig2: control 93.29, caffeine 85.29, taurine 85.98 and caffeine + taurine 84.69; Figure 3C).

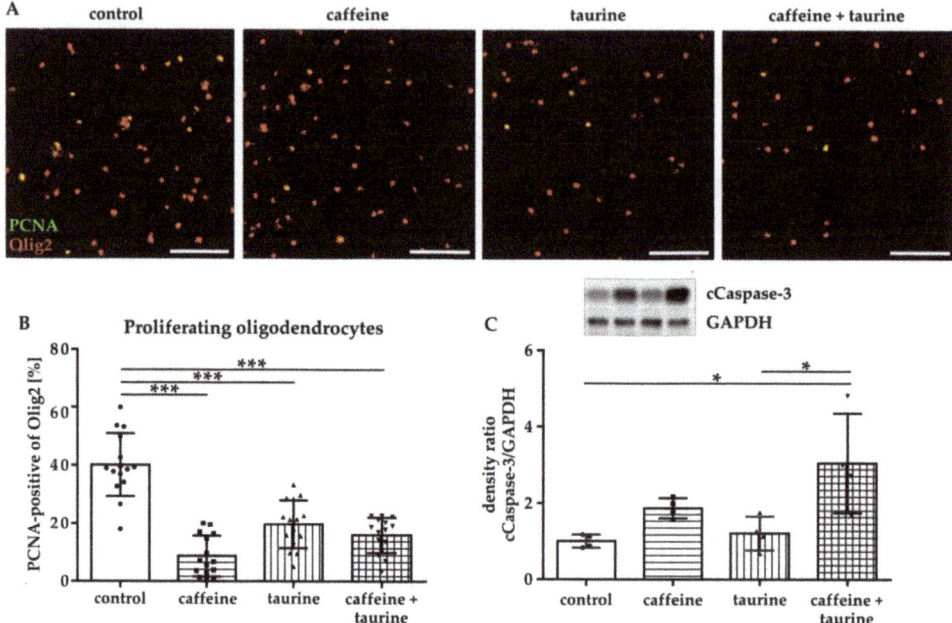

Figure 2. Immature oligodendrocyte cell loss is caused by a decreased proliferation and increased degeneration induced by caffeine and taurine. After treatment with or without 0.3 mg/mL caffeine and 4 mg/mL taurine alone or in combination, cells were analysed for proliferation via immunocytochemistry and for apoptosis via western blot. (**A**) Representative images of immunofluorescence staining of proliferating oligodendrocytes (PCNA green, Olig2 red). The number of proliferating oligodendrocytes was quantified in 15 images per group derived from three independent experiments (**B**) Scale bar 400 μm. Ratio of cCaspase-3 and GAPDH protein expression was analyzed in protein lysates of cultured oligodendrocytes derived from four independent experiments (**C**), depicted by circle = control, square = caffeine, triangle up = taurine, triangle down = caffeine + taurine). * $p < 0.05$, *** $p < 0.001$, one-way ANOVA followed by a Bonferroni post hoc test.

3.3. Caffeine and Taurine Reduce Dendrite Branching Immediately after Treatment

The effect of energy drink components on neuronal network formation was analysed in primary hippocampal neurons. Immediately after treatment with caffeine and taurine alone or in combination, the number of Map2-positive neurons was significantly reduced (Supplementary Figure S1). To get further insight into potential effects on neuronal network formation, neuronal dendrites were analysed (Figure 4A). Two types of dendrites were analysed, primary dendrites attached to the soma and higher dendrites, branching directly from primary dendrites using the NeuronJ plugin [21] of ImageJ software (Figure 4A). We detected a significantly reduced number of total dendrites in all treatment groups compared to controls ($F_{3, 370} = 25.07$; mean: control 5.76, caffeine 3.94, taurine 3.31 and caffeine + taurine 3.83, Figure 4B). The reduction of total dendrites was mainly caused by a reduction of higher dendrites, demonstrated by a significant reduction by 20–40% in treated cells compared to controls ($F_{3, 160} = 9.70$; mean: control 3.87, caffeine 2.51, taurine 2.09 and caffeine + taurine 2.62; Figure 4D). In addition to the number of dendrites their length was similarly reduced (Figure 4E). Again, higher dendrites were primarily affected, as shown by significantly reduced lengths to 55–60% compared to controls, while no significant differences were observed for primary dendrites (Figure 4F,G).

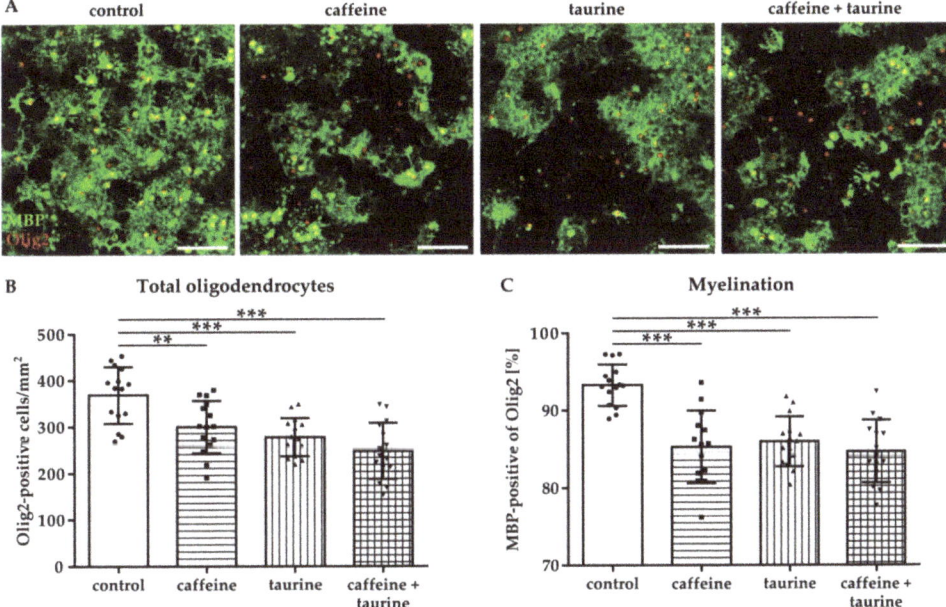

Figure 3. Myelination capacity of immature oligodendrocytes is decreased by caffeine and taurine. Primary immature oligodendrocytes were treated with or without 0.3 mg/mL caffeine, 4 mg/mL taurine, and the combination of both for 24 h followed by media exchange to differentiating conditions for another three days. (**A**) Representative images of immunofluorescence staining for the pan-oligodendrocyte marker Olig2 (red) and the myelination marker MBP (green) to visualize mature oligodendrocytes. The density of oligodendrocytes was quantified by counting Olig2 positive cells (**B**). MBP-positive oligodendrocytes were quantified by subtracting MBP-negative cells from the total Olig2-positive cell number. (**C**). Data are derived from 15 images per group out of three independent experiments, depicted by circle = control, square = caffeine, triangle up = taurine, triangle down = caffeine + taurine. Scale bar 400 µm. ** $p < 0.01$, *** $p < 0.001$, one-way ANOVA followed by a Bonferroni post hoc test.

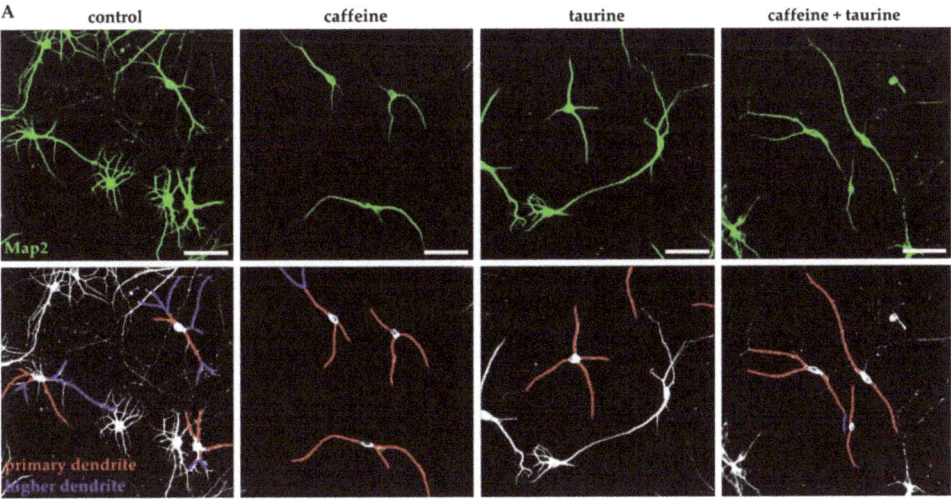

Figure 4. *Cont.*

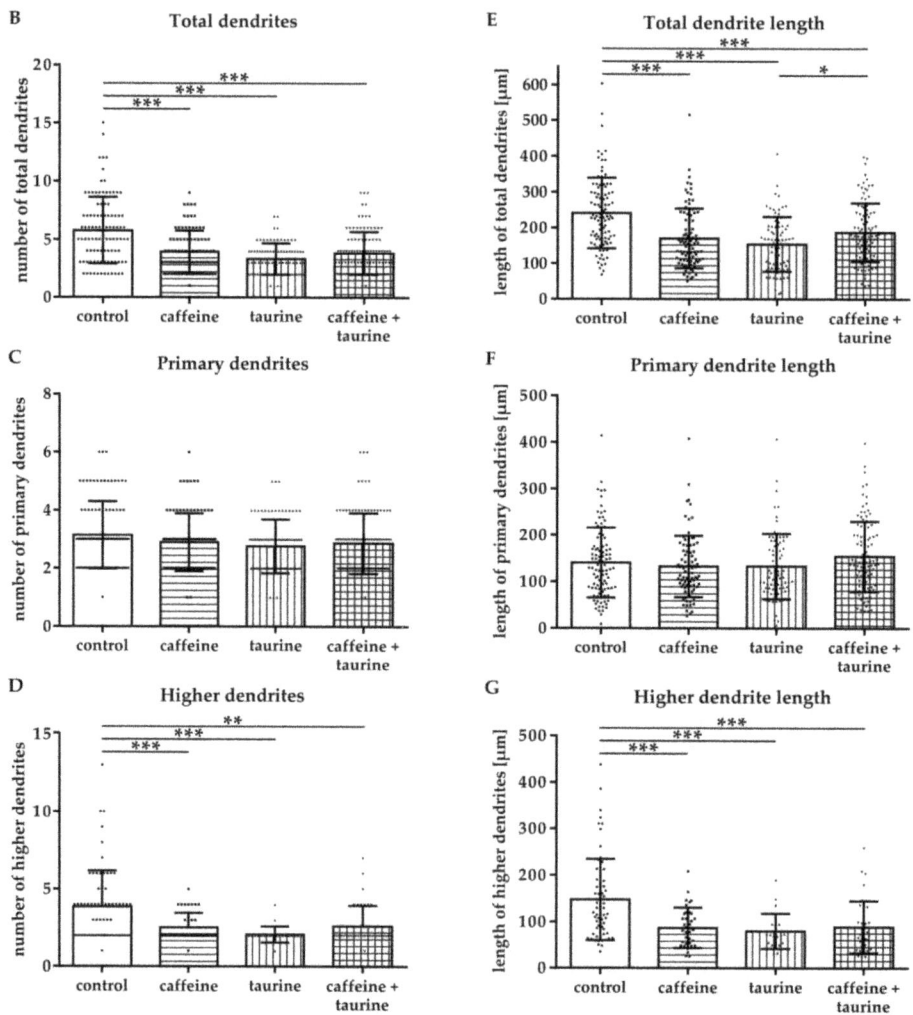

Figure 4. Caffeine and taurine alone or in combination reduce branching of dendrites in primary hippocampal neurons. Following three days in culture primary hippocampal neurons were incubated with or without 0.3 mg/mL caffeine, 4 mg/mL taurine and the combination of both for 24 h. (**A**) Dendrites were visualized by immunofluorescence staining for microtubule-associated protein 2 (Map2, green). Morphological changes were measured by defining primary dendrites (**A**, bottom row, red) and higher dendrites (**A**, bottom row, blue). The amount of total (**B**), primary (**C**), and higher (**D**) dendrites was quantified; subfigures (**E–G**) represent results of quantification of dendritic lengths, respectively. Data are derived from 25–30 images per group out of three independent experiments (n = 83–103 cells per group, depicted by circle = control, square = caffeine, triangle up = taurine, triangle down = caffeine + taurine). Scale bar 100 µm. * $p < 0.05$, ** $p < 0.01$, *** $p < 0.001$, one-way ANOVA followed by a Bonferroni post hoc test.

3.4. Prolonged Disturbance of Dendrite and Axonal Morphology Following Short-Term Caffeine and Taurine Treatment

To investigate whether the acute effect of caffeine and taurine on dendrite morphology correlates with changes in neuronal development and network formation, neurons were cultivated under standard culture conditions for another three days following substance treatment. According to results after immediate analysis at the acute time point, the number of Map2-positive higher dendrites and their length were significantly reduced to an average of 50% compared to controls ($F_{3, 211} = 21.75$; mean: control 6.73, caffeine 3.35, taurine 3.73 and caffeine + taurine 3.41; Figure 5A–G). To verify whether disturbed dendrite branching was associated with changes in axonal morphology we analysed TAU-expression by immunocytochemistry. While we observed a densely packed network of intact axons without or occasionally appearing breaks in the control group, caffeine and taurine treated neurons demonstrated more axon breaks and pearl-like structures (Figure 5H), previously described as accumulations of microtubule associated and molecular motor proteins as well as organelles and vesicles, as an indicator for defective and damaged neurons [12,24].

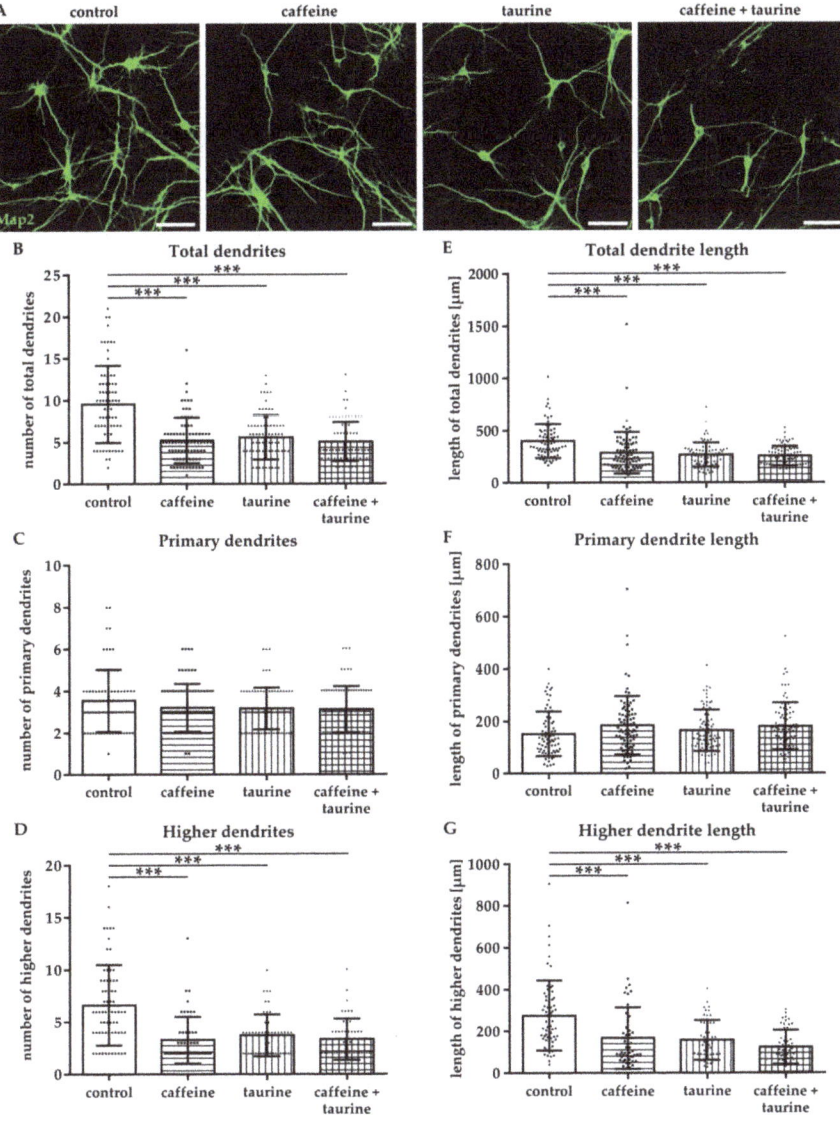

Figure 5. Cont.

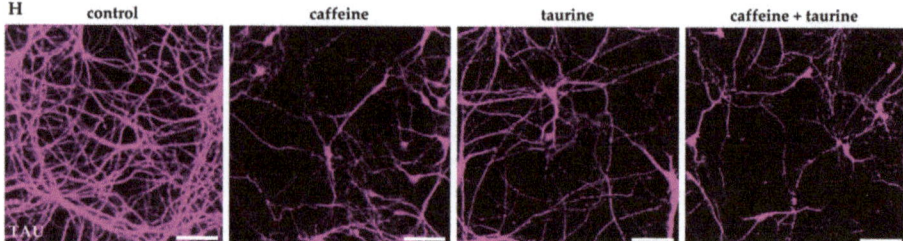

Figure 5. Caffeine and taurine lead to sustained reduced dendritic branching and disturbed axonal network formation. After three days in culture primary hippocampal neurons were treated with or without 0.3 mg/mL caffeine, 4 mg/mL taurine and the combination of both for 24 h followed by cultivation under standard culture conditions for another three days. (**A**) Representative images of Map2 (green) stained dendrites. Quantifications of the amount of total, primary and higher dendrites, as well as their lengths are shown in subfigures (**B–G**). Data are derived from 25–30 images per group out of three independent experiments (n = 75–82 cells per group, depicted by circle = control, square = caffeine, triangle up = taurine, triangle down = caffeine + taurine). Morphological changes of axons were visualized by immunofluorescence staining for TAU (**H**). Scale bar 100 μm. *** $p < 0.001$, one-way ANOVA followed by a Bonferroni post hoc test.

4. Discussion

The widespread consumption of energy drinks became popular among adolescents below the age of 25 in recent years. Taking the fact that brain development in childhood/adolescence is not completed [9], neuronal and glial cell types might be particularly vulnerable to high doses of energy drink ingredients. The goal of the present study was to investigate the effects of the main energy drink components caffeine and taurine on neuronal cells and immature oligodendrocytes. Using purified primary cell cultures, we demonstrated that the energy drink ingredients caffeine and taurine induce degeneration and reduce proliferation of immature oligodendrocytes, accompanied by a decreased myelination capacity. Furthermore, caffeine and taurine impaired neuronal network formation revealed by reduced dendrite branching and fragmented axons. The present study suggests detrimental effects of increased energy drink consumption particularly during brain development which lasts into early adulthood.

The observed adverse health effects of excessive energy drink consumption have been mainly attributed to high caffeine concentrations. We demonstrated that caffeine inhibits proliferation and myelination capacity of primary oligodendrocytes. These results seem to contradict previous findings in models of adult neurodegenerative diseases like Parkinson and Alzheimer's disease [25]. Furthermore, in vitro studies on hypoxia-induced degeneration of oligodendrocytes demonstrated protective effects by caffeine treatment [26]. In the context of brain injury to the developing brain, Endesfelder et al. also described neuroprotective effects of caffeine revealed by reduced oxidative stress, decreased neuronal degeneration, and diminished inflammation after oxygen-induced toxicity in vivo [27,28]. However, caffeine concentrations, used in these previous studies, have been much lower than the ones used in the present in vitro study, i.e., Endesfelder et al. used a 30-fold lower concentration [28].

Besides differences in dose, long duration of caffeine exposure might explain our findings. This is supported by recent studies in mouse epidermal cells and human neuroblastoma cells that suggested that even low caffeine concentrations for 24 h may induce apoptotic cell degeneration through caspase 3-induced signalling-pathways [29,30]. In the present study we decided for 24 h exposure according to the previous studies by Zeidán-Chuliá et al. and Doyle et al. [12,31]. Furthermore, caffeine is absorbed very fast, reaching peak plasma concentrations after 30–120 min [32]. Based on its hydrophobic structure it can easily pass the blood–brain barrier [33]; and CSF levels are described to be similar to plasma concentrations [34]. The different half-life times of caffeine with 100 h in preterms, compared to

3–5 h in adults [34], suggest an exponential decrease of the caffeine half-life time during development. Therefore, we decided for 24 h substance exposure. Nevertheless, further studies are needed on in vivo pharmacokinetics of caffeine in childhood and adolescence. Interestingly, effects of single taurine treatment on immature oligodendrocyte degeneration were less pronounced compared to caffeine single and combined treatment. However, proliferation of A2B5-positive oligodendrocytes was significantly reduced, resulting in an overall decreased cell number. These results indicate that detrimental effects of taurine on developing oligodendrocytes might be rather attributed to inhibition of proliferation than induction of degeneration. This seems to be in contrast to previous reports where taurine was described as a putative neuromodulator, improving neurological dysfunctions, especially cognitive function [35,36]. On the other hand, in human lung cancer cells taurine treatment with different concentrations for 24 h, 48 h, and 72 h inhibited cell proliferation [37], which is in accordance to our observations in the present study. Further research will be needed to delineate positive and negative effects of taurine in cell- and disease-specific experimental settings.

The combined treatment of caffeine and taurine induced the most pronounced increase of oligodendrocyte degeneration compared to single treatments, which may indicate interactions between both compounds. Additive effects of caffeine and taurine have already been described in a study analysing cardiac parameters in athletes demonstrating exacerbated effects of single compounds after simultaneous uptake [38]. Furthermore, mice treated with caffeine and taurine for 2 weeks demonstrated a significantly enhanced endurance performance after a combined treatment compared to single treatments [39]. Even though an increased calcium-release in muscles or competitive inhibition of adenosine receptors expressed by different neuronal cells in the CNS has been discussed [39], the detailed underlying mechanisms of a potential interaction remain elusive and require further investigation.

Brain development is strongly dependent on oligodendrocyte maturation into myelinating cells. Therefore, we analysed differentiation capacity of immature oligodendrocytes demonstrating a significantly decreased number of mature MBP-positive oligodendrocytes three days after treatment. These results suggest that energy compounds not only induce acute cellular degeneration but that biological programs of surviving oligodendrocytes are severely disturbed. This is of particular importance, as myelination is the key for neuronal network formation [40,41]. Even though neurogenesis in most cortical and subcortical regions is supposed to be completed by postnatal-day 15 in rats and by 2.5 years in humans [9], neurogenesis lasts into adulthood in other brain regions, i.e., the hippocampus and olfactory bulbs [42,43]. Furthermore, during puberty neuronal network formation and integration is reorganized requiring competent oligodendrocytes to myelinate axons and to enable formation of new synapses [41].

In addition to competent myelinating oligodendrocytes, neuronal reorganisation during puberty depends on neuronal integrity, e.g., axonal network formation and dendritic branching [44]. Therefore, we analysed the effects of caffeine and taurine on neurons isolated from the hippocampus, the main structure of learning and memory formation involving adult neurogenesis and synaptogenesis [18]. In addition to neuronal cell loss immediately after treatment with caffeine and taurine, a significant reduction in number and length of total dendrites mainly caused by a reduction of higher dendrite branching was observed. These effects persisted for several days, which is of particular importance considering that dendritic arborisation coordinates with synaptic activity and is important for neural network integrity [45]. Furthermore, disturbed maintenance and disruption of dendrites and synapses has been associated with psychiatric illnesses, such as schizophrenia and major depressive disorders, as well as neurodegenerative diseases, such as Alzheimer's disease [46]. Nevertheless, similarly as for oligodendrocytes, these results appear contradicting to previous findings, describing enhanced dendrite outgrowth in primary hippocampal neurons after taurine and caffeine treatment [47,48]. However, again concentrations applied, seem to be decisive. For example, protective effects of taurine on dendrite outgrowth were observed at 100 µM, while 2.7 mM, approximately equivalent to 0.34 mg/mL, was described to decrease neurite length and number [47,49] supporting our observations. Besides dendritic branching, axonal integrity is important for functionality and activity of neurons [50]. Analysis of axonal morphology demonstrated an increased number of axonal breaks and pearl-like structures three days after treatment with caffeine and taurine and especially in the combined treatment. Similar structures were also described in human neuronal SH-SY5Y cells incubated with caffeine and in an experimental model of Alzheimer's disease [12,24]. This abnormal morphology was suggested to be caused by accumulation of proteins, organelles, and vesicles and to result in axonal defects and impaired axonal transport. In view of these previous studies, our observations suggest that high concentrations of caffeine and taurine in energy drinks do not only inhibit the capacity of dendritic branching but also disturb axonal function.

We have chosen high concentrations of caffeine and taurine corresponding to that of commercially available energy drinks. We are aware of the fact that concentrations applied in the present and previous [12] in vitro studies are higher than concentrations determined in plasma of humans and rodents after oral consumption/administration [32,33,51]. However, translation of in vitro doses to humans is always limited considering the complex variables, one cannot control for in vitro, e.g., co-consumption of other drugs like alcohol and smoking or of sugar provided in energy drinks which may affect pharmacokinetics. Our rationale was mainly based on the fact that consumption, especially in adolescents and young adults, is still rising. Twelve percent of adolescents and 13.4% of young adults have been identified as high acute consumers, with at least 1 L of energy drink consumption per session, and high chronic consumers, with 13.3% of young adults consuming an average volume of 4.5 L/month, as well as 12% of adolescents being high chronic consumers, with 4–5 sessions/week and an average volume of 7 L/month [22].

In the present study we provide evidence that an increased consumption of energy drinks may negatively influence neurodevelopment during childhood and adolescence, reducing immature oligodendrocyte survival and their differentiation capacity, which is accompanied by direct effects on neuronal integrity. Effects were analyzed in purified primary cell cultures. Even though pharmacokinetics of single energy drink compounds after oral intake can hardly be modeled in vitro, the rapid absorption of caffeine and taurine and unproblematic passing of the blood–brain barrier [52,53], indicate that high concentrations of caffeine and taurine reach the brain. In view of the continuous rise of teens and children consuming energy drinks further studies are needed to confirm these effects in vivo considering the complex interactions between different CNS cell types needed for oligodendrocyte development, myelination and axonal network formation during puberty.

Supplementary Materials: The following are available online at http://www.mdpi.com/2073-4409/8/11/1381/s1, Figure S1: Caffeine and taurine reduce the number of hippocampal neurons. Table S1: Detailed results of statistical analyses for effects on oligodendrocytes. Table S2: Detailed results of statistical analyses for effects on hippocampal neurons.

Author Contributions: Conceptualization, M.S., K.M., U.F.-M., and I.B.; Data Curation, M.S., A.M., K.K., J.H., and I.B.; Formal Analysis, M.S., A.M., K.M., J.H., and I.B.; Funding Acquisition, U.F.-M., J.H., and I.B.; Investigation, M.S., A.M., and K.K.; Methodology, M.S., A.M., K.M., K.K., J.H., and I.B.; Validation, M.S., A.M., K.K., J.H., and I.B.; Writing original draft and revised manuscript, M.S., U.F.-M., J.H. and I.B.

Funding: This research was funded by C.D. Stiftung (T228-23.816). We acknowledge support by the Open Access Publication Fund of the University of Duisburg-Essen.

Acknowledgments: The authors thank Mandana Rizazad and Christian Köster for ongoing excellent technical assistance.

Conflicts of Interest: The authors declare no conflict of interest.

References

1. Gallimberti, L.; Buja, A.; Chindamo, S.; Vinelli, A.; Lazzarin, G.; Terraneo, A.; Scafato, E.; Baldo, V. Energy drink consumption in children and early adolescents. *Eur. J. Pediatr.* **2013**, *172*, 1335–1340. [CrossRef] [PubMed]
2. Seifert, S.M.; Schaechter, J.L.; Hershorin, E.R.; Lipshultz, S.E. Health effects of energy drinks on children, adolescents, and young adults. *Pediatrics* **2011**, *127*, 511–528. [CrossRef] [PubMed]
3. Ehlers, A.; Marakis, G.; Lampen, A.; Hirsch-Ernst, K.I. Risk assessment of energy drinks with focus on cardiovascular parameters and energy drink consumption in Europe. *Food Chem. Toxicol.* **2019**, *130*, 109–121. [CrossRef] [PubMed]

4. Al-Basher, G.I.; Aljabal, H.; Almeer, R.S.; Allam, A.A.; Mahmoud, A.M. Perinatal exposure to energy drink induces oxidative damage in the liver, kidney and brain, and behavioral alterations in mice offspring. *Biomed. Pharmacother.* **2018**, *102*, 798–811. [CrossRef] [PubMed]
5. Grasser, E.K.; Yepuri, G.; Dulloo, A.G.; Montani, J.P. Cardio- and cerebrovascular responses to the energy drink Red Bull in young adults: A randomized cross-over study. *Eur. J. Nutr.* **2014**, *53*, 1561–1571. [CrossRef] [PubMed]
6. Holubcikova, J.; Kolarcik, P.; Madarasova Geckova, A.; Reijneveld, S.A.; van Dijk, J.P. Regular energy drink consumption is associated with the risk of health and behavioural problems in adolescents. *Eur. J. Pediatr.* **2017**, *176*, 599–605. [CrossRef] [PubMed]
7. Hammond, D.; Reid, J.L.; Zukowski, S. Adverse effects of caffeinated energy drinks among youth and young adults in Canada: A Web-based survey. *CMAJ Open* **2018**, *6*, e19–e25. [CrossRef]
8. Giedd, J.N.; Blumenthal, J.; Jeffries, N.O.; Castellanos, F.X.; Liu, H.; Zijdenbos, A.; Paus, T.; Evans, A.C.; Rapoport, J.L. Brain development during childhood and adolescence: A longitudinal MRI study. *Nat. Neurosci.* **1999**, *2*, 861–863. [CrossRef]
9. Semple, B.D.; Blomgren, K.; Gimlin, K.; Ferriero, D.M.; Noble-Haeusslein, L.J. Brain development in rodents and humans: Identifying benchmarks of maturation and vulnerability to injury across species. *Prog. Neurobiol.* **2013**, *106*, 1–16. [CrossRef]
10. Geeraert, B.L.; Lebel, R.M.; Lebel, C. A multiparametric analysis of white matter maturation during late childhood and adolescence. *Hum. Brain Mapp.* **2019**, *40*, 4345–4356. [CrossRef]
11. Reis, R.; Charehsaz, M.; Sipahi, H.; Ekici, A.I.; Macit, C.; Akkaya, H.; Aydin, A. Energy Drink Induced Lipid Peroxidation and Oxidative Damage in Rat Liver and Brain When Used Alone or Combined with Alcohol. *J. Food Sci.* **2017**, *82*, 1037–1043. [CrossRef] [PubMed]
12. Zeidan-Chulia, F.; Gelain, D.P.; Kolling, E.A.; Rybarczyk-Filho, J.L.; Ambrosi, P.; Terra, S.R.; Pires, A.S.; da Rocha, J.B.; Behr, G.A.; Moreira, J.C. Major components of energy drinks (caffeine, taurine, and guarana) exert cytotoxic effects on human neuronal SH-SY5Y cells by decreasing reactive oxygen species production. *Oxid. Med. Cell. Longev.* **2013**, *2013*, 791–795. [CrossRef] [PubMed]
13. Brehmer, F.; Bendix, I.; Prager, S.; van de Looij, Y.; Reinboth, B.S.; Zimmermanns, J.; Schlager, G.W.; Brait, D.; Sifringer, M.; Endesfelder, S.; et al. Interaction of inflammation and hyperoxia in a rat model of neonatal white matter damage. *PLoS ONE* **2012**, *7*, e49023. [CrossRef] [PubMed]
14. McCarthy, K.D.; de Vellis, J. Preparation of separate astroglial and oligodendroglial cell cultures from rat cerebral tissue. *J. Cell Biol.* **1980**, *85*, 890–902. [CrossRef]
15. Serdar, M.; Herz, J.; Kempe, K.; Lumpe, K.; Reinboth, B.S.; Sizonenko, S.V.; Hou, X.; Herrmann, R.; Hadamitzky, M.; Heumann, R.; et al. Fingolimod protects against neonatal white matter damage and long-term cognitive deficits caused by hyperoxia. *Brain Behav. Immun.* **2016**, *52*, 106–119. [CrossRef]
16. Janowska, J.; Ziemka-Nalecz, M.; Sypecka, J. The Differentiation of Rat Oligodendroglial Cells Is Highly Influenced by the Oxygen Tension: In Vitro Model Mimicking Physiologically Normoxic Conditions. *Int. J. Mol. Sci.* **2018**, *19*, 331. [CrossRef]
17. Pfeiffer, S.E.; Warrington, A.E.; Bansal, R. The oligodendrocyte and its many cellular processes. *Trends Cell Biol.* **1993**, *3*, 191–197. [CrossRef]
18. Stuchlik, A. Dynamic learning and memory, synaptic plasticity and neurogenesis: An update. *Front. Behav. Neurosci.* **2014**, *8*, 106. [CrossRef]
19. Persad, L.A.B. Energy drinks and the neurophysiological impact of caffeine. *Front. Neurosci.* **2011**, *5*, 116. [CrossRef]
20. Beaudoin, G.M., III; Lee, S.H.; Singh, D.; Yuan, Y.; Ng, Y.G.; Reichardt, L.F.; Arikkath, J. Culturing pyramidal neurons from the early postnatal mouse hippocampus and cortex. *Nat. Protoc.* **2012**, *7*, 1741–1754. [CrossRef]
21. Meijering, E.; Jacob, M.; Sarria, J.-C.; Steiner, P.; Hirling, H.; Unser, M.; Sarria, J. Design and validation of a tool for neurite tracing and analysis in fluorescence microscopy images. *Cytometry* **2004**, *58*, 167–176. [CrossRef]
22. Zucconi, S.; Volpato, C.; Adinolfi, F.; Gandini, E.; Gentile, E.; Loi, A.; Fioriti, L. Gathering consumption data on specific consumer groups of energy drinks. *EFSA Support. Publ.* **2013**, *10*. [CrossRef]
23. Crowley, L.C.; Waterhouse, N.J. Detecting Cleaved Caspase-3 in Apoptotic Cells by Flow Cytometry. *Cold Spring Harb. Protoc.* **2016**, *2016*. [CrossRef] [PubMed]

24. Stokin, G.B.; Lillo, C.; Falzone, T.L.; Brusch, R.G.; Rockenstein, E.; Mount, S.L.; Raman, R.; Davies, P.; Masliah, E.; Williams, D.S.; et al. Axonopathy and transport deficits early in the pathogenesis of Alzheimer's disease. *Science* **2005**, *307*, 1282–1288. [CrossRef] [PubMed]
25. Kolahdouzan, M.; Hamadeh, M.J. The neuroprotective effects of caffeine in neurodegenerative diseases. *CNS Neurosci. Ther.* **2017**, *23*, 272–290. [CrossRef] [PubMed]
26. Cao, T.; Ma, T.; Xu, Y.; Tian, Y.; Cai, Q.; Li, B.; Li, H. Caffeine Treatment Promotes Differentiation and Maturation of Hypoxic Oligodendrocytes via Counterbalancing Adenosine 1 Adenosine Receptor-Induced Calcium Overload. *Med. Sci. Monit.* **2019**, *25*, 1729–1739. [CrossRef]
27. Endesfelder, S.; Weichelt, U.; Strauß, E.; Schlör, A.; Sifringer, M.; Scheuer, T.; Bührer, C.; Schmitz, T. Neuroprotection by Caffeine in Hyperoxia-Induced Neonatal Brain Injury. *Int. J. Mol. Sci.* **2017**, *18*, 187. [CrossRef]
28. Endesfelder, S.; Zaak, I.; Weichelt, U.; Bührer, C.; Schmitz, T. Caffeine protects neuronal cells against injury caused by hyperoxia in the immature brain. *Free. Radic. Biol. Med.* **2014**, *67*, 221–234. [CrossRef]
29. He, Z.; Ma, W.-Y.; Hashimoto, T.; Bode, A.M.; Yang, C.S.; Dong, Z. Induction of apoptosis by caffeine is mediated by the p53, Bax, and caspase 3 pathways. *Cancer Res.* **2003**, *63*, 4396–4401.
30. Jang, M.H.; Shin, M.C.; Kang, I.S.; Baik, H.H.; Cho, Y.H.; Chu, J.P.; Kim, E.H.; Kim, C.J. Caffeine induces apoptosis in human neuroblastoma cell line SK-N-MC. *J. Korean Med. Sci.* **2002**, *17*, 674–678. [CrossRef]
31. Doyle, W.; Shide, E.; Thapa, S.; Chandrasekaran, V. The effects of energy beverages on cultured cells. *Food Chem. Toxicol.* **2012**, *50*, 3759–3768. [CrossRef] [PubMed]
32. White, J.R.; Padowski, J.M.; Zhong, Y.; Chen, G.; Luo, S.; Lazarus, P.; Layton, M.E.; McPherson, S. Pharmacokinetic analysis and comparison of caffeine administered rapidly or slowly in coffee chilled or hot versus chilled energy drink in healthy young adults. *Clin. Toxicol.* **2016**, *54*, 308–312. [CrossRef] [PubMed]
33. Kaplan, G.B.; Greenblatt, D.J.; Leduc, B.W.; Thompson, M.L.; Shader, R.I. Relationship of plasma and brain concentrations of caffeine and metabolites to benzodiazepine receptor binding and locomotor activity. *J. Pharmacol. Exp. Ther.* **1989**, *248*, 1078–1083. [PubMed]
34. Abdel-Hady, H.; Nasef, N.; Shabaan, A.E.; Nour, I. Caffeine therapy in preterm infants. *World J. Clin. Pediatr.* **2015**, *4*, 81–93. [CrossRef]
35. Curran, C.P.; Marczinski, C.A. Taurine, caffeine, and energy drinks: Reviewing the risks to the adolescent brain. *Birth Defects Res.* **2017**, *109*, 1640–1648. [CrossRef]
36. Kilb, W. Putative Role of Taurine as Neurotransmitter During Perinatal Cortical Development. In *Advances in Experimental Medicine and Biology*; Lee, D.H., Schaffer, S.W., Eds.; Springer: Dordrecht, The Netherlands, 2017. [CrossRef]
37. Tu, S.; Zhang, X.L.; Wan, H.F.; Xia, Y.Q.; Liu, Z.Q.; Yang, X.H.; Wan, F.S. Effect of taurine on cell proliferation and apoptosis human lung cancer A549 cells. *Oncol. Lett.* **2018**, *15*, 5473–5480. [CrossRef]
38. Baum, M.; Weiss, M. The influence of a taurine containing drink on cardiac parameters before and after exercise measured by echocardiography. *Amino Acids* **2001**, *20*, 75–82. [CrossRef]
39. Imagawa, T.F.; Hirano, I.; Utsuki, K.; Horie, M.; Naka, A.; Matsumoto, K.; Imagawa, S. Caffeine and taurine enhance endurance performance. *Int. J. Sports Med.* **2009**, *30*, 485–488. [CrossRef]
40. De Hoz, L.; Simons, M. The emerging functions of oligodendrocytes in regulating neuronal network behaviour. *Bioessays* **2015**, *37*, 60–69. [CrossRef]
41. Wang, F.; Yang, Y.-J.; Yang, N.; Chen, X.-J.; Huang, N.-X.; Zhang, J.; Wu, Y.; Liu, Z.; Gao, X.; Li, T.; et al. Enhancing Oligodendrocyte Myelination Rescues Synaptic Loss and Improves Functional Recovery after Chronic Hypoxia. *Neuron* **2018**, *99*, 689–701. [CrossRef]
42. Altman, J.; Das, G.D. Autoradiographic and histological evidence of postnatal hippocampal neurogenesis in rats. *J. Comp. Neurol.* **1965**, *124*, 319–335. [CrossRef] [PubMed]
43. Shors, T.J.; Miesegaes, G.; Beylin, A.; Zhao, M.; Rydel, T.; Gould, E. Neurogenesis in the adult is involved in the formation of trace memories. *Nature* **2001**, *410*, 372–376. [CrossRef] [PubMed]
44. Tavosanis, G. Dendritic structural plasticity. *Dev. Neurobiol.* **2012**, *72*, 73–86. [CrossRef] [PubMed]
45. Arikkath, J. Molecular mechanisms of dendrite morphogenesis. *Front. Cell. Neurosci.* **2012**, *6*, 61. [CrossRef]
46. Lin, Y.-C.; Koleske, A.J. Mechanisms of synapse and dendrite maintenance and their disruption in psychiatric and neurodegenerative disorders. *Annu. Rev. Neurosci.* **2010**, *33*, 349–378. [CrossRef]
47. Shivaraj, M.C.; Marcy, G.; Low, G.; Ryu, J.R.; Zhao, X.; Rosales, F.J.; Goh, E.L.K. Taurine Induces Proliferation of Neural Stem Cells and Synapse Development in the Developing Mouse Brain. *PLoS ONE* **2012**, *7*, e42935. [CrossRef]

48. Yu, N.Y.; Bieder, A.; Raman, A.; Mileti, E.; Katayama, S.; Einarsdottir, E.; Fredholm, B.B.; Falk, A.; Tapia-Páez, I.; Daub, C.O.; et al. Acute doses of caffeine shift nervous system cell expression profiles toward promotion of neuronal projection growth. *Sci. Rep.* **2017**, *7*, 11458. [CrossRef]
49. Nusetti, S.; Obregón, F.; Quintal, M.; Benzo, Z.; Lima, L. Taurine and Zinc Modulate Outgrowth from Goldfish Retinal Explants. *Neurochem. Res.* **2005**, *30*, 1483–1492. [CrossRef]
50. Beirowski, B. Concepts for regulation of axon integrity by enwrapping glia. *Front. Cell. Neurosci.* **2013**, *7*, 256. [CrossRef]
51. Catalán-Latorre, A.; Nacher, A.; Merino, V.; Diez, O.; Sanjuán, M.M. A preclinical study to model taurine pharmokinetics in the undernourished rat. *Br. J. Nutr.* **2018**, *119*, 826–835. [CrossRef]
52. Kang, Y.-S.; Ohtsuki, S.; Takanaga, H.; Tomi, M.; Hosoya, K.-I.; Terasaki, T. Regulation of taurine transport at the blood-brain barrier by tumor necrosis factor-α, taurine and hypertonicity. *J. Neurochem.* **2002**, *83*, 1188–1195. [CrossRef] [PubMed]
53. Lachance, M.; Marlowe, C.; Waddell, W. Autoradiographic disposition of [1-methyl-14C]- and [2-14C] caffeine in mice. *Toxicol. Appl. Pharmacol.* **1983**, *71*, 237–241. [CrossRef]

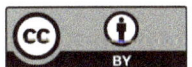

© 2019 by the authors. Licensee MDPI, Basel, Switzerland. This article is an open access article distributed under the terms and conditions of the Creative Commons Attribution (CC BY) license (http://creativecommons.org/licenses/by/4.0/).

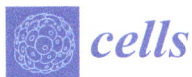

Review

Oligodendrocytes in Development, Myelin Generation and Beyond

Sarah Kuhn [†], Laura Gritti [†], Daniel Crooks and Yvonne Dombrowski *

Wellcome-Wolfson Institute for Experimental Medicine, Queen's University Belfast, Belfast BT9 7BL, UK; skuhn01@qub.ac.uk (S.K.); l.gritti@qub.ac.uk (L.G.); dcrooks03@qub.ac.uk (D.C.)
* Correspondence: y.dombrowski@qub.ac.uk; Tel.: +0044-28-9097-6127
† These authors contributed equally.

Received: 15 October 2019; Accepted: 7 November 2019; Published: 12 November 2019

Abstract: Oligodendrocytes are the myelinating cells of the central nervous system (CNS) that are generated from oligodendrocyte progenitor cells (OPC). OPC are distributed throughout the CNS and represent a pool of migratory and proliferative adult progenitor cells that can differentiate into oligodendrocytes. The central function of oligodendrocytes is to generate myelin, which is an extended membrane from the cell that wraps tightly around axons. Due to this energy consuming process and the associated high metabolic turnover oligodendrocytes are vulnerable to cytotoxic and excitotoxic factors. Oligodendrocyte pathology is therefore evident in a range of disorders including multiple sclerosis, schizophrenia and Alzheimer's disease. Deceased oligodendrocytes can be replenished from the adult OPC pool and lost myelin can be regenerated during remyelination, which can prevent axonal degeneration and can restore function. Cell population studies have recently identified novel immunomodulatory functions of oligodendrocytes, the implications of which, e.g., for diseases with primary oligodendrocyte pathology, are not yet clear. Here, we review the journey of oligodendrocytes from the embryonic stage to their role in homeostasis and their fate in disease. We will also discuss the most common models used to study oligodendrocytes and describe newly discovered functions of oligodendrocytes.

Keywords: oligodendrocytes; OPC; oligodendrocyte progenitor cells; myelin; myelination; remyelination; multiple sclerosis

---

1. Introduction

Oligodendrocytes are the myelinating cells of the central nervous system (CNS). They are generated from oligodendrocyte progenitor cells following tightly orchestrated processes of migration, proliferation and differentiation [1]. Oligodendrocytes are fundamental to myelin formation in the developing CNS and critical for myelin regeneration following injury including in the most common demyelinating disease multiple sclerosis (MS) [2,3]. In this review, we discuss the journey of oligodendrocytes in development from the embryonic stage to oligodendrocyte function in health and their fate in disease. We will also review the most common models used to study oligodendrocyte behaviour and function and discuss recent advances in our knowledge of oligodendrocytes.

2. Oligodendrocyte Progenitor Cells (OPC) and Oligodendrocytes in Development

2.1. OPC and Oligodendrocytes during Embryonic Development

Oligodendrocytes are one of the major glial cell types in the CNS besides microglia and astroglia. Oligodendrocytes were first described by Virchow [4], Deiters [5] and Golgi [6] in the 19th century. While neurons had been well characterised at that time, an abundant unknown cell type called "neuroglia" became the focus of attention. Analysing the fine structure of the brain led Virchow to introduce the term "Nervenkitt" (German: nerve glue) as cells appeared in between nerves [4,7]. Distinct from neurons, these cells could not grow axons [5] and were able to proliferate even postnatally. Initially, they were not thought to have a role other than being connective tissue. Pio del Rio-Hortega eventually differentiated neuroglia into microglia and four types of oligodendroglia by using more advanced staining techniques, including silver carbonate [8,9].

Amongst the glial populations, bipolar cells were found to be highly proliferative and migratory, whereas filamentous myelin-producing glia were mainly found in white matter suggesting a bipolar precursor cell type, later termed oligodendrocyte progenitor cell (OPC), and a distinct, differentiated cell type, the oligodendrocyte [10].

The origin of neurons was well characterised within the CNS yet less was known about the origin of oligodendrocytes and microglia [11,12]. Microglia originate from the yolk sack [13], while oligodendrocytes develop from multiple origins in the brain and anterior spinal cord with radial glial cells, the ventral ventricular zone and dorsal spinal cord as sources [14–19]. Neural progenitor cells (NPC) arising in the neural tube during embryonic development are the common precursors for oligodendrocytes, astrocytes and neurons [20,21].

Murine OPC in brain and spinal cord are characterised by the expression of DM-20 mRNA [16,22]. Using this marker, three temporal waves of OPC development were identified starting in the ventral ventricular zone after neural tube closure from E9.5 [16]. Rat OPC first appeared at around E14 [17] and human OPC at E45, reflecting the gestational week 6.5 [23]. Across species, several waves of OPC generation were identified. The first wave of OPC generation in the forebrain is followed by a smaller second wave from the dorsal ventricular zone and by a third postnatal wave originating in the cortex [24]. In the spinal cord, ventrally-derived OPC are followed by a wave of dorsally-derived OPC [25,26], which make up to 20% of total OPC [19,25].

These waves subsequently lead to an overproduction of progenitor cells, which compete for space and survival factors provided by astrocytes and axons [24,27–29]. It was shown that most OPC from the first cortical wave die [24,27]. However, Orduz et al. recently demonstrated that a subpopulation of first-wave cortical OPC not only survive but have non-redundant functions [30].

In the adult normal CNS, the majority of proliferating cells are of oligodendroglial lineage origin, which by dividing self-renew and generate mature oligodendrocytes, whereas little evidence exists that neurons are able to proliferate in adulthood [31–34].

During vertebrate development, one of the major and best-established morphogens is the Sonic hedgehog (Shh) protein, required for most OPC to originate during early embryogenesis [26,35]. Shh is produced by the notochord, which is essential for the CNS dorsal–ventral axis development [36,37]. OPC as well as motor neurons originate from similar areas in the ventral neural tube during development and need equal amounts of Shh in order to arise, which suggests an interlinked generation of both cell types [38–40]. However, in vitro experiments with Shh deficient cells indicated that Shh is not an absolute requirement for OPC origination [41], while mice lacking a notochord did not develop any OPC [38]. Cai et al. corroborated these findings in vivo demonstrating *Nkx6*- and *Shh*-independent generation of an OPC subpopulation, which suggests the involvement of other molecular pathways [26]. Indeed, *Shh* is important for the timing of OPC generation as a recent study has shown [42].

Tightly regulated epigenetic mechanisms, such as DNA methylation and histone modification, have recently been discovered in the regulation of OPC differentiation that are distinct in the different developmental stages and in myelin regeneration (reviewed in detail in [43]).

More recently, activated neurons were shown to play a role in the origination and proliferation of OPC, and oligodendrocytes to myelinate [44–47].

2.2. Distribution of OPC and Oligodendrocytes within the CNS

Only 5%–8% of total glial cells are OPC [48], which are evenly distributed in white (WM) and grey matter (GM), with OPC being slightly less abundant in GM [48]. The location gives rise to behavioural differences between WM and GM OPC; while WM NG2$^+$ OPC in organotypic brain slices had a greater proliferative response to PDGF-A, GM OPC were less responsive to PDGF-A and morphologically and genetically less mature than WM OPC [49,50]. In vivo, more WM OPC differentiate into myelinating oligodendrocytes than GM OPC, many of which remain NG2$^+$ progenitors as shown by Dimou et al. [51,52], suggesting a potential backup pool of OPC during adulthood. In the adult CNS, oligodendrocyte generation from OPC is slowed down and WM OPC generate about 20% of total differentiated and myelinating oligodendrocytes in the murine corpus callosum vs. 5% in the cortex [53]. However, 20% of cortical GM oligodendroglial lineage cells are differentiated CNP$^+$ NG2$^-$ oligodendrocytes yet these cells do not myelinate [53]. Recently, Hughes et al. demonstrated that cortical NG2$^+$ cells are highly dynamic, balancing their population by proliferation, differentiation and self-repulsion to maintain homeostasis [54].

In order for axonal myelination to occur, migration of OPC from their site of origin into the developing WM tracts of the CNS is required [55]. To overcome this spatial distance, OPC migrate in a jumping or crawling mode along blood vessels within the CNS, which is dependent on WNT signalling [56,57]. Their subsequent excessive proliferation, especially in the WM, leads to an abundant pool of progenitors throughout the brain and spinal cord [58].

2.3. Developmental Markers of OPC and Oligodendrocytes

New-born OPC are characterised by the expression of DM-20 mRNA, an isoform of protein proteolipid protein (PLP), the most abundant myelin protein [16]. There are numerous additional markers that determine the oligodendroglial cell lineage and reflect their developmental stage, the most prominent are summarised in Figure 1. Once committed to the oligodendroglial lineage, cell surface antigens can be recognized by specific antibodies such as A2B5 [59]. In vitro, A2B5 positive cells can differentiate into both oligodendrocytes and astrocytes, which were therefore termed oligodendrocyte-type-2 astrocyte (O-2A) progenitor cells [60]. O-2A progenitor cells constitutively differentiate into oligodendrocytes unless specific environmental cues redirect differentiation into astrocytes [61].

The best characterised marker for OPC is PDGFR-α, the receptor for PDGF-A, the most potent OPC mitogen and survival factor, which is produced by both astrocytes and neurons [15,62–64]. Consequently, overexpression of this growth factor, e.g., during development, leads to increase in OPC numbers [64].

Pre-oligodendrocytes engage with a target axon, thereby losing their bipolarity, and start to build filamentous myelin outgrowths. At this differentiation stage, pre-oligodendrocytes are characterised by the expression of three main myelin associated markers, 2′, 3′-cyclic-nucleotide 3′-phosphodiesterase (CNPase) and the cell surface markers O4 and O1 [65,66]. CNPase has two different isoforms which are differentially expressed: oligodendrocyte precursors only seem to express the larger isoform, whereas myelinating oligodendrocytes were shown to express both isoforms [67]. O4 is already expressed in late progenitors, whereas O1 is typical for pre-myelinating oligodendrocytes [68] (Figure 1).

Mature, differentiated oligodendrocytes are characterised by the production of myelin and myelin proteins, and in combination with a cell lineage specific marker such as Olig2 can be used to identify this maturation stage (Figure 1). The myelin proteins include myelin basic protein (MBP) [69,70], which is expressed on the cytoplasmic surface of the plasma membrane [71], the transmembrane protein PLP [16,72], myelin associated glycoprotein (MAG) [73] as well as the membrane marker galactocerebroside (GalC) [74] and surface marker myelin-oligodendrocyte glycoprotein (MOG) [69]. MBP and MAG first appear between postnatal day 5 and 7 in murine CNS-derived oligodendrocytes, whereas MOG emerges one to two days later [75]. Interestingly, PLP was recently described to be expressed in murine Olig2$^+$PDGFR-α$^+$ cells, which makes it an early marker for OPC with a role in process extension [76].

Two genetically related, but functionally different, transcription factors Olig1 and Olig2 are present throughout the oligodendroglial lineage [77,78]. Olig2 is essential for NPC to develop into OPC [79] and Olig2 gain of function in OPC can promote remyelination in mice [80]. The role of

Olig1 is less well known. Olig1 has a non-redundant role in OPC differentiation and myelination in murine brain development; however, spinal cord OPC are less dependent on Olig1 for differentiation and myelination [81,82]. In repair, however, Olig1 deficient mice showed delayed oligodendrocyte differentiation and impaired remyelination of demyelinated CNS lesions [83]. Another transcription factor involved in oligodendrocyte development that characterises the entire oligodendroglial lineage is SOX10 [84]. SOX10 is essential for NPC derived oligodendroglial lineage specification during early development and for OPC differentiation [85–87], while transcription factor Nkx2.2 promotes and regulates timing of oligodendrocyte differentiation [88,89]. A marker for early oligodendroglial lineage cells is the proteoglycan NG2, however, NG2$^+$ cells are able to differentiate into oligodendrocytes but also into astrocytes [90]. Antibodies against the markers described here are commercially available.

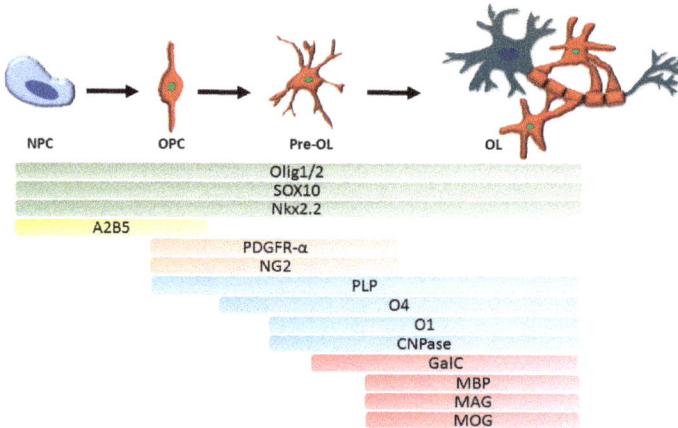

Figure 1. Schematic depiction of oligodendroglial lineage markers specific for different developmental stages from neuronal progenitor cells (NPC) to myelinating oligodendrocyte (OL). A2B5 recognises progenitor cells, NPC and oligodendrocyte progenitor cells (OPC), while oligodendroglial cell lineage markers Olig1 and 2 as well as Sox10 and Nkx2.2 are expressed in all cells of the lineage, OPC and pre-oligodendrocytes (pre-OL) are characterised by PDGFR-α and NG2 expression. PLP, O4, O1 and CNPase are expressed during transition from progenitor to differentiated oligodendrocytes, while differentiated, axon-myelinating oligodendrocytes are characterised by myelin protein expression (MBP, MAG, MOG, GalC). NPC: neuronal progenitor cell; OPC: oligodendrocyte progenitor cell; OL: oligodendrocyte; PDGFR-α: platelet-derived growth factor receptor A; NG2: neuron-glial antigen 2; PLP: proteolipid protein; CNPase: 2′,3′-Cyclic-nucleotide 3′-phosphodiesterase; MBP: myelin basic protein; MAG: myelin associated glycoprotein; MOG: myelin-oligodendrocyte glycoprotein; GalC: galactocerebroside.

2.4. Other Myelin-Producing Cells

Schwann cells are the oligodendrocyte counterpart in the peripheral nervous system (PNS), derived from the neural crest [91]. Oligodendrocytes and Schwann cells share main functions in providing support and insulation for axons. However, Schwann cells are only able to myelinate single axons rather than multiple axons contrary to oligodendrocytes (reviewed in [92,93]). This feature is dependent on an E3 ligase component, deficiency of which leads to increased myelination potential in murine Schwann cells in vivo [94].

Schwann cells as well as oligodendrocytes are region specific for the CNS and the peripheral nervous system and a glial barrier at the motor exit points was found to prevent oligodendrocytes exiting from the CNS. The cells forming this barrier are motor exit point (MEP) glia, which were recently described as the third cell type capable of producing myelin [95,96]. MEP glia share communalities with both oligodendrocytes and Schwann cells; like OPC, they are derived from the ventral neural tube and they express Olig2 as do oligodendroglial lineage cells. MEP glia are also characterised by the expression of SOX10 and WIF1. This, combined with Olig2 and Foxd3 expression, identifies this population [96]. Similar to Schwann cells, MEP glia express Foxd3 and they are able to myelinate just one axon, although the molecular mechanism underlying the process is different. MEP glia lack *krox20*, a key initiator of myelination for Schwann cells, and are also not affected by *gpr126* deficiency as opposed to Schwann cells. Moreover, MEP glia selectively myelinate spinal motor root axons [95–97] and were described to have a role in preventing the migration of OPC into the periphery by blocking off OPC in the CNS via direct contact [96].

3. Oligodendrocyte Function in Health

3.1. Myelination of Axons

The myelin sheath is an extension of the oligodendrocyte and Schwann cell plasma membrane that wraps around nerve axons in a concentric fashion [98] as shown in Figure 2. In 1717, Leeuwenhoek described a 'nervule' with 'fatty parts' around it, likely being the first ever description of myelin [99].

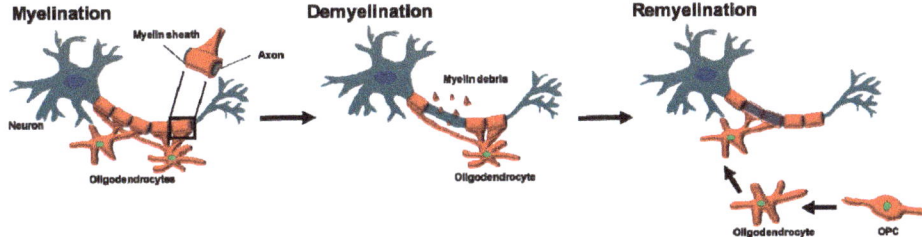

Figure 2. Oligodendrocytes in myelination, demyelination and remyelination. Oligodendrocytes myelinate large diameter axons in the CNS and provide trophic support for the underlying axon. Oligodendrocytes are highly vulnerable and insults such as trauma, immune-mediated attacks or ischaemia can lead to oligodendrocyte death and demyelination. Newly differentiated oligodendrocytes derived from an adult OPC pool can replace deceased oligodendrocytes, which can reinstate the myelin sheath around demyelinated axons (remyelination). Regenerated myelin is thinner than the original myelin sheath.

Since then, technical advances in histology and optical techniques have allowed for both the structure and function of the myelin sheath to be explored in detail [3,98,100]. For example, high-resolution time-lapse live imaging, electron microscopy and magnetic resonance imaging of the dynamic processes of myelination and remyelination in vivo have been hugely beneficial to the advancement of our understanding of oligodendrocyte biology in health and disease [3,98,101].

Myelination is a complex and tightly regulated process (reviewed in [102]). In vivo time-lapse imaging in transgenic zebrafish revealed that oligodendrocytes continually extend and retract their processes towards axons before settling into their final positions [103]. The oligodendrocyte processes also sense neighbouring cells to ensure uniform spacing of myelin segments with evenly spaced nodes [104]. Once a mature oligodendrocyte connects with an axon, the oligodendrocyte plasma membrane architecture changes rapidly. Numerous hypotheses have been suggested to explain how the oligodendrocyte extends its plasma membrane to wrap axons and form a compact myelin sheath [99]. Two of the most prominent hypotheses suggest that myelin either extends an inner tongue repeatedly around the axon [105] or alternatively that 'croissant-like' layers of myelin sheath are formed on top of pre-existing ones [106]. Sophisticated studies that combined high resolution in vivo imaging and 3D reconstructions of optic nerve fibres fixed with high pressure freezing facilitated improved visualisation of the dynamic process of myelination [107]. These studies revealed that myelination occurs via plasma membrane extension laterally down the axon to form the paranodal loops [107], a discovery consistent with the original mechanism proposed by Geren and Schmitt [105].

Myelination is a highly regulated process that is governed by several molecular cues. Only axons with a large diameter are myelinated [108–110], and myelination itself increases the axonal diameter not just simply by the extra myelin sheaths around the axon, but also due to localised neurofilament accumulation and phosphorylation [111,112].

Myelin sheath formation is regulated by several factors such as neuregulin 1 in Schwann cells [113] and Ca^{2+} activity in oligodendrocytes [101], as well as by neuronal activity, which can identify axons for myelination [46]. Intriguingly, neuronal activity regulates also OPC proliferation, differentiation and survival [44–47].

3.2. Functions of the Myelin Sheath

Functionally, the myelin sheath facilitates rapid transmission of axon potentials and provides metabolic support to the axons it ensheaths [3,100]. Sodium channels are located at the intermittent interruptions (nodes of Ranvier), where short portions of the axon are left unwrapped [100,114]. Myelin is an electrical insulator and when the membrane at the node is excited, the axon potential 'jumps' from one node of Ranvier to the next, due to the low capacitance of the sheath, in a process called saltatory conduction. Little energy is required to depolarise the remaining membrane between the nodes given the low capacitance of the sheath, which results in transmission of the action potential [100,115]. This form of transmission is much faster than in non-myelinated axons [3].

Oligodendrocytes and the myelin sheath metabolically support axons. Oligodendrocytes can generate lactate, which can then be transferred to axons to generate metabolic energy in the form of ATP [116]. In the brain, lactate is shuttled through the most abundant lactate transporter MCT1, and both MCT2 and MCT4 [117]. MCT1 expression has been detected in endothelial cells, however oligodendrocytes and the myelin sheath also harness MCT1 to transport lactate to axons [117,118]. Lee et al. depleted *MCT1* gene expression in spinal cord cultures, which led to extensive neuronal death; an effect that could be rescued with exogenous lactate supplementation [117]. Indeed, a number of glycolytic and Krebs cycle enzymes such as succinate dehydrogenase and fumarase are expressed in the myelin sheath, which contribute to glucose catabolism and ATP production [119].

The central function of oligodendrocytes in the CNS is the generation of myelin during development, adaptive myelination in adulthood and remyelination after damage, while OPC predominantly serve as a backup pool to generate new oligodendrocytes. However, CNS remyelination can also be mediated by infiltrating Schwann cells, which was described for multiple conditions including MS and traumatic brain injury [2]. Post-developmental OPC can also differentiate into other neural lineage cells such as astrocytes and Schwann cells [120]. OPC-derived Schwann cells reside in CNS regions deficient in astrocytes, suggesting that severely demyelinated lesions that are partially necrotic may inhibit astrogliosis, and that a lack of astrocytic scarring may encourage Schwann cell infiltration [120,121]. The factors governing transition from OPC to Schwann cells remain elusive [2], but these data suggest that an astrocyte-derived factor is necessary for OPC differentiation into oligodendrocytes [120].

3.3. Non-Myelinating Functions of Oligodendrocytes and OPC

Emerging evidence suggests OPC have an immunomodulatory capacity. OPC express cytokine receptors [122–124] and assess their microenvironment through filopodia extension [103]. In response to inflammatory cues, OPC can migrate to sites of injury, in a manner similar to that of microglia [54,125]. Upon exposure to IFNγ, OPC cross-present antigen to cytotoxic $CD8^+$ T cells in vitro and in vivo, leading to their cytotoxic death [126,127]. This newly discovered pro-inflammatory OPC phenotype promotes tissue damage and blocks remyelination. This suggests that suppression of OPC-mediated inflammation may ameliorate cell death in favour of promoting OPC differentiation into myelin-producing oligodendrocytes [127].

4. Models to Study Oligodendrocytes and OPC

4.1. Rodent and Human In Vitro Models

Several protocols have been developed to isolate and culture oligodendrocytes from rodent brains at different stages from embryonic into adulthood [128–130]. The isolation of OPC and oligodendrocytes from murine CNS tissue is based on the expression of markers typical of this maturation stage, for example PDGFR-α or A2B5 for OPC or O4 or GalC for oligodendrocytes [129,130]. These primary cultures are suitable for studying the proliferation, survival and differentiation of OPC as well as the effect of molecules of interest on OPC and oligodendrocyte biology. Moreover, different protocols have been developed to study myelination by co-culturing oligodendrocytes with neurons or synthetic nanofibers [110,131]. Primary OPC cultures derived from e.g., rodents, are particularly interesting for studying the proliferation and differentiation of OPC and are suitable for high throughput screening of pharmacological compounds that may interfere with these processes [132].

However, primary OPC cultures are restricted by the availability of animals and related ethical issues. To overcome these limitations, several laboratories developed spontaneously immortalised cell lines derived from O-2A rat precursors, such as CG-4 or OLN-93 immortalised OPC [133,134], or primary murine OPC immortalised by viral infection, such as Oli-neu [135]. These cell lines are karyotypically normal, express the marker typical of their developmental stages and they can be differentiated into mature oligodendrocytes by withdrawing mitogenic factors, such as in CG-4, or by adding factors, such as dibutyryl cAMP for Oli-neu and OLN-93 [133–135]. Immortalised cell lines have undeniable advantages, such as the consistency, the robustness and the low costs related to the model, but because of the unpredictable nature of mutations that lead to the immortalisation, any assumption and translation to any physiological function need to be corroborated by an additional model.

Although the biology of oligodendroglial cells is conserved between rodents and humans, there are some differences between species that should be considered for any translation from murine models to the human physiology (reviewed in [136,137]). The peculiar structure and position of the brain and spinal cord reduces the possibilities of obtaining cells directly from human CNS tissue. One strategy that can be adopted is to isolate OPC from surgery biopsies, e.g., from healthy resection margin of brain tumours (excluding the tumour itself), resected tissue from epileptic or traumatic brain tissue [138]. Another strategy involves the use of post mortem brains or spinal cords; as cells can be isolated up to 12 h after death, from any area of the CNS [139]. Adult human oligodendrocytes can be cultured for 2–3 weeks or directly used for further analysis (for example for mRNA or protein analysis). Although these approaches are precious to unravel the differences between rodent and human biology, the availability of these tissues and the possibility to isolate only oligodendrocytes are a limiting factor.

In recent years, the establishment of induced pluripotent stem cells (iPSC) overcame the restricted availability of human CNS biopsies [140]. iPSC are reprogrammed from somatic cells (e.g., fibroblasts, peripheral blood mononuclear cells) that can be obtained in a non-invasive way. iPSC can subsequently be differentiated to any cell type of interest by inducing their differentiation via specific growth factors (e.g., T3, NT3, IGF, PDGF-A for inducing OPC) or inducing the expression of transcription factors necessary for the transition (e.g., SOX10, Olig2 and NKX6.2 for OPC/oligodendrocytes) [141–143]. Recently, protocols with increasing efficiency and reduced time to obtain oligodendrocytes from human iPSC (iOL) were developed; from 170 days in vitro to 20 days to obtain a culture with mature oligodendrocytes (around 70% efficiency of which 20% expressing MBP) ([141–143] and reviewed in [137]). The possibility of having OPC and oligodendrocytes derived from healthy donors and patients with neurological diseases as a model of study made iPSC popular in the last decade as proven by the variety of protocols developed. Moreover, the possibility of following the differentiation of OPC into iOL is a valuable tool to study this process in a human system. iOL can also represent a precious model to screen drugs promoting differentiation and/or myelin production directly on human cells, possibly directly derived from patients, as exemplified by Ehrlich et al. [142]. Unfortunately, the elevated costs and the time necessary to obtain iOL reduce the accessibility to this technique on a routine basis in the majority of laboratories. More efficient and cheaper protocols to obtain iOL are desirable for the future to broaden our knowledge in human oligodendrocyte biology.

The methods described above (summarised in Table 1) entail the use of an isolated population. Other methods have been developed to mimic the complexity of the environment in which OPC and oligodendrocytes reside, such as mixed glia cultures [144], organotypic brain slices [145], and iPSC derived organoids [146]. These models are useful to study the impact of other cell types on OPC and oligodendrocytes, to decipher any indirect effect exerted by other CNS cells and to complement in vivo studies.

Table 1. Summary of animal and human models listed in Sections 4.1 and 4.2. This list provides examples of a variety of models available to study OPC and oligodendrocyte (OL) biology.

In vitro Animal Models	In vitro Human Models	In Vivo Animal Models
OPC/OL cultures [128–130]	OPC derived from biopsies [138] or post mortem CNS [139]	Reporter mice (e.g., Sox10-Venus mice, CNP-EGFP mice, PLP-EGFP mice) [147–149]
Immortalized oligodendroglial cells lines (e.g., CG-4, OLN-93, Oli-neu) [133–135]	iOL derived from human iPSC [137,141–143]	Reporter zebrafish (e.g., Tg(sox10:mRFP), Tg(olig2:EGFP), Tg(mbp:EGFP)) [103,150,151]

OPC: Oligodendrocyte Progenitor Cell, OL: oligodendrocyte, CNS: Central Nervous System, iOL: induced Oligodendrocyte, iPSC: induced Pluripotent Stem Cell.

4.2. In Vivo Models

One of the most used strategies to study oligodendroglial lineage cells is to genetically label markers typical of the lineage or of the maturation stage of interest with fluorescent proteins (see Table 1). These are particular suitable models to study the biology of oligodendrocytes in the context of a complex biological system. The most used species used for this purpose are mice or zebrafish. Mice generated to detect OPC during development and maturation are for example Sox10-Venus [147] or CNP-EGFP mice [148]. Other mice were generated targeting specific proteins, such as PLP-EGFP mice [149]. In recent years, zebrafish became popular as a model to study remyelination, due to some unique features: large numbers of offspring that develop quickly and outside of the mother, the transparency and small size of the animals that make live imaging of genetically modified zebrafish possible, the reduced costs and reduced level of self-consciousness compared to mammalian models. In fact, zebrafish share 70% of the genome with humans and most of the genes related to myelin are conserved [152,153]. Different transgenic zebrafish have been developed to study different stages and function of OPC and oligodendrocytes such as Tg(sox10:mRFP), Tg(olig2:EGFP) and Tg(mbp:EGFP) [103,150,151]. Given the consistency of the model, transgenic zebrafish are also suitable for high-throughput screening: recently, Early et al. developed an automatic analysis tool where zebrafish larvae are automatically delivered to a spinning disk confocal microscope and the images handled by an image analysis pipeline, facilitating the screening of pro-myelinating compounds [154].

4.3. Animal Models to study Oligodendrocytes and Remyelination in Multiple Sclerosis

There are no animal models that entirely recapitulate all of the features of MS, but different murine models are established to investigate different aspects of the pathology [155]. Experimental autoimmune encephalomyelitis (EAE) is an acute demyelinating episode triggered by the immune system stimulated by myelin protein with adjuvants [156]. EAE is a reproducible, well established model with a defined clinical pattern making it suitable to investigate the relevance of different molecular pathways for MS progression or the efficacy of new treatments.

Two models of non-immune-mediated demyelination use either dietary given cuprizone (a copper chelator) or injected lysolecithin (a lipidolitic detergent) [157,158]. Although the initiation of these models lacks immune engagement, immune cells are recruited to the demyelinated areas, indicating the importance of these cells also in the repair phase [159,160]. These models do not recapitulate any of the typical symptoms that patients with MS experience, but are very useful to investigate molecular and cellular mechanisms involved in the damage and repair phase. Cuprizone is a toxin that induces acute demyelination and is characterised by a peak of OPC infiltration 4 weeks after the start of the cuprizone diet in the corpus callosum, one of the most demyelinated areas in this model [161,162]. The infiltrated OPC are able to differentiate into oligodendrocytes in the following 2 weeks, representing the most abundant population after 6 weeks of cuprizone diet [162]. However, remyelination starts only after cuprizone is withdrawn: in one week, indeed, it is possible to observe an increased expression of myelin associated markers in the corpus callosum that stabilises upon complete remyelination 5 weeks after the re-establishment of a normal diet [162]. Interestingly, Sachs et al. recently developed a modified protocol able to slow down remyelination by the administration of rapamycin, an mTOR inhibitor, to the cuprizone treated mice, giving an extended temporal window to study the processes involved in myelin regeneration [162].

Lysolecithin induced demyelination is also a valuable model to study the remyelination process given the well described and distinct phases of OPC recruitment and proliferation in the lesion site between day five and 10 after the lesion induction, OPC differentiation between day 10 and 14 followed by myelin regeneration [83,158,163,164]. This well-established model is suitable for distinguishing the effect of molecules and cells of interest, including oligodendrocytes, in the different phases of myelin regeneration in an accurate manner.

The aforementioned models are able to recapitulate some features of MS; a comprehensive in vivo model reflecting the complexity of the disease is still lacking. Combination models have been developed to align animal models closer with human disease. For example, Rüther et al. combined cuprizone induced demyelination with EAE to induce a chronic model with persistent clinical signs and chronic lesions even in the forebrain, a region that is not usually affected in EAE, and with a robust immune component [165].

5. Oligodendrocytes in Disease

5.1. Oligodendrocytes in Diseases with Myelin Pathology

Oligodendrocyte death is not necessarily a sign of disease. Oligodendrocytes can die throughout development and adulthood without underlying pathology to enable neuronal plasticity and lifelong learning [166,167]. However, OPC and particularly oligodendrocytes are highly vulnerable to oxidative stress due to low antioxidant levels, for instance glutathione, and high iron content, which is required for enzyme activity. Iron in combination with hydrogen peroxide, from dismutation of superoxide, can produce highly reactive hydroxyl radicals via the Fenton reaction [168].

Especially during myelination oligodendrocytes are vulnerable to cytotoxic by-products from a high metabolic turnover (e.g., reactive oxygen species (ROS), hydrogen peroxide) [169,170]. Likewise, oligodendrocytes are susceptible to excitotoxicity from high glutamate and ATP concentrations [171,172]. Due to this vulnerability oligodendrocytes are affected in a range of disorders.

The most common pathological causes of oligodendrocyte death in the CNS are trauma, ischaemia or autoimmune attacks. Oligodendrocyte death can lead to subsequent demyelination or it can follow as a result of primary myelin damage [173]. In traumatic injuries and ischaemia, oligodendrocyte death and demyelination can follow the original injury [120,174], whereas in autoimmune diseases such as MS, oligodendrocytes are a primary target of an immune attack against myelin and oligodendrocyte specific proteins.

Much rarer are genetic defects that lead to oligodendrocyte damage as seen in some leukodystrophies [175]. The main cause of oligodendrocyte death in these diseases seem to be the accumulation of mutated PLP1, a prevalent protein in the myelin sheath, that fails to be transported to the plasma membrane leading to apoptosis of the cell [176].

White matter pathology is a characteristic of Alzheimer's disease (AD), however oligodendrocyte death and demyelination are believed to occur secondary to neurodegeneration [177]. In post mortem AD tissue Olig2+ oligodendrocyte lineage cells were decreased [178] as were myelinating oligodendrocytes in a mouse model of AD [179]. The underlying cause is not established; however toxicity of beta-amyloid is likely a contributing factor [179,180]. Yet, oligodendrocyte pathology can be evident even before any neurodegenerative events materialise as a study by Fischer showed [181]. Intriguingly, WM pathology in AD is predominately affecting those CNS regions that were myelinated last during development (neuropathologic retrogenesis) [182,183], suggesting a connection between late myelin development and AD.

While oligodendrocyte pathology is not regarded as the primary cause, oligodendrocytes are downstream targets in some neuropsychiatric disorders including schizophrenia, bipolar disorders, autism, ADHD, mood disorders and depression (reviewed in [184] and [185]). For instance, oligodendrocyte density was region-specifically reduced in patients with bipolar disorders and schizophrenia [186–188], and animal models to study demyelination, such as the cuprizone model, have also been used to model aspects of schizophrenia and anxiety disorders (reviewed in [189]). In a chronic stress model oligodendrocyte specific genes were downregulated in the amygdala and prefrontal cortex [190], while dysregulation of oligodendrocytes and nodes of Ranvier is associated with depression [191].

5.2. Oligodendrocytes in Demyelination

Demyelinating diseases are the most common pathologies affecting oligodendrocytes. The most common demyelinating disease is MS [192]. MS is characterised by an immune-mediated attack against myelin sheaths and oligodendrocytes, primarily by myelin-specific CD8+ T cells [193]. This results in demyelination, which is characterised by destruction of the myelin sheath and death of oligodendrocytes [194] leaving axons denuded and vulnerable to neurodegeneration [1].

Genetic fate-mapping studies allowed adult OPC differentiation fates to be tracked after demyelination. This confirmed that adult OPC that represent approximately 6% of the total CNS cell numbers [48] are the main source of new oligodendrocytes after myelin damage [195]. In response to demyelination, adult OPC undergo a switch to an activated state that is characterised by an increased expression of numerous transcription factors [196,197]. These include SOX2 and TCF7L2, the latter of which is central to WNT signalling and maintains OPC in the cell cycle to enable proliferation and colonisation of areas of demyelination [2,197]. OPC migrate to the lesion, guided by microglia and astrocyte-derived factors including fibroblast growth factor and brain-derived neurotrophic factor [2,198,199], before differentiating into mature oligodendrocytes by exiting the cell cycle [200], a conversion led by the transcription factor E2F1 and proto-oncogene MYC [201,202]. The new oligodendrocyte is able to replace the destroyed myelin with a shorter and thinner myelin sheath [157] as shown in Figure 2.

5.3. Oligodendrocytes in Ageing

Ageing is associated with increased white matter atrophy, a decline in motor learning and diminished remyelination capacity [203,204]. The latter is due to changes in the ageing CNS environment [204] and to the decreased ability to recruit OPC that subsequently fail to differentiate into oligodendrocytes [205,206]. Rejuvenation can restore the reparative capacity in the CNS as the Franklin lab has shown: in a parabiosis experiment with young and old mice that were subjected to demyelination macrophages were key to restore the remyelination capacity in old animals by clearing myelin debris [204].

Due to their high metabolic rate during myelination, for the maintenance of myelin and for the trophic support of axons [117] oligodendrocytes are exposed to prolonged periods of cytotoxic by-products such as ROS; for instance, cholesterol synthesis is highly energy intensive [207] and also declines with age [208]. Additionally, compared to astrocytes oligodendrocytes have reduced antioxidants levels [169,209], which further decline with age [210]. Oligodendrocytes are highly vulnerable to oxidative stress, which can result in DNA damage [211]. With age, DNA repair mechanisms are either not efficient or are disturbed thus leading to oligodendrocyte apoptosis. As OPC recruitment and differentiation into oligodendrocytes is diminished with age [205,212], dead oligodendrocytes are not as efficiently replaced in old age as they were in younger age leading to white matter atrophy over time.

6. Oligodendrocytes in Myelin Regeneration

Remyelination is a natural regenerative process, which is believed to prevent neurodegeneration and restore function [2,213]. In MS and animal models of MS, the ability to remyelinate efficiently declines with age and disease progression (reviewed in [214]). Our knowledge about the mechanisms involved is mainly based on animal studies, which although powerful, deliver a simplified picture of what occurs in humans. This becomes increasingly clear with results from recent cell population studies in human healthy and MS brain tissue demonstrating the existence of different oligodendrocyte lineage cells, dependent on location, origin, disease phenotype and age [215–217]. New functions of oligodendrocyte lineage cells beyond their central roles in myelination and trophic support were recently identified including immunomodulatory properties as shown by Falcao et al. [126]. Given that MS is an immune-mediated disease, it would be striking if oligodendrocytes are not just the targets of an immune attack in MS but are actively involved in disease pathology.

OPC are central to remyelination by generating new oligodendrocytes that replace those lost after injury [218,219]. In contrast, surviving adult oligodendrocytes were long thought to not be involved in remyelination. This dogma has recently been revised for both rodents and humans as studies by Duncan et al. and Yeung et al. demonstrated [215,220]. Using rodent and non-human primate animal models, Duncan et al. showed that oligodendrocytes are connected to both myelinated and remyelinated myelin sheaths indicating that existing oligodendrocytes contribute to remyelination [220]. Comparing C14 in genomic DNA with atmospheric C14, Yeung et al. calculated the age of oligodendrocytes in MS lesions. The authors concluded that rather than newly formed oligodendrocytes from OPC old 'spared' oligodendrocytes regenerated myelin in remyelinated MS lesions [215].

Remyelination seems to replicate aspects of developmental myelination, at least in parts. For instance, similar transcription factors are involved in both processes, such as Myrf and Zfp488 [221,222]. Conversely, while Klf9 and Stat3 seem non-essential in developmental myelination they are critical for efficient remyelination [223,224] and Arnett et al. showed that the transcription factor Olig1 is more important than Olig2 in remyelination suggesting their role is reversed compared to developmental myelination [83].

In human MS lesions, Chang et al. and Kuhlmann et al. identified a block in OPC differentiation into oligodendrocytes as the bottleneck for efficient remyelination in MS [225,226]. In early MS and in successfully remyelinated lesions, differentiated oligodendrocytes are found within WM lesions, while in chronic stages of the disease, which is characterised by predominantly non-remyelinating lesions, differentiated oligodendrocyte are rare [225]. Albeit in lower numbers, OPC are still found in these chronic MS lesions indicating that OPC deficiency is not the primary cause for remyelination failure; it can, however, contribute to the impaired differentiation of OPC into remyelinating oligodendrocytes [225,227].

A study by Boyd et al. showed that deficiency of OPC within lesions either due to impaired recruitment and/or proliferation is another cause of remyelination failure for 37% of MS lesions, predominantly chronic active lesions. OPC deficiency in these lesions is linked to Semaphorin 3A that prevents OPC migration into the lesion area [205,228].

To overcome remyelination failure in MS new targets to enhance remyelination therapeutically are currently examined. Originally thought to only contribute to the pathology of MS, the immune system is now recognised in facilitating remyelination. Depletion of macrophages or lymphocytes leads to impaired remyelination following toxin-induced demyelination in animal models [159,229]. For instance, M2 macrophages and microglia promote oligodendrocyte differentiation via activin-A [230] and we showed that regulatory T cells promote oligodendrocyte differentiation and remyelination via CCN3 secretion [231].

7. Concluding Remarks

Oligodendrocytes have come a long way from the original description as 'Nervenkitt' to their central importance as the myelinating cells of the CNS. Adding to this key function, oligodendrocytes provide trophic support to axons and more recently, likely have additional immunomodulatory capacity. While we have a good understanding of the role of oligodendrocytes in myelination and remyelination, there is still a gap of knowledge of the molecular mechanisms involved in these processes. Given the similarities between myelination and remyelination, a better understanding of myelination can provide clues that can be harnessed to improve myelin regeneration, an unmet need for the treatment of demyelinating diseases, such as MS.

Only recently, new roles of oligodendrocytes have been uncovered such as potential immunomodulatory functions, which warrant further investigation, particularly in disease context. For instance, the question of whether oligodendrocytes are actively participating in disease progression e.g., in MS, by perpetuating inflammation would be interesting to address.

Advances in the models to study oligodendrocyte biology and function, such as cell population-based approaches, has broadened our knowledge beyond their classical roles.

Despite the mechanistic similarities between animals and humans in development and maturation of OPC and oligodendrocytes, there are differences that need to be accounted for when translating results to the human system. Different in vitro approaches based, e.g., on human iPSC will help to overcome the intrinsic interspecies differences that can complement and validate the discoveries from animal models.

In conclusion, oligodendrocytes have long left behind the 'Nervenkitt' attribute and are recognised as critical regulators of neuronal functions in CNS development, homeostasis and regeneration.

Author Contributions: Conceptualization, Y.D., L.G., S.K. and D.C.; Writing—Original Draft Preparation, S.K., L.G., D.C. and Y.D.; Writing—Review & Editing, S.K., L.G., D.C. and Y.D.; Visualization, S.K.; Supervision, Y.D.; Project Administration, L.G. and Y.D.; Funding Acquisition, Y.D.

Funding: Part of this work was supported by a grant to Y.D. from the Medical Research Foundation of the Freemasons of Ireland (PhD studentship D.C.).

Conflicts of Interest: The authors declare no conflict of interest.

References

1. Bradl, M.; Lassmann, H. Oligodendrocytes: Biology and pathology. *Acta Neuropathol.* **2010**, *119*, 37–53. [CrossRef] [PubMed]
2. Franklin, R.J.M.; Ffrench-Constant, C. Regenerating CNS myelin-from mechanisms to experimental medicines. *Nat. Rev. Neurosci* **2017**, *18*, 753–769. [CrossRef] [PubMed]
3. Nave, K.A. Myelination and support of axonal integrity by glia. *Nature* **2010**, *468*, 244–252. [CrossRef] [PubMed]
4. Virchow, R. Gesammelte Abhandlungen zur Wissenschaftlichen Medicin; Hamm, Frankfurt a.M. 1856. Available online: https://archive.org/details/b21462161 (accessed on 9 November 2019).
5. Deiters, O.F.C. Untersuchungen über Gehirn und Rückenmark des Menschen und der Säugetiere; Braunschweig. 1865. Available online: https://archive.org/details/untersuchungen00deit/page/n8 (accessed on 9 November 2019).
6. Golgi, C. Sulla Fina Anatomia Degli Organi Centrali del Sistema Nervoso. Milano, 1885. Available online: https://archive.org/details/b21978724/page/n8 (accessed on 9 November 2019).
7. Virchow, R. Die Cellularpathologie in ihrer Begründung auf physiologische und pathologische Gewebelehre. Berlin, 1858. Available online: https://archive.org/details/diecellularpatho00virc/page/n8 (accessed on 9 November 2019).

8. Del Rio-Hortega, P. La microglia y su transformacíon en células en bastoncito y cuerpos gránulo-adiposos. *Trab. Lab. Invest. Biol. Madrid.* **1920**, *18*, 37–82.
9. Del Rio-Hortega, P. Arte y artificio de la ciencia histológica. *Residencia Revista de la Residencia de Estudiantes IV.* **1933**, *4*, 191–206.
10. Hardy, R.; Reynolds, R. Proliferation and differentiation potential of rat forebrain oligodendroglial progenitors both in vitro and in vivo. *Development* **1991**, *111*, 1061–1080. [PubMed]
11. Rexed, B. The cytoarchitectonic organization of the spinal cord in the cat. *J. Comp. Neurol.* **1952**, *96*, 415–495. [CrossRef] [PubMed]
12. Nornes, H.O.; Das, G.D. Temporal pattern of neurogenesis in spinal cord of rat. I. An autoradiographic study — time and sites of origin and migration and settling patterns of neuroblasts. *Brain Res.* **1974**, *73*, 121–138. [CrossRef]
13. Ginhoux, F.; Prinz, M. Origin of microglia: Current concepts and past controversies. *Cold Spring Harb. Perspect. Biol.* **2015**, *7*, 1–15. [CrossRef] [PubMed]
14. Raff, M.C.; Miller, R.H.; Noble, M. A glial progenitor cell that develops in vitro into an astrocyte or an oligodendrocyte depending on culture medium. *Nature* **1983**, *303*, 390–396. [CrossRef] [PubMed]
15. Pringle, N.P.; Richardson, W.D. A singularity of PDGF alpha-receptor expression in the dorsoventral axis of the neural tube may define the origin of the oligodendrocyte lineage. *Development* **1993**, *117*.
16. Timsit, S.; Martinez, S.; Allinquant, B.; Peyron, F.; Puelles, L.; Zalc, B. Oligodendrocytes originate in a restricted zone of the embryonic ventral neural tube defined by DM-20 mRNA expression. *J. Neurosci.* **1995**, *15*, 1012–1024. [CrossRef] [PubMed]
17. Warf, B.C.; Fok-Seang, J.; Miller, R.H. Evidence for the ventral origin of oligodendrocyte precursors in the rat spinal cord. *J. Neurosci.* **1991**, *11*, 2477–2488. [CrossRef] [PubMed]
18. Vallstedt, A.; Klos, J.M.; Ericson, J. Multiple dorsoventral origins of oligodendrocyte generation in the spinal cord and hindbrain. *Neuron* **2005**, *45*, 55–67. [CrossRef] [PubMed]
19. Fogarty, M.; Richardson, W.D.; Kessaris, N. A subset of oligodendrocytes generated from radial glia in the dorsal spinal cord. *Development* **2005**, *132*, 1951–1959. [CrossRef] [PubMed]
20. Davis, A.A.; Temple, S. A self-renewing multipotential stem cell in embryonic rat cerebral cortex. *Nature* **1994**, *372*, 263–266. [CrossRef] [PubMed]
21. Rogister, B.; Ben-Hur, T.; Dubois-Dalcq, M. From neural stem cells to myelinating oligodendrocytes. *Mol. Cell. Neurosci.* **1999**, *14*, 287–300. [CrossRef] [PubMed]
22. Spassky, N.; Goujet-Zalc, C.; Parmantier, E.; Olivier, C.; Martinez, S.; Ivanova, A.; Ikenaka, K.; Macklin, W.; Cerruti, I.; Zalc, B.; et al. Multiple restricted origin of oligodendrocytes. *J. Neurosci.* **1998**, *18*, 8331–8343. [CrossRef] [PubMed]
23. Hajihosseini, M.; Tham, T.N.; Dubois-Dalcq, M. Origin of oligodendrocytes within the human spinal cord. *J. Neurosci.* **1996**, *16*, 7981–7994. [CrossRef] [PubMed]
24. Kessaris, N.; Fogarty, M.; Iannarelli, P.; Grist, M.; Wegner, M.; Richardson, W.D. Competing waves of oligodendrocytes in the forebrain and postnatal elimination of an embryonic lineage. *Nat. Neurosci.* **2006**, *9*, 173–179. [CrossRef] [PubMed]
25. Tripathi, R.B.; Clarke, L.E.; Burzomato, V.; Kessaris, N.; Anderson, P.N.; Attwell, D.; Richardson, W.D. Dorsally and Ventrally Derived Oligodendrocytes Have Similar Electrical Properties but Myelinate Preferred Tracts. *J. Neurosci.* **2011**, *31*, 6809–6819. [CrossRef] [PubMed]
26. Cai, J.; Qi, Y.; Hu, X.; Tan, M.; Liu, Z.; Zhang, J.; Li, Q.; Sander, M.; Qiu, M. Generation of oligodendrocyte precursor cells from mouse dorsal spinal cord independent of Nkx6 regulation and Shh signaling. *Neuron* **2005**, *45*, 41–53. [CrossRef] [PubMed]
27. Barres, B.A.; Hart, I.K.; Coles, H.S.; Burne, J.F.; Voyvodic, J.T.; Richardson, W.D.; Raff, M.C. Cell death and control of cell survival in the oligodendrocyte lineage. *Cell* **1992**, *70*, 31–46. [CrossRef]
28. Trapp, B.D.; Nishiyama, A.; Cheng, D.; Macklin, W. Differentiation and death of premyelinating oligodendrocytes in developing rodent brain. *J. Cell Biol.* **1997**, *137*, 459–468. [CrossRef] [PubMed]
29. Barres, B.A.; Raff, M.C. Axonal control of oligodendrocyte development. *J. Cell Biol.* **1999**, *147*, 1123–1128. [CrossRef] [PubMed]
30. Orduz, D.; Benamer, N.; Ortolani, D.; Coppola, E.; Vigier, L.; Pierani, A.; Angulo, M.C. Developmental cell death regulates lineage-related interneuron-oligodendroglia functional clusters and oligodendrocyte homeostasis. *Nat. Commun.* **2019**, *10*. [CrossRef] [PubMed]

31. Bhardwaj, R.D.; Curtis, M.A.; Spalding, K.L.; Buchholz, B.A.; Fink, D.; Björk-Eriksson, T.; Nordborg, C.; Gage, F.H.; Druid, H.; Eriksson, P.S.; et al. Neocortical neurogenesis in humans is restricted to development. *Proc. Natl. Acad. Sci. USA* **2006**, *103*, 12564–12568. [CrossRef] [PubMed]
32. Bandeira, F.; Lent, R.; Herculano-Houzel, S. Changing numbers of neuronal and non-neuronal cells underlie postnatal brain growth in the rat. *Proc. Natl. Acad. Sci. USA* **2009**, *106*, 14108–14113. [CrossRef] [PubMed]
33. Barnabé-Heider, F.; Göritz, C.; Sabelström, H.; Takebayashi, H.; Pfrieger, F.W.; Meletis, K.; Frisén, J. Origin of New Glial Cells in Intact and Injured Adult Spinal Cord. *Cell Stem Cell* **2010**, *7*, 470–482. [CrossRef] [PubMed]
34. Inta, D.; Alfonso, J.; von Engelhardt, J.; Kreuzberg, M.M.; Meyer, A.H.; van Hooft, J.A.; Monyer, H. Neurogenesis and widespread forebrain migration of distinct GABAergic neurons from the postnatal subventricular zone. *Proc. Natl. Acad. Sci. USA* **2008**, *105*, 20994–20999. [CrossRef] [PubMed]
35. Orentas, D.M.; Hayes, J.E.; Dyer, K.L.; Miller, R.H. Sonic hedgehog signaling is required during the appearance of spinal cord oligodendrocyte precursors. *Development* **1999**, *126*, 2419–2429. [PubMed]
36. Van Straaten, H.W.M.; Hekking, J.W.M.; Beursgens, J.P.W.M.; Terwindt-Rouwenhorst, E.; Drukker, J. Effect of the notochord on proliferation and differentiation in the neural tube of the chick embryo. *Development* **1989**, *107*, 793–803. [CrossRef]
37. Echelard, Y.; Epstein, D.J.; St-Jacques, B.; Shen, L.; Mohler, J.; McMahon, J.A.; McMahon, A.P. Sonic hedgehog, a member of a family of putative signaling molecules, is implicated in the regulation of CNS polarity. *Cell* **1993**, *75*, 1417–1430. [CrossRef]
38. Pringle, N.P.; Yu, W.-P.; Guthrie, S.; Roelink, H.; Lumsden, A.; Peterson, A.C.; Richardson, W.D. Determination of Neuroepithelial Cell Fate: Induction of the Oligodendrocyte Lineage by Ventral Midline Cells and Sonic Hedgehog. *Dev. Biol.* **1996**, *177*, 30–42. [CrossRef] [PubMed]
39. Richardson, M.K.; Hanken, J.; Gooneratne, M.L.; Pieau, C.; Raynaud, A.; Selwood, L.; Wright, G.M. There is no highly conserved embryonic stage in the vertebrates: Implications for current theories of evolution and development. *Anat. Embryol.* **1997**, *196*, 91–106. [CrossRef] [PubMed]
40. Roelink, H.; Augsburger, A.; Heemskerk, J.; Korzh, V.; Norlin, S.; Ruiz i Altaba, A.; Tanabe, Y.; Placzek, M.; Edlund, T.; Jessell, T.M.; et al. Floor plate and motor neuron induction by vhh-1, a vertebrate homolog of hedgehog expressed by the notochord. *Cell* **1994**, *76*, 761–775. [CrossRef]
41. Nery, S.; Wichterle, H.; Fishell, G. Sonic hedgehog contributes to oligodendrocyte specification in the mammalian forebrain. *Development* **2001**, *128*, 527–540. [PubMed]
42. Hashimoto, H.; Jiang, W.; Yoshimura, T.; Moon, K.H.; Bok, J.; Ikenaka, K. Strong sonic hedgehog signaling in the mouse ventral spinal cord is not required for oligodendrocyte precursor cell (OPC) generation but is necessary for correct timing of its generation. *Neurochem. Int.* **2018**, *119*, 178–183. [CrossRef] [PubMed]
43. Tiane, A.; Schepers, M.; Rombaut, B.; Hupperts, R.; Prickaerts, J.; Hellings, N.; van den Hove, D.; Vanmierlo, T. From OPC to Oligodendrocyte: An Epigenetic Journey. *Cells* **2019**, *8*, 1236. [CrossRef] [PubMed]
44. Barres, B.A.; Raff, M.C. Proliferation of oligodendrocyte precursor cells depends on electrical activity in axons. *Nature* **1993**, *361*, 258–260. [CrossRef] [PubMed]
45. Hughes, E.G.; Orthmann-Murphy, J.L.; Langseth, A.J.; Bergles, D.E. Myelin remodeling through experience-dependent oligodendrogenesis in the adult somatosensory cortex. *Nat. Neurosci.* **2018**, *21*, 696–706. [CrossRef] [PubMed]
46. Gibson, E.M.; Purger, D.; Mount, C.W.; Goldstein, A.K.; Lin, G.L.; Wood, L.S.; Inema, I.; Miller, S.E.; Bieri, G.; Zuchero, J.B.; et al. Neuronal Activity Promotes Oligodendrogenesis and Adaptive Myelination in the Mammalian Brain. *Science* **2014**, *344*, 1252304. [CrossRef] [PubMed]
47. Mitew, S.; Gobius, I.; Fenlon, L.R.; McDougall, S.J.; Hawkes, D.; Xing, Y.L.; Bujalka, H.; Gundlach, A.L.; Richards, L.J.; Kilpatrick, T.J.; et al. Pharmacogenetic stimulation of neuronal activity increases myelination in an axon-specific manner. *Nat. Commun.* **2018**, *9*, 306. [CrossRef] [PubMed]
48. Dawson, M.R.L.; Polito, A.; Levine, J.M.; Reynolds, R. NG2-expressing glial progenitor cells: An abundant and widespread population of cycling cells in the adult rat CNS. *Mol. Cell. Neurosci.* **2003**, *24*, 476–488. [CrossRef]
49. Hill, R.A.; Patel, K.D.; Medved, J.; Reiss, A.M.; Nishiyama, A. NG2 cells in white matter but not gray matter proliferate in response to PDGF. *J. Neurosci.* **2013**, *33*, 14558–14566. [CrossRef] [PubMed]
50. Lentferink, D.H.; Jongsma, J.M.; Werkman, I.; Baron, W. Grey matter OPCs are less mature and less sensitive to IFNγ than white matter OPCs: consequences for remyelination. *Sci. Rep.* **2018**, *8*, 2113. [CrossRef] [PubMed]

51. Dimou, L.; Simon, C.; Kirchhoff, F.; Takebayashi, H.; Götz, M. Progeny of Olig2-expressing progenitors in the gray and white matter of the adult mouse cerebral cortex. *J. Neurosci.* **2008**, *28*, 10434–10442. [CrossRef] [PubMed]
52. Kang, S.H.; Fukaya, M.; Yang, J.K.; Rothstein, J.D.; Bergles, D.E. NG2+ CNS glial progenitors remain committed to the oligodendrocyte lineage in postnatal life and following neurodegeneration. *Neuron* **2010**, *68*, 668–681. [CrossRef] [PubMed]
53. Rivers, L.E.; Young, K.M.; Rizzi, M.; Jamen, F. PDGFRA/NG2 glia generate myelinating oligodendrocytes and piriform projection neurons in adult mice. *Nat. Neurosci.* **2008**, *11*, 1–24. [CrossRef] [PubMed]
54. Hughes, E.G.; Kang, S.H.; Fukaya, M.; Bergles, D.E. Oligodendrocyte progenitors balance growth with self-repulsion to achieve homeostasis in the adult brain. *Nat. Neurosci.* **2013**, *16*, 668–676. [CrossRef] [PubMed]
55. Lachapelle, F.; Gumpel, M.; Baulac, M.; Jacque, C.; Duc, P.; Baumann, N. Transplantation of CNS Fragments into the Brain of Shiverer Mutant Mice: Extensive Myelination by Implanted Oligodendrocytes. *Dev. Neurosci.* **1983**, *6*, 325–334. [CrossRef] [PubMed]
56. Tsai, H.H.; Niu, J.; Munji, R.; Davalos, D.; Chang, J.; Zhang, H.; Tien, A.C.; Kuo, C.J.; Chan, J.R.; Daneman, R.; et al. Oligodendrocyte precursors migrate along vasculature in the developing nervous system. *Science* **2016**, *351*, 379–384. [CrossRef] [PubMed]
57. Niu, J.; Tsai, H.H.; Hoi, K.K.; Huang, N.; Yu, G.; Kim, K.; Baranzini, S.E.; Xiao, L.; Chan, J.R.; Fancy, S.P.J. Aberrant oligodendroglial–vascular interactions disrupt the blood–brain barrier, triggering CNS inflammation. *Nat. Neurosci.* **2019**, *22*, 709–718. [CrossRef] [PubMed]
58. Miller, R.H.; Payne, J.; Milner, L.; Zhang, H.; Orentas, D.M. Spinal cord oligodendrocytes develop from a limited number of migratory, highly proliferative precursors. *J. Neurosci. Res.* **1997**, *50*, 157–168. [CrossRef]
59. Fok-Seang, J.; Miller, R.H. Distribution and differentiation of A2B5+ glial precursors in the developing rat spinal cord. *J Neurosci Res* **1994**, *37*, 219–235. [CrossRef] [PubMed]
60. Raff, M.C.; Abney, E.R.; Miller, R.H. Two glial cell lineages diverge prenatally in rat optic nerve. *Dev. Biol.* **1984**, *106*, 53–60. [CrossRef]
61. Hughes, S.M.; Lillien, L.E.; Raff, M.C.; Rohrer, H.; Sendtner, M. Ciliary neurotrophic factor induces type-2 astrocyte differentiation in culture. *Nature* **1988**, *335*, 70–73. [CrossRef] [PubMed]
62. Noble, M.; Murray, K.; Stroobant, P.; Waterfield, M.D.; Riddle, P. Platelet-derived growth factor promotes division and motility and inhibits premature differentiation of the oligodendrocyte/type-2 astrocyte progenitor cell. *Nature* **1988**, *333*, 560–562. [CrossRef] [PubMed]
63. Yeh, H.J.; Ruit, K.G.; Wang, Y.X.; Parks, W.C.; Snider, W.D.; Deuel, T.F. PDGF A-chain gene is expressed by mammalian neurons during development and in maturity. *Cell* **1991**, *64*, 209–216. [CrossRef]
64. Calver, A.R.; Hall, A.C.; Yu, W.P.; Walsh, F.S.; Heath, J.K.; Betsholtz, C.; Richardson, W.D. Oligodendrocyte population dynamics and the role of PDGF in vivo. *Neuron* **1998**, *20*, 869–882. [CrossRef]
65. Sommer, I.; Schachner, M. Monoclonal antibodies (O1 to O4) to oligodendrocyte cell surfaces: An immunocytological study in the central nervous system. *Dev. Biol.* **1981**, *83*, 311–327. [CrossRef]
66. Braun, P.E.; Sandillon, F.; Edwards, A.; Matthieu, J.-M.; Privat, A. Immunocytochemical Localization by Electron Microscopy of 2′,3′-Cyclic Nucleotide 3′-Phosphodiesterase in Developing Oligodendrocytes of Normal and Mutant Brain. *J. Neurosci.* **1988**, *8*, 3057–3066. [CrossRef] [PubMed]
67. Scherer, S.S.; Braun, P.E.; Grinspan, J.; Collarini, E.; Wang, D.Y.; Kamholz, J. Differential regulation of the 2′,3′-cyclic nucleotide 3′-phosphodiesterase gene during oligodendrocyte development. *Neuron* **1994**, *12*, 1363–1375. [CrossRef]
68. Jakovcevski, I.; Filipovic, R.; Mo, Z.; Rakic, S.; Zecevic, N. Oligodendrocyte development and the onset of myelination in the human fetal brain. *Front. Neuroanat.* **2009**, *3*. [CrossRef] [PubMed]
69. Brunner, C.; Lassmann, H.; Waehneldt, T.V.; Matthieu, J.-M.; Linington, C. Differential Ultrastructural Localization of Myelin Basic Protein, Myelin/Oligodendroglial Glycoprotein, and 2′,3′-Cyclic Nucleotide 3′-Phosphodiesterase in the CNS of Adult Rats. *J. Neurochem.* **1989**, *52*, 296–304. [CrossRef] [PubMed]
70. Linnington, C.; Webb, M.; Woodhams, P.L. A novel myelin-associated glycoprotein defined by a mouse monoclonal antibody. *J. Neuroimmunol.* **1984**, *6*, 387–396. [CrossRef]
71. Barbarese, E.; Barry, C.; Chou, C.J.; Goldstein, D.J.; Nakos, G.A.; Hyde-DeRuyscher, R.; Scheld, K.; Carson, J.H. Expression and Localization of Myelin Basic Protein in Oligodendrocytes and Transfected Fibroblasts. *J. Neurochem.* **1988**, *51*, 1737–1745. [CrossRef] [PubMed]

72. Michalski, J.P.; Anderson, C.; Beauvais, A.; de Repentigny, Y.; Kothary, R. The proteolipid protein promoter drives expression outside of the oligodendrocyte lineage during embryonic and early postnatal development. *PLoS ONE* **2011**, *6*. [CrossRef] [PubMed]
73. Trapp, B.D. Myelin-Associated Glycoprotein Location and Potential Functions. *Ann. N. Y. Acad. Sci.* **1990**, *605*, 29–43. [CrossRef] [PubMed]
74. Raff, M.C.; Mirsky, R.; Fields, K.L.; Lisak, R.P.; Dorfman, S.H.; Silberberg, D.H.; Gregson, N.A.; Leibowitz, S.; Kennedy, M.C. Galactocerebroside is a specific cell-surface antigenic marker for oligodendrocytes in culture. *Nature* **1978**, *274*, 813–816. [CrossRef] [PubMed]
75. Dubois-Dalcq, M.; Behar, T.; Hudson, L.; Lazzarini, R.A. Emergence of three myelin proteins in oligodendrocytes cultured without neurons. *J. Cell Biol.* **1986**, *102*, 384–392. [CrossRef] [PubMed]
76. Harlow, D.E.; Saul, K.E.; Culp, C.M.; Vesely, E.M.; Macklin, W.B. Expression of proteolipid protein gene in spinal cord stem cells and early oligodendrocyte progenitor cells is dispensable for normal cell migration and myelination. *J. Neurosci.* **2014**, *34*, 1333–1343. [CrossRef] [PubMed]
77. Zhou, Q.; Wang, S.; Anderson, D.J. Identification of a novel family of oligodendrocyte lineage-specific basic helix-loop-helix transcription factors. *Neuron* **2000**, *25*, 331–343. [CrossRef]
78. Zhou, Q.; Anderson, D.J. The bHLH transcription factors OLIG2 and OLIG1 couple neuronal and glial subtype specification. *Cell* **2002**, *109*, 61–73. [CrossRef]
79. Rowitch, D.H. Glial specification in the vertebrate neural tube. *Nat. Rev. Neurosci.* **2004**, *5*, 409–419. [CrossRef] [PubMed]
80. Wegener, A.; Deboux, C.; Bachelin, C.; Frah, M.; Kerninon, C.; Seilhean, D.; Weider, M.; Wegner, M.; Nait-Oumesmar, B. Gain of Olig2 function in oligodendrocyte progenitors promotes remyelination. *Brain* **2015**, *138*, 120–135. [CrossRef] [PubMed]
81. Xin, M.; Yue, T.; Ma, Z.; Wu, F.; Gow, A.; Lu, Q.R. Myelinogenesis and axonal recognition by oligodendrocytes in brain are uncoupled in Olig1-null mice. *J. Neurosci.* **2005**, *25*, 1354–1365. [CrossRef] [PubMed]
82. Dai, J.; Bercury, K.K.; Ahrendsen, J.T.; Macklin, W.B. Olig1 function is required for oligodendrocyte differentiation in the mouse brain. *J. Neurosci.* **2015**, *35*, 4386–4402. [CrossRef] [PubMed]
83. Arnett, H.A.; Fancy, S.P.J.; Alberta, J.A.; Zhao, C.; Plant, S.R.; Kaing, S.; Raine, C.S.; Rowitch, D.H.; Franklin, R.J.M.; Stiles, C.D. bHLH Transcription Factor Olig1 Is Required to Repair Demyelinated Lesions in the CNS. *Science* **2004**, *306*, 2111–2115. [CrossRef] [PubMed]
84. Kuhlbrodt, K.; Herbarth, B.; Sock, E.; Hermans-Borgmeyer, I.; Wegner, M. Sox10, a novel transcriptional modulator in glial cells. *J. Neurosci.* **1998**, *18*, 237–250. [CrossRef] [PubMed]
85. Pozniak, C.D.; Langseth, A.J.; Dijkgraaf, G.J.P.; Choe, Y.; Werb, Z.; Pleasure, S.J. Sox10 directs neural stem cells toward the oligodendrocyte lineage by decreasing Suppressor of Fused expression. *Proc. Natl. Acad. Sci. USA* **2010**, *107*, 21795–21800. [CrossRef] [PubMed]
86. Stolt, C.C.; Rehberg, S.; Ader, M.; Lommes, P.; Riethmacher, D.; Schachner, M.; Bartsch, U.; Wegner, M. Terminal differentiation of myelin-forming oligodendrocytes depends on the transcription factor Sox10. *Genes Dev.* **2002**, *16*, 165–170. [CrossRef] [PubMed]
87. Stolt, C.C.; Lommes, P.; Friedrich, R.P.; Wegner, M. Transcription factors Sox8 and Sox10 perform non-equivalent roles during oligodendrocyte development despite functional redundancy. *Development* **2004**, *131*, 2349–2358. [CrossRef] [PubMed]
88. Qi, Y.; Cai, J.; Wu, Y.; Wu, R.; Lee, J.; Fu, H.; Rao, M.; Sussel, L.; Rubenstein, J.; Qiu, M. Control of oligodendrocyte differentiation by the Nkx2.2 homeodomain transcription factor. *Development* **2001**, *128*, 2723–2733. [PubMed]
89. Zhu, Q.; Zhao, X.; Zheng, K.; Li, H.; Huang, H.; Zhang, Z.; Mastracci, T.; Wegner, M.; Chen, Y.; Sussel, L.; et al. Genetic evidence that Nkx2.2 and Pdgfra are major determinants of the timing of oligodendrocyte differentiation in the developing CNS. *Development* **2014**, *141*, 548–555. [CrossRef] [PubMed]
90. Zhu, X.; Bergles, D.E.; Nishiyama, A. NG2 cells generate both oligodendrocytes and gray matter astrocytes. *Development* **2008**, *135*, 145–157. [CrossRef] [PubMed]
91. Woodhoo, A.; Sommer, L. Development of the Schwann cell lineage: From the neural crest to the myelinated nerve. *Glia* **2008**, *56*, 1481–1490. [CrossRef] [PubMed]
92. Jessen, K.R.; Mirsky, R. The origin and development of glial cells in peripheral nerves. *Nat. Rev. Neurosci.* **2005**, *6*, 671–682. [CrossRef] [PubMed]
93. Salzer, J.L. Schwann cell myelination. *Cold Spring Harb. Perspect. Biol.* **2015**, *7*, a020529. [CrossRef] [PubMed]

94. Harty, B.L.; Coelho, F.; Pease-Raissi, S.E.; Mogha, A.; Ackerman, S.D.; Herbert, A.L.; Gereau, R.W.; Golden, J.P.; Lyons, D.A.; Chan, J.R.; et al. Myelinating Schwann cells ensheath multiple axons in the absence of E3 ligase component Fbxw7. *Nat. Commun.* **2019**, *10*, 2976. [CrossRef] [PubMed]
95. Kucenas, S.; Wang, W.-D.; Knapik, E.W.; Appel, B. A selective glial barrier at motor axon exit points prevents oligodendrocyte migration from the spinal cord. *J. Neurosci.* **2009**, *29*, 15187–15194. [CrossRef] [PubMed]
96. Smith, C.J.; Morris, A.D.; Welsh, T.G.; Kucenas, S. Contact-Mediated Inhibition Between Oligodendrocyte Progenitor Cells and Motor Exit Point Glia Establishes the Spinal Cord Transition Zone. *PLoS Biol.* **2014**, *12*, e1001961. [CrossRef] [PubMed]
97. Fontenas, L.; Welsh, T.G.; Piller, M.; Coughenour, P.; Gandhi, A.V.; Prober, D.A.; Kucenas, S. The Neuromodulator Adenosine Regulates Oligodendrocyte Migration at Motor Exit Point Transition Zones. *Cell Rep.* **2019**, *27*, 115–128.e5. [CrossRef] [PubMed]
98. Raine, C.S. Morphology of Myelin and Myelination. In *Myelin*; Springer US: Boston, MA, USA, 1984; pp. 1–50.
99. Rosenbluth, J. A brief history of myelinated nerve fibers: one hundred and fifty years of controversy. *J. Neurocytol.* **1999**, *28*, 251–262. [CrossRef] [PubMed]
100. Morell, P.; Quarles, R.H. The Myelin Sheath. 1999. Available online: https://www.ncbi.nlm.nih.gov/books/NBK27954/ (accessed on 9 November 2019).
101. Baraban, M.; Koudelka, S.; Lyons, D.A. Ca2+ activity signatures of myelin sheath formation and growth in vivo. *Nat. Neurosci.* **2018**, *21*, 19–23. [CrossRef] [PubMed]
102. Nave, K.-A.; Werner, H.B. Myelination of the Nervous System: Mechanisms and Functions. *Annu. Rev. Cell Dev. Biol.* **2014**, *30*, 503–533. [CrossRef] [PubMed]
103. Kirby, B.B.; Takada, N.; Latimer, A.J.; Shin, J.; Carney, T.J.; Kelsh, R.N.; Appel, B. In vivo time-lapse imaging shows dynamic oligodendrocyte progenitor behavior during zebrafish development. *Nat. Neurosci.* **2006**, *9*, 1506–1511. [CrossRef] [PubMed]
104. Simons, M.; Trotter, J. Wrapping it up: The cell biology of myelination. *Curr. Opin. Neurobiol.* **2007**, *17*, 533–540. [CrossRef] [PubMed]
105. Geren, B.B.; Schmitt, F.O. The structure of the Schwann cell and its relation to the axon in certain invertebrate nerve fibers. *Proc. Natl. Acad. Sci. USA* **1954**, *40*, 863–870. [CrossRef] [PubMed]
106. Sobottka, B.; Ziegler, U.; Kaech, A.; Becher, B.; Goebels, N. CNS live imaging reveals a new mechanism of myelination: The liquid croissant model. *Glia* **2011**, *59*, 1841–1849. [CrossRef] [PubMed]
107. Snaidero, N.; Möbius, W.; Czopka, T.; Hekking, L.H.P.; Mathisen, C.; Verkleij, D.; Goebbels, S.; Edgar, J.; Merkler, D.; Lyons, D.A.; et al. Myelin Membrane Wrapping of CNS Axons by PI(3,4,5)P3-Dependent Polarized Growth at the Inner Tongue. *Cell* **2014**, *156*, 277–290. [CrossRef] [PubMed]
108. Friede, R.L. Control of myelin formation by axon caliber. (With a model of the control mechanism). *J. Comp. Neurol.* **1972**, *144*, 233–252. [CrossRef] [PubMed]
109. Windebank, A.J.; Wood, P.; Bunge, R.P.; Dyck, P.J. Myelination determines the caliber of dorsal root ganglion neurons in culture. *J. Neurosci.* **1985**, *5*, 1563–1569. [CrossRef] [PubMed]
110. Lee, S.; Leach, M.K.; Redmond, S.A.; Chong, S.Y.C.; Mellon, S.H.; Tuck, S.J.; Feng, Z.-Q.; Corey, J.M.; Chan, J.R. A culture system to study oligodendrocyte myelination processes using engineered nanofibers. *Nat. Methods* **2012**, *9*, 917–922. [CrossRef] [PubMed]
111. Sánchez, I.; Hassinger, L.; Paskevich, P.A.; Shine, H.D.; Nixon, R.A. Oligodendroglia regulate the regional expansion of axon caliber and local accumulation of neurofilaments during development independently of myelin formation. *J. Neurosci.* **1996**, *16*, 5095–5105. [CrossRef] [PubMed]
112. Sánchez, I.; Hassinger, L.; Sihag, R.K.; Cleveland, D.W.; Mohan, P.; Nixon, R.A. Local Control of Neurofilament Accumulation during Radial Growth of Myelinating Axons in Vivo. *J. Cell Biol.* **2000**, *151*, 1013–1024. [CrossRef] [PubMed]
113. Nave, K.-A.; Salzer, J.L. Axonal regulation of myelination by neuregulin 1. *Curr. Opin. Neurobiol.* **2006**, *16*, 492–500. [CrossRef] [PubMed]
114. Waxman, S.G.; Ritchie, J.M. Molecular dissection of the myelinated axon. *Ann. Neurol.* **1993**, *33*, 121–136. [CrossRef] [PubMed]
115. Seidl, A.H. Regulation of conduction time along axons. *Neuroscience* **2014**, *276*, 126–134. [CrossRef] [PubMed]
116. Bercury, K.K.; Macklin, W.B. Dynamics and Mechanisms of CNS Myelination. *Dev. Cell* **2015**, *32*, 447–458. [CrossRef] [PubMed]

117. Lee, Y.; Morrison, B.M.; Li, Y.; Lengacher, S.; Farah, M.H.; Hoffman, P.N.; Liu, Y.; Tsingalia, A.; Jin, L.; Zhang, P.-W.; et al. Oligodendroglia metabolically support axons and contribute to neurodegeneration. *Nature* **2012**, *487*, 443–448. [CrossRef] [PubMed]
118. Fünfschilling, U.; Supplie, L.M.; Mahad, D.; Boretius, S.; Saab, A.S.; Edgar, J.; Brinkmann, B.G.; Kassmann, C.M.; Tzvetanova, I.D.; Möbius, W.; et al. Glycolytic oligodendrocytes maintain myelin and long-term axonal integrity. *Nature* **2012**, *485*, 517–521. [CrossRef] [PubMed]
119. Ravera, S.; Bartolucci, M.; Calzia, D.; Aluigi, M.G.; Ramoino, P.; Morelli, A.; Panfoli, I. Tricarboxylic acid cycle-sustained oxidative phosphorylation in isolated myelin vesicles. *Biochimie* **2013**, *95*, 1991–1998. [CrossRef] [PubMed]
120. Assinck, P.; Duncan, G.J.; Plemel, J.R.; Lee, M.J.; Stratton, J.A.; Manesh, S.B.; Liu, J.; Ramer, L.M.; Kang, S.H.; Bergles, D.E.; et al. Myelinogenic Plasticity of Oligodendrocyte Precursor Cells following Spinal Cord Contusion Injury. *J. Neurosci.* **2017**, *37*, 8635–8654. [CrossRef] [PubMed]
121. Itoyama, Y.; Ohnishi, A.; Tateishi, J.; Kuroiwa, Y.; Webster, H.D. Spinal cord multiple sclerosis lesions in Japanese patients: Schwann cell remyelination occurs in areas that lack glial fibrillary acidic protein (GFAP). *Acta Neuropathol.* **1985**, *65*, 217–223. [CrossRef] [PubMed]
122. Baerwald, K.D.; Popko, B. Developing and mature oligodendrocytes respond differently to the immune cytokine interferon-gamma. *J. Neurosci. Res.* **1998**, *52*, 230–239. [CrossRef]
123. Arnett, H.A.; Mason, J.; Marino, M.; Suzuki, K.; Matsushima, G.K.; Ting, J.P.-Y. TNFα promotes proliferation of oligodendrocyte progenitors and remyelination. *Nat. Neurosci.* **2001**, *4*, 1116–1122. [CrossRef] [PubMed]
124. Bonora, M.; De Marchi, E.; Patergnani, S.; Suski, J.M.; Celsi, F.; Bononi, A.; Giorgi, C.; Marchi, S.; Rimessi, A.; Duszyński, J.; et al. Tumor necrosis factor-α impairs oligodendroglial differentiation through a mitochondria-dependent process. *Cell Death Differ.* **2014**, *21*, 1198–1208. [CrossRef] [PubMed]
125. Kang, Z.; Wang, C.; Zepp, J.; Wu, L.; Sun, K.; Zhao, J.; Chandrasekharan, U.; DiCorleto, P.E.; Trapp, B.D.; Ransohoff, R.M.; et al. Act1 mediates IL-17–induced EAE pathogenesis selectively in NG2+ glial cells. *Nat. Neurosci.* **2013**, *16*, 1401–1408. [CrossRef] [PubMed]
126. Falcão, A.M.; van Bruggen, D.; Marques, S.; Meijer, M.; Jäkel, S.; Agirre, E.; Samudyata; Floriddia, E.M.; Vanichkina, D.P.; ffrench-Constant, C.; et al. Disease-specific oligodendrocyte lineage cells arise in multiple sclerosis. *Nat. Med.* **2018**, *24*, 1837–1844.
127. Kirby, L.; Jin, J.; Cardona, J.G.; Smith, M.D.; Martin, K.A.; Wang, J.; Strasburger, H.; Herbst, L.; Alexis, M.; Karnell, J.; et al. Oligodendrocyte precursor cells present antigen and are cytotoxic targets in inflammatory demyelination. *Nat. Commun.* **2019**, *10*, 3887. [CrossRef] [PubMed]
128. Dincman, T.A.; Beare, J.E.; Ohri, S.S.; Whittemore, S.R. Isolation of cortical mouse oligodendrocyte precursor cells. *J. Neurosci. Methods* **2012**, *209*, 219–226. [CrossRef] [PubMed]
129. Emery, B.; Dugas, J.C. Purification of oligodendrocyte lineage cells from mouse cortices by immunopanning. *Cold Spring Harb. Protoc.* **2013**, *2013*, 854–868. [CrossRef] [PubMed]
130. Flores-Obando, R.E.; Freidin, M.M.; Abrams, C.K. Rapid and specific immunomagnetic isolation of mouse primary oligodendrocytes. *J. Vis. Exp.* **2018**, *2018*. [CrossRef] [PubMed]
131. Pang, Y.; Zheng, B.; Kimberly, S.L.; Cai, Z.; Rhodes, P.G.; Lin, R.C.S. Neuron-oligodendrocyte myelination co-culture derived from embryonic rat spinal cord and cerebral cortex. *Brain Behav.* **2012**, *2*, 53–67. [CrossRef] [PubMed]
132. Mei, F.; Fancy, S.P.J.; Shen, Y.A.A.; Niu, J.; Zhao, C.; Presley, B.; Miao, E.; Lee, S.; Mayoral, S.R.; Redmond, S.A.; et al. Micropillar arrays as a high-throughput screening platform for therapeutics in multiple sclerosis. *Nat. Med.* **2014**, *20*, 954–960. [CrossRef] [PubMed]
133. Louis, J.C.; Magal, E.; Muir, D.; Manthorpe, M.; Varon, S. CG-4, A new bipotential glial cell line from rat brain, is capable of differentiating in vitro into either mature oligodendrocytes or type-2 astrocytes. *J. Neurosci. Res.* **1992**, *31*, 193–204. [CrossRef] [PubMed]
134. Richter-Landsberg, C.; Heinrich, M. OLN-93: A new permanent oligodendroglia cell line derived from primary rat brain glial cultures. *J. Neurosci. Res.* **1996**, *45*, 161–173. [CrossRef]
135. Jungl, M.; Kramer', E.; Grzenkowskil, M.; Tang2, K.; Biakemore2, W.; Aguzzi3, A.; Khazaie4, K.; Chiichlia4, K.; Von Blankenfeld5, G.; Kettenmann5, H.; et al. Lines of Murine Oligodendroglial Precursor Cells Immortalized by an Activated neu Tvrosine Kinase Show Distinct Degrees of Interaction with Axons In Wtro and In Wvo. *EJN* **1995**, *7*, 1245–1265.

136. Van Tilborg, E.; de Theije, C.G.M.; van Hal, M.; Wagenaar, N.; de Vries, L.S.; Benders, M.J.; Rowitch, D.H.; Nijboer, C.H. Origin and dynamics of oligodendrocytes in the developing brain: Implications for perinatal white matter injury. *Glia* **2018**, *66*, 221–238. [CrossRef] [PubMed]
137. Chanoumidou, K.; Mozafari, S.; Baron-Van Evercooren, A.; Kuhlmann, T. Stem cell derived oligodendrocytes to study myelin diseases. *Glia* **2019**, glia.23733. [CrossRef] [PubMed]
138. Medina-Rodríguez, E.M.; Arenzana, F.J.; Bribián, A.; De Castro, F. Protocol to isolate a large amount of functional oligodendrocyte precursor cells from the cerebral cortex of adult mice and humans. *PLoS ONE* **2013**, *8*, e81620.
139. De Groot, J.A.; Montagne, L.; Janssen, I.; Ravid, R.; Van Der Valk, P.; Veerhuis, R. Isolation and characterization of adult microglial cells and oligodendrocytes derived from postmortem human brain tissue. *Brain Res. Protoc.* **2000**, *5*, 85–94. [CrossRef]
140. Takahashi, K.; Yamanaka, S. Induction of Pluripotent Stem Cells from Mouse Embryonic and Adult Fibroblast Cultures by Defined Factors. *Cell* **2006**, *126*, 663–676. [CrossRef] [PubMed]
141. Wang, S.; Bates, J.; Li, X.; Schanz, S.; Chandler-Militello, D.; Levine, C.; Maherali, N.; Studer, L.; Hochedlinger, K.; Windrem, M.; et al. Human iPSC-derived oligodendrocyte progenitor cells can myelinate and rescue a mouse model of congenital hypomyelination. *Cell Stem Cell* **2013**, *12*, 252–264. [CrossRef] [PubMed]
142. Ehrlich, M.; Mozafari, S.; Glatza, M.; Starost, L.; Velychko, S.; Hallmann, A.L.; Cui, Q.L.; Schambach, A.; Kim, K.P.; Bachelin, C.; et al. Rapid and efficient generation of oligodendrocytes from human induced pluripotent stem cells using transcription factors. *Proc. Natl. Acad. Sci. USA* **2017**, *114*, E2243–E2252. [CrossRef] [PubMed]
143. García-León, J.A.; Kumar, M.; Boon, R.; Chau, D.; One, J.; Wolfs, E.; Eggermont, K.; Berckmans, P.; Gunhanlar, N.; de Vrij, F.; et al. SOX10 Single Transcription Factor-Based Fast and Efficient Generation of Oligodendrocytes from Human Pluripotent Stem Cells. *Stem Cell Rep.* **2018**, *10*, 655–672.
144. Dittmer, M.; Young, A.; O'Hagan, T.; Eleftheriadis, G.; Bankhead, P.; Dombrowski, Y.; Medina, R.J.; Fitzgerald, D.C. Characterization of a murine mixed neuron-glia model and cellular responses to regulatory T cell-derived factors. *Mol Brain* **2018**, *11*, 25. [CrossRef] [PubMed]
145. Harrer, M.D.; von Büdingen, H.C.; Stoppini, L.; Alliod, C.; Pouly, S.; Fischer, K.; Goebels, N. Live imaging of remyelination after antibody-mediated demyelination in an ex-vivo model for immune mediated CNS damage. *Exp. Neurol.* **2009**, *216*, 431–438. [CrossRef] [PubMed]
146. Marton, R.M.; Miura, Y.; Sloan, S.A.; Li, Q.; Revah, O.; Levy, R.J.; Huguenard, J.R.; Pașca, S.P. Differentiation and maturation of oligodendrocytes in human three-dimensional neural cultures. *Nat. Neurosci.* **2019**, *22*, 484–491. [CrossRef] [PubMed]
147. Shibata, S.; Yasuda, A.; Renault-Mihara, F.; Suyama, S.; Katoh, H.; Inoue, T.; Inoue, Y.U.; Nagoshi, N.; Sato, M.; Nakamura, M.; et al. Sox10-Venus mice: A new tool for real-time labeling of neural crest lineage cells and oligodendrocytes. *Mol. Brain* **2010**, *3*. [CrossRef] [PubMed]
148. Yuan, X.; Chittajallu, R.; Belachew, S.; Anderson, S.; McBain, C.J.; Gallo, V. Expression of the green fluorescent protein in the oligodendrocyte lineage: A transgenic mouse for developmental and physiological studies. *J. Neurosci. Res.* **2002**, *70*, 529–545. [CrossRef] [PubMed]
149. Mallon, B.S.; Shick, H.E.; Kidd, G.J.; Macklin, W.B. Proteolipid Promoter Activity Distinguishes Two Populations of NG2-Positive Cells throughout Neonatal Cortical Development. *J. Neurosci.* **2002**, *22*, 876–885. [CrossRef] [PubMed]
150. Almeida, R.G.; Czopka, T.; Ffrench-Constant, C.; Lyons, D.A. Individual axons regulate the myelinating potential of single oligodendrocytes in vivo. *Development* **2011**, *138*, 4443–4450. [CrossRef] [PubMed]
151. Shin, J.; Park, H.-C.; Topczewska, J.M.; Mawdsley, D.J.; Appel, B. Neural cell fate analysis in zebrafish using olig2 BAC transgenics. *Methods Cell Sci.* **2003**, *25*, 7–14. [CrossRef] [PubMed]
152. Howe, K.; Clark, M.D.; Torroja, C.F.; Torrance, J.; Berthelot, C.; Muffato, M.; Collins, J.E.; Humphray, S.; McLaren, K.; Matthews, L.; et al. The zebrafish reference genome sequence and its relationship to the human genome. *Nature* **2013**, *496*, 498–503. [CrossRef] [PubMed]
153. Nawaz, S.; Schweitzer, J.; Jahn, O.; Werner, H.B. Molecular evolution of myelin basic protein, an abundant structural myelin component. *Glia* **2013**, *61*, 1364–1377. [CrossRef] [PubMed]

154. Early, J.J.; Cole, K.L.; Williamson, J.M.; Swire, M.; Kamadurai, H.; Muskavitch, M.; Lyons, D.A. An automated high-resolution in vivo screen in zebrafish to identify chemical regulators of myelination. *Elife* **2018**, *7*. [CrossRef] [PubMed]
155. Ransohoff, R.M. Animal models of multiple sclerosis: The good, the bad and the bottom line. *Nat. Neurosci.* **2012**, *15*, 1074–1077. [CrossRef] [PubMed]
156. Croxford, A.L.; Kurschus, F.C.; Waisman, A. Mouse models for multiple sclerosis: Historical facts and future implications. *Biochim. Biophys. Acta Mol. Basis Dis.* **2011**, *1812*, 177–183. [CrossRef] [PubMed]
157. Blakemore, W.F. Pattern of remyelination in the CNS. *Nature* **1974**, *249*, 577–578. [CrossRef] [PubMed]
158. Hall, S.M. The effect of injections of lysophosphatidyl choline into white matter of the adult mouse spinal cord. *J. Cell Sci.* **1972**, *10*, 535–546. [PubMed]
159. Kotter, M.R.; Setzu, A.; Sim, F.J.; Van Rooijen, N.; Franklin, R.J.M. Macrophage depletion impairs oligodendrocyte remyelination following lysolecithin-induced demyelination. *Glia* **2001**, *35*, 204–212. [CrossRef] [PubMed]
160. Kipp, M.; Clarner, T.; Dang, J.; Copray, S.; Beyer, C. The cuprizone animal model: New insights into an old story. *Acta Neuropathol.* **2009**, *118*, 723–736. [CrossRef] [PubMed]
161. Matsushima, G.K.; Morell, P. The Neurotoxicant, Cuprizone, as a Model to Study Demyelination and Remyelination in the Central Nervous System. *Brain Pathol.* **2006**, *11*, 107–116. [CrossRef] [PubMed]
162. Sachs, H.H.; Bercury, K.K.; Popescu, D.C.; Narayanan, S.P.; Macklin, W.B. A new model of Cuprizone-Mediated demyelination/remyelination. *ASN Neuro.* **2014**, *6*. [CrossRef] [PubMed]
163. Woodruff, R.H.; Fruttiger, M.; Richardson, W.D.; Franklin, R.J.M. Platelet-derived growth factor regulates oligodendrocyte progenitor numbers in adult CNS and their response following CNS demyelination. *Mol. Cell. Neurosci.* **2004**, *25*, 252–262. [CrossRef] [PubMed]
164. Fancy, S.P.J.; Baranzini, S.E.; Zhao, C.; Yuk, D.I.; Irvine, K.A.; Kaing, S.; Sanai, N.; Franklin, R.J.M.; Rowitch, D.H. Dysregulation of the Wnt pathway inhibits timely myelination and remyelination in the mammalian CNS. *Genes Dev.* **2009**, *23*, 1571–1585. [CrossRef] [PubMed]
165. Rüther, B.J.; Scheld, M.; Dreymueller, D.; Clarner, T.; Kress, E.; Brandenburg, L.O.; Swartenbroekx, T.; Hoornaert, C.; Ponsaerts, P.; Fallier-Becker, P.; et al. Combination of cuprizone and experimental autoimmune encephalomyelitis to study inflammatory brain lesion formation and progression. *Glia* **2017**, *65*, 1900–1913. [CrossRef] [PubMed]
166. Sampaio-Baptista, C.; Johansen-Berg, H. White Matter Plasticity in the Adult Brain. *Neuron* **2017**, *96*, 1239–1251. [CrossRef] [PubMed]
167. McKenzie, I.A.; Ohayon, D.; Li, H.; Paes de Faria, J.; Emery, B.; Tohyama, K.; Richardson, W.D. Motor skill learning requires active central myelination. *Science* **2014**, *346*, 318–322. [CrossRef] [PubMed]
168. Butts, B.D.; Houde, C.; Mehmet, H. Maturation-dependent sensitivity of oligodendrocyte lineage cells to apoptosis: Implications for normal development and disease. *Cell Death Differ.* **2008**, *15*, 1178–1186. [CrossRef] [PubMed]
169. Juurlink, B.H.J.; Thorburne, S.K.; Hertz, L. Peroxide-scavenging deficit underlies oligodendrocyte susceptibility to oxidative stress. *Glia* **1998**, *22*, 371–378. [CrossRef]
170. McTigue, D.M.; Tripathi, R.B. The life, death, and replacement of oligodendrocytes in the adult CNS. *J. Neurochem.* **2008**, *107*, 1–19. [CrossRef] [PubMed]
171. Matute, C.; Torre, I.; Pérez-Cerdá, F.; Pérez-Samartín, A.; Alberdi, E.; Etxebarria, E.; Arranz, A.M.; Ravid, R.; Rodríguez-Antigüedad, A.; Sánchez-Gómez, M.V.; et al. P2X 7 receptor blockade prevents ATP excitotoxicity in oligodendrocytes and ameliorates experimental autoimmune encephalomyelitis. *J. Neurosci.* **2007**, *27*, 9525–9533. [CrossRef] [PubMed]
172. Matute, C.; Sánchez-Gómez, M.V.; Martínez-Millán, L.; Miledi, R. Glutamate receptor-mediated toxicity in optic nerve oligodendrocytes. *Proc. Natl. Acad. Sci. USA* **1997**, *94*, 8830–8835. [CrossRef] [PubMed]
173. Traka, M.; Podojil, J.R.; McCarthy, D.P.; Miller, S.D.; Popko, B. Oligodendrocyte death results in immune-mediated CNS demyelination. *Nat. Neurosci.* **2016**, *19*, 65–74. [CrossRef] [PubMed]
174. Fancy, S.P.J.; Harrington, E.P.; Yuen, T.J.; Silbereis, J.C.; Zhao, C.; Baranzini, S.E.; Bruce, C.C.; Otero, J.J.; Huang, E.J.; Nusse, R.; et al. Axin2 as regulatory and therapeutic target in newborn brain injury and remyelination. *Nat. Neurosci.* **2011**, *14*, 1009–1016. [CrossRef] [PubMed]
175. Torii, T.; Miyamoto, Y.; Yamauchi, J.; Tanoue, A. Pelizaeus-Merzbacher disease: Cellular pathogenesis and pharmacologic therapy. *Pediatr. Int.* **2014**, *56*, 659–666. [CrossRef] [PubMed]

176. Simons, M.; Krämer, E.M.; Macchi, P.; Rathke-Hartlieb, S.; Trotter, J.; Nave, K.A.; Schulz, J.B. Overexpression of the myelin proteolipid protein leads to accumulation of cholesterol and proteolipid protein in endosomes/lysosomes: Implications for Pelizaeus-Merzbacher disease. *J. Cell Biol.* **2002**, *157*, 327–336. [CrossRef] [PubMed]
177. McAleese, K.E.; Walker, L.; Graham, S.; Moya, E.L.J.; Johnson, M.; Erskine, D.; Colloby, S.J.; Dey, M.; Martin-Ruiz, C.; Taylor, J.P.; et al. Parietal white matter lesions in Alzheimer's disease are associated with cortical neurodegenerative pathology, but not with small vessel disease. *Acta Neuropathol.* **2017**, *134*, 459–473. [CrossRef] [PubMed]
178. Behrendt, G.; Baer, K.; Buffo, A.; Curtis, M.A.; Faull, R.L.; Rees, M.I.; Götz, M.; Dimou, L. Dynamic changes in myelin aberrations and oligodendrocyte generation in chronic amyloidosis in mice and men. *Glia* **2013**, *61*, 273–286. [CrossRef] [PubMed]
179. Desai, M.K.; Mastrangelo, M.A.; Ryan, D.A.; Sudol, K.L.; Narrow, W.C.; Bowers, W.J. Early oligodendrocyte/myelin pathology in Alzheimer's disease mice constitutes a novel therapeutic target. *Am. J. Pathol.* **2010**, *177*, 1422–1435. [CrossRef] [PubMed]
180. Xu, J.; Chen, S.; Ahmed, S.H.; Chen, H.; Ku, G.; Goldberg, M.P.; Hsu, C.Y. Amyloid-beta peptides are cytotoxic to oligodendrocytes. *J. Neurosci.* **2001**, *21*, 1–5. [CrossRef]
181. Fischer, F.U.; Wolf, D.; Scheurich, A.; Fellgiebel, A. Altered whole-brain white matter networks in preclinical Alzheimer's disease. *NeuroImage Clin.* **2015**, *8*, 660–666. [CrossRef] [PubMed]
182. Braak, H.; Braak, E. Development of Alzheimer-related neurofibrillary changes in the neocortex inversely recapitulates cortical myelogenesis. *Acta Neuropathol.* **1996**, *92*, 197–201. [CrossRef] [PubMed]
183. Reisberg, B.; Franssen, E.H.; Souren, L.E.M.; Auer, S.R.; Akram, I.; Kenowsky, S. Evidence and mechanisms of retrogenesis in Alzheimer's and other dementias: Management and treatment import. *Am. J. Alzheimers. Dis. Other Demen.* **2002**, *17*, 202–212. [CrossRef] [PubMed]
184. Fields, R.D. ScienceDirect-Trends in Neurosciences: White matter in learning, cognition and psychiatric disorders. *Trends Neurosci.* **2009**, *31*, 361–370. [CrossRef] [PubMed]
185. Edgar, N.; Sibille, E. A putative functional role for oligodendrocytes in mood regulation. *Transl. Psychiatry* **2012**, *2*, e109. [CrossRef] [PubMed]
186. Rajkowska, G. Cell pathology in bipolar disorder. *Bipolar Disord.* **2002**, *4*, 105–116. [CrossRef] [PubMed]
187. Vostrikov, V.M.; Uranova, N.A.; Orlovskaya, D.D. Deficit of perineuronal oligodendrocytes in the prefrontal cortex in schizophrenia and mood disorders. *Schizophr. Res.* **2007**, *94*, 273–280. [CrossRef] [PubMed]
188. Tkachev, D.; Mimmack, M.L.; Ryan, M.M.; Wayland, M.; Freeman, T.; Jones, P.B.; Starkey, M.; Webster, M.J.; Yolken, R.H.; Bahn, S. Oligodendrocyte dysfunction in schizophrenia and bipolar disorder. *Lancet* **2003**, *362*, 798–805. [CrossRef]
189. Herring, N.R.; Konradi, C. Myelin, copper, and the cuprizone model of schizophrenia. *Front. Biosci. Sch.* **2011**, *3 S*, 23–40.
190. Cathomas, F.; Azzinnari, D.; Bergamini, G.; Sigrist, H.; Buerge, M.; Hoop, V.; Wicki, B.; Goetze, L.; Soares, S.; Kukelova, D.; et al. Oligodendrocyte gene expression is reduced by and influences effects of chronic social stress in mice. *Genes, Brain Behav.* **2019**, *18*, 1–14. [CrossRef] [PubMed]
191. Miyata, S.; Taniguchi, M.; Koyama, Y.; Shimizu, S.; Tanaka, T.; Yasuno, F.; Yamamoto, A.; Iida, H.; Kudo, T.; Katayama, T.; et al. Association between chronic stress-induced structural abnormalities in Ranvier nodes and reduced oligodendrocyte activity in major depression. *Sci. Rep.* **2016**, *6*, 1–12. [CrossRef] [PubMed]
192. Love, S. Demyelinating diseases. *J. Clin. Pathol.* **2006**, *59*, 1151–1159. [CrossRef] [PubMed]
193. Saxena, A.; Bauer, J.; Scheikl, T.; Zappulla, J.; Audebert, M.; Desbois, S.; Waisman, A.; Lassmann, H.; Liblau, R.S.; Mars, L.T. Cutting Edge: Multiple Sclerosis-Like Lesions Induced by Effector CD8 T Cells Recognizing a Sequestered Antigen on Oligodendrocytes. *J. Immunol.* **2008**, *181*, 1617–1621. [CrossRef] [PubMed]
194. Duncan, I.D.; Radcliff, A.B. Inherited and acquired disorders of myelin: The underlying myelin pathology. *Exp. Neurol.* **2016**, *283*, 452–475. [CrossRef] [PubMed]
195. Hesp, Z.C.; Goldstein, E.A.; Miranda, C.J.; Kaspar, B.K.; McTigue, D.M.; Kaspar, B.K.; McTigue, D.M. Chronic Oligodendrogenesis and Remyelination after Spinal Cord Injury in Mice and Rats. *J. Neurosci.* **2015**, *35*, 1274–1290. [CrossRef] [PubMed]
196. Levine, J.M.; Reynolds, R. Activation and Proliferation of Endogenous Oligodendrocyte Precursor Cells during Ethidium Bromide-Induced Demyelination. *Exp. Neurol.* **1999**, *160*, 333–347. [CrossRef] [PubMed]

197. Fancy, S.P.J.; Zhao, C.; Franklin, R.J.M. Increased expression of Nkx2.2 and Olig2 identifies reactive oligodendrocyte progenitor cells responding to demyelination in the adult CNS. *Mol. Cell. Neurosci.* **2004**, *27*, 247–254. [CrossRef] [PubMed]
198. Arai, K.; Lo, E.H. An oligovascular niche: Cerebral endothelial cells promote the survival and proliferation of oligodendrocyte precursor cells. *J. Neurosci.* **2009**, *29*, 4351–4355. [CrossRef] [PubMed]
199. Hammond, T.R.; Gadea, A.; Dupree, J.; Kerninon, C.; Nait-Oumesmar, B.; Aguirre, A.; Gallo, V. Astrocyte-Derived Endothelin-1 Inhibits Remyelination through Notch Activation. *Neuron* **2014**, *81*, 588–602. [CrossRef] [PubMed]
200. Casaccia-Bonnefil, P.; Tikoo, R.; Kiyokawa, H.; Friedrich, V.; Chao, M.V.; Koff, A. Oligodendrocyte precursor differentiation is perturbed in the absence of the cyclin-dependent kinase inhibitor p27Kip1. *Genes Dev.* **1997**, *11*, 2335–2346. [CrossRef] [PubMed]
201. Magri, L.; Gacias, M.; Wu, M.; Swiss, V.A.; Janssen, W.G.; Casaccia, P. c-Myc-dependent transcriptional regulation of cell cycle and nucleosomal histones during oligodendrocyte differentiation. *Neuroscience* **2014**, *276*, 72–86. [CrossRef] [PubMed]
202. Magri, L.; Swiss, V.A.; Jablonska, B.; Lei, L.; Pedre, X.; Walsh, M.; Zhang, W.; Gallo, V.; Canoll, P.; Casaccia, P. E2F1 coregulates cell cycle genes and chromatin components during the transition of oligodendrocyte progenitors from proliferation to differentiation. *J. Neurosci.* **2014**, *34*, 1481–1493. [CrossRef] [PubMed]
203. Habes, M.; Erus, G.; Toledo, J.B.; Zhang, T.; Bryan, N.; Launer, L.J.; Rosseel, Y.; Janowitz, D.; Doshi, J.; Van Der Auwera, S.; et al. White matter hyperintensities and imaging patterns of brain ageing in the general population. *Brain* **2016**, *139*, 1164–1179. [CrossRef] [PubMed]
204. Ruckh, J.M.; Zhao, J.W.; Shadrach, J.L.; Van Wijngaarden, P.; Rao, T.N.; Wagers, A.J.; Franklin, R.J.M. Rejuvenation of regeneration in the aging central nervous system. *Cell Stem Cell* **2012**, *10*, 96–103. [CrossRef] [PubMed]
205. Sim, F.J.; Zhao, C.; Penderis, J.; Franklin, R.J.M. The age-related decrease in CNS remyelination efficiency is attributable to an impairment of both oligodendrocyte progenitor recruitment and differentiation. *J. Neurosci.* **2002**, *22*, 2451–2459. [CrossRef] [PubMed]
206. Zhu, X.; Hill, R.A.; Dietrich, D.; Komitova, M.; Suzuki, R.; Nishiyama, A. Age-dependent fate and lineage restriction of single NG2 cells. *Development* **2011**, *138*, 745–753. [CrossRef] [PubMed]
207. Saher, G.; Brügger, B.; Lappe-Siefke, C.; Möbius, W.; Tozawa, R.I.; Wehr, M.C.; Wieland, F.; Ishibashi, S.; Nave, K.A. High cholesterol level is essential for myelin membrane growth. *Nat. Neurosci.* **2005**, *8*, 468–475. [CrossRef] [PubMed]
208. Thelen, K.M.; Falkai, P.; Bayer, T.A.; Lütjohann, D. Cholesterol synthesis rate in human hippocampus declines with aging. *Neurosci. Lett.* **2006**, *403*, 15–19. [CrossRef] [PubMed]
209. Thorburne, S.K.; Juurlink, B.H.J. Low Glutathione and High Iron Govern the Susceptibility of Oligodendroglial Precursors to Oxidative Stress. *J. Neurochem.* **1996**, *67*, 1014–1022. [CrossRef] [PubMed]
210. Liu, R.M.; Choi, J. Age-associated decline in γ-glutamylcysteine synthetase gene expression in rats. *Free Radic. Biol. Med.* **2000**, *28*, 566–574. [CrossRef]
211. Back, S.A.; Luo, N.L.; Borenstein, N.S.; Levine, J.M.; Volpe, J.J.; Kinney, H.C. Late oligodendrocyte progenitors coincide with the developmental window of vulnerability for human perinatal white matter injury. *J. Neurosci.* **2001**, *21*, 1302–1312. [CrossRef] [PubMed]
212. Shields, S.A.; Gilson, J.M.; Blakemore, W.F.; Franklin, R.J.M. Remyelination occurs as extensively but more slowly in old rats compared to young rats following gliotoxin-induced CNS demyelination. *Glia* **1999**, *28*, 77–83. [CrossRef]
213. Duncan, I.D.; Brower, A.; Kondo, Y.; Curlee, J.F.; Schultz, R.D. Extensive remyelination of the CNS leads to functional recovery. *Proc. Natl. Acad. Sci. USA* **2009**, *106*, 6832–6836. [CrossRef] [PubMed]
214. Gruchot, J.; Weyers, V.; Göttle, P.; Förster, M.; Hartung, H.-P.; Küry, P.; Kremer, D. The Molecular Basis for Remyelination Failure in Multiple Sclerosis. *Cells* **2019**, *8*, 825. [CrossRef] [PubMed]
215. Yeung, M.S.; Djelloul, M.; Steiner, E.; Bernard, S.; Salehpour, M.; Possnert, G.; Brundin, L.; Frisén, J. Oligodendrocyte generation dynamics in multiple sclerosis. *Nature* **2019**, *24*, 1837–1844. [CrossRef] [PubMed]
216. Marques, S.; Zeisel, A.; Codeluppi, S.; van Bruggen, D.; Falcão, A.M.; Xiao, L.; Li, H.; Häring, M.; Hochgerner, H.; Romanov, R.A.; et al. Oligodendrocyte heterogeneity in the mouse juvenile and adult central nervous system. *Science* **2016**, *352*, 1326–1329. [CrossRef] [PubMed]

217. Viganò, F.; Möbius, W.; Götz, M.; Dimou, L. Transplantation reveals regional differences in oligodendrocyte differentiation in the adult brain. *Nat. Neurosci.* **2013**, *16*, 1370–1372. [CrossRef] [PubMed]
218. Crawford, A.H.; Tripathi, R.B.; Foerster, S.; McKenzie, I.; Kougioumtzidou, E.; Grist, M.; Richardson, W.D.; Franklin, R.J.M. Pre-existing mature oligodendrocytes do not contribute to remyelination following toxin-induced spinal cord demyelination. *Am. J. Pathol.* **2016**, *186*, 511–516. [CrossRef] [PubMed]
219. Targett, M.P.; Sussman, J.; Scolding, N.; O'Leary, M.T.; Compston, D.A.; Blakemore, W.F. Failure to achieve remyelination of demyelinated rat axons following transplantation of glial cells obtained from the adult human brain. *Neuropathol. Appl. Neurobiol.* **1996**, *22*, 199–206. [CrossRef] [PubMed]
220. Duncan, I.D.; Radcliff, A.B.; Heidari, M.; Kidd, G.; August, B.K.; Wierenga, L.A. The adult oligodendrocyte can participate in remyelination. *Proc. Natl. Acad. Sci. USA* **2018**, *115*, E11807–E11816. [CrossRef] [PubMed]
221. Soundarapandian, M.M.; Selvaraj, V.; Lo, U.G.; Golub, M.S.; Feldman, D.H.; Pleasure, D.E.; Deng, W. Zfp488 promotes oligodendrocyte differentiation of neural progenitor cells in adult mice after demyelination. *Sci. Rep.* **2011**, *1*, 1–9. [CrossRef] [PubMed]
222. Duncan, G.J.; Plemel, J.R.; Assinck, P.; Manesh, S.B.; Muir, F.G.W.; Hirata, R.; Berson, M.; Liu, J.; Wegner, M.; Emery, B.; et al. Myelin regulatory factor drives remyelination in multiple sclerosis. *Acta Neuropathol.* **2017**, *134*, 403–422. [CrossRef] [PubMed]
223. Dugas, J.C.; Ibrahim, A.; Barres, B.A. The T3-induced gene KLF9 regulates oligodendrocyte differentiation and myelin regeneration. *Mol. Cell. Neurosci.* **2012**, *50*, 45–57. [CrossRef] [PubMed]
224. Steelman, A.J.; Zhou, Y.; Koito, H.; Kim, S.J.; Payne, H.R.; Lu, Q.R.; Li, J. Activation of oligodendroglial Stat3 is required for efficient remyelination. *Neurobiol. Dis.* **2016**, *91*, 336–346. [CrossRef] [PubMed]
225. Kuhlmann, T.; Miron, V.; Cuo, Q.; Wegner, C.; Antel, J.; Brü«Ck, W.; Kuhlmann, T. Differentiation block of oligodendroglial progenitor cells as a cause for remyelination failure in chronic multiple sclerosis. *Brain* **2008**, *131*, 1749–1758. [CrossRef] [PubMed]
226. Chang, A.; Tourtellotte, W.W.; Rudick, R.; Trapp, B.D. Premyelinating oligodendrocytes in chronic lesions of multiple sclerosis. *N. Engl. J. Med.* **2002**, *346*, 165–173. [CrossRef] [PubMed]
227. Mason, J.L.; Toews, A.; Hostettler, J.D.; Morell, P.; Suzuki, K.; Goldman, J.E.; Matsushima, G.K. Oligodendrocytes and Progenitors Become Progressively Depleted within Chronically Demyelinated Lesions. *Am. J. Pathol.* **2004**, *164*, 1673–1682. [CrossRef]
228. Boyd, A.; Zhang, H.; Williams, A. Insufficient OPC migration into demyelinated lesions is a cause of poor remyelination in MS and mouse models. *Acta Neuropathol.* **2013**, *125*, 841–859. [CrossRef] [PubMed]
229. Bieber, A.J.; Kerr, S.; Rodriguez, M. Efficient central nervous system remyelination requires T cells. *Ann. Neurol.* **2003**, *53*, 680–684. [CrossRef] [PubMed]
230. Miron, V.E.; Boyd, A.; Zhao, J.-W.; Yuen, T.J.; Ruckh, J.M.; Shadrach, J.L.; van Wijngaarden, P.; Wagers, A.J.; Williams, A.; Franklin, R.J.M.; et al. M2 microglia and macrophages drive oligodendrocyte differentiation during CNS remyelination. *Nat. Neurosci.* **2013**, *16*, 1211–1218. [CrossRef] [PubMed]
231. Dombrowski, Y.; O'Hagan, T.; Dittmer, M.; Penalva, R.; Mayoral, S.R.; Bankhead, P.; Fleville, S.; Eleftheriadis, G.; Zhao, C.; Naughton, M.; et al. Regulatory T cells promote myelin regeneration in the central nervous system. *Nat. Neurosci.* **2017**, *20*, 674–680. [CrossRef] [PubMed]

© 2019 by the authors. Licensee MDPI, Basel, Switzerland. This article is an open access article distributed under the terms and conditions of the Creative Commons Attribution (CC BY) license (http://creativecommons.org/licenses/by/4.0/).

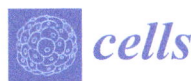

Article

Combinatory Multifactor Treatment Effects on Primary Nanofiber Oligodendrocyte Cultures

Lukas S. Enz [1], Thomas Zeis [1], Annalisa Hauck [1], Christopher Linington [2] and Nicole Schaeren-Wiemers [1,*]

[1] Neurobiology, Department of Biomedicine, University Hospital Basel, University Basel, Zentrum für Lehre und Forschung, 4031 Basel, Switzerland; lukas.enz@unibas.ch (L.S.E.); thomas.zeis@unibas.ch (T.Z.); annalisa.hauck@unibas.ch (A.H.)
[2] Institute of Infection, Immunity and Inflammation, College of Medical Veterinary and Life Sciences, University of Glasgow, Glasgow G12 8TA, UK; christopher.linington@glasgow.ac.uk
* Correspondence: nicole.schaeren-wiemers@unibas.ch; Tel.: +41-61-328-7394

Received: 30 September 2019; Accepted: 5 November 2019; Published: 12 November 2019

Abstract: Multiple sclerosis (MS) is a chronic inflammatory demyelinating and neurodegenerative disease of the central nervous system. Neurological deficits are attributed to inflammatory demyelination, which compromises axonal function and survival. These are mitigated in experimental models by rapid and often complete remyelination of affected axons, but in MS this endogenous repair mechanism frequently fails, leaving axons increasingly vulnerable to the detrimental effects of inflammatory and metabolic stress. Understanding the molecular basis of remyelination and remyelination failure is essential to develop improved therapies for this devastating disease. However, recent studies suggest that this is not due to a single dominant mechanism, but rather represents the biological outcome of multiple changes in the lesion microenvironment that combine to disrupt oligodendrocyte differentiation. This identifies a pressing need to develop technical platforms to investigate combinatory and/or synergistic effects of factors differentially expressed in MS lesions on oligodendrocyte proliferation and differentiation. Here we describe protocols using primary oligodendrocyte cultures from Bl6 mice on 384-well nanofiber plates to model changes affecting oligodendrogenesis and differentiation in the complex signaling environment associated with multiple sclerosis lesions. Using platelet-derived growth factor (PDGF–AA), fibroblast growth factor 2 (FGF2), bone morphogenetic protein 2 (BMP2) and bone morphogenetic protein 4 (BMP4) as representative targets, we demonstrate that we can assess their combinatory effects across a wide range of concentrations in a single experiment. This in vitro model is ideal for assessing the combinatory effects of changes in availability of multiple factors, thus more closely modelling the situation in vivo and furthering high-throughput screening possibilities.

Keywords: oligodendrocyte; myelin; remyelination; screening; nanofibers; multiple sclerosis

1. Introduction

Multiple Sclerosis (MS) is a chronic inflammatory, demyelinating disease of the central nervous system (CNS) with diverse clinical presentations and a heterogeneous histopathology. It is suggested that demyelination and failure of remyelination lead to axonal degeneration and functional impairment. This axonal pathology is the underlying cause of disability in patients with MS and is attributed to the detrimental effects of inflammatory demyelination on the functional and structural integrity of affected axons [1,2]. In this context, demyelination not only disrupts axonal conduction per se but also disrupts metabolic support provided via the myelin sheath whilst simultaneously enhancing axonal susceptibility to damage by inflammatory mediators, a combination of effects predicted to exacerbate axonal loss and result in irreversible neurological deficits. These effects of demyelination on axonal health are mitigated in animal models by rapid and often complete remyelination by oligodendrocytes derived from an endogenous pool of oligodendrocyte progenitor cells (OPCs). However, in MS, this repair mechanism frequently fails, leaving affected axons increasingly vulnerable to inflammatory and metabolic stress [3].

Why remyelination fails in MS remains poorly understood, but it is attributed to changes in the lesion microenvironment that compromise OPC recruitment, survival and/or differentiation, and axon function [4–9], which are compounded by factors including disease chronicity [10] and factors not related to the disease, such as gender and age [11].

Developmental myelination is under tight spatial and temporal control and is coordinated by factors including neuronal activity, changes affecting growth factor availability, and stage specific expression of their receptors within the oligodendrocyte lineage. It is assumed that remyelination recapitulates many features of this complex developmental program [12]. It is therefore not surprising that remyelination can be disrupted experimentally by many different mechanisms, including inappropriate re-expression of developmental cues and continuing presence of myelin debris as well as changes affecting growth factor availability, progenitor cell migration, and composition of the extracellular matrix [13]. Strong circumstantial arguments can be made for each of these mechanisms contributing to remyelination failure in MS, but their relative importance is unclear. To resolve this question, several groups performed comparative transcriptomic studies on normal-appearing white matter, active inflammatory demyelinating lesions, remyelinating lesions, and inactive chronically demyelinated lesions with the aim of identifying specific molecules or signaling pathways that may provide targets for treatment strategies designed to enhance remyelination [14–17]. However, these studies have failed to identify any single factor or pathway consistently associated with remyelination failure. Instead they demonstrate there is significant intra-study and -lesion heterogeneity with regard to the expression of genes predicted to influence oligodendrogenesis and myelination between different lesion types. An observation that has led us to speculate failure of remyelination is the net result of dysregulation of multiple pathways.

To understand the consequences of this heterogeneity, an experimental platform is required in which we can rapidly assess concentration dependent effects of multiple factors on OPC proliferation, differentiation, and myelination. Primary co-culture systems are suitable to investigate specific questions on oligodendrocyte development and myelination, but due to the complexity of these systems, direct effects on proliferation, differentiation, and myelination can hardly be discerned from indirect effects. Quantitative approaches are often handicapped due to the cell heterogeneity in these co-culture systems. In 2012, the research group of Jonah Chan demonstrated oligodendrocytes are capable of myelinating engineered nanofibers [18]. This technique has enormous potential to evaluate the effect of single molecules on oligodendrocyte myelination, and to identify potential therapeutic targets [19].

To demonstrate the effectiveness of this platform we focused on four factors differentially regulated in MS lesions that influence OPC proliferation, differentiation, and myelination: platelet-derived growth factor subunit A dimer (PDGF–AA [20]), fibroblast growth factor 2 (FGF2 [15,21]), bone morphogenetic protein 2 (BMP2 [22]), and bone morphogenetic protein 4 (BMP4 [22,23]). We were able to show that our model system is an efficient way of screening effects in a multifactor treatment paradigm. A major application of this model system may be the modeling of the complex environment in a demyelinated lesion.

2. Materials and Methods

2.1. Oligodendrocyte Cell Culture

Primary oligodendrocyte cultures were prepared from post-natal day 0–2 C57Bl/6 mice, as described before [24]. Briefly, forebrains were collected aseptically and after removal of the meninges, the cortices were triturated 35 times through a 1 mL pipet in "DBGFP" medium (Table 1) and filtered through a 70 μm cell strainer. Cells were grown in suspension culture in DBGFP at 37 °C, 5% CO_2, and 95% air in DBGFP to generate oligospheres. After two weeks, cultures from multiple donors were pooled, centrifuged at 300× g for five minutes, and resuspended in plating medium (Table 1). After gentle trituration through a G27 needle, cells were plated at a density of 10,000 oligodendrocytes/well in 384-well nanofiber plates (Z694568–1EA, Sigma–Aldrich Chemie GmbH, Buchs, Switzerland) coated with poly–L–lysine (P4707–50ML, Sigma–Aldrich Chemie GmbH, Buchs, Switzerland).

Table 1. Composition of used cell culture media.

	Product	Product Number	Company	Dilution/Concentration
DBGFP:	Dulbecco's Modified Eagle's Medium/Nutrient Mixture F-12 Ham with (4-(2-hydroxyethyl)-1-piperazineethanesulfonic acid) (HEPES)	31330095	Gibco/ThermoFisher Scientific, USA	-
	B–27 Supplement (50×)	17504001	Gibco/ThermoFisher Scientific, USA	1:50
	L–Glutamine (200 mM)	25030024	ThermoFisher Scientific, USA	1:100
	Fibroblast growth factor 2 (FGF2)	100-18B	PeproTech EC, Ltd., UK	20 ng/mL
	Platelet-derived growth factor (PDGF)	100–13A	PeproTech EC, Ltd., UK	20 ng/mL
	Antibiotic–Antimycotic	15240062	Gibco/ThermoFisher Scientific, USA	1:100
Plating: Treatment:	DBGFP medium without PDGF–AA and FGF2. DBGFP medium without PDGF–AA and FGF2 and one/two/three of the following:			
	PDGF–AA	100–13A	PeproTech EC, Ltd., UK	0–20 ng/mL
	FGF2	100–18B	PeproTech EC, Ltd., UK	0–20 ng/mL
	Bone morphogenetic protein 2 (BMP2)	120–02	PeproTech EC, Ltd., UK	0–100 ng/mL
	BMP4	315–27	PeproTech EC, Ltd., UK	0–100 ng/mL

2.2. Immune Fluorescence Stainings

Immunofluorescent stainings were either performed with 4′,6-diamidin-2-phenylindol (DAPI) and against galactosylceramide (O1), platelet-derived growth factor alpha (PDGFRa) and myelin basic protein (MBP) or with DAPI and against myelin oligodendrocyte glycoprotein (MOG), oligodendrocyte lineage factor 2 (OLIG2), and glial fibrillary acidic protein (GFAP) (Table 2).

Table 2. Dyes and antibodies used for the stainings.

Dye/Antibody	Type/Species	Company	Cat. Nr.	Dilution
4′,6-Diamidin-2-phenylindol (DAPI)	-	Sigma Aldrich		1:15,000
O1	Monoclonal/Mouse	Kindly provided by Prof. M. Schwab, Zürich, CH	D9542-10 mg	1:250
Platelet derived growth factor alpha (PDGFRa)	Polyclonal/Rabbit	Kindly provided by Prof. William B. Stallcup, La Jolla, CA, US		1:4000
Myelin basic protein (MBP)	Monoclonal/Rat	Merck Millipore		1:250
Myelin oligodendrocyte glycoprotein (MOG)	Monoclonal/Mouse	Kindly provided by Prof. R. Reynolds, London, UK	MAB386	1:250
Oligodendrocyte linear factor 2 (OLIG2)	Polyclonal/Rabbit	Merck Millipore	Clone Z12	1:2000
Glial fibrillary acidic protein (GFAP)	Polyclonal/Chicken	Aves Labs	AB9610	1:2000
dk–a–m–488	Monoclonal/Donkey	Jackson ImmunoResearch	AB_2313547	1:700
dk–a–rb–594	Monoclonal/Donkey	Jackson ImmunoResearch		1:700
dk–a–rt–647	Monoclonal/Donkey	Jackson ImmunoResearch	715-545-140 711-585-152	1:700
dk–a–ck–647	Monoclonal/Donkey	Jackson ImmunoResearch	712-605-150 703-605-155	1:700

First, for staining of living cells (O1 staining), the cultured cells were blocked in 10% fetal bovine serum in DMEM/F12 medium at 37 °C for 30 min, and thereafter the cells were incubated for 30 min with O1 supernatant at room temperature. All wells were then washed twice with phosphate buffered saline (PBS), and fixed with 4% paraformaldehyde for 15 min at room temperature. Thereafter, the cells were washed three times with PBS for five minutes and incubated for 1 h with blocking solution (5% bovine serum albumin, 1% normal donkey serum, 0.2% Triton-X100 in PBS). Primary antibodies were diluted in blocking solution and applied overnight at 4 °C (Table 2). The cells were washed three times with PBS (15 min each at room temperature). The secondary antibody (Table 2) was then applied for one hour in PBS with DAPI at room temperature. The cells were washed three times with PBS again and then rinsed twice with tap water and covered with ibidi mounting medium (ibidi GmbH, Gräfelfing, Germany, Cat. No. 50001).

2.3. Image Analysis

384-well plates were imaged using a Nikon Ti2 microscope (Nikon, Tokyo, Japan) fitted with a Prime 95B camera (Teledyne Photometrics, Tucson, AZ, USA). The center of each well was scanned (6 × 6 fields of view) with z-stacks over 27.2 µm with 1.7 µm per slice and a resolution of 0.28 micrometer per pixel. This resulted in images of 2.37 × 2.37 mm or about 51% of the total well area. For the illustrative images of Figure 1, an Olympus IX83 microscope was used. All image analysis was then performed with ImageJ (Version 1.51s, FIJI distribution, NIH, Bethesda, MD, USA). Stacks were first compressed to single images with Z-Project by maximum intensity. For quality control, every DAPI image was reviewed for proper focusing and wells were rescanned if more than 5% of the image was out of focus. All images were then converted to 8-bit images and thresholded at values of 125/255 (DAPI), 160/255 (PDGFRa) or 75/255 (MBP). The percentage of pixels above the threshold was considered as the percent of area positive for the respective marker and used for further analysis.

2.4. Statistical Analysis

All statistical analysis was performed using R (R Development Core Team, Vienna, Austria, 2010). The experiments were performed on three 384-well plates, leading to a total of six wells per treatment condition for DAPI and three wells per treatment condition for all other stainings (Figure 1B). Each plate was normalized to the average measurement per plate, the measurements and treatments were log-transformed, and a pseudo count was added to the treatment values to avoid log of zero. Obvious outliers were removed from the analysis and data from all three plates was pooled for the analysis. Two different linear models were fitted: one with PDGF–AA, FGF2, and BMP2 and all possible interaction terms as independent variables and the other with BMP4 instead of BMP2. p-values smaller than 0.01 were considered to be statistically significant.

2.5. Data Availability

All original greyscale microscopy images used for image analysis are deposited on the BioStudies database of the European Bioinformatics Institute (EMBL-EBI, Hinxton, Cambridge, UK, accession number S-BIAD10, link: https://www.ebi.ac.uk/biostudies/BioImages/studies/S-BIAD10). All original image analysis data may be found in the supplements (Supplementary Data 1).

3. Results

3.1. The Nanofiber Cell Cultures Give Rise to Highly Pure Proliferating and Differentiating Oligodendrocytes

Primary mouse oligodendrocytes were cultivated as spheres and plated on three 384-well nanofiber plates for 14 days with PDGF–AA and FGF2 in combination or independently concentrated at 0, 0.625, 1.25, 2.5, 5, 10, or 20 ng/mL and BMP2 or BMP4 concentrated at 0, 10, 50, or 100 ng/mL (Figure 1a,b). The cells were then stained for PDGFRa, O1, MBP, OLIG2, MOG, or GFAP and scanned with a microscope. A total of 911 of 912 wells were correctly focused and could be used for further analysis.

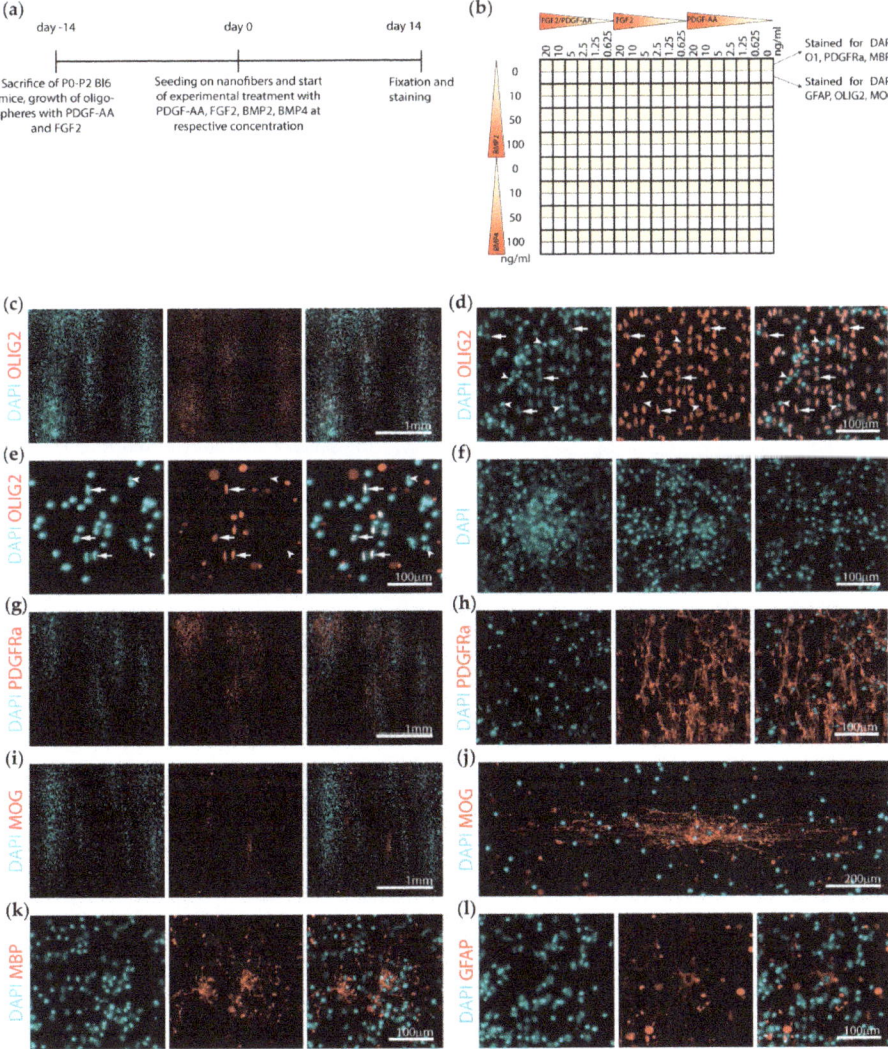

Figure 1. Experimental set up and cell culture characterization. (**a**) Illustration of the experimental timeline showing the sacrifice of the mice, two-week growth of the oligospheres, and plating on the nanofibers. (**b**) Schematic drawing of the experimental set-up of the 384-nanofiber plates. (**c–l**) Representative images of the different stainings. (**c**) The cells proliferated in clusters growing along the nanofibers. (**d**) Most of the nuclei (stained with DAPI) colocalized with the oligodendrocyte lineage marker OLIG2 (arrows, well treated with 20 ng/mL platelet-derived growth factor subunit A dimer (PDGF–AA) and fibroblast growth factor 2 (FGF2)). (**e**) Note, some nuclei showed a dense and sometimes fragmented morphology and were not positive for oligodendrocyte lineage factor 2 (OLIG2) (arrowheads, (**d** and **e**)). This was more pronounced in the wells with less PDGF–AA and FGF2 and more bone morphogenetic protein 2 (BMP2) (well treated with 0.625 ng/mL PDGF–AA and FGF2). (**f**) Dense cell clusters were not eligible for accurate counting of the nuclei. (**g**, **h**, and **k**) PDGFRa and MBP were mainly expressed within the clusters, while (**i** and **j**) the larger MOG positive cells were usually situated in proximity but not within the clusters. (**l**) Possible contamination with glial fibrillary acidic protein (GFAP) positive astrocytes was very rare, with most wells showing no staining for GFAP.

Image inspection revealed clusters of cells oriented along the nanofibers expressing the oligodendrocyte lineage marker OLIG2 (Figure 1c, arrows). Some nuclei did not show colocalization with OLIG2, these nuclei were however most often dense or fragmented, suggestive of cell death (Figure 1d, arrowheads). This phenomenon was more pronounced in the wells treated without or with only relatively low concentrations of PDGF–AA and FGF2 (Figure 1e). Initial efforts to quantify the number of cells by counting the DAPI nuclei demonstrated cell numbers between 3000 (e.g., upon 100 ng/mL BMP2 treatment) and 12,000 cells (e.g., upon 20 ng/mL PDGF-AA and FGF2 treatment) per imaged area to be present, clearly indicating that proliferation and cell death occurred after plating of the initial 10,000 cells per well. However, in particular, the dense cell clusters were not eligible for automated cell counting, and thus a more simplified approach of evaluating the area stained for DAPI was chosen as a surrogate marker for the number of cells present (Figure 1f).

PDGFRa was mostly expressed in the densely populated areas, with only little expression between the clusters (Figure 1c). Expression of the myelin protein MOG was most often detected at the border of the dense cell clusters (Figure 1c), whereas MBP signal was both detected in smaller cells within the clusters and in larger cells between the clusters (Figure 1c). Staining for astrocytes with GFAP revealed only very few astrocytes being present, while most wells showed no GFAP-positive cell (Figure 1c).

3.2. Cell Density Is Strongly Increased by Platelet-Derived Growth Factor Subunit A Dimer (PDGF–AA), While Fibroblast Growth Factor 2 (FGF2) Potentiated the Effect of PDGF–AA and Bone Morphogenetic Protein 2 (BMP2) Overrides the Effects of PDGF–AA

After 14 days in culture, the OPCs have proliferated to cover on average 1.7% of the area with DAPI (range: 0.5–19.3%). We detected a gradient of increased cell density with rising levels of PDGF–AA as detected by the area stained positive for DAPI, independent of the FGF2 concentration (Figure 2a,b). FGF2 in absence of PDGF–AA did not show an effect on cell density, but enhanced cell density with increasing concentrations if a certain amount of PDGF–AA was simultaneously present (Figure 2a,b). The effect of PDGF–AA on cell density and the interaction with FGF2 was statistically significant (Table 3).

Table 3. Significant estimates and p-values derived from the linear model.

	Factor	DAPI	p-Value	Platelet-Derived Growth Factor Alpha (PDGFRa)	p-Value
BMP2 Models	platelet-derived growth factor subunit A dimer (PDGF–AA)	0.26	$<10^{-8}$	0.49	$<10^{-13}$
	Fibroblast growth factor 2 (FGF2)		ns		ns
	PDGF–AA:FGF2	0.19	$<10^{-15}$	0.11	$<10^{-5}$
	Bone morphogenetic protein 2 (BMP2)	0.11	$<10^{-5}$		ns
	PDGF–AA:BMP2	−0.05	$<10^{-7}$	−0.08	$<10^{-6}$
	FGF2:BMP2		ns		ns
	PDGF–AA:FGF2:BMP2	−0.02	$<10^{-8}$	−0.02	$<10^{-3}$
BMP4 Models	PDGF–AA	0.21	$<10^{-5}$	0.41	$<10^{-8}$
	FGF2		ns		ns
	PDGF–AA:FGF2	0.18	$<10^{-15}$	0.11	$<10^{-5}$
	BMP4		ns		ns
	PDGF–AA:BMP4		ns		ns
	FGF2:BMP4		ns		ns
	PDGF–AA:FGF2:BMP4		ns		ns

The colon ":" depicts interaction terms between the factors, ns: not significant.

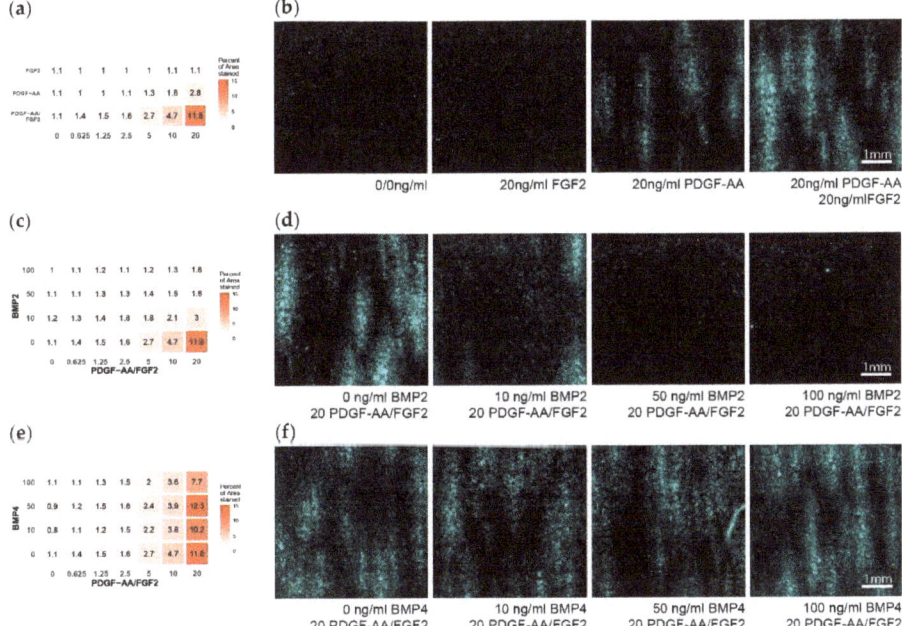

Figure 2. Oligodendrocyte progenitor cells (OPC) cell density after 14 days of multifactor treatment. (**a**) Heatmap showing the percent of area positive for DAPI, as a measure for OPC cell density, dependent on the platelet-derived growth factor subunit A dimer (PDGF–AA) and fibroblast growth factor 2 (FGF2) treatment. (**b**) Representative microscopy images showing the DAPI signal upon different PDGF–AA and FGF2 treatments. (**c**) Heatmap showing the percent of area positive for DAPI dependent on the PDGF–AA/FGF2 and bone morphogenetic protein 2 (BMP2) treatment. (**d**) Representative microscopy images of PDGF–AA and FGF2 concentrated at 20 ng/mL and with BMP2 levels of 0–100 ng/mL. (**e**) Heatmap showing the percent of area positive for DAPI dependent on the PDGF–AA/FGF2 and BMP4 treatment. (**f**) Representative microscopy images of PDGF–AA and FGF2 concentrated at 20 ng/mL and with BMP4 levels of 0–100 ng/mL.

Already, relatively low concentrations of 10 ng/mL of BMP2 over 14 days were able to nullify the cell density effect of PDGF–AA and FGF2, with higher concentrations of BMP2 showing no additional effect. BMP2 showed no effect if PDGF–AA was not present, and the calculated positive main effect of BMP2 from the linear model should not be interpreted due to the detected interactions with PDGF–AA and FGF2 (Figure 2c,d, Table 3). BMP4 showed no effect on cell density for all concentrations tested (Figure 2e,f, Table 3).

3.3. Early Differentiation Is Promoted by Platelet-Derived Growth Factor Subunit A Dimer (PDGF–AA), Enhanced by Fibroblast Growth Factor 2 (FGF2) and Inhibited by Bone Morphogenetic Protein 2 (BMP2)

14 days after seeding the cells have differentiated to cover an average of about 43.3% with PDGFRa signal (range: 28.4–77.8%). A gradient of PDGFRa expression is detected with increasing levels of PDGF–AA independent of the FGF2 concentration (Figure 3a,b). With increasing levels of FGF2, a gradient of PDGFRa signal is only detected if minimal concentrations of PDGF–AA are present. Both the effect of PDGF–AA and the interaction of PDGF–AA and FGF2 reached statistical significance (Table 3).

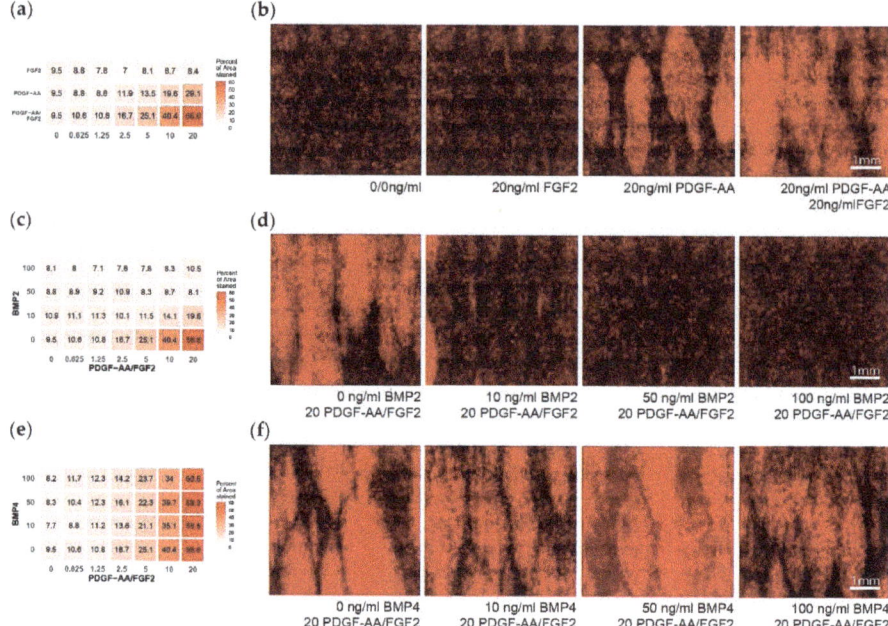

Figure 3. Early oligodendrocyte progenitor cells (OPC) differentiation after 14 days of multifactor treatment. (**a**) Heatmap showing the percent of area positive for platelet-derived growth factor alpha (PDGFRa), as a measure for early OPC differentiation, dependent on the platelet-derived growth factor subunit A dimer (PDGF–AA) and fibroblast growth factor 2 (FGF2) treatment. (**b**) Representative microscopy images showing the PDGFRa expression upon different PDGF–AA and FGF2 treatments. (**c**) Heatmap showing the PDGFRa expression in dependency of the PDGF–AA/FGF2 and bone morphogenetic protein 2 (BMP2) treatment. (**d**) Representative microscopy images of PDGF–AA and FGF2 concentrated at 20 ng/mL and with BMP2 levels of 0–100 ng/mL. (**e**) Heatmap showing the PDGFRa expression in dependency of the PDGF–AA/FGF2 and BMP4 treatment. (**f**) Representative microscopy images of PDGF and FGF2 concentrated at 20 ng/mL and with BMP4 levels of 0–100 ng/mL.

This gradient disappears with increasing levels of BMP2 dose dependent between 0–50 ng/mL with only minimal additional effect of 100 ng/mL BMP2 (Figure 3c,d). While the main effect of BMP2 did not reach significance, the interaction of BMP2 with PDGF–AA and with PDGF–AA and FGF2 reached statistical significance (Table 3). BMP4 did not show any effect on PDGFRa expression, independent of its concentration (Figure 3e,f, Table 3).

3.4. Late Differentiation is Unaffected by Platelet-Derived Growth Factor Subunit A Dimer (PDGF–AA), Fibroblast Growth Factor 2 (FGF2), Bone Morphogenetic Protein 2 (BMP2) and BMP4

The treatments with PDGF–AA, FGF2, BMP2, and BMP4 did not demonstrate statistically significant effects on MBP expression (Figure 4a–e, Table 3). Though BMP2 seemed to inhibit late differentiation with high concentrations, this effect was not linear and did not reach statistical significance (Figure 4c,d). Upon visual investigation, we observed no apparent change in the length, processes, or area of the MBP expressing cells.

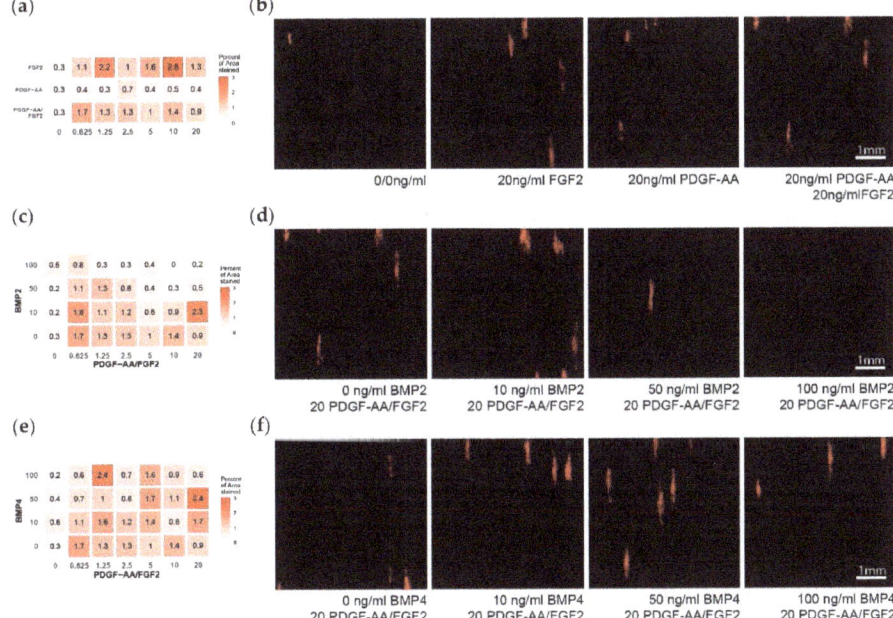

Figure 4. Late oligodendrocyte progenitor cells (OPC) differentiation after 14 days of multifactor treatment. (**a**) Heatmap showing the influence of platelet-derived growth factor subunit A dimer (PDGF–AA) and fibroblast growth factor 2 (FGF2) on late differentiation measured as percent of area positive for myelin basic protein (MBP). (**b**) Representative microscopy images showing the MBP expression. (**c**) Heatmap showing the influence of bone morphogenetic protein 2 (BMP2) on MBP expression. (**d**) Representative microscopy images of PDGF–AA and FGF2 concentrated at 20 ng/mL and with BMP2 levels of 0–100 ng/mL. (**e**) Heatmap showing the influence of BMP4 on MBP expression. (**f**) Representative microscopy images of PDGF–AA and FGF2 concentrated at 20 ng/mL and with BMP4 levels of 0–100 ng/mL.

4. Discussion

Recently, high-throughput screening studies have identified several compounds that promote remyelination [25–28], including clemastine, which is currently being investigated in a phase II clinical trial in optic neuritis (Clinical trials identifier NCT02521311). However, these screens focused on screening individual factors under culture conditions that do not replicate the complex pathologic environment of an MS lesion. To address this question, we elected to build on existing technologies to develop a platform in which we could rapidly screen for multiparametric effects that mimic the lesion microenvironment and its effects on cells of the oligodendrocyte lineage.

We successfully established a cell culture system in which highly purified oligodendrocytes myelinate nanofibers in 384-well nanofiber plates to reliably and efficiently quantify the effects of multi-factor treatments on oligodendrocyte development and myelination. We implemented a standardized operating procedure for cell culturing, imaging, and image analysis that optimizes reproducibility and mapped combinatory, concentration-dependent effects of PDGF–AA, FGF2, BMP2 and BMP4 on oligodendrocytes and myelination.

PDGF–AA is known to be essential for oligodendrocyte generation and survival [29] and differentiation [30]. We detected a positive effect of PDGF–AA on the number of cells as reported before [31–33]. We also detected a positive effect of PDGF–AA on early OPC differentiation into PDGFRa positive cells. This simultaneous positive effect on differentiation is controversial, however, as a factor promoting proliferation effectively keeps a cell in the cell-cycle, while promoting differentiation requires the cell to exit the cell-cycle. Cell culture experiments have demonstrated that proliferation may cause mechanical restraint, which then induces OPC differentiation indirectly [34]. We interpret the expression of PDGFRa mainly within the more densely populated clusters in this manner. In our cell culture system, FGF2 showed no effect on cell density and early OPC differentiation in absence of PDGF–AA. However, FGF2 showed an increasing effect on both cell density and differentiation with rising levels of PDGF–AA being present, thus enhancing the effect of PDGF–AA. As suggested by our own observations, FGF2 has been shown to not be essential for OPC development, in contrast to PDGF–AA [30]. FGF2 is further known to stimulate OPC proliferation and migration and to increase oligodendrocyte process elongation [35,36], but also to have a negative effect on differentiation [30] and myelination [37], by keeping the OPC in the cell-cycle.

BMPs were reported to inhibit OPC proliferation, oligodendrocyte maturation, and myelin protein expression and to push OPCs into the astrocyte lineage, if thyroid hormone is present as well [38–41]. In line with these previous data, our results demonstrate a strong reduction of OPC cell density and differentiation caused by BMP2. We further demonstrated that BMP2 effectively overwrites the effect of PDGF–AA and FGF2 already at low concentrations, irrespective of the concentrations of PDGF–AA and FGF2. As only very few GFAP expressing cells developed within our culture systems, we did not expect and did not detect an increase in astrocytes when adding BMP2. In our study, BMP4 had no effect on cell density and differentiation. This may be explained by the fact that BMP4 only acts in a certain time frame of OPC development, mainly during the GalC positive phase. In our culture system, this phase may have already been passed during the two weeks the cells were kept as oligospheres prior to seeding on the nanofibers.

As our system was intended to model the signaling environment of a demyelinated lesion by expressing factors known to be expressed there, we did not expect to detect many cells showing late differentiation. Accordingly, we detected few MBP positive cells, statistically irrespective of the treatment. This may be suggestive of a fate determination prior to treatment beginning, possibly already within the brain or during the oligosphere stage. These cells differentiated remarkably despite high BMP2 levels, which otherwise efficiently inhibit both proliferation and early differentiation. Our treatments however are not optimized for assessing late differentiation and myelination, as this would require for example a withdrawal of PDGF–AA and FGF2, which keep the OPCs within proliferation.

Even though the dysregulation of the factors tested here has been demonstrated on RNA and protein level in MS lesions, there is currently no data available concerning the local concentrations of these factors. While the concentrations of PDGF–AA and FGF2 have been measured in the cerebrospinal fluid [42–44], BMP levels have so far only been determined within blood serum samples of MS patients [45]. However, this data cannot easily be extrapolated to the local situation within lesions, where concentrations could potentially reach much higher levels.

We may conclude that our cell culture system is suitable for studying more complex effects of multifactor treatments on oligodendrocytes. This approach enables to better model the signaling environment of MS lesions, where the decision is made, whether lesions are chronically demyelinated or remyelination and thus functional recovery may occur. To this end, any improved mapping and quantification of the factors present in vivo in MS lesions may improve the in vitro model system. This model may then serve as an alternative platform to screen novel therapeutic approaches in the ongoing research on remyelination therapy.

Supplementary Materials: The following are available online at http://www.mdpi.com/2073-4409/8/11/1422/s1, Data 1: Image analysis data.

Author Contributions: Conceptualization, T.Z., C.L. and N.S.-W.; Methodology, T.Z.; Software, L.S.E.; Validation, L.S.E.; Formal Analysis, L.S.E.; Investigation, L.S.E. and T.Z.; Resources, T.Z. and N.S.W.; Data Curation, L.S.E.; Writing Original Draft Preparation, L.S.E., T.Z. and N.S.-W.; Writing Review & Editing, L.S.E., T.Z., A.H., C.L. and N.S.W.; Visualization, L.S.E.; Supervision, N.S.-W.; Project Administration, N.S.-W.; Funding Acquisition, N.S.-W.

Funding: This study was supported by the Schweizerischer Nationalfonds zur Förderung der Wissenschaftlichen Forschung (31003A_159528) and by the Freiwillige Akademische Gesellschaft (FAG) both to N.S.W., by the Schweizerischer Nationalfonds zur Förderung der Wissenschaftlichen Forschung (323530_171139) to L.E. and the United Kingdom Multiple Sclerosis Society (C.L).

Acknowledgments: Jonah Chan for helpful discussions. Robert Ivanek for statistical consulting.

Conflicts of Interest: The authors declare no conflict of interest.

References

1. Kuhlmann, T.; Lingfeld, G.; Bitsch, A.; Schuchardt, J.; Bruck, W. Acute axonal damage in multiple sclerosis is most extensive in early disease stages and decreases over time. *Brain* **2002**, *125*, 2202–2212. [CrossRef] [PubMed]
2. Trapp, B.D.; Peterson, J.; Ransohoff, R.M.; Rudick, R.; Mork, S.; Bo, L. Axonal transection in the lesions of multiple sclerosis. *N. Engl. J. Med.* **1998**, *338*, 278–285. [CrossRef] [PubMed]
3. Franklin, R.J. Why does remyelination fail in multiple sclerosis? *Nat. Rev. Neurosci.* **2002**, *3*, 705–714. [CrossRef] [PubMed]
4. Boyd, A.; Zhang, H.; Williams, A. Insufficient OPC migration into demyelinated lesions is a cause of poor remyelination in MS and mouse models. *Acta Neuropathol.* **2013**, *125*, 841–859. [CrossRef] [PubMed]
5. Kuhlmann, T.; Miron, V.; Cui, Q.; Wegner, C.; Antel, J.; Bruck, W. Differentiation block of oligodendroglial progenitor cells as a cause for remyelination failure in chronic multiple sclerosis. *Brain* **2008**, *131*, 1749–1758. [CrossRef] [PubMed]
6. Mason, J.L.; Toews, A.; Hostettler, J.D.; Morell, P.; Suzuki, K.; Goldman, J.E.; Matsushima, G.K. Oligodendrocytes and progenitors become progressively depleted within chronically demyelinated lesions. *Am. J. Pathol.* **2004**, *164*, 1673–1682. [CrossRef]
7. Chang, A.; Tourtellotte, W.W.; Rudick, R.; Trapp, B.D. Premyelinating oligodendrocytes in chronic lesions of multiple sclerosis. *N. Engl. J. Med.* **2002**, *346*, 165–173. [CrossRef] [PubMed]
8. Wolswijk, G. Chronic stage multiple sclerosis lesions contain a relatively quiescent population of oligodendrocyte precursor cells. *J. Neurosci.* **1998**, *18*, 601–609. [CrossRef] [PubMed]
9. Ludwin, S.K. Chronic demyelination inhibits remyelination in the central nervous system. An analysis of contributing factors. *Lab. Investig.* **1980**, *43*, 382–387. [PubMed]
10. Goldschmidt, T.; Antel, J.; Konig, F.B.; Bruck, W.; Kuhlmann, T. Remyelination capacity of the MS brain decreases with disease chronicity. *Neurology* **2009**, *72*, 1914–1921. [CrossRef] [PubMed]
11. Franklin, R.J.; Ffrench-Constant, C. Remyelination in the CNS: From biology to therapy. *Nat. Rev. Neurosci.* **2008**, *9*, 839–855. [CrossRef] [PubMed]
12. Franklin, R.J.; Hinks, G.L. Understanding CNS remyelination: Clues from developmental and regeneration biology. *J. Neurosci. Res.* **1999**, *58*, 207–213. [CrossRef]
13. Kotter, M.R.; Stadelmann, C.; Hartung, H.P. Enhancing remyelination in disease—Can we wrap it up? *Brain* **2011**, *134*, 1882–1900. [CrossRef] [PubMed]
14. Zeis, T.; Howell, O.W.; Reynolds, R.; Schaeren-Wiemers, N. Molecular pathology of Multiple Sclerosis lesions reveals a heterogeneous expression pattern of genes involved in oligodendrogliogenesis. *Exp. Neurol.* **2018**, *305*, 76–88. [CrossRef] [PubMed]
15. Mohan, H.; Friese, A.; Albrecht, S.; Krumbholz, M.; Elliott, C.L.; Arthur, A.; Menon, R.; Farina, C.; Junker, A.; Stadelmann, C.; et al. Transcript profiling of different types of multiple sclerosis lesions yields FGF1 as a promoter of remyelination. *Acta Neuropathol. Commun.* **2014**, *2*, 168. [CrossRef] [PubMed]
16. Mycko, M.P.; Papoian, R.; Boschert, U.; Raine, C.S.; Selmaj, K.W. cDNA microarray analysis in multiple sclerosis lesions: Detection of genes associated with disease activity. *Brain* **2003**, *126*, 1048–1057. [CrossRef] [PubMed]
17. Tajouri, L.; Mellick, A.S.; Ashton, K.J.; Tannenberg, A.E.; Nagra, R.M.; Tourtellotte, W.W.; Griffiths, L.R. Quantitative and qualitative changes in gene expression patterns characterize the activity of plaques in multiple sclerosis. *Brain Research. Mol. Brain Res.* **2003**, *119*, 170–183. [CrossRef] [PubMed]
18. Lee, S.; Leach, M.K.; Redmond, S.A.; Chong, S.Y.; Mellon, S.H.; Tuck, S.J.; Feng, Z.Q.; Corey, J.M.; Chan, J.R. A culture system to study oligodendrocyte myelination processes using engineered nanofibers. *Nat. Methods* **2012**, *9*, 917–922. [CrossRef] [PubMed]

19. Hauser, S.L.; Chan, J.R.; Oksenberg, J.R. Multiple sclerosis: Prospects and promise. *Ann. Neurol.* **2013**, *74*, 317–327. [CrossRef] [PubMed]
20. Scolding, N.; Franklin, R.; Stevens, S.; Heldin, C.H.; Compston, A.; Newcombe, J. Oligodendrocyte progenitors are present in the normal adult human CNS and in the lesions of multiple sclerosis. *Brain* **1998**, *121*, 2221–2228. [CrossRef] [PubMed]
21. Clemente, D.; Ortega, M.C.; Arenzana, F.J.; de Castro, F. FGF-2 and Anosmin-1 are selectively expressed in different types of multiple sclerosis lesions. *J. Neurosci.* **2011**, *31*, 14899–14909. [CrossRef] [PubMed]
22. Costa, C.; Eixarch, H.; Martínez-Sáez, E.; Calvo-Barreiro, L.; Calucho, M.; Castro, Z.; Ortega-Aznar, A.; Ramón y Cajal, S.; Montalban, X.; Espejo, C. Expression of Bone Morphogenetic Proteins in Multiple Sclerosis Lesions. *Am. J. Pathol.* **2019**, *189*, 665–676. [CrossRef] [PubMed]
23. Harnisch, K.; Teuber-Hanselmann, S.; Macha, N.; Mairinger, F.; Fritsche, L.; Soub, D.; Meinl, E.; Junker, A. Myelination in Multiple Sclerosis Lesions Is Associated with Regulation of Bone Morphogenetic Protein 4 and Its Antagonist Noggin. *Int. J. Mol. Sci.* **2019**, *20*, 154. [CrossRef] [PubMed]
24. Pedraza, C.E.; Monk, R.; Lei, J.; Hao, Q.; Macklin, W.B. Production, characterization, and efficient transfection of highly pure oligodendrocyte precursor cultures from mouse embryonic neural progenitors. *Glia* **2008**, *56*, 1339–1352. [CrossRef] [PubMed]
25. Deshmukh, V.A.; Tardif, V.; Lyssiotis, C.A.; Green, C.C.; Kerman, B.; Kim, H.J.; Padmanabhan, K.; Swoboda, J.G.; Ahmad, I.; Kondo, T.; et al. A regenerative approach to the treatment of multiple sclerosis. *Nature* **2013**, *502*, 327–332. [CrossRef] [PubMed]
26. Mei, F.; Fancy, S.P.J.; Shen, Y.A.; Niu, J.; Zhao, C.; Presley, B.; Miao, E.; Lee, S.; Mayoral, S.R.; Redmond, S.A.; et al. Micropillar arrays as a high-throughput screening platform for therapeutics in multiple sclerosis. *Nat. Med.* **2014**, *20*, 954–960. [CrossRef] [PubMed]
27. Mei, F.; Mayoral, S.R.; Nobuta, H.; Wang, F.; Desponts, C.; Lorrain, D.S.; Xiao, L.; Green, A.J.; Rowitch, D.; Whistler, J.; et al. Identification of the Kappa-Opioid Receptor as a Therapeutic Target for Oligodendrocyte Remyelination. *J. Neurosci.* **2016**, *36*, 7925–7935. [CrossRef] [PubMed]
28. Najm, F.J.; Madhavan, M.; Zaremba, A.; Shick, E.; Karl, R.T.; Factor, D.C.; Miller, T.E.; Nevin, Z.S.; Kantor, C.; Sargent, A.; et al. Drug-based modulation of endogenous stem cells promotes functional remyelination in vivo. *Nature* **2015**, *522*, 216–220. [CrossRef] [PubMed]
29. Vana, A.C.; Flint, N.C.; Harwood, N.E.; Le, T.Q.; Fruttiger, M.; Armstrong, R.C. Platelet-derived growth factor promotes repair of chronically demyelinated white matter. *J. Neuropathol. Exp. Neurol.* **2007**, *66*, 975–988. [CrossRef] [PubMed]
30. Murtie, J.C.; Zhou, Y.X.; Le, T.Q.; Vana, A.C.; Armstrong, R.C. PDGF and FGF2 pathways regulate distinct oligodendrocyte lineage responses in experimental demyelination with spontaneous remyelination. *Neurobiol. Dis.* **2005**, *19*, 171–182. [CrossRef] [PubMed]
31. Furusho, M.; Dupree, J.L.; Nave, K.A.; Bansal, R. Fibroblast growth factor receptor signaling in oligodendrocytes regulates myelin sheath thickness. *J. Neurosci.* **2012**, *32*, 6631–6641. [CrossRef] [PubMed]
32. Furusho, M.; Ishii, A.; Bansal, R. Signaling by FGF Receptor 2, Not FGF Receptor 1, Regulates Myelin Thickness through Activation of ERK1/2-MAPK, Which Promotes mTORC1 Activity in an Akt-Independent Manner. *J. Neurosci.* **2017**, *37*, 2931–2946. [CrossRef] [PubMed]
33. McKinnon, R.D.; Matsui, T.; Dubois-Dalcq, M.; Aaronson, S.A. FGF modulates the PDGF-driven pathway of oligodendrocyte development. *Neuron* **1990**, *5*, 603–614. [CrossRef]
34. Rosenberg, S.S.; Kelland, E.E.; Tokar, E.; De la Torre, A.R.; Chan, J.R. The geometric and spatial constraints of the microenvironment induce oligodendrocyte differentiation. *Proc. Natl. Acad. Sci. USA* **2008**, *105*, 14662–14667. [CrossRef] [PubMed]
35. Fortin, D.; Rom, E.; Sun, H.; Yayon, A.; Bansal, R. Distinct fibroblast growth factor (FGF)/FGF receptor signaling pairs initiate diverse cellular responses in the oligodendrocyte lineage. *J. Neurosci.* **2005**, *25*, 7470–7479. [CrossRef] [PubMed]
36. Akiyama, M.; Hasegawa, H.; Hongu, T.; Frohman, M.A.; Harada, A.; Sakagami, H.; Kanaho, Y. Trans-regulation of oligodendrocyte myelination by neurons through small GTPase Arf6-regulated secretion of fibroblast growth factor-2. *Nat. Commun.* **2014**, *5*, 4744. [CrossRef] [PubMed]
37. Wang, Z.; Colognato, H.; Ffrench-Constant, C. Contrasting effects of mitogenic growth factors on myelination in neuron-oligodendrocyte co-cultures. *Glia* **2007**, *55*, 537–545. [CrossRef] [PubMed]

38. See, J.; Zhang, X.; Eraydin, N.; Mun, S.B.; Mamontov, P.; Golden, J.A.; Grinspan, J.B. Oligodendrocyte maturation is inhibited by bone morphogenetic protein. *Mol. Cell Neurosci.* **2004**, *26*, 481–492. [CrossRef] [PubMed]
39. Grinspan, J.B.; Edell, E.; Carpio, D.F.; Beesley, J.S.; Lavy, L.; Pleasure, D.; Golden, J.A. Stage-specific effects of bone morphogenetic proteins on the oligodendrocyte lineage. *J. Neurobiol.* **2000**, *43*, 1–17. [CrossRef]
40. Sabo, J.K.; Aumann, T.D.; Merlo, D.; Kilpatrick, T.J.; Cate, H.S. Remyelination is altered by bone morphogenic protein signaling in demyelinated lesions. *J. Neurosci.* **2011**, *31*, 4504–4510. [CrossRef] [PubMed]
41. Cheng, X.; Wang, Y.; He, Q.; Qiu, M.; Whittemore, S.R.; Cao, Q. Bone morphogenetic protein signaling and olig1/2 interact to regulate the differentiation and maturation of adult oligodendrocyte precursor cells. *Stem Cells* **2007**, *25*, 3204–3214. [CrossRef] [PubMed]
42. Harirchian, M.H.; Tekieh, A.H.; Modabbernia, A.; Aghamollaii, V.; Tafakhori, A.; Ghaffarpour, M.; Sahraian, M.A.; Naji, M.; Yazdankhah, M. Serum and CSF PDGF-AA and FGF-2 in relapsing-remitting multiple sclerosis: A case-control study. *Eur. J. Neurol.* **2012**, *19*, 241–247. [CrossRef] [PubMed]
43. Su, J.J.; Osoegawa, M.; Matsuoka, T.; Minohara, M.; Tanaka, M.; Ishizu, T.; Mihara, F.; Taniwaki, T.; Kira, J. Upregulation of vascular growth factors in multiple sclerosis: Correlation with MRI findings. *J. Neurol. Sci.* **2006**, *243*, 21–30. [CrossRef] [PubMed]
44. Sarchielli, P.; Di Filippo, M.; Ercolani, M.V.; Chiasserini, D.; Mattioni, A.; Bonucci, M.; Tenaglia, S.; Eusebi, P.; Calabresi, P. Fibroblast growth factor-2 levels are elevated in the cerebrospinal fluid of multiple sclerosis patients. *Neurosci. Lett.* **2008**, *435*, 223–228. [CrossRef] [PubMed]
45. Penn, M.; Mausner-Fainberg, K.; Golan, M.; Karni, A. High serum levels of BMP-2 correlate with BMP-4 and BMP-5 levels and induce reduced neuronal phenotype in patients with relapsing-remitting multiple sclerosis. *J. Neuroimmunol.* **2017**, *310*, 120–128. [CrossRef] [PubMed]

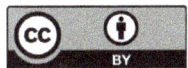

© 2019 by the authors. Licensee MDPI, Basel, Switzerland. This article is an open access article distributed under the terms and conditions of the Creative Commons Attribution (CC BY) license (http://creativecommons.org/licenses/by/4.0/).

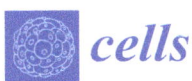

Article

High Speed Ventral Plane Videography as a Convenient Tool to Quantify Motor Deficits during Pre-Clinical Experimental Autoimmune Encephalomyelitis

Jiangshan Zhan [1,2], Vladislav Yakimov [1,2], Sebastian Rühling [1,2], Felix Fischbach [1,2], Elena Nikolova [1,2], Sarah Joost [1], Hannes Kaddatz [1], Theresa Greiner [1], Julia Frenz [1], Carsten Holzmann [1] and Markus Kipp [1,*]

1. Institute of Anatomy, Rostock University Medical Center, 18057 Rostock, Germany; jiangshan.zhan@campus.lmu.de (J.Z.); vladislavvd15@gmail.com (V.Y.); sebastian.ruehling@tum.de (S.R.); felix@famfischbach.de (F.F.); evladimirovanikolova@gmail.com (E.N.); sarah.joost@med.uni-rostock.de (S.J.); hannes.kaddatz@uni-rostock.de (H.K.); theresa.greiner@uni-rostock.de (T.G.); julia.frenz97@gmx.de (J.F.); carsten.holzmann@med.uni-rostock.de (C.H.)
2. Institute of Anatomy II, Faculty of Medicine, LMU Munich, 80336 Munich, Germany
* Correspondence: markus.kipp@med.uni-rostock.de; Tel.: +49-381-494-8401

Received: 23 August 2019; Accepted: 11 November 2019; Published: 14 November 2019

Abstract: Experimental autoimmune encephalomyelitis (EAE) is the most commonly used multiple sclerosis animal model. EAE mice typically develop motor deficits in a caudal-to-rostral pattern when inflammatory lesions have already developed. However, to monitor more subtle behavioral deficits during lesion development (i.e., pre-clinical phase), more sophisticated methods are needed. Here, we investigated whether high speed ventral plane videography can be applied to monitor early motor deficits during 'pre-clinical' EAE. For this purpose, EAE was induced in C57BL/6 mice and gait abnormalities were quantified using the DigiGait™ apparatus. Gait deficits were related to histopathological changes. 10 out of 10 control (100%), and 14 out of 18 (77.8%) pre-clinical EAE mice could be evaluated using DigiGait™. EAE severity was not influenced by DigiGait™-related mice handlings. Most gait parameters recorded from day 6 post-immunization until the end of the experiment were found to be stable in control mice. During the pre-clinical phase, when conventional EAE scorings failed to detect any functional impairment, EAE mice showed an increased *Swing Time*, increased *%Swing Stride*, decreased *%Stance Stride*, decreased *Stance/Swing*, and an increased *Absolute Paw Angle*. In summary, DigiGait™ is more sensitive than conventional scoring approaches to study motor deficits during the EAE pre-clinical phase.

Keywords: DigiGait™; experimental autoimmune encephalomyelitis; multiple sclerosis; gait analysis

1. Introduction

Multiple sclerosis (MS) is an autoimmune, inflammatory, demyelinating disease of the central nervous system (CNS). On the histopathological level, MS lesions are characterized by large inflammatory plaques of white matter demyelination. Such focal inflammatory lesions are associated with oligodendrocyte destruction, reactive gliosis and axonal degeneration. The composition of established inflammatory infiltrates varies between patients and/or lesion stages but commonly includes CD8[+] T-lymphocytes and macrophages. In addition to focal white matter lesions, gray matter demyelination and/or atrophy and diffuse white matter injury are frequently observed [1–3]. While the characteristics of established lesions are well investigated, how such lesions develop is less well understood. On one hand, it is discussed that early during the development of inflammatory MS lesions, autoreactive T- and B-cells invade the brain parenchyma, get reactivated, and promote the development of inflammatory demyelination. Other authors suggest, however, that the recruitment of peripheral immune cells is a secondary phenomenon, triggered by a local, brain intrinsic degenerative event [4,5]. For example, one post-mortem study has shown that early MS lesions are characterized by oligodendrocyte degeneration and microglia activation in the absence of overt peripheral immune cells [6]. Whatever is true, imaging studies clearly demonstrate that subtle CNS pathologies can be observed before symptoms become evident [7–9].

For the development of new therapeutic options in MS, several models are available and can be roughly broken down into the categories of autoimmune and non-autoimmune animal models. Experimental autoimmune encephalomyelitis (EAE) is the most commonly used animal model to study autoimmune-mediated aspects of the disease. In this model, experimental animals (commonly rodents) are immunized with a CNS-related antigen administered in a strong adjuvant, usually complete Freund's adjuvant (CFA). Following immunization, antigens are phagocytized by local professional antigen-presenting cells, transported to local lymph nodes or the spleen, where they trigger the development of encephalitogenic T_{h1}- and T_{h17}-cell immune responses. This finally leads to inflammation within different CNS regions, mainly the spinal cord and the cerebellum [10]. On the behavioral level, this model is characterized by an ascending paralysis that begins in the tail and spreads to involve the hind limbs and, finally, fore limbs. Although different grading systems exist, the disease is usually rated on a scale ranging from grades 0–5. Grade 1 is assigned to mice that have lost tail tonicity, whereas grade 2 is assigned to mice that additionally show hind limb weakness. As the disease progresses, through grade 3 and 4, fore limb motor dysfunction additionally develops.

In MS, especially the early stages of lesion pathophysiology are poorly understood. Several studies were able to demonstrate that discrete histopathological changes occur within the brain parenchyma before acute inflammatory lesions become visible. Such changes include fibrinogen deposition [11], oligodendrocyte injury [6], focal microglia activation [12], and the downregulation of neuronal and oligodendrocyte marker gene expression [13]. In EAE, clinical symptoms are generally applied to mark the onset of disease, because this coincides with autoimmune effector $CD4^+$ T-cell infiltration into the CNS parenchyma [14,15]. However, recent reports show that structural and functional changes take place within CNS tissues before the development of clinically overt symptoms. Such observed changes include, among others, the activation of endothelial cells and astrocytes [16], reductions in myelin gene expression [13], or altered glutamate transmission [17]. Furthermore, in vivo imaging studies nicely demonstrate intraluminal crawling of encephalitogenic T-cells [14] and perivascular clustering of microglia [18] prior to the onset of clinical symptoms. In line with the observation of changes in brain homeostasis prior to the development of overt, inflammatory lesions our group recently demonstrated that toxic damage to the oligodendrocyte-myelin unit not just leads to glia activation but at the same time triggers the recruitment of peripheral immune cells into the CNS in the predisposed host [4,5,19]. Together, these data strongly implicate that subclinical alterations take place in the CNS tissue during the development of EAE that might predispose it to immunopathology.

In recent years, an extensive body of literature has demonstrated benefits of early treatment of MS with disease modifying drugs. Specifically, research has shown that early treatment in relation to disease onset is associated with significantly improved physical and mental outcomes, including lower relapse rates and lower expanded disability status scale (EDSS) scores, both in the short- and long-term [20–23]. A better understanding of the pre-clinical pathological processes would allow the development of early and probably effective therapeutic options. This requires mechanistic studies during the largely invisible pre-clinical disease stage. While novel and sensitive imaging modalities are currently available to visualize pathological changes during pre-symptomatic EAE, appropriate modalities to measure functional deficits are still missing.

In this work, we aimed to investigate whether high speed ventral plane videography is appropriate for the quantification of pre-clinical functional deficits in EAE.

2. Materials and Methods

2.1. Animals

For this study, 10-week-old C57BL/6 female mice (n = 40) were purchased from Janvier Labs, Le Genest-Saint-Isle, France. All experimental procedures were approved by the Review Board for the Care of Animal Subjects of the district government (Regierung Oberbayern; reference number 55.2-154-2532-73-15; Germany). The mice were maintained in a pathogen-free environment with a maximum of five animals per cage and with *ad libitum* food and water. Cages were changed once per week and microbiological monitoring was performed according to the Federation of European Laboratory Animal Science Associations recommendations. Mice were acclimated at the housing conditions for at least one week before EAE induction.

2.2. EAE Induction, Disease Scoring, and Experimental Groups

To induce the formation of encephalitogenic T-cells in peripheral lymphatic tissues, the mice were subcutaneously immunized with an emulsion of myelin oligodendrocyte glycoprotein (MOG_{35-55}) peptide dissolved in complete Freund's adjuvant followed by intraperitoneal injections of pertussis toxin (PTx) in PBS on the day of and the day after immunization (Hooke Laboratories, Inc., Lawrence, USA) as previously published [4]. Disease severity was scored as follows: 1, The entire tail drops over the observer's finger when the mouse is picked up by the base of the tail; 2, the legs are not spread apart but held close together when the mouse is picked up by the base of the tail, and mice exhibit a clearly apparent wobbly gait; 3, the tail is limp and mice show complete paralysis of hind legs (a score of 3.5 is given if the mouse is unable to raise itself when placed on its side); 4, the tail is limp and mice show complete hind leg paralysis and partial front leg paresis, and the mouse is minimally moving around the cage but appears alert and feeding; 5, the mouse is euthanized due to severe paralysis. The parameter *"disease onset"* was defined as the day post immunization when the first clinical deficit (see above) was observed. The parameter *"maximum disease score"* was defined as the highest clinical score, reached by a mouse at any time-point during the experiment. The parameter *"cumulative disease score"* was calculated by adding all clinical scores, registered during the experiment for a single mouse.

The following treatment groups were included: $Control^{DigiGait}$ mice: Non-immunized mice were subjected to gait analyses; EAE^{Only} mice: EAE was induced by MOG_{35-55} immunization + CFA/PTx, but mice were not subjected to gait analyses; $EAE^{DigiGait}$ mice: EAE was induced by MOG_{35-55} immunization + CFA/PTx, and mice were subjected to gait analyses starting at day 6 post immunization; $PTx^{DigiGait}$ mice: Mice were injected with CFA and PTx, and mice were subjected to gait analyses starting at day 6 post immunization.

2.3. High Speed Ventral Plane Videography and Evaluation

Gait parameters were assessed using the DigiGait™ imaging system along with the DigiGait™ 15.0 analysis software (Mouse Specifics, Inc.; Quincy, MA, USA) [24]. The DigiGait™ apparatus consists of a clear plastic treadmill with a high speed under-mounted digital camera (Basler Technologies Inc.) used for imaging paw prints. The treadmill belt was accelerated gradually to 15 cm/s. Images were collected at a rate of 140 frames/s. and stored as audio video interleaved (AVI) files for later blinded analyses. To improve the contrast for automated foot print analysis, the tails of the mice were colored with black dye. The treadmill belt was cleaned with 70% (*v/v*) ethanol between each animal testing. Animals were habituated to the machine one day prior to testing. Data obtained from the training day were not included in the final data evaluation. The image analysis software digitally encoded the individual paw area and position relative to the tread-belt. Each paw of the animal was treated as a unique signature so that later analyses of foot movements could be performed on separate limbs. Following this strategy, the DigiGait™ analysis software computes 39 gait parameters for the fore limbs and 43 for the hind limbs of each animal. The minimal duration of each video sequence required for subsequent foot-print analyses was 5 s. Runs where mice could not run at 15 cm/s for a minimum of 5 s were excluded from subsequent analyses. This number of strides has been validated as being sufficient to analyze treadmill walking behavior in mice [25]. Figure 1 illustrates the principal setup of the performed gait analyses.

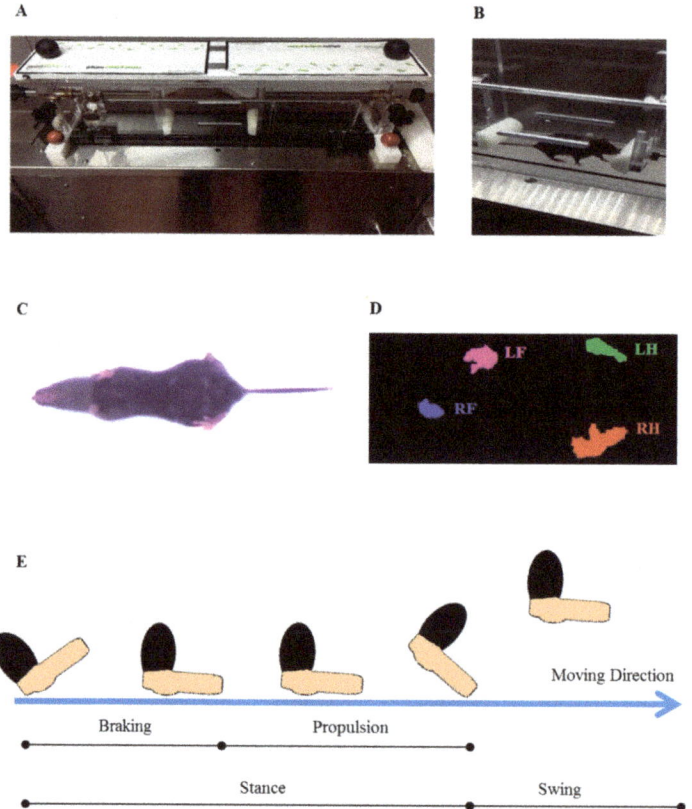

Figure 1. High speed ventral plane videography using the DigiGait™ setup. (**A**) Setup of the DigiGait™ imaging system. (**B**) DigiGait™ setup with a mouse in the running chamber during ventral plane videography recordings. (**C**) Representative image of a mouse during ventral plane videography recordings. (**D**) Representative image of the position of the single paws extracted from the ventral plane videography recordings by the provided analysis tool. (**E**) A graphical depiction of various aspects of a single mouse stride. Each stride can be subdivided into a stance and swing part. The stance part can be further subdivided into a braking and propulsion phase. LF: Left Fore; LH: Left Hind; RF: Right Fore; RH: Right Hind.

To analyze gait abnormalities during the pre-clinical disease stage, we first quantified fore limb and hind limb gait patterns in five control and 10 EAE-induced mice. This first group is referred to as Cohort#1. To verify results of this first experiment, hind limb gait patterns were analyzed in another cohort of five control and 10 EAE-induced mice, referred to as Cohort#2. Both cohorts were finally evaluated by a second evaluator blinded to the treatment groups (i.e., Evaluator 2).

2.4. Rotarod Analysis

To determine balance and motor coordination in control (Control^{Rotarod}; n = 10) and EAE (EAE^{Rotarod}; n = 8) mice, an accelerod system (TSE Systems, Bad Homburg, Germany) for small rodents was used (TSE Systems, Bad Homburg, Germany) as previously published by our group [26]. The apparatus consists of a base platform and a rotating rod (30 mm diameter, 114 mm width) with a non-skid surface. Each experimental mouse was subjected to three training sessions at a constant rotation speed of 5 rpm (rounds per min) for 2 min. These training sessions were conducted from day 3 to day 5 post immunization. Data obtained from the training sessions were not included in the data evaluation. During the testing session, an accelerating modus was used, which began at 4 rpm and accelerated to 40 rpm over a period of 300 s (i.e., 5 min). Two trials per test day were carried out, with a 60 min rest in between each trial. For each trial and each animal, latency, maximum speed, and walking distance before falling off were automatically recorded. The testing sessions were repeated from day 6 to day 13 post immunization. Only data obtained during pre-clinical disease stages were included for the final data evaluation.

2.5. Tissue Preparation and Histological Evaluation

For (immuno-) histological studies, mice were deeply anaesthetized with ketamine (100 mg·kg^{-1} i.p.) and xylazine (10 mg·kg^{-1} i.p.), and transcardially perfused with ice-cold phosphate-buffered saline (PBS) followed by a 3.7% formaldehyde solution (pH = 7.4). Tissues were postfixed overnight in a 3.7% formaldehyde solution, dissected, and embedded in paraffin. 5 μm thick sections were prepared using a slide microtome, dried at ambient temperature for at least 3 h, and subsequently dried overnight at 48 °C before starting the different staining procedures. For immunohistochemistry, sections were rehydrated and, if necessary, antigens were unmasked by heating in a Tris/EDTA (pH 9.0) buffer. After washing in PBS, sections were blocked in blocking solution (serum of the species in which the secondary antibody was produced) for 1 h. Then, sections were incubated overnight (4 °C) with primary antibodies diluted in blocking solution. The next day, slides were incubated in 0.3% hydrogen peroxide/PBS for 1 h and then incubated with biotinylated secondary antibodies for 1 h followed by peroxidase-coupled avidin-biotin complex (ABC kit; Vector Laboratories, Peterborough, UK). Sections were finally exposed to 3,3′-diaminobenzidine (DAKO, Santa Clara, CA, USA) as a peroxidase substrate. To visualize cell nuclei, sections were briefly stained with hematoxylin solution if appropriate. Negative control sections without primary antibodies were processed in parallel to ensure specificity of the staining. For microglia labelling anti-ionized calcium-binding adapter molecule 1 antibodies ([IBA1] 1:5000; Wako; #019-19741) were combined with anti-rabbit secondary antibodies (1:200; Vector; #BA-1000). For lymphocyte labelling, anti-CD3 antibodies ([CD3] 1:500; Abcam; ab11089) were combined with anti-rat secondary antibodies (1:200; Vector; #BA 9400). Luxol fast blue (LFB)/periodic acid-Schiff (PAS) stains were performed following standard protocols. Stained and processed sections were digitalized using a Leica DM6 B automated microscope (Leica Microsystems CMS GmbH, Wetzlar, Germany) equipped with a DMC6200 camera.

To analyse the extent of inflammatory demyelination in the spinal cord among Control^{DigiGait}, EAE^{Only}, and EAE^{DigiGait} mice, the entire white matter was outlined in the digitalized images of LFB/PAS stained sections, and the areas of infiltrated white matter were measured using the open source program ImageJ 1.50. The measurements were conducted by one evaluator (J.Z.), blinded to the treatment groups. The areas of infiltrated white matter were then divided by the entire white matter area of the respective spinal cord section, and the result is given as relative infiltrated white matter area (in %). Representative images are shown in Figure 2C.

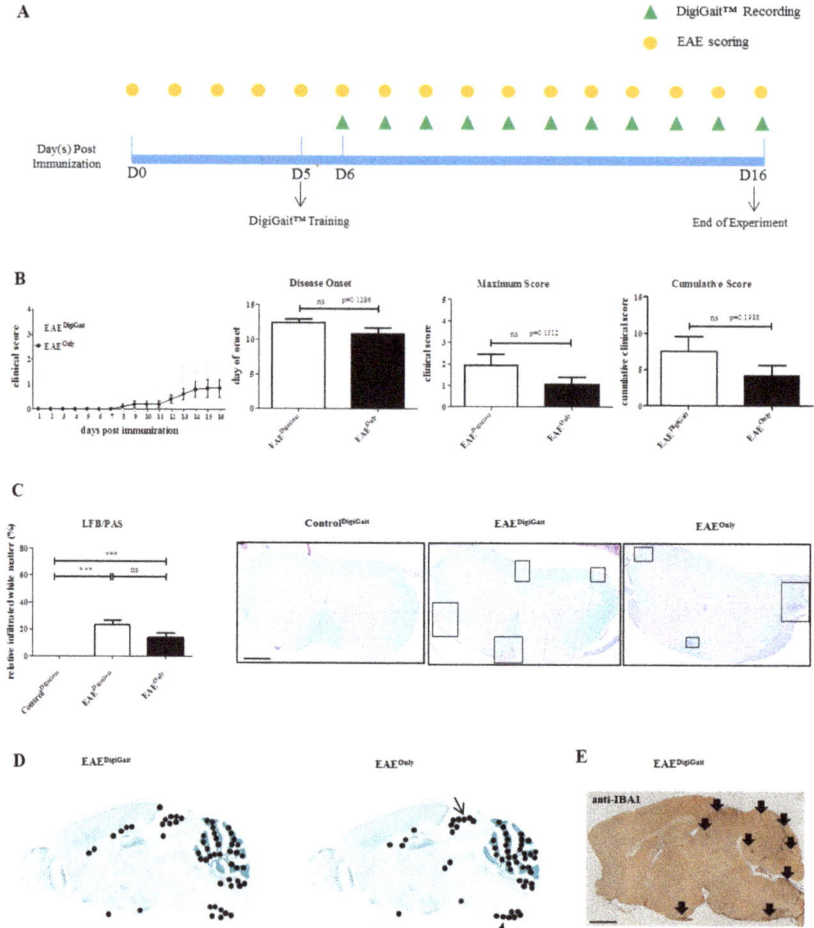

Figure 2. Manipulation during DigiGait™ recordings does not ameliorate EAE severity. (**A**) Schematic depiction of the experimental setup. D = days post immunization. The yellow circles indicate time points when EAE scoring was performed. The green triangles indicate time points when DigiGait™-measurements were performed. Note that at day 5 post immunization (D5), one DigiGait™ training session was conducted. (**B**) Clinical course and evaluation of the disease parameters *disease onset*, *maximum score*, and *cumulative score* in EAE^{DigiGait} (n = 10) and EAE^{Only} (n = 10) mice. Note that 8 EAE^{DigiGait} and 6 EAE^{Only} mice, which developed clinical disease, were included to calculate the parameter *disease onset*. Data from all mice were included to calculate the parameters *maximum score* and *cumulative score*. Statistical comparison was done using an unpaired t-test. (**C**) Extent of inflammatory demyelination among Control^{DigiGait}, EAE^{DigiGait}, and EAE^{Only} mice evaluated in LFB/PAS stained sections (n = 72 sections). Black boxes highlight the inflammatory foci. Statistical comparison was done using a one-way analysis of variance with the obtained *p*-values corrected for multiple testing using the Dunnett's post hoc test. (**D**) Cumulative map of the spatial distribution of microgliosis in the CNS of EAE^{DigiGait} and EAE^{Only} mice, visualized by anti-IBA1 stains. Twenty sections from 10 individual animals were included per group. Each black dot shows the position of a focal IBA1$^+$ lesion which was identified by both evaluators (J.Z. and H.K.). (**E**) Representative anti-IBA1 stain demonstrating IBA1$^+$ lesions in an EAE^{DigiGait} mouse. Scale bar (**C**) = 300 μm; Scale bar (**E**) = 1 mm. EAE: Experimental Autoimmune Encephalomyelitis; LFB/PAS: Luxol fast blue/periodic acid-Schiff; CNS: Central Nervous System; IBA1: ionized calcium-binding adapter molecule 1. *** $p \leq 0.001$, ns = not significant.

To analyse the spatial distribution of microgliosis in mid-sagittal brain sections from EAE^{Only} and EAE^{DigiGait} mice, sections were stained with anti-IBA1 antibodies and microgliosis sites were highlighted in a brain-template adopted from the Allen Mouse Brain Atlas [27]. Each black dot represents a single lesion per individual mouse (Figure 2D). These analyses were conducted by two evaluators blinded to the treatment groups (J.Z. and H.K.).

2.6. Statistical Analyses

All data are given as the arithmetic means ± SEM. Differences between groups were statistically tested using the software package GraphPad Prism 5 (GraphPad Software Inc., San Diego, CA, USA). The D'Agostino and Pearson test was applied to test for Gaussian distribution of the data. The definite statistical procedure applied for the different analyses is provided in the figure legends. p-value ≤ 0.05 were considered statistically significant. The following symbols are used to indicate the level of significance: * $p ≤ 0.05$, ** $p ≤ 0.01$, *** $p ≤ 0.001$, ns = not significant.

3. Results

3.1. Manipulation of DigiGait™ Does Not Decrease EAE Severity

Previous studies have shown that stress might impact on EAE disease development [28]. Since the handling of the mice during DigiGait™ recordings might lead to additional stress, in a first step we systematically compared EAE severity in MOG$_{35-55}$-induced EAE mice which were subjected to DigiGait™ (n = 10; EAE^{DigiGait}) recordings or not (n = 10; EAE^{Only}). After immunization, the mice were evaluated daily for the occurrence and severity of clinical symptoms based on conventional evaluation protocols (see materials and methods section). The gait patterns were recorded daily starting six days post immunization until the mice reached an EAE score of ≥ 2 (equals hind limb paresis), or until day 16 post immunization (i.e., end of the experiment). A schematic depiction of the experimental setup is shown in Figure 2A.

As demonstrated in Figure 2B, both, EAE^{Only} and EAE^{DigiGait} mice, exhibited motor behavioral deficits which are typical for MOG$_{35-55}$-induced EAE in C57BL/6 mice, starting with a limp tail and progressing towards hind limb paralysis. In the EAE^{Only} group, 6 out of 10 and in the EAE^{DigiGait} group 8 out of 10 mice developed clinical deficits, respectively. Although the clinical symptoms in EAE^{DigiGait} mice tended to be more severe compared to EAE^{Only} mice, no significant differences were observed for the parameters *time of disease onset* (EAE^{DigiGait}, 12.38 ± 0.5650 days versus EAE^{Only}, 10.83 ± 0.7923 days; p = 0.1286, just including mice which developed clinical disease), *maximum disease score* (EAE^{DigiGait}, 1.950 ± 0.4913 days versus EAE^{Only}, 1.050 ± 0.3452; p = 0.1512), and *cumulative disease score* (EAE^{DigiGait}, 7.500 ± 2.053 days versus EAE^{Only}, 4.200 ± 1.379 days; p = 0.1988) (Figure 2B). Next, we analyzed the extent of inflammatory infiltrates in EAE^{DigiGait} and EAE^{Only} mice to correlate functional deficits with histopathological changes. For this purpose, three spinal cord sections (cervical to lumbar level) were collected in a random fashion for each mouse and the inflamed white matter area in relation to the entire spinal cord white matter area was quantified in LFB/PAS stained sections.

As demonstrated in Figure 2C, no significant difference was observed in the extent of inflammatory demyelination between EAE^{DigiGait} and EAE^{Only} mice (EAE^{DigiGait}, 23.28% ± 3.549% versus EAE^{Only}, 13.99% ± 3.205%). Spearman's correlation analysis, including data from both experimental groups, revealed a highly significant correlation between spinal cord white matter inflammation and the extent of clinical deficits (r = 0.7221; r^2 = 0,52; 95% confidence interval = 0.59 to 0.82; p-value (two-tailed) ≤ 0.0001). Furthermore, we analyzed the spatial distribution of microgliosis in the brains of EAE^{DigiGait} and EAE^{Only} mice. As demonstrated in Figure 2D,E, focal microgliosis was found in diverse brain regions such as the cerebellum, dorsal midbrain (arrow in Figure 2D), ventral medulla oblongata around the inferior olivary complex (arrowhead in Figure 2D), and to some extent around the third ventricle. In summary, both cohorts demonstrate widespread CNS inflammation with no quantitative differences in the extent of CNS lesion formation.

Beyond, we analyzed the densities of CD3$^+$ lymphocytes in the spinal cord dorsal column and the white matter of the cerebellum. As demonstrated in Figure 3, lymphocyte densities were low in Control^{DigiGait}, but high in EAE^{DigiGait} and EAE^{Only} mice (Spinal cord dorsal column, Control^{DigiGait} 10.87 ± 4.180 cells/mm^2, versus EAE^{DigiGait}, 134.5 ± 19.20 cells/mm^2 versus EAE^{Only}, 129.9 ± 21.00 cells/mm^2: Cerebellum white matter, Control^{DigiGait} 1.367 ± 0.7197 cells/mm^2, versus EAE^{DigiGait}, 292.9 ± 56.61 cells/mm^2 versus EAE^{Only}, 225.9 ± 65.31 cells/mm^2). Of note, no significant differences were observed between EAE^{DigiGait} and EAE^{Only} mice.

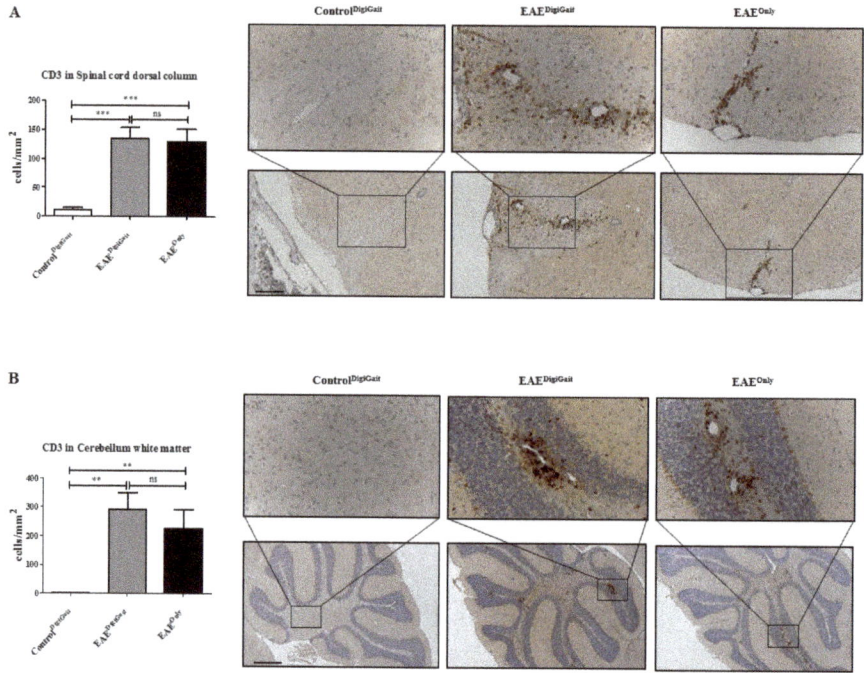

Figure 3. Lymphocyte densities in the spinal cord and cerebellar white matter. (**A**) Numbers of CD3$^+$ lymphocytes in the dorsal column of the spinal cord (n = 75 sections) in Control^{DigiGait}, EAE^{DigiGait}, and EAE^{Only} mice. (**B**) Numbers of CD3$^+$ lymphocytes in the white matter of the cerebellum (n = 25 sections) in Control^{DigiGait}, EAE^{DigiGait}, and EAE^{Only} mice. Statistical comparison was done using a one-way analysis of variance with the obtained p-values corrected for multiple testing using the Dunnett's post hoc test. Note that no significant difference has been observed between EAE^{DigiGait} and EAE^{Only} mice. Scale bar (**A**) = 150 μm; Scale bar (**B**) = 300 μm. ** $p \leq 0.01$, *** $p \leq 0.001$, ns = not significant.

3.2. Most Gait Parameters Are Stable in Control Mice

Next, we investigated the reliability of the gait analysis procedure. To this end, gait analyses were conducted in control mice (n = 10, two separate experiments), and the coefficient of variation (CV), which is defined as the ratio of the standard deviation to the mean (SD/mean), was calculated. The term "high variability parameters" was defined as gait parameters which had a CV of higher than 30% [29]. As described in the materials and method section of this manuscript, the DigiGait™ computes 39 gait parameters for the fore limbs and 43 for the hind limbs, respectively. As listed in Table 1, 10 out of 39 (25.6%) fore limb, and 13 out of 43 (30.2%) hind limb parameters showed a high variability in control mice. This, on the one hand, indicates that not all of the gait parameters evaluated by the DigiGait™ software are adequate for the detection of a pathological gate, at least in mice at the applied experimental settings. However, a significant proportion of gait parameters (i.e., 30) can reliably be measured using the DigiGait™ apparatus.

Table 1. High variability parameters in control mice. List of gait parameters which were found to be highly variable in control animals. High variability parameters were defined as gait metrics which show a coefficient of variation (CV) of more than 30% in control mice [29]. For more information, see the materials and methods section of this manuscript.

	Parameters with High Variability
Fore Limbs (10 out of 39 parameters) 25.6%	Absolute Paw Angle (Sum) Stride Width Variability Step Angle Variability Stance Width CV Step Angle CV Paw Area Variability at Peak Stance (Average) Overlap Distance (Average) Paw Placement Positioning (Average) Paw Angle (Left fore limb) Paw Angle (Right fore limb)
Hind Limbs (13 out of 43 parameters) 30.2%	Stride Length Variability (Average) Stride Width Variability Stride Length CV (Average) Stance Width CV Step Angle CV Paw Area Variability at Peak Stance (Average) Paw Placement Positioning (Average) Tau-Propulsion (Average) Overlap Distance (Average) Ataxia Coefficient (Average) Paw Angle (Left hind limb) Paw Angle (Right hind limb) Paw Drag (Average)

3.3. Mice Show Gait Abnormalities in Hind Limbs during the EAE Pre-Clinical Phase

In a next step, we asked whether gait abnormalities can be quantified during the pre-clinical EAE phase. For this purpose, we systematically compared changes of the gait parameters in control (referred to as Control^{DigiGait}; n = 10) and MOG$_{35-55}$-immunized (referred to as EAE^{DigiGait}; n = 18) mice. As it has been shown that the running speed can influence gait parameters in rodents [30], we used a constant speed of 15 cm/s.

As demonstrated in Figure 4, 18 out of 20 immunized animals developed clinical EAE. EAE was severe in some animals (#2 and #9 with a score of five) but moderate in others (for example, #6 with a transient score of one). MOG$_{35-55}$ immunization severely influenced the success rate of gait analysis recordings. Just 3 out of 18 animals could be daily evaluated until the day of disease onset (i.e., mice #7, #17, and #18), whereas 6 out of 18 animals could be daily evaluated until the day BEFORE disease onset (#3, #11, and #12, additionally to the mice #7, #17, #18). Four animals could not be evaluated at any time point after MOG$_{35-55}$ immunization (#4, #5, #9, and #14).

Mouse Number	Treatment	d6	d7	d8	d9	d10	d11	d12	d13	d14	d15	d16
#1	EAE^{DigiGait}	0	0	0	0	0	0	0	0	0	1	1.5
#2		0	0	0	0	0	2	2.5	2.5	2.5	4	5
#3		0	0	0	0	0	1	1	3	3	3	3
#4		0	0	0	0	1	1	2	2	2.5	2.5	2.5
#5		0	0	0	0	0	0	0	2	3	2.5	2.5
#6		0	0	0	0	0	0	0	1	1	1	0
#7		0	0	0	0	0	0	0	1	1	1	1
#8		0	0	0	0	0	0	0	2	2.5	2.5	2.5
#9		0	0	2.5	3	3	2.5	4	5	5	5	
#10		0	0	0	0	0	0	2.5	2.5	2.5	3	
#11		0	0	0	0	0	0	2	2.5	3	3	
#12		0	0	0	2.5	3	2.5	2.5	2.5	2.5	1.5	
#13		0	0	0	0	0.5	1.5	2.5	2.5	2.5	2.5	
#14		0	0	2.5	3	3	2.5	2.5	2.5	2.5		
#15		0	0	0	0	0	0	0	0	2.5	2.5	
#16		0	0	0	0	1	1.5	1.5	2.5	2.5	2.5	
#17		0	0	0	0	0	0	0	1.5	2	2.5	
#18		0	0	0	0	0	0	1.5	3	3	3	
#19	PTx^{DigiGait}	0	0	0	0	0	0	0	0	0	0	
#20		0	0	0	0	0	0	0	0	0	0	
#21		0	0	0	0	0	0	0	0	0	0	
#22		0	0	0	0	0	0	0	0	0	0	
#23		0	0	0	0	0	0	0	0	0	0	
#24		0	0	0	0	0	0	0	0	0	0	
#25		0	0	0	0	0	0	0	0	0	0	
#26		0	0	0	0	0	0	0	0	0	0	
#27		0	0	0	0	0	0	0	0	0	0	
#28		0	0	0	0	0.5	0	0	0	0		
#29	Control^{DigiGait}	0	0	0	0	0	0	0	0	0	0	0
#30		0	0	0	0	0	0	0	0	0	0	0
#31		0	0	0	0	0	0	0	0	0	0	0
#32		0	0	0	0	0	0	0	0	0	0	0
#33		0	0	0	0	0	0	0	0	0	0	0
#34		0	0	0	0	0	0	0	0	0	0	
#35		0	0	0	0	0	0	0	0	0	0	
#36		0	0	0	0	0	0	0	0	0	0	
#37		0	0	0	0	0	0	0	0	0	0	
#38		0	0	0	0	0	0	0	0	0	0	

Pattern	Illustration	Control^{DigiGait} (n=10)	PTx^{DigiGait} (n=10)	EAE^{DigiGait} (n=18)
	Time points included for data analyses	105	66	55
	Completed DigiGait assessments at 15cm/s	105	69	62
	Failed DigiGait assessments at 15cm/s	0	31	59
	Completed Ratio (%)	100	69	51

Figure 4. Summary of gait analyses experiments. Days with successfully conducted DigiGait^{TM} recordings are highlighted in green, whereas days on which no DigiGait^{TM} recordings could be performed are highlighted in red. Numbers in the boxes indicate the level of motor behavior deficits evaluated by classical EAE scoring. Yellow crosses indicate time points included for data analyses.

As outlined in the materials and method section, gait analyses were initiated at day 6 post immunization and continued daily until the animals (i) either reached a score of ≥ 2, (ii) were not able to run on the treadmill at the given velocity (i.e., 15 cm/s), or (iii) until day 16 post immunization. Following this strategy and pooling the data from two independent experiments, 105 gait analyses were performed in control animals for the different time points with a success rate of 100%. 121 gait analyses were performed in MOG_{35-55}-immunized mice with a success rate of 51% (equals 62 completed gait analyses). These results already suggest that although conventional EAE scoring protocols fail to detect overt changes (i.e., paralysis of the tail), the motor performance is already impaired at this 'pre-clinical' disease stage.

Blinded evaluations of the high speed ventral plane videography recordings were performed in two separate cohorts of animals, referred to as cohort#1 (five control animals and eight EAE animals) and cohort#2 (five control animals and 10 EAE animals). Only data obtained during the pre-clinical disease stages were included. In a first step, fore limb and hind limb gait parameters were evaluated in the cohort#1 mice and statistically compared. As one would expect in a model of ascending paralysis [31,32], more gait parameters were altered in the hind limbs (n = 15) compared to the fore limbs (n = 9) during the pre-clinical disease stage. As demonstrated in Table 2, 15 distinct hind limb gait metrics were found to be increased or decreased in $EAE^{DigiGait}$ compared to $Control^{DigiGait}$ mice during the pre-clinical disease stage. To verify these findings, the gait parameters which were found to be significantly different in the cohort#1 mice were re-evaluated in our cohort#2 mice. For the fore limb parameters, none of the 9 parameters were verified in the cohort#2 mice. In contrast, from the 15 gait parameters found to be different in the hind limbs of cohort#1 mice, 7 were verified in the second cohort. These were the gait metrics *Swing Time (Average), %Swing Stride (Average), %Stance Stride (Average), Stance/Swing (Average), Paw Angle-Left Hind, Paw Angle-Right Hind,* and *Absolute Paw Angle (Sum)*.

As demonstrated in the materials and methods section, the gait signals provided by the software requires some manual, thus subjective, adjustments. To verify that our results are indeed valid, another independent evaluator performed the analyses of cohort#1 and cohort#2 video sequences in a blinded manner. As demonstrated in Table 2, all 7 gait parameters were approved by the second evaluator.

Next, we were interested whether gait abnormalities during pre-clinical EAE can as well be detected using the Rotarod test which is widely used to evaluate the motor coordination of rodents [33,34]. To this end, performance in the rotarod test was compared between 10 control ($Control^{Rotarod}$) mice and 8 pre-clinical EAE mice ($EAE^{Rotarod}$). As demonstrated in Figure 5, $EAE^{Rotarod}$ mice showed comparable values in the Rotarod parameters *latency* ($EAE^{Rotarod}$, 212.7 ± 8.617 s versus $Control^{Rotarod}$, 195.7 ± 7.033 s; $p = 0.1106$), *maximum speed* ($EAE^{Rotarod}$, 29.39 ± 1.036 rpm. versus $Control^{Rotarod}$, 27.41 ± 0.8427 rpm.; $p = 0.1367$), and *walking distance* ($EAE^{Rotarod}$, 5.935 ± 0.3887 m versus $Control^{Rotarod}$, 5.239 ± 0.3128 m; $p = 0.1169$) when compared with $Control^{Rotarod}$ mice.

Table 2. Gait abnormalities during pre-clinical EAE. Summary of gait parameters found to be altered during pre-clinical EAE. Two independent experiments were performed, referred to as Cohort#1 and Cohort#2. Gait parameters were evaluated by two independent observers, referred to as Evaluator 1 and Evaluator 2. Arrows indicate whether gait metrics were increased or decreased during the pre-clinical EAE phase. During pre-clinical EAE, 9 fore limb gait parameters were found to be different in Cohort#1 mice, but not in Cohort#2 mice (indicated by ns = not significant). In contrast, 15 hind limb gait parameters were found to be different in Cohort#1 mice, and 7 of these were found to be as well different in the Cohort#2 mice (indicated by the respective p-value). All of these 7 parameters were verified by the Evaluator 2 (last column). The D'Agostino and Pearson test was applied to test for normal distribution of the data. p-values for the effect of EAE treatment were calculated using t-test or Mann–Whitney test according to data distribution. All videos were analyzed by two evaluators (J.Z. and V.Y.) blinded for the experimental groups. * $p \leq 0.05$, ** $p \leq 0.01$, *** $p \leq 0.001$, ns = not significant; ↑: increased; ↓: decreased.

	Parameter Number	Parameters	Evaluator 1 Cohort#1 (Change, Significance, p-Value)	Evaluator 1 Cohort#2 (Change, Significance, p-Value)	Evaluator 2 Cohort#1 and Cohort#2 (Change, Significance, p-Value)
Fore Limbs	#1	Paw Angle Variability (Average)	↓, *, 0.0483	↓, ns, 0.7092	
	#2	Stance Width	↑, *, 0.0241	↑, ns, 0.8720	
	#3	Stride Length Variability (Average)	↓, ***, 0.0008	↑, ns, 0.5670	
	#4	Stride Width Variability	↓, ***, 0.0001	↓, ns, 0.5056	
	#5	Stride Length CV (Average)	↓, *, 0.0101	↓, ns, 0.3456	
	#6	Stance Width CV	↓, ***, <0.0001	↓, ns, 0.6412	
	#7	Paw Area at Peak Stance (Average)	↑, *, 0.0486	↑, ns, 0.1747	
	#8	Paw Area Variability at Peak Stance (Average)	↓, **, 0.0097	↓, ns, 0.2705	
	#9	Ataxia Coefficient (Average)	↓, **, 0.0082	↓, ns, 0.2659	
Hind Limbs	#1	Swing Time (Average)	↑, *, 0.0239	↑, ***, <0.0001	↑, ***, <0.0001
	#2	%Swing Stride (Average)	↑, *, 0.0278	↑, ***, <0.0001	↑, ***, <0.0001
	#3	%Stance Stride (Average)	↓, *, 0.0278	↓, ***, <0.0001	↓, ***, <0.0001
	#4	Stance/Swing (Average)	↓, *, 0.0274	↓, ***, <0.0001	↓, ***, 0.0002
	#5	Paw Angle–Left Hind	↑, ***, 0.0006	↑, ns, 0.0006	
	#6	Paw Angle–Right Hind	↑, ***, <0.0001	↑, **, 0.005	
	#7	Absolute Paw Angle (Sum)	↑, ***, <0.0001	↑, ***, 0.0002	↑, ***, <0.0001
	#8	Stride Width Variability	↓, **, 0.0071	↓, ns, 0.5056	
	#9	Stance Width CV	↓, **, 0.0073	↑, ns, 0.6412	
	#10	Paw Area at Peak Stance (Average)	↓, ***, 0.0005	↑, ns, 0.4922	
	#11	Paw Area Variability at Peak Stance (Average)	↓, *, 0.0403	↑, ns, 0.2317	
	#12	MAX dA/dT (Average)	↓, **, 0.0010	↑, ns, 0.2313	
	#13	Tau-Propulsion (Average)	↓, *, 0.0198	↓, ns, 0.2448	
	#14	Midline Distance (Sum)	↑, ***, <0.0001	↓, *, 0.0442	↑, ***, <0.0001
	#15	Paw Drag (Average)	↑, ***, 0.0001	↑, ns, 0.7821	

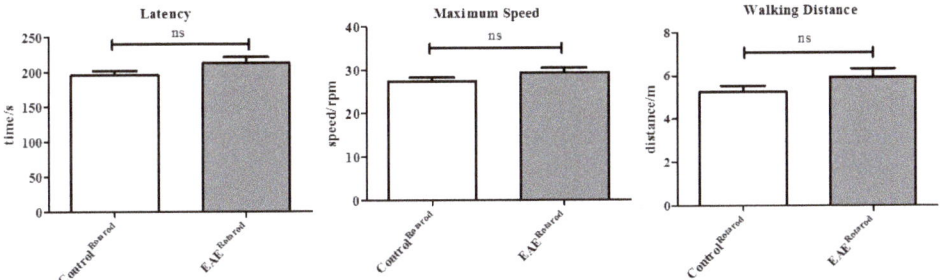

Figure 5. Gross locomotor ability in the Rotarod assay during pre-clinical EAE. Gait parameters were assessed in Control^{Rotarod} (n = 10) and EAE^{Rotarod} (n = 8) mice. Both cohorts were tested for their ability to run on a rotating cylinder that accelerated its speed with time (4–40 rpm in 300 s). Latencies to fall from the accelerating cylinder (i.e., *latency*), the *maximum speed* mice were able to run, and the *walking distance* on the rotating cylinder are presented as mean ± SEM. The D'Agostino and Pearson test was applied to test for normal distribution of the data. *p*-values for the effect of EAE treatment were calculated using t-test or Mann-Whitney test according to data distribution. ns = not significant.

3.4. Gait Abrnoramilties in Mice Sub-Immunized with CFA and PTx

Our analyses so far suggest that during pre-clinical EAE, motor abnormalities can be quantified using high speed ventral plane videography. Severe inflammation is characteristic for the clinical but not pre-clinical EAE phase. We, thus, assumed that diffuse, innate immune driven pathological processes account at least in part for the observed gait abnormalities. To mimic diffuse innate immune activation, we systematically investigated gait abnormalities in control mice and mice injected with CFA and PTx without the MOG$_{35-55}$ peptide (referred to as sub-immunization). Various studies have shown that the administration of CFA and PTx without the MOG$_{35-55}$ peptide induces diffuse innate immune activation in the CNS of mice [35–38]. In particular, we analyzed whether or not the identified gait metrics found to be altered during pre-clinical EAE are as well different in sub-immunized mice. We excluded the two parameters "paw-angle of the left hind limb" and "paw angle of the right hind limb" because both were found to be highly variable in control animals (see Table 1). Among the remaining five abnormal gait parameters during the EAE pre-clinical phase, we found that *Swing Time (Average)* was significantly different between sub-immunized (PTx^{DigiGait}) and fully immunized (EAE^{DigiGait}) mice. In contrast, such a difference was not observed for the other 4 gait parameters suggesting that most of the observed gait differences are due to diffuse innate immune system activation (Figure 6).

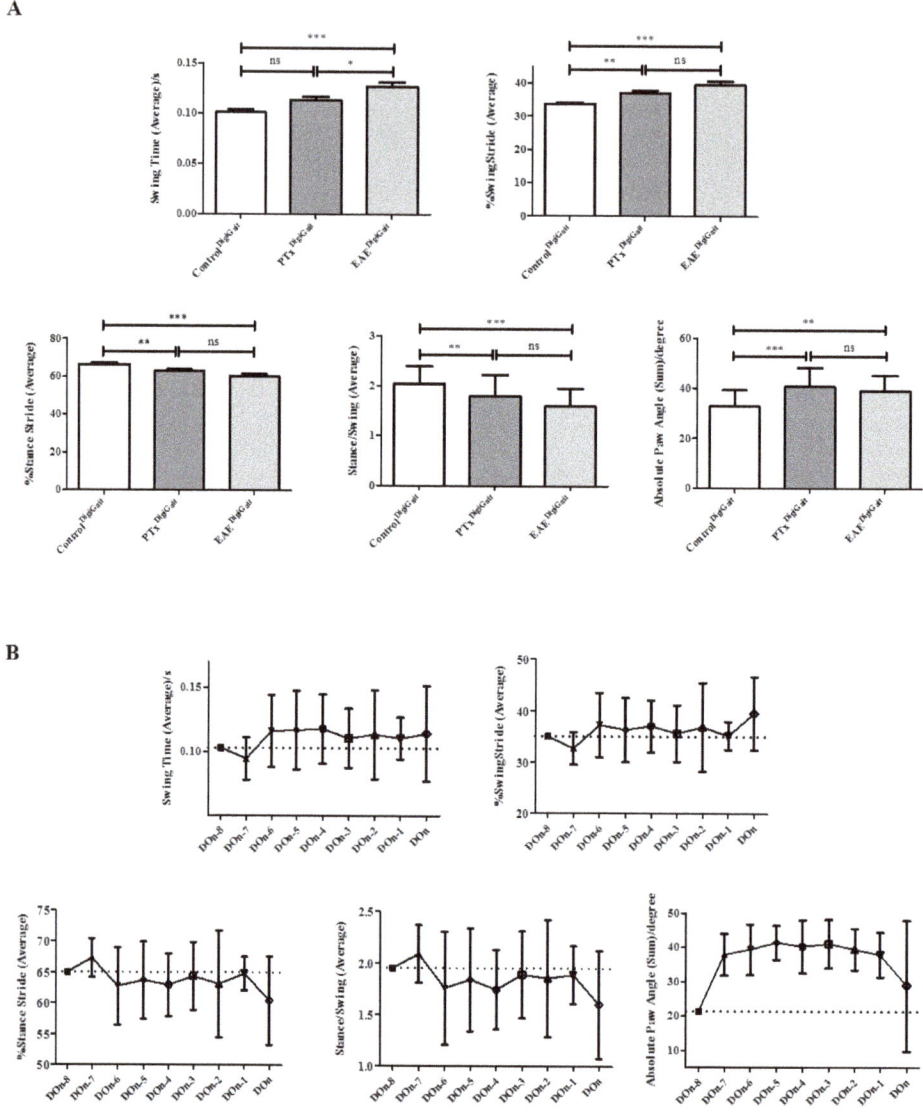

Figure 6. Effect of EAE sub-immunization on gait parameters. (**A**) Differences of the gait metrics in Control^{DigiGait}, PTx^{DigiGait}, and EAE^{DigiGait} mice. D'Agostino and Pearson test was applied to test for normal distribution of the data. *p*-values generated using one-way ANOVA with Bonferroni post-test for multiple comparisons of individual pairs of treatment. Note that the gait parameter *Swing Time* is significantly different between sub-immunized (PTx^{DigiGait}) and fully immunized (EAE^{DigiGait}) mice. (**B**) Gait parameters over time in fully immunized (EAE^{DigiGait}) mice. Don = day of onset, Don-1 = 1 day before onset, etc. * $p \leq 0.05$, ** $p \leq 0.01$, *** $p \leq 0.001$, ns = not significant.

4. Discussion

The most commonly used behavioral evaluation method in EAE is based on the severity of motor deficits, which is mainly driven by spinal cord pathology. In most studies, each mouse is graded daily and given a score ranging from 0 to 5 [39–41]. Parameters include limp tail or hind limb weakness when

EAE is mild and partial or complete hind limb and fore limb paralysis in severe EAE cases. Of note, this evaluation approach is neither very sensitive nor objective. Therefore, in order to detect minor motor deficits, more accurate and reliable EAE evaluation methods are urgently needed. In this study, we used the high speed ventral plane videography system DigiGait™ to characterize and quantify a set of different gait metrics during pre-clinical EAE. We were able to show (1) that manipulation during DigiGait™ measurements does not decrease EAE severity; (2) that many gait parameters are stable in control mice; (3) that the mice show hind limb gait abnormalities during pre-clinical EAE and, (4) that most of the observed gait abnormalities during pre-clinical EAE are probably driven by an interplay of innate and adaptive immune activation.

The expanded disability status scale (EDSS), which is the most commonly used measure of disability for MS, ranges from 0 to 10 in 0.5 unit increments that represent higher levels of disability and is based on the individual, subjective examination by a neurologist. EDSS steps 1.0 to 4.5 refer to people with MS who are able to walk without any aid and are based on measures of impairment in eight functional systems, among motor disturbances. Other measures of motor disability in MS include the timed 25 foot walk, which assesses ambulatory function, or walking [42], and the 9 hole peg test, which measures upper body function and manual dexterity [43]. Indeed, gait impairment is a hallmark of MS which significantly impacts on the quality of life of the individual [44]. Comparable to the human disease, MS models are characterized by gait abnormalities [4,5]. As already stated above, there is no standard EAE scoring system which research groups would use to measure EAE severity [45]. The use of different EAE scoring systems prohibits direct comparison of clinical EAE data published from different laboratories. Furthermore, the applied scoring systems rely on subjective rather than objective evaluations. An objective and quantitative approach would, therefore, be of great interest for pre-clinical trials using the EAE model.

Different automatic or semi-automatic systems have been applied to quantify gait abnormalities in different EAE models, among the CatWalk™ XT system. The CatWalk™ System consists of a glass walkway that is illuminated by fluorescent light. When the paw is in contact with the upper surface of the walkway, the print light is reflected, which is detected by an appropriate high speed color camera and detection software. Of note, the animal walks across the glass plate voluntarily which is different to the system applied in the current study. This method has been performed in the EAE model using different species such as Lewis rats [46], Brown Norway rats [47], or C57BL/6 mice [48]. In our study, we observed that MOG_{35-55} immunization severely influenced the success rate of gait analysis recordings. Just 3 out of 18 animals could be daily evaluated until the day of disease onset, whereas 6 out of 18 animals could be daily evaluated until the day BEFORE disease onset. This result clearly demonstrates that running at a velocity of 15 cm/s displays a motor-performance challenge which cannot be met by most of the mice during pre-clinical EAE. Bernardes et al. noted in their study that with disease progression, some animals were not able to cross the CatWalk™ walkway after established EAE [48]. During pre-clinical EAE all animals were able to perform the gait analysis task which is in contrast to our results. However, one major difference between the CatWalk™ and the DigiGait™ system is that in the former, mice gait is voluntary whereas in the latter, mice are forced to walk by the motorized treadmill. It is, thus, possible that forced movements are more demanding compared to voluntary ones. Nevertheless, in line with our results the authors found a decrease in *Swing Speed* which equals the observed increase of the *Swing Time* in our study.

In this study, we applied high speed ventral plane videography to analyze gait abnormalities during pre-clinical EAE. High speed ventral plane videography has been shown to be a useful approach to quantify subtle locomotors abnormalities in mouse models of neurodegenerative movement disorders, such as Amyotrophic lateral sclerosis (ALS), Huntington or cerebellar ataxia [49]. For example, altered hind limb movement, accompanied by some changes in coordination and stability characterized the gait abnormalities in SOD1 G93A transgenic mice, which is a model of ALS [49], whereas *Stride Length* and *Stride Frequencies* were found to be altered in a model of Parkinson's disease [50]. Gait analyses were as well found to be useful in non-neurological disorders such as in collagen-induced arthritis [51] or in a model of muscular dystrophy [52]. We followed an exploratory approach (analyzing 39 different gait parameters for the fore limbs and 43 for the hind limbs) to study gait abnormalities during pre-clinical EAE. As many gait parameters change with running speed [30], the analyses were performed in this study at a constant speed of 15 cm/s (see Materials and Methods Section). Based on this extensive dataset, we identified a small set of relevant gait parameters which were different in pre-clinical EAE compared to control mice. These parameters, namely *Swing Time, %Swing Stride, %Stance Stride, Stance/Swing, Paw Angle-Left Hind, Paw Angle-Right Hind,* and *Absolute Paw Angle*, may be used in following studies to assess potential therapeutic effects during pre-clinical EAE. The definition of these parameters, as provided by the manufacturer of the DigiGait™ system are as follow: *Swing Time*—Time duration of the swing phase (no paw contact with belt) given in seconds; *%Swing Stride*—Percent of the total stride duration that the paw is in the air (swing phase); *%Stance Stride*—% of the total stride duration that the paw is in any contact with the belt; *Stance/Swing*—Ratio of stance phase time to swing phase time; *Paw Angle-Left or Right Hind*—The angle that the paw makes with the long axis of the direction of motion of the animal; *Absolute Paw Angle*—Absolute value of the paw angle. Having these definitions in mind it is not surprising to find the parameters *Swing Time* and *%Swing Stride* to be increased while the gait parameter *%Stance Stride* is decreased. However, this particular finding nicely demonstrates the reliability of the used evaluation method. Worth to note that, in line with our findings of an increased *Paw Angle*, these gait deficits were found to be associated with ataxia, spinal cord injury, and demyelinating disease [53].

One major finding of the present study is that gait abnormalities during the pre-clinical EAE phase can be quantified. Such alterations have as well been observed by others. For example, Leva et al. found in SJL/J mice immunized with proteolipid protein ($PLP_{139-151}$) that the CatWalk™ gait parameter *Maximum Contact Area* decreased three days post immunization, at a time point were conventional disease scoring protocols failed to detect any disease activity [54]. Similar observations were reported by Silva et al. [46], as well using the CatWalk™ System in Lewis rats [46]. Of note, the gait parameter *Maximum Contact Area*, which is called *Paw Area at Peak Stance* in the DigiGait™ environment, was found to be decreased for the hind limbs in Cohort#1 animals, however, we were not able to reproduce this finding in Cohort#2 mice. In the later study, Silva et al. observed, besides a reduced *Maximum Contact Area* of the paw, reductions of the so-called *Regularity Index (RI)* during pre-clinical EAE. *RI* represents a gait metrics for motor coordination. For fully coordinated locomotion, each paw is placed exactly once every four steps. There are a total of six possible step sequence patterns that can be used by a rodent while walking. These patterns can be categorized into three groups: Alternate (Aa: [RF: Right front-RH: Right hind-LF: Left front-LH: Left hind]: RF-RH-LF-LH, Ab: LF-RH-RF-LH); cruciate (Ca: RF-LF-RH-LH, Cb: LF-RF-LH-RH); and rotary (Ra: RF-LF-LH-RH, Rb: LF-RF-RH-LH). The Ab pattern is the most commonly observed. The larger the number of missteps intersperse between regular step patterns, the lower is the *RI* [55]. The same gait parameter is not evaluated by the DigiGait™ software. However, it includes the metrics *Gait Symmetry* which computes the ratio of forelimb stepping frequency to hind limb stepping frequency. It has been shown that the parameter *Gait Symmetry* declines with age and treadmill training counteracted the decline of *Gait Symmetry* [56]. Of note, no differences with respect to the parameter *Gait Symmetry* were found during the pre-clinical EAE phase in our current study.

In a recent study, Kappos et al. analyzed the validity and reliability of the CatWalk™ system as a static and dynamic gait analysis tool for the assessment of functional nerve recovery in small animal models [55]. They found that among different gait parameters, *Swing Duration* was the most reliable and valid gait parameter. In our study, *Swing Time*, which is essentially the same as *Swing Duration*, was found to be increased in both experimental cohorts and the difference was verified by two independent observers. Of note, it has been shown that *Swing Duration* increases with pain [57–59], and pain, which is a frequent and disabling symptom in MS patients, as well characterizes EAE animals to some extent [60]. Of note, a recent study showed that pain can as well be observed during the pre-clinical EAE phase [61]. It is, thus, possible that pain is the underlying mechanism of the observed increased *Swing Time* in our EAE mice. Further studies are needed to verify or reject this hypothesis.

Another important finding of our study is that sub-immunization of the mice with CFA and PTx is sufficient to induce moderate gait abnormalities in the experimental mice. In animal models of EAE, the disease is induced actively by immunization with myelin protein peptides, such as MOG or PLP peptide dissolved in CFA, or passively by activated neuroantigen-specific T-cells transfer. The incidence and severity of the disease induced by neuroantigens in CFA is promoted by PTx co-injection [62]. Although PTx has been widely used in EAE induction of rodents, the exact role of PTx in initiating EAE remains controversial. Historically, it was thought that this microbial product facilitates EAE by breaking down the blood-brain barrier and thereby helps pathogenic T-cells to migrate into the CNS. Further studies have shown that PTx increases the expression of endothelial adhesion molecules which triggers leukocyte infiltration into the brain [37]. PTx could also facilitate EAE induction through modulating the interaction between the innate and adaptive immune system in the response to self-antigens [36]. Moreover, PTx has other biological functions that could contribute to its activity in EAE such as inducing maturation of dendritic cells [38], enhancing T effector cells' cytokine production as well as reducing T regulatory cells' activity [63,64]. Murugesan et al. showed that CFA/PTx alone could cause widespread gene alterations that could prime the choroid plexus to unlock the CNS to T-cell infiltration during neuroinflammatory disease [65]. In this study, we used sub-immunization to uncover whether autoreactive T-cells are required to induce the observed gait abnormalities. As demonstrated in Figure 6A, the extent of gait alterations was found to be more severe in fully immunized mice compared to sub-immunized animals. These results suggest that both, innate and adaptive immunity, act in concert to induce gait abnormalities during pre-clinical EAE.

One major advantage of semi-automated gait analyses in EAE and other neurodegenerative diseases is that such metrics can be directly compared with measurement obtained during clinical trials. In a recent trial, Liparoti et al. investigated gait patterns in minimally disabled RRMS patients applying a three dimensional-gait analysis approach. They could show that, compared to healthy controls, RRMS show an increase of *Swing Time* [66]. Beyond, Novotna et al. were able to show that MS patients with no apparent disability (EDSS 0-1.5) showed abnormalities in the GAITRite gait analysis instrument [67], suggesting that particular aspects of human gait abnormalities can be investigated in mice.

Another important advantage of the DigiGait™ analysis system is the semi-automated analysis approach. Although some manual adjustments have to be performed during the video analysis procedure, false negative or positive results due to experimenter bias are less likely to occur. Nevertheless, blinding during the video analysis procedure is mandatory.

5. Conclusions

In summary, DigiGait™ is more sensitive than conventional scoring approaches to study motor deficits during the EAE pre-clinical phase. To evaluate such abnormalities we suggest to either quantify the numbers of successful runs on the treadmill and/or to quantify the gait parameters *Swing Time*, *% Swing Stride*, *%Stance Stride*, *Stance/Swing* ratio, or *Absolute Paw Angle*. Early detection of gait abnormalities in the EAE model may accelerate the development of therapies for MS.

Author Contributions: M.K. and J.Z. designed the concept of the present study and supervised it. J.Z., V.Y., and S.R. performed high speed ventral plane videography in mice. J.Z., V.Y., and F.F. performed data analyses. J.Z., E.N., S.J., T.G., J.F., and H.K. performed (immuno-) histochemistry and related analyses. J.Z., T.G., J.F., and C.H. performed Rotarod test and related analyses. J.Z. drafted the manuscript. M.K. critically revised the article for important intellectual content. All authors read and approved the final version of the manuscript.

Funding: This research was funded by the Deutsche Forschungsgemeinschaft (KI 1469/8-1; #398138584; M.K.).

Acknowledgments: J.Z. is financially supported by the China Scholarship Council for living stipend (CSC201706010354). We thank Frauke Winzer, Astrid Baltruschat, Sarah Wübbel, Beate Aschauer, Barbara Mosler, and Sabine Tost for their excellent and valuable technical assistance.

Conflicts of Interest: The authors declare no conflict of interest.

References

1. Elkjaer, M.L.; Frisch, T.; Reynolds, R.; Kacprowski, T.; Burton, M.; Kruse, T.A.; Thomassen, M.; Baumbach, J.; Illes, Z. Unique RNA signature of different lesion types in the brain white matter in progressive multiple sclerosis. *Acta Neuropathol. Commun.* **2019**, *7*, 58. [CrossRef]
2. Van der Poel, M.; Ulas, T.; Mizee, M.R.; Hsiao, C.C.; Miedema, S.S.M.; Adelia; Schuurman, K.G.; Helder, B.; Tas, S.W.; Schultze, J.L.; et al. Transcriptional profiling of human microglia reveals grey-white matter heterogeneity and multiple sclerosis-associated changes. *Nat. Commun.* **2019**, *10*, 1139. [CrossRef]
3. Vercellino, M.; Trebini, C.; Capello, E.; Mancardi, G.L.; Giordana, M.T.; Cavalla, P. Inflammatory responses in Multiple Sclerosis normal-appearing white matter and in non-immune mediated neurological conditions with wallerian axonal degeneration: A comparative study. *J. Neuroimmunol.* **2017**, *312*, 49–58. [CrossRef]
4. Ruther, B.J.; Scheld, M.; Dreymueller, D.; Clarner, T.; Kress, E.; Brandenburg, L.O.; Swartenbroekx, T.; Hoornaert, C.; Ponsaerts, P.; Fallier-Becker, P.; et al. Combination of cuprizone and experimental autoimmune encephalomyelitis to study inflammatory brain lesion formation and progression. *Glia* **2017**, *65*, 1900–1913. [CrossRef]
5. Scheld, M.; Ruther, B.J.; Grosse-Veldmann, R.; Ohl, K.; Tenbrock, K.; Dreymuller, D.; Fallier-Becker, P.; Zendedel, A.; Beyer, C.; Clarner, T.; et al. Neurodegeneration Triggers Peripheral Immune Cell Recruitment into the Forebrain. *J. Neurosci.* **2016**, *36*, 1410–1415. [CrossRef]
6. Barnett, M.H.; Prineas, J.W. Relapsing and remitting multiple sclerosis: Pathology of the newly forming lesion. *Ann. Neurol.* **2004**, *55*, 458–468. [CrossRef]
7. McDonnell, G.V.; Cabrera-Gomez, J.; Calne, D.B.; Li, D.K.; Oger, J. Clinical presentation of primary progressive multiple sclerosis 10 years after the incidental finding of typical magnetic resonance imaging brain lesions: The subclinical stage of primary progressive multiple sclerosis may last 10 years. *Mult. Scler.* **2003**, *9*, 204–209. [CrossRef]
8. De Groot, C.J.; Bergers, E.; Kamphorst, W.; Ravid, R.; Polman, C.H.; Barkhof, F.; van der Valk, P. Post-mortem MRI-guided sampling of multiple sclerosis brain lesions: Increased yield of active demyelinating and (p)reactive lesions. *Brain* **2001**, *124*, 1635–1645. [CrossRef]
9. Laule, C.; Vavasour, I.M.; Whittall, K.P.; Oger, J.; Paty, D.W.; Li, D.K.; MacKay, A.L.; Arnold, D.L. Evolution of focal and diffuse magnetisation transfer abnormalities in multiple sclerosis. *J. Neurol.* **2003**, *250*, 924–931. [CrossRef]
10. Kipp, M.; Nyamoya, S.; Hochstrasser, T.; Amor, S. Multiple sclerosis animal models: A clinical and histopathological perspective. *Brain Pathol.* **2017**, *27*, 123–137. [CrossRef]
11. Lee, N.J.; Ha, S.K.; Sati, P.; Absinta, M.; Luciano, N.J.; Lefeuvre, J.A.; Schindler, M.K.; Leibovitch, E.C.; Ryu, J.K.; Petersen, M.A.; et al. Spatiotemporal distribution of fibrinogen in marmoset and human inflammatory demyelination. *Brain* **2018**, *141*, 1637–1649. [CrossRef]
12. Van der Valk, P.; Amor, S. Preactive lesions in multiple sclerosis. *Curr. Opin. Neurol.* **2009**, *22*, 207–213. [CrossRef]
13. Evangelidou, M.; Karamita, M.; Vamvakas, S.S.; Szymkowski, D.E.; Probert, L. Altered expression of oligodendrocyte and neuronal marker genes predicts the clinical onset of autoimmune encephalomyelitis and indicates the effectiveness of multiple sclerosis-directed therapeutics. *J. Immunol.* **2014**, *192*, 4122–4133. [CrossRef]
14. Bartholomaus, I.; Kawakami, N.; Odoardi, F.; Schlager, C.; Miljkovic, D.; Ellwart, J.W.; Klinkert, W.E.; Flugel-Koch, C.; Issekutz, T.B.; Wekerle, H.; et al. Effector T cell interactions with meningeal vascular structures in nascent autoimmune CNS lesions. *Nature* **2009**, *462*, 94–98. [CrossRef]
15. Flugel, A.; Berkowicz, T.; Ritter, T.; Labeur, M.; Jenne, D.E.; Li, Z.; Ellwart, J.W.; Willem, M.; Lassmann, H.; Wekerle, H. Migratory activity and functional changes of green fluorescent effector cells before and during experimental autoimmune encephalomyelitis. *Immunity* **2001**, *14*, 547–560. [CrossRef]
16. Alvarez, J.I.; Saint-Laurent, O.; Godschalk, A.; Terouz, S.; Briels, C.; Larouche, S.; Bourbonniere, L.; Larochelle, C.; Prat, A. Focal disturbances in the blood-brain barrier are associated with formation of neuroinflammatory lesions. *Neurobiol. Dis.* **2015**, *74*, 14–24. [CrossRef]

17. Centonze, D.; Muzio, L.; Rossi, S.; Cavasinni, F.; De Chiara, V.; Bergami, A.; Musella, A.; D'Amelio, M.; Cavallucci, V.; Martorana, A.; et al. Inflammation triggers synaptic alteration and degeneration in experimental autoimmune encephalomyelitis. *J. Neurosci.* **2009**, *29*, 3442–3452. [CrossRef]
18. Baranzini, S.E.; Bernard, C.C.; Oksenberg, J.R. Modular transcriptional activity characterizes the initiation and progression of autoimmune encephalomyelitis. *J. Immunol.* **2005**, *174*, 7412–7422. [CrossRef]
19. Chrzanowski, U.; Bhattarai, S.; Scheld, M.; Clarner, T.; Fallier-Becker, P.; Beyer, C.; Rohr, S.O.; Schmitz, C.; Hochstrasser, T.; Schweiger, F.; et al. Oligodendrocyte degeneration and concomitant microglia activation directs peripheral immune cells into the forebrain. *Neurochem. Int.* **2019**, *126*, 139–153. [CrossRef]
20. Masuda, H.; Mori, M.; Hirano, S.; Kojima, K.; Uzawa, A.; Uchida, T.; Ohtani, R.; Kuwabara, S. Relapse numbers and earlier intervention by disease modifying drugs are related with progression of less brain atrophy in patients with multiple sclerosis. *J. Neurol. Sci.* **2019**, *403*, 78–84. [CrossRef]
21. Landfeldt, E.; Castelo-Branco, A.; Svedbom, A.; Lofroth, E.; Kavaliunas, A.; Hillert, J. The long-term impact of early treatment of multiple sclerosis on the risk of disability pension. *J. Neurol.* **2018**, *265*, 701–707. [CrossRef]
22. PRISMS Study Group; The University of British Columbia MS/MRI Analysis Group. PRISMS-4: Long-term efficacy of interferon-beta-1a in relapsing MS. *Neurology* **2001**, *56*, 1628–1636. [CrossRef]
23. Kavaliunas, A.; Manouchehrinia, A.; Stawiarz, L.; Ramanujam, R.; Agholme, J.; Hedstrom, A.K.; Beiki, O.; Glaser, A.; Hillert, J. Importance of early treatment initiation in the clinical course of multiple sclerosis. *Mult. Scler.* **2017**, *23*, 1233–1240. [CrossRef]
24. Hampton, T.G.; Stasko, M.R.; Kale, A.; Amende, I.; Costa, A.C. Gait dynamics in trisomic mice: Quantitative neurological traits of Down syndrome. *Physiol. Behav.* **2004**, *82*, 381–389. [CrossRef]
25. Kale, A.; Amende, I.; Meyer, G.P.; Crabbe, J.C.; Hampton, T.G. Ethanol's effects on gait dynamics in mice investigated by ventral plane videography. *Alcohol. Clin. Exp. Res.* **2004**, *28*, 1839–1848. [CrossRef]
26. Schlegel, V.; Thieme, M.; Holzmann, C.; Witt, M.; Grittner, U.; Rolfs, A.; Wree, A. Pharmacologic Treatment Assigned for Niemann Pick Type C1 Disease Partly Changes Behavioral Traits in Wild-Type Mice. *Int. J. Mol. Sci.* **2016**, *17*, 1866. [CrossRef]
27. Lein, E.S.; Hawrylycz, M.J.; Ao, N.; Ayres, M.; Bensinger, A.; Bernard, A.; Boe, A.F.; Boguski, M.S.; Brockway, K.S.; Byrnes, E.J.; et al. Genome-wide atlas of gene expression in the adult mouse brain. *Nature* **2007**, *445*, 168–176. [CrossRef]
28. Perez-Nievas, B.G.; Garcia-Bueno, B.; Madrigal, J.L.; Leza, J.C. Chronic immobilisation stress ameliorates clinical score and neuroinflammation in a MOG-induced EAE in Dark Agouti rats: Mechanisms implicated. *J. Neuroinflamm.* **2010**, *7*, 60. [CrossRef]
29. Brown, C.E. *Applied Multivariate Statistics in Geohydrology and Related Sciences*; Springer Science & Business Media: Berlin, Germany, 2012.
30. Hruska, R.E.; Kennedy, S.; Silbergeld, E.K. Quantitative aspects of normal locomotion in rats. *Life Sci.* **1979**, *25*, 171–179. [CrossRef]
31. Butter, C.; Baker, D.; O'Neill, J.K.; Turk, J.L. Mononuclear cell trafficking and plasma protein extravasation into the CNS during chronic relapsing experimental allergic encephalomyelitis in Biozzi AB/H mice. *J. Neurol. Sci.* **1991**, *104*, 9–12. [CrossRef]
32. Oldendorf, W.H.; Towner, H.F. Blood-brain barrier and DNA changes during the evolution of experimental allergic encephalomyelitis. *J. Neuropathol. Exp. Neurol.* **1974**, *33*, 616–631. [CrossRef] [PubMed]
33. Nampoothiri, S.S.; Potluri, T.; Subramanian, H.; Krishnamurthy, R.G. Rodent Gymnastics: Neurobehavioral Assays in Ischemic Stroke. *Mol. Neurobiol.* **2017**, *54*, 6750–6761. [CrossRef] [PubMed]
34. Curzon, P.; Zhang, M.; Radek, R.J.; Fox, G.B. The Behavioral Assessment of Sensorimotor Processes in the Mouse: Acoustic Startle, Sensory Gating, Locomotor Activity, Rotarod, and Beam Walking. In *Methods of Behavior Analysis in Neuroscience*, 2nd ed.; Buccafusco, J.J., Ed.; CRC Press/Taylor & Francis: Boca Raton, FL, USA, 2009.
35. Munoz, J.J.; Bernard, C.C.; Mackay, I.R. Elicitation of experimental allergic encephalomyelitis (EAE) in mice with the aid of pertussigen. *Cell Immunol.* **1984**, *83*, 92–100. [CrossRef]
36. Hofstetter, H.H.; Shive, C.L.; Forsthuber, T.G. Pertussis toxin modulates the immune response to neuroantigens injected in incomplete Freund's adjuvant: Induction of Th1 cells and experimental autoimmune encephalomyelitis in the presence of high frequencies of Th2 cells. *J. Immunol.* **2002**, *169*, 117–125. [CrossRef]

37. Kerfoot, S.M.; Long, E.M.; Hickey, M.J.; Andonegui, G.; Lapointe, B.M.; Zanardo, R.C.; Bonder, C.; James, W.G.; Robbins, S.M.; Kubes, P. TLR4 contributes to disease-inducing mechanisms resulting in central nervous system autoimmune disease. *J. Immunol.* **2004**, *173*, 7070–7077. [CrossRef]
38. Shive, C.L.; Hofstetter, H.; Arredondo, L.; Shaw, C.; Forsthuber, T.G. The enhanced antigen-specific production of cytokines induced by pertussis toxin is due to clonal expansion of T cells and not to altered effector functions of long-term memory cells. *Eur. J. Immunol.* **2000**, *30*, 2422–2431. [CrossRef]
39. Bittner, S.; Afzali, A.M.; Wiendl, H.; Meuth, S.G. Myelin oligodendrocyte glycoprotein (MOG35-55) induced experimental autoimmune encephalomyelitis (EAE) in C57BL/6 mice. *J. Vis. Exp.* **2014**. [CrossRef]
40. Miller, S.D.; Karpus, W.J. Experimental autoimmune encephalomyelitis in the mouse. *Curr. Protoc. Immunol.* **2007**. [CrossRef]
41. Stromnes, I.M.; Goverman, J.M. Active induction of experimental allergic encephalomyelitis. *Nat. Protoc.* **2006**, *1*, 1810–1819. [CrossRef]
42. Motl, R.W.; Cohen, J.A.; Benedict, R.; Phillips, G.; LaRocca, N.; Hudson, L.D.; Rudick, R.; Multiple Sclerosis Outcome Assessments, C. Validity of the timed 25-foot walk as an ambulatory performance outcome measure for multiple sclerosis. *Mult. Scler.* **2017**, *23*, 704–710. [CrossRef]
43. Feys, P.; Lamers, I.; Francis, G.; Benedict, R.; Phillips, G.; LaRocca, N.; Hudson, L.D.; Rudick, R.; Multiple Sclerosis Outcome Assessments, C. The Nine-Hole Peg Test as a manual dexterity performance measure for multiple sclerosis. *Mult. Scler.* **2017**, *23*, 711–720. [CrossRef] [PubMed]
44. Heesen, C.; Bohm, J.; Reich, C.; Kasper, J.; Goebel, M.; Gold, S.M. Patient perception of bodily functions in multiple sclerosis: Gait and visual function are the most valuable. *Mult. Scler.* **2008**, *14*, 988–991. [CrossRef] [PubMed]
45. Fiander, M.D.; Stifani, N.; Nichols, M.; Akay, T.; Robertson, G.S. Kinematic gait parameters are highly sensitive measures of motor deficits and spinal cord injury in mice subjected to experimental autoimmune encephalomyelitis. *Behav. Brain Res.* **2017**, *317*, 95–108. [CrossRef] [PubMed]
46. Silva, G.A.; Pradella, F.; Moraes, A.; Farias, A.; dos Santos, L.M.; de Oliveira, A.L. Impact of pregabalin treatment on synaptic plasticity and glial reactivity during the course of experimental autoimmune encephalomyelitis. *Brain Behav.* **2014**, *4*, 925–935. [CrossRef]
47. Herold, S.; Kumar, P.; Jung, K.; Graf, I.; Menkhoff, H.; Schulz, X.; Bahr, M.; Hein, K. CatWalk gait analysis in a rat model of multiple sclerosis. *BMC Neurosci.* **2016**, *17*, 78. [CrossRef]
48. Bernardes, D.; Oliveira, A.L.R. Comprehensive catwalk gait analysis in a chronic model of multiple sclerosis subjected to treadmill exercise training. *BMC Neurol.* **2017**, *17*, 160. [CrossRef]
49. Preisig, D.F.; Kulic, L.; Kruger, M.; Wirth, F.; McAfoose, J.; Spani, C.; Gantenbein, P.; Derungs, R.; Nitsch, R.M.; Welt, T. High-speed video gait analysis reveals early and characteristic locomotor phenotypes in mouse models of neurodegenerative movement disorders. *Behav. Brain Res.* **2016**, *311*, 340–353. [CrossRef]
50. Amende, I.; Kale, A.; McCue, S.; Glazier, S.; Morgan, J.P.; Hampton, T.G. Gait dynamics in mouse models of Parkinson's disease and Huntington's disease. *J. Neuroeng. Rehabil.* **2005**, *2*, 20. [CrossRef]
51. Vincelette, J.; Xu, Y.; Zhang, L.N.; Schaefer, C.J.; Vergona, R.; Sullivan, M.E.; Hampton, T.G.; Wang, Y.X. Gait analysis in a murine model of collagen-induced arthritis. *Arthritis Res. Ther.* **2007**, *9*, R123. [CrossRef]
52. Hampton, T.G.; Kale, A.; Amende, I.; Tang, W.; McCue, S.; Bhagavan, H.N.; VanDongen, C.G. Gait disturbances in dystrophic hamsters. *J. Biomed. Biotechnol.* **2011**, *2011*, 235354. [CrossRef]
53. Powell, E.; Anch, A.M.; Dyche, J.; Bloom, C.; Richtert, R.R. The splay angle: A new measure for assessing neuromuscular dysfunction in rats. *Physiol. Behav.* **1999**, *67*, 819–821. [CrossRef]
54. Leva, G.; Klein, C.; Benyounes, J.; Halle, F.; Bihel, F.; Collongues, N.; De Seze, J.; Mensah-Nyagan, A.G.; Patte-Mensah, C. The translocator protein ligand XBD173 improves clinical symptoms and neuropathological markers in the SJL/J mouse model of multiple sclerosis. *Biochim. Et Biophys. Acta Mol. Basis Dis.* **2017**, *1863*, 3016–3027. [CrossRef] [PubMed]
55. Kappos, E.A.; Sieber, P.K.; Engels, P.E.; Mariolo, A.V.; D'Arpa, S.; Schaefer, D.J.; Kalbermatten, D.F. Validity and reliability of the CatWalk system as a static and dynamic gait analysis tool for the assessment of functional nerve recovery in small animal models. *Brain Behav.* **2017**, *7*, e00723. [CrossRef] [PubMed]
56. Dorner, H.; Otte, P.; Platt, D. Training influence on age-dependent changes in the gait of rats. *Gerontology* **1996**, *42*, 7–13. [CrossRef] [PubMed]
57. Vrinten, D.H.; Hamers, F.F. 'CatWalk' automated quantitative gait analysis as a novel method to assess mechanical allodynia in the rat; a comparison with von Frey testing. *Pain* **2003**, *102*, 203–209. [CrossRef]

58. Duffy, S.S.; Keating, B.A.; Perera, C.J.; Lees, J.G.; Tonkin, R.S.; Makker, P.G.S.; Carrive, P.; Butovsky, O.; Moalem-Taylor, G. Regulatory T Cells and Their Derived Cytokine, Interleukin-35, Reduce Pain in Experimental Autoimmune Encephalomyelitis. *J. Neurosci.* **2019**, *39*, 2326–2346. [CrossRef]
59. Catuneanu, A.; Paylor, J.W.; Winship, I.; Colbourne, F.; Kerr, B.J. Sex differences in central nervous system plasticity and pain in experimental autoimmune encephalomyelitis. *Pain* **2019**, *160*, 1037–1049. [CrossRef]
60. Harada, Y.; Zhang, J.; Imari, K.; Yamasaki, R.; Ni, J.; Wu, Z.; Yamamoto, K.; Kira, J.I.; Nakanishi, H.; Hayashi, Y. Cathepsin E in neutrophils contributes to the generation of neuropathic pain in experimental autoimmune encephalomyelitis. *Pain* **2019**. [CrossRef]
61. Serizawa, K.; Tomizawa-Shinohara, H.; Yasuno, H.; Yogo, K.; Matsumoto, Y. Anti-IL-6 Receptor Antibody Inhibits Spontaneous Pain at the Pre-onset of Experimental Autoimmune Encephalomyelitis in Mice. *Front. Neurol.* **2019**, *10*, 341. [CrossRef]
62. Lee, J.M.; Olitsky, P.K. Simple method for enhancing development of acute disseminated encephalomyelitis in mice. *Proc. Soc. Exp. Biol. Med.* **1955**, *89*, 263–266. [CrossRef]
63. Chen, X.; Winkler-Pickett, R.T.; Carbonetti, N.H.; Ortaldo, J.R.; Oppenheim, J.J.; Howard, O.M. Pertussis toxin as an adjuvant suppresses the number and function of CD4+CD25+ T regulatory cells. *Eur. J. Immunol.* **2006**, *36*, 671–680. [CrossRef] [PubMed]
64. Wakatsuki, A.; Borrow, P.; Rigley, K.; Beverley, P.C. Cell-surface bound pertussis toxin induces polyclonal T cell responses with high levels of interferon-gamma in the absence of interleukin-12. *Eur. J. Immunol.* **2003**, *33*, 1859–1868. [CrossRef] [PubMed]
65. Murugesan, N.; Paul, D.; Lemire, Y.; Shrestha, B.; Ge, S.; Pachter, J.S. Active induction of experimental autoimmune encephalomyelitis by MOG35-55 peptide immunization is associated with differential responses in separate compartments of the choroid plexus. *Fluids Barriers CNS* **2012**, *9*, 15. [CrossRef] [PubMed]
66. Liparoti, M.; Della Corte, M.; Rucco, R.; Sorrentino, P.; Sparaco, M.; Capuano, R.; Minino, R.; Lavorgna, L.; Agosti, V.; Sorrentino, G.; et al. Gait abnormalities in minimally disabled people with Multiple Sclerosis: A 3D-motion analysis study. *Mult. Scler. Relat. Disord.* **2019**, *29*, 100–107. [CrossRef] [PubMed]
67. Novotna, K.; Sobisek, L.; Horakova, D.; Havrdova, E.; Lizrova Preiningerova, J. Quantification of Gait Abnormalities in Healthy-Looking Multiple Sclerosis Patients (with Expanded Disability Status Scale 0-1.5). *Eur. Neurol.* **2016**, *76*, 99–104. [CrossRef] [PubMed]

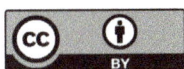

© 2019 by the authors. Licensee MDPI, Basel, Switzerland. This article is an open access article distributed under the terms and conditions of the Creative Commons Attribution (CC BY) license (http://creativecommons.org/licenses/by/4.0/).

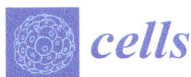

Review

Oligodendrocytes as A New Therapeutic Target in Schizophrenia: From Histopathological Findings to Neuron-Oligodendrocyte Interaction

Florian J. Raabe [1,2,3], Lenka Slapakova [1,2], Moritz J. Rossner [3], Ludovico Cantuti-Castelvetri [4], Mikael Simons [4,5,6], Peter G. Falkai [1] and Andrea Schmitt [1,3,7,*]

1. Department of Psychiatry and Psychotherapy, University Hospital, LMU Munich, Nussbaumstrasse 7, 80336 Munich, Germany; Florian.Raabe@med.uni-muenchen.de (F.J.R.); Lenka.Slapakova@med.uni-muenchen.de (L.S.); Peter.Falkai@med.uni-muenchen.de (P.G.F.)
2. International Max Planck Research School for Translational Psychiatry (IMPRS-TP), Kraepelinstr. 2-10, 80804 Munich, Germany
3. Molecular and Behavioural Neurobiology, Department of Psychiatry and Psychotherapy, University Hospital, LMU Munich, 80336 Munich, Germany; Moritz.Rossner@med.uni-muenchen.de
4. German Center for Neurodegenerative Diseases (DZNE), Feodor-Lynen Str. 17, 81377 Munich, Germany; Ludovico.Cantuti-Castelvetri@dzne.de (L.C.-C.); Mikael.Simons@dzne.de (M.S.)
5. Munich Cluster for Systems Neurology (SyNergy), 81377 Munich, Germany
6. Institute of Neuronal Cell Biology, Technical University Munich, 80805 Munich, Germany
7. Laboratory of Neuroscience (LIM27), Institute of Psychiatry, University of Sao Paulo, 05453-010 São Paulo, Brazil
* Correspondence: andrea.schmitt@med.uni-muenchen.de; Tel.: +49-(0)89-4400-52761; Fax: +49-(0)89-4400-55530

Received: 22 October 2019; Accepted: 21 November 2019; Published: 23 November 2019

Abstract: Imaging and postmortem studies have revealed disturbed oligodendroglia-related processes in patients with schizophrenia and provided much evidence for disturbed myelination, irregular gene expression, and altered numbers of oligodendrocytes in the brains of schizophrenia patients. Oligodendrocyte deficits in schizophrenia might be a result of failed maturation and disturbed regeneration and may underlie the cognitive deficits of the disease, which are strongly associated with impaired long-term outcome. Cognition depends on the coordinated activity of neurons and interneurons and intact connectivity. Oligodendrocyte precursors form a synaptic network with parvalbuminergic interneurons, and disturbed crosstalk between these cells may be a cellular basis of pathology in schizophrenia. However, very little is known about the exact axon-glial cellular and molecular processes that may be disturbed in schizophrenia. Until now, investigations were restricted to peripheral tissues, such as blood, correlative imaging studies, genetics, and molecular and histological analyses of postmortem brain samples. The advent of human-induced pluripotent stem cells (hiPSCs) will enable functional analysis in patient-derived living cells and holds great potential for understanding the molecular mechanisms of disturbed oligodendroglial function in schizophrenia. Targeting such mechanisms may contribute to new treatment strategies for previously treatment-resistant cognitive symptoms.

Keywords: schizophrenia; oligodendrocytes; myelin; interneuron; pluripotent stem cells; cognition; treatment

1. Introduction

Over 40% of patients with schizophrenia (SZ) have an unfavorable outcome, and only 16% of patients recover with a reduction of symptoms and improvement of social functioning. Cognitive deficits and negative symptoms are the most important predictors for poor social and functional outcome in SZ and major contributors to disability [1,2]. To date, no treatment—including antipsychotics—has shown satisfactory efficacy in improving cognitive deficits and negative symptoms in SZ [3,4], and innovative treatment strategies that target underlying pathological processes are urgently needed.

SZ is regarded as a neurodevelopmental disorder, and risk factors include childhood trauma [5] and birth and obstetric complications [6], all of which may influence brain development. In humans, myelination and white matter development occur at a high rate in the first years of childhood [7], continue at a slightly slower rate during adolescence, and enter another dynamic phase in cortical areas during young adulthood [8], a vulnerable period of brain development that coincides with the average age of onset of SZ [9]. In some cortical areas, myelination contributes to lifelong brain plasticity, an adaptive process to "learning," and only reaches its maximum level after decades [10].

2. Findings of the Relationship of Myelination Deficits, Impaired White Matter, and Cognition from Human Brain Imaging Studies

Diffusion tensor imaging (DTI) examines brain white matter microarchitecture on the basis of free water diffusion properties within a certain three-dimensional area (voxel). Different DTI indices, or their combinations, are associated (to different extents) with the degree of fiber tract organization and myelination and with axonal integrity. The most important DTI indices are fractional anisotropy (FA), mean diffusivity (MD), axial diffusivity (AD), and radial diffusivity (RD) [11]. A pioneer study performed DTI imaging and CLARITY immunolabeling of whole-brain myelin basic protein (MBP), which is essential for myelination and represents 30% of total myelin brain protein [12], in the same mouse brain, and revealed that DTI-derived FA significantly correlated with MBP expression, whereas MD, AD, and RD did not [13]. Previous meta-analyses of voxel-based DTI studies in SZ and first-episode SZ found reduced FA, in particular in fronto-temporal-limbic pathways [14–16].

Recently, the ENIGMA Schizophrenia DTI Working Group performed the largest international multicenter study to date, in 4322 individuals, which revealed broad white matter microstructural differences in SZ [17]. Widespread FA reductions were significant in 19 of 25 regions and, remarkably, were driven more by peripheral white matter disturbances than by disturbances in specific core regions of interest. The group also found a widespread increase in MD and RD and consequently suggested that lower FA was most likely driven by aberrant myelination in most regions [17]. The group concluded that lower FA in SZ is not due to the potential impact of antipsychotic treatment on white matter because it did not find significant associations between FA and antipsychotic treatment [17]. This conclusion is supported by a meta-analysis in minimally treated first-episode SZ patients that also showed a reduction in FA in the fronto-limbic circuitry [15].

Disturbances of white matter integrity within the fornix, which contains the white matter tracts of the hippocampus, correlate with impairments in episodic memory in SZ [18,19]. Oligodendrocyte dysfunction leads to disturbances in myelination and consequently to deficient propagation of nerve impulses and impaired cognition [20]. Moreover, in SZ patients and controls, oligodendrocyte-related gene variants, such as myelin-associated glycoprotein (MAG) and cyclic nucleotide phosphodiesterase (CNP), are related to cognitive performance and this relationship is mediated by white matter tract integrity [21]. Interestingly, a single nucleotide polymorphism of the oligodendrocyte transcription factor Olig2, which is necessary for maturation of oligodendrocyte progenitor cells, has also been associated with impaired cognition, mediated by reduced white matter FA in healthy controls [21]. FA and cognition are also reduced in individuals at ultra-high risk for psychosis, and lower FA, accompanied by higher RD, was linked to demyelination [22]. Moreover, widespread higher FA was associated with improved cognitive performance in people at ultra-high risk for psychosis, but not in healthy controls [22].

3. Histopathological Studies of Oligodendrocytes in Schizophrenia (SZ)

A reduction of perineuronal oligodendrocytes in the gray matter of the prefrontal cortex has been reported in SZ [23]. Stereological analyses have found a reduced number of oligodendrocytes in the dorsolateral prefrontal cortex (DLPFC) [24] but not in the anterior cingulate cortex [25]. In design-based stereological postmortem studies of Nissl (cresyl violet) and myelin (luxol fast-blue) stained sections, our group showed a decreased oligodendrocyte number in the left CA4 region of the anterior and posterior hippocampus in SZ [26,27]. The stereologically estimated loss of oligodendrocytes in this region was associated with cognitive deficits [28]. A study that aimed to validate the loss of oligodendrocytes by using immunohistochemical markers found a trend for decreased oligodendrocyte transcription factor Olig1 immuno-positive oligodendrocyte density in the left CA4, but no reduction of the transcription factor Olig2 [28]. Olig1 antibodies stain precursor forms and mature oligodendrocyte populations, and both Olig1 and Olig2 are needed for progenitor development and repair of myelin [29]. Moreover, the finding by Schmitt et al. (2009) [26] and Falkai et al. (2016) [27] of decreased oligodendrocyte number and Falkai et al. (2016) [28] of association with cognitive deficits led to the hypothesis that the decreased number of oligodendrocytes is related to a failure of maturation and indicates a disturbed regenerative recovery process in the CA4/dentate region [30]. Interestingly, the loss of oligodendrocytes is confined to the CA4 region, a region that is now regarded as the polymorph layer of the dentate gyrus. This region connects the dentate gyrus, where neurogenesis can be observed, with the CA3 region [31]. We found evidence for disturbed neurogenesis in SZ in that the volume and number of granule neurons in the left dentate gyrus were reduced [28]. These findings replicated those of former studies [32] that described such thinning and were interpreted as a sign for disturbed neurodevelopment in SZ. Furthermore, the CA4/dentate gyrus region is the neuroanatomical basis for the cognitive domain "pattern separation" and other neurocognitive functions such as declarative memory, which have been shown to be disturbed in SZ [33].

When interpreting histopathology studies in SZ, one must also consider their limitations. Design-based stereological studies are superior to cell density studies because the two-dimensional assessment of Olig1 or Olig2 immunostained cells may be confounded by volume differences that are due to tissue shrinkage associated with formalin fixation or staining procedures, cutting of cells during sectioning, non-random orientation, and irregular cell shape and size [34]. Moreover, long-term treatment with antipsychotics may confound results. Using design-based stereology in histologically stained serial brain sections, we performed a count of the different cell types based on morphological criteria (neurons, astrocytes, oligodendrocytes) that come into focus within unbiased virtual counting spaces distributed in a systematic-random fashion throughout the different regions of the hippocampus. Estimated cell numbers were calculated from the numbers of counted cells and the sampling probability according to Schmitz and Hof (2005) [35]. Our group showed that the dose of antipsychotics in chlorpromazine equivalents had no influence on oligodendrocyte numbers [26,27].

4. Evidence of Oligodendrocyte Deficits from Molecular Studies

In SZ, genome-wide microarray studies have shown that expression of myelin- and oligodendrocyte-related genes is profoundly affected in the prefrontal, temporal, and occipital cortex, hippocampus, and basal ganglia [36].

In a microarray study, in the temporal cortex, our group showed decreased mRNA expression of contactin-associated protein, which mediates contact between oligodendrocytes and the synapse, thus indicating dysfunctional oligodendrocyte-neuronal interactions in SZ (Schmitt et al. 2012). In a series of proteomic studies in frozen postmortem tissue, we showed that in SZ myelination-related proteins, such as MBP and myelin oligodendrocyte glycoprotein (MOG), are downregulated in the DLPFC, anterior temporal lobe, and corpus callosum (e.g., [37,38]). In an immunohistochemistry study, we detected a decreased intensity of myelin-related MBP staining in the entorhinal cortex of SZ patients and found a correlation between decreased myelination and disorganization of pre-alpha cells [39]. Single-cell transcriptome analysis of gene expression in different cell populations [40], such as oligodendrocytes in the hippocampal region and prefrontal cortex, has not yet been performed in postmortem brains from patients with SZ.

5. The "Defective Maturation" Hypothesis of SZ

To date, it is unclear whether a loss of oligodendrocyte progenitors or of mature oligodendrocytes, and therefore a failure in differentiation or apoptosis, contributes to the reduced number of oligodendrocytes in patients with SZ. The cause of reduced oligodendrocyte numbers may be important for the development of future treatment strategies targeting deficits in oligodendrocyte-related pathological processes. For example, one potential treatment may be to improve the differentiation of oligodendrocyte progenitor cells to myelinating oligodendrocytes, thereby promoting remyelination and possibly contributing to improvement of treatment-resistant cognitive and negative symptoms.

Animal models have shown that oligodendrocyte progenitor cell proliferation and differentiation is required for remyelination [41]. However, in multiple sclerosis, remyelination is often incomplete. Besides a loss of mature oligodendrocytes, reductions in oligodendrocyte progenitor cells have been reported [42], as well as increased death of these progenitor cells and reduced process extension under stress conditions [43]. It has been hypothesized that oligodendrocyte progenitor cells, which are capable of myelination, are reduced in brain regions of SZ patients, resulting in decreased plasticity and remyelination capacity. Progenitor cells can be labeled by using antibodies that bind to oligodendrocyte proteins, which are expressed during specific stages of oligodendrocyte development [41]. However, a first cell density study of the prefrontal cortex in SZ detected no loss of early NG2-immunopositive oligodendrocyte progenitor cells [44]. This study did detect a loss of oligodendrocytes positive for Olig2, a transcription factor expressed in oligodendrocyte progenitors at later stages and in mature oligodendrocytes [44], but Olig2 is not suitable for identifying progenitor cells specifically. Additional labeling with neurite outgrowth inhibitor (Nogo)-A, which reliably identifies mature oligodendrocytes, has been shown to be a way to identify specific stages of oligodendrocytes in human brain regions from patients with multiple sclerosis [45]. Nogo is known to regulate cellular processes and has three isoforms, Nogo-A, -B, and -C. Specifically, Nogo-A is highly expressed in oligodendrocytes. Mature oligodendrocytes derived from surgery tissue specimens from adult patients express both Nogo-A and Olig2. Double immunohistochemistry with anti-Nogo-A, a marker that reliably identifies mature oligodendrocytes in human CNS tissue [45], revealed that almost all of the weakly positive Olig2 cells were also Nogo-A positive and were identified as mature oligodendrocytes. In contrast, Olig2-strong cells were negative for Nogo-A. Therefore, double-staining immunohistochemistry allows oligodendrocyte progenitors to be reliably identified and studies identified oligodendrocytes with weak Olig2 and strong NogoA staining as mature oligodendrocytes, but those with strong Olig2 and negative NogoA staining as progenitors [43,46]. Other immunohistochemical markers, such as PDFαR and NG2, have also been used to identify oligodendrocyte progenitor cells [41]. In SZ, however, stereological studies investigating the number and apoptosis of mature oligodendrocytes or progenitors are still lacking.

6. The Intercellular Interactions of Oligodendrocytes with Microglia and Neurons

A meta-analysis reported mild inflammation of the brain in SZ with activation of microglia [47], which may contribute to the oligodendrocyte deficit [48]. Ultrastructural analysis revealed activated microglia near dystrophic and apoptotic oligodendrocytes and demyelinating and dysmyelinating axons [49,50]. Oligodendrocytes have glutamatergic n-methyl-D-aspartate (NMDA) receptors, and our group showed that NMDA receptor hypofunction after MK-801 treatment of human cell cultures causes oligodendrocyte dysfunction by inducing deficits in glycolysis [51]. MK-801 is a potent NMDA receptor antagonist, and treatment with this class of antagonists represents the most reliable pharmacological model of the cognitive, positive, and negative symptoms of SZ [52,53]. Therefore, NMDAR antibodies, as part of an inflammatory process, may influence oligodendrocyte pathology.

In SZ, a dysfunction of γ-amino-butyric acid (GABA)ergic interneurons has been proposed to play a role in the pathophysiology of cognitive deficits [54]. More specifically, mRNA and protein levels of parvalbumin-positive interneurons were shown to be affected in SZ, while cell number and density were not consistently reduced [55]. However, a dysfunction of inhibitory interneurons may contribute to a hypofunction of the NMDA receptor and a glutamatergic imbalance, leading to cognitive deficits and negative and positive symptoms [52]. Recently, it has become evident that, besides the well-known myelination of glutamatergic projection neurons, a large fraction of myelin ensheathes axons of cortical inhibitory neurons, especially of parvalbumin-positive basket cells [56]. These findings have relevance for oligodendrocyte pathology in SZ [55] because synaptic signaling between interneurons and oligodendrocyte precursor cells is known to influence the differentiation of oligodendrocyte progenitors in the hippocampus [57].

The dysfunction of parvalbuminergic interneurons may be a result of impaired myelin plasticity. Fast-spiking parvalbuminergic interneurons are essential in generating cortical oscillations in the gamma range (30–120 Hz), mediated by synchronized inhibition of pyramidal neurons [58,59]. Through rhythmic perisomatic inhibition of pyramidal neurons, synchronous ensembles of parvalbuminergic interneurons evoke high-frequency gamma oscillations in the cortex and hippocampus [60,61]. These gamma oscillations can be determined by electroencephalographic (EEG) recordings [62]. In SZ, dysfunctional gamma oscillations are the basis of deficits in cognitive functions, such as attention and working memory [63–65]. Impaired maturation of interneuron-related gamma oscillations may be a fundamental link between the cognitive and memory deficits associated with early life stress and the etiologies of SZ, which are based on aberrant neurodevelopment [66].

The relationship between oligodendrocytes and interneuron pathology in SZ is unknown [67]. A large fraction of myelinating oligodendrocytes ensheath fast-spiking parvalbuminergic interneurons. The fast-spiking parvalbumin-positive inhibitory interneurons of the basket cell class, which have very high tonic activity, may require myelin to support their high-energy demands [68], and it is presumed that myelin regulates extracellular potassium buffering [69,70]. Glycolytic oligodendrocytes support the energy demands of axonal intermediate metabolism by delivering lactate to the encapsulated axonal compartment, so that neuronal mitochondria can generate ATP [71,72]. Moreover, optogenetic activation of parvalbumin-positive interneurons in the mouse primary visual cortex (V1) sharpens neuronal feature selectivity and improves perceptual discrimination, and therefore, parvalbuminergic activation has functional and behavioral impact [73]. Lactate needs to be delivered because myelin prevents axons from having rapid access to extracellular metabolites. This concept of metabolic coupling of myelin and axons is an important new development in neuroscience [74]. Besides myelination and metabolic support, electrically coupled perisomatic oligodendrocytes buffer K+ currents and influence high-frequency neuronal excitability, e.g., of excitatory pyramidal [69] and hippocampal inhibitory interneurons [75].

7. The Role of Environmental Risk Factors in Oligodendrocyte Differentiation

Myelination of the brain has been shown to depend on experiences, and neurodevelopmental stress-related disturbances in social experience-dependent myelination have been proposed to play a role in SZ [76]. The mouse model of social isolation immediately after weaning (postnatal day 21–50) presents with a deficit in oligodendrocyte morphology, reduced myelin thickness, decreased MBP and MAG expression, a deficit in SZ-related behavior (PPI, working memory), and decreased social exploration [77,78]. Importantly, in contrast to the effects of adult social isolation, this early induced phenotype could not be rescued by later social re-integration [78]. In adult mice exposed to social isolation, clemastine, a muscarinic receptor antagonist, enhanced oligodendrocyte differentiation and myelination and improved social avoidance behavior [79].

Epidemiological studies have proven that exposure to early stress in the form of abuse and neglect in childhood increases the risk for later development of SZ [5,80,81]. Childhood abuse and neglect are known to have a negative influence on cognition in patients with SZ [5]. However, to date, no specific treatment exists for SZ-related cognitive deficits, negative symptoms, and underlying myelination and oligodendrocyte deficits. In this context, drug repurposing is a promising way to address new treatment targets aimed at improving outcome in SZ. Miconazole (an antifungal agent) and clobetasol (a corticosteroid) are known to improve remyelination and maturation of oligodendrocytes, and the latter is also an immunosuppressant. In the lysolecithin lesion model, a multiple sclerosis mouse model, both substances enhanced remyelination and increased the number of new oligodendrocytes. Moreover, these drugs enhanced differentiation and maturation of oligodendrocytes in mouse pluripotent epiblast stem cell-derived oligodendrocyte progenitor cells [82].

8. The Impact of Genetic Schizophrenia Risk on the Oligodendroglial Linage

Genome-wide association studies (GWAS) and exome sequencing approaches have provided solid evidence of common and rare genetic variations in complex psychiatric disorders such as SZ. So far, around 150 genetic risk single nucleotide polymorphisms (SNPs) have been unequivocally identified [83], and more loci will be revealed by the most recent GWAS studies with increased sample sizes. GWAS have validated the polygenic architecture of SZ, which was postulated decades before [84]. Further analysis identified several risk SNPs associated with genes of known regulatory function in neurons and also SNPs associated with genes relevant for glial cells, oligodendrocyte progenitor cells, and mature oligodendrocytes [85–87]. Remarkably, the expert-curated glia-oligodendrocyte pathway (comprising 52 genes) is associated more strongly with the genetic risk for SZ than with that for bipolar disorder [86]. In a study of uncurated but computed cell type-specific gene expression based on mice scRNA-seq and human snRNAseq data, SZ risk genes identified in GWAS were most significantly associated with a dedicated set of mature neuronal cell types (medium spiny neurons, cortical and hippocampal glutamatergic projection neurons, and cortical GABAergic interneurons) than with other neuronal or glial cell types [87]. However, based on only human cell-type specific gene expression profiles, oligodendrocyte progenitor cells and oligodendrocytes also showed enrichment in genes associated with SZ. In this study, the cell-type association of astrocytes or microglia was much lower [87]. Interestingly, increasing evidence indicates that aerobic exercise increases hippocampal volume and improves cognition in SZ patients [88–90]. Previous studies showed that the effects of exercise on the hippocampus might be connected to the polygenic burden of SZ risk variants [89]. The modulatory role of cell type-specific SZ polygenic risk scores (PRS) on exercise-induced volume changes in the CA1, CA2/3, and CA4/dentate gyrus subfields was recently assessed. These analyses showed that the polygenic burden associated with oligodendrocyte precursor cells and radial glia significantly influenced the volume changes between baseline and three months in the CA4/dentate gyrus subfield in SZ patients performing endurance training. A higher oligodendrocyte precursor cell- or RG-associated genetic risk burden was associated with a less pronounced volume increase or even a decrease in CA4/dentate gyrus during the exercise intervention. Therefore, it was hypothesized that SZ cell type-specific polygenic risk modulates the aerobic exercise-induced neuroplastic processes in CA4/dentate gyrus of the hippocampus [91].

9. Patient-Derived Neurobiological Test Systems Indicate Oligodendroglial Contribution to SZ

Until recently, most insights into SZ have been generated from postmortem tissue samples and imaging, genetic, pharmacological, and animal studies. Cellular reprogramming methods to generate induced pluripotent stem cells (iPSC) now provide a new opportunity to model the complex polygenetic conditions of SZ by generating patient-derived human iPSC (hiPSC)-based neurobiological test systems [92,93]. The pioneer work of Brennand et al. (2011) first characterized hiPSC-derived neurons from SZ patients and revealed decreased neuronal connectivity, decreased neurites, and decreased levels of post-synaptic protein PSD95 [94]. Subsequent studies focused on specific neuronal subtypes, such as pyramidal cortical interneurons and dentate gyrus granule neurons, and a series of studies revealed cell-autonomous neuronal disturbances in SZ [92,95]. Although pioneer studies confirmed postmortem findings and revealed additional aspects of the molecular mechanisms of

SZ, hiPSC-based disease modeling has several limitations. Economical and technical limitations include high costs, biological intra- and inter-individual variability, robustness of applied protocols, affordability, and scalability. Most studies included fewer than five individuals per group, and only a few included more than 10 individuals per group. However, the field of hiPSC is rapidly evolving and is addressing the above-mentioned challenges. Nevertheless, several conceptual limitations will remain, at least in the medium term. Examples of such conceptual limitations are as follows: (1) hiPSC-based systems cannot fully mimic the human gene x real world environment interactions that are part of the etiology of SZ [96], although aspects of known environmental risk factors (e.g., infection, stress, inflammation) can be modeled [95]; (2) hiPSC-based models are more powerful models of genetic risk for SZ than of SZ as a disease entity; (3) hiPSC models do not mimic network macro connectivity, which is assumed to be disturbed in SZ [97]; and, (4) long-lasting processes, such as aging and maturation over many years, are disturbed in SZ [98] but are difficult to mimic in vitro.

In contrast to investigations on hiPSC-derived neurons, only very few studies have investigated the impact of oligodendroglial cells in SZ-related hiPSC models. Expression of the SZ risk gene FEZ1 is regulated by SZ-relevant pathways, and knockdown of FEZ1 in murine and human iPSC-derived oligodendroglial cells was found to disturb oligodendrocyte development [99]. A family-based approach used hiPSC oligodendrocyte progenitor cells to investigate the contribution to SZ of two rare missense mutations in CSPG4, which codes for NG2, a prominent marker for proliferating oligodendrocyte progenitor cells [100]. The study found that hiPSC oligodendrocyte progenitor cells with one of the CSPG4 mutations showed dysregulated posttranslational processing, subcellular localization of mutant NG2, and impaired oligodendrocyte progenitor cell survival, with reduced differentiation to mature oligodendrocytes. Carrier-derived hiPSC neurons were not pathological, underlining the oligodendroglial cell-autonomous effect of the CSPG4 mutations. Remarkably, DTI-detectable impairments of white matter integrity were found in affected mutation carriers but not in their unaffected siblings or the general population [100]. In a pioneer study by Windrem and colleagues [101] in hiPSC from patients with childhood-onset SZ, glial precursor cells, which could mature into both oligodendroglial and astroglial lineage cells, showed altered transcriptomic signatures and impaired astroglial maturation and hypomyelination. Moreover, immune-deficient mice that received human precursor cells from SZ patients showed psychosis-related behaviors and cognitive impairments compared with control mice that received cells from healthy individuals [101]. Another study revealed reduced differentiation of hiPSC-derived marker O4 of the oligodendrocyte lineage (O4-positive cells) late oligodendrocyte progenitor cells and oligodendrocytes in SZ patient-derived hiPSC lines compared with control lines. Moreover, white matter myelin content correlated with the number of O4-positive cells [102]. The above studies underline the cell-autonomous contribution of the oligodendroglial lineage to SZ. However, they have several limitations. Family-based studies investigated single, rare SZ variants with large effects [99,100], but the genetic reality of most SZ patients is a polygenic accumulation of common variants with low individual effect sizes [83]. Windrem et al. studied glial progenitor cells (GPCs) in a very limited number of individuals with childhood-onset SZ (a rare disorder) with a very time-consuming experimental protocol (>200 days to generate GPCs) [101], which limits subsequent functional analysis or rescue experiments. McPhie et al. found evidence for impaired development of oligodendrocytes in SZ, but their analysis was limited to immunocytochemistry and did not dissect possible underlying mechanisms [102]. All these pioneering studies used different approaches that needed 65 to more than 200 days. Therefore, studies are needed that pave the way for modeling diseases within a shorter time and thus enable the cell-type specific dissection of disturbed pathways, gene regulation, and molecular mechanisms in a more systematic and potentially scalable manner.

Technically, and similar to the case with neurons, two different strategies are available to generate hiPSC-derived oligodendrocyte progenitor cells/oligodendrocytes (for details, we refer the reader to detailed reviews [103,104]). The first and older strategy is to mimic the embryological and "natural" development of oligodendrocyte progenitor cells/oligodendrocytes by in vitro patterning with chemical stimulation. The advantage of this method is that researchers can investigate the developmental aspect of a disease. The disadvantages are the time (it takes 55 to more than 200 days to generate O4+ late-stage oligodendrocyte progenitor cells) and costs of generating oligodendrocyte progenitor cells/oligodendrocytes. Recent developments have tried to accelerate extracellular lineage pattering by adding ectopic expression of cell-type determining transcription factors [105,106]. This approach allows hiPSCs to be differentiated to MBP+ oligodendrocytes within 22 days [106]. An additional advantage is the reduced cellular heterogeneity. Probably the most important disadvantages of directed differentiation approaches are their limitations in studying the early developmental aspects of SZ [93]. Oligodendrocyte progenitor cells and oligodendrocytes are heterogeneous across brain regions and vary with age [107], so investigations are needed that address this diversity.

10. The Road to New Therapies

Imaging, postmortem, and pioneer hiPSC studies have provided evidence for cell-autonomous deficits of the oligodendroglial lineage in SZ (Table 1). Despite the tremendous progress in two- and three-dimensional hiPSC-derived myelinating neurobiological test systems, these systems are always limited by their construct validity in brain disorders, where circuit levels contribute to behavioral and cognitive deficits. Nevertheless, patient-specific cellular systems enable the study of disease-associated endophenotypes, such as axonal support or multiple aspects of myelination, and expand the experimental repertoire in psychiatric research [93].

Table 1. Summary of disturbed oligodendrocyte function in schizophrenia. CA4: cornu ammonis 4; DLPFC: dorsolateral prefrontal cortex; hiPSC: human induced pluripotent stem cells; iPSC: induced pluripotent stem cells; MAG: myelin-associated glycoprotein; MBP: myelin basic protein; MOG: myelin oligodendrocyte glycoprotein; SZ: schizophrenia.

In vivo brain imaging studies	• Decreased fractional anisotropy as a sign of impaired white matter tract integrity [14,17] • Deficits in connectivity in relevant neuronal networks [108] • Single nucleotide polymorphisms in the *MAG* and *Olig2* genes are related to white matter tract integrity and cognitive performance [21]
Histopathology (postmortem)	• Decreased oligodendrocyte number in DLPFC and CA4 of the hippocampus [24,26,27] • Decreased MBP immunohistochemical staining intensity [39] • Reduced density of perineuronal oligodendrocytes [23]
Transcriptomic studies	• Decreased expression of myelin- and oligodendrocyte-related genes, such as *MAG* and *MBP*, in several relevant brain regions [109,110]
Proteomic studies	• Decreased expression of myelin- and oligodendrocyte-related proteins, such as MOG and MBP, in several relevant gray and white matter brain regions [37,38]
hiPSC studies	• Impaired oligodendrocyte maturation and hypomyelinization after neonatal implantation into mice of iPSC-derived oligodendrocyte progenitor cells from SZ patients [101] • Reduced differentiation of O4-positive late oligodendrocyte precursor cells and oligodendrocytes from SZ hiPSC lines compared with control hiPSC lines. Correlation between white matter myelin content and number of O4-positive cells [102]

Besides technical and conceptual limitations of hiPSC-based disease modeling of a complex disease such as SZ, a major challenge in generating useful patient-derived neurobiological test systems is meaningful patient stratification [93]. Future translational studies need to investigate the characteristics of such stratification. A stringent, at best hypothesis-driven pre-selection of relevant patient subgroups might allow corresponding molecular mechanisms to be identified in SZ. In addition to human and animal in vivo studies, hiPSC technology might be a key method to identify diseases-relevant cellular and molecular profiles and to perform subsequent genetic and pharmacological rescue experiments

(Figure 1). Despite important limitations, hiPSC-based disease modeling represents a new and potentially powerful option to study cellular phenotypes in SZ. hiPSC technology allows researchers to use personalized strategies to address old questions and might help identify different molecular pathways as potential targets for new treatment strategies.

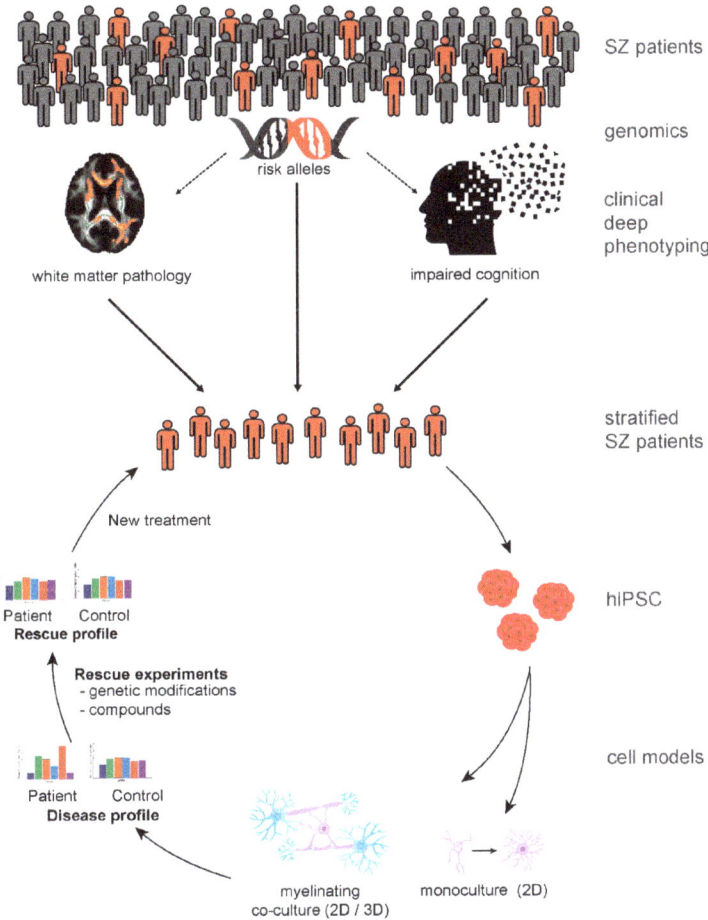

Figure 1. Principals of patient stratification for subsequent human-induced pluripotent stem cell (hiPSC)-based cellular disease modeling and new treatment strategies. Stratification of schizophrenia (SZ) patients could be based on genetics or endophenotypes or a combination of the two. Recent evidence suggests that patients with oligodendrocyte dysfunction and white matter pathology have cognitive impairments. Red human icons illustrate patients who are risk gene carriers with the shared endophenotypes of disturbed white matter pathology and impaired cognition. Meaningful patient stratification based on genomics and clinical deep phenotyping enables subsequent investigations of underlining cellular and molecular mechanisms. hiPSC technology enables the generation of a toolbox of patient-derived cell models. Monocultures of glial cells and myelinating co-culture systems could simulate disease-relevant endophenotype profiles of SZ in vitro. Moreover, hiPSC-derived models can be used for genetic and pharmacological rescue experiments and pave the way for new treatment options. Aspects or parts of the illustrations have been published previously [93,111].

Author Contributions: Conceptualization of the review, F.J.R. and A.S.; Writing—Original Draft Preparation, F.J.R. and A.S.; Writing—Review and Editing, F.J.R., L.S., M.J.R., L.C.-C., M.S., P.G.F., and A.S.; Visualization, F.J.R.

Funding: This work was supported by grants from the German Research Foundation (SPP Glia RO 4076/3-1 and PsyCourse, FKZ RO 4076/5-1, RO 241/16-1 and FA 241/16-1) to M.J.R. and P.G.F. Furthermore, it was funded by the Else Kröner-Fresenius Foundation (A.S., F.J.R. and P.G.F.).

Acknowledgments: We thank Jacquie Klesing, board-certified Editor in the Life Sciences (ELS), for editing assistance with the manuscript.

Conflicts of Interest: The authors declare no conflict of interest. The funding sponsors were not involved in the conceptualization or writing of this review.

References

1. Green, M.F. What are the functional consequences of neurocognitive deficits in schizophrenia? *Am. J. Psychiatry* **1996**, *153*, 321–330. [CrossRef]
2. Green, M.F.; Horan, W.P.; Lee, J. Nonsocial and social cognition in schizophrenia: Current evidence and future directions. *World Psychiatry* **2019**, *18*, 146–161. [CrossRef]
3. Goff, D.C.; Hill, M.; Barch, D. The treatment of cognitive impairment in schizophrenia. *Pharm. Biochem. Behav.* **2011**, *99*, 245–253. [CrossRef]
4. Hasan, A.; Falkai, P.; Wobrock, T.; Lieberman, J.; Glenthoj, B.; Gattaz, W.F.; Thibaut, F.; Moller, H.J. World Federation of Societies of Biological Psychiatry (WFSBP) Guidelines for Biological Treatment of Schizophrenia, part 1: Update 2012 on the acute treatment of schizophrenia and the management of treatment resistance. *World J. Biol. Psychia.* **2012**, *13*, 318–378. [CrossRef] [PubMed]
5. Popovic, D.; Schmitt, A.; Kaurani, L.; Senner, F.; Papiol, S.; Malchow, B.; Fischer, A.; Schulze, T.G.; Koutsouleris, N.; Falkai, P. Childhood Trauma in Schizophrenia: Current Findings and Research Perspectives. *Front. Neurosci.* **2019**, *13*, 274. [CrossRef] [PubMed]
6. Schmitt, A.; Malchow, B.; Hasan, A.; Falkai, P. The impact of environmental factors in severe psychiatric disorders. *Front. Neurosci.* **2014**, *8*, 19. [CrossRef] [PubMed]
7. Hermoye, L.; Saint-Martin, C.; Cosnard, G.; Lee, S.K.; Kim, J.; Nassogne, M.C.; Menten, R.; Clapuyt, P.; Donohue, P.K.; Hua, K.; et al. Pediatric diffusion tensor imaging: Normal database and observation of the white matter maturation in early childhood. *Neuroimage* **2006**, *29*, 493–504. [CrossRef] [PubMed]
8. Miller, D.J.; Duka, T.; Stimpson, C.D.; Schapiro, S.J.; Baze, W.B.; McArthur, M.J.; Fobbs, A.J.; Sousa, A.M.; Sestan, N.; Wildman, D.E.; et al. Prolonged myelination in human neocortical evolution. *Proc. Natl. Acad. Sci. USA* **2012**, *109*, 16480–16485. [CrossRef]
9. Hoistad, M.; Segal, D.; Takahashi, N.; Sakurai, T.; Buxbaum, J.D.; Hof, P.R. Linking white and grey matter in schizophrenia: Oligodendrocyte and neuron pathology in the prefrontal cortex. *Front. Neuroanat* **2009**, *3*, 9. [CrossRef]
10. Timmler, S.; Simons, M. Grey matter myelination. *Glia* **2019**, *67*, 2063–2070. [CrossRef]
11. Alba-Ferrara, L.M.; de Erausquin, G.A. What does anisotropy measure? Insights from increased and decreased anisotropy in selective fiber tracts in schizophrenia. *Front. Integr. Neurosci.* **2013**, *7*, 9. [CrossRef] [PubMed]
12. Boggs, J.M. Myelin basic protein: A multifunctional protein. *Cell. Mol. Life Sci.* **2006**, *63*, 1945–1961. [CrossRef] [PubMed]
13. Chang, E.H.; Argyelan, M.; Aggarwal, M.; Chandon, T.S.; Karlsgodt, K.H.; Mori, S.; Malhotra, A.K. The role of myelination in measures of white matter integrity: Combination of diffusion tensor imaging and two-photon microscopy of CLARITY intact brains. *Neuroimage* **2017**, *147*, 253–261. [CrossRef] [PubMed]
14. Ellison-Wright, I.; Bullmore, E. Meta-analysis of diffusion tensor imaging studies in schizophrenia. *Schizophr Res.* **2009**, *108*, 3–10. [CrossRef] [PubMed]
15. Yao, L.; Lui, S.; Liao, Y.; Du, M.Y.; Hu, N.; Thomas, J.A.; Gong, Q.Y. White matter deficits in first episode schizophrenia: An activation likelihood estimation meta-analysis. *Prog. Neuro-Psychoph.* **2013**, *45*, 100–106. [CrossRef]
16. Vitolo, E.; Tatu, M.K.; Pignolo, C.; Cauda, F.; Costa, T.; Ando, A.; Zennaro, A. White matter and schizophrenia: A meta-analysis of voxel-based morphometry and diffusion tensor imaging studies. *Psychiat. Res. Neuroim.* **2017**, *270*, 8–21. [CrossRef]

17. Kelly, S.; Jahanshad, N.; Zalesky, A.; Kochunov, P.; Agartz, I.; Alloza, C.; Andreassen, O.A.; Arango, C.; Banaj, N.; Bouix, S.; et al. Widespread white matter microstructural differences in schizophrenia across 4322 individuals: Results from the ENIGMA Schizophrenia DTI Working Group. *Mol. Psychiatr.* **2018**, *23*, 1261–1269. [CrossRef]
18. Kuroki, N.; Kubicki, M.; Nestor, P.G.; Salisbury, D.F.; Park, H.J.; Levitt, J.J.; Woolston, S.; Frumin, M.; Niznikiewicz, M.; Westin, C.F.; et al. Fornix integrity and hippocampal volume in male schizophrenic patients. *Biol. Psychiatry* **2006**, *60*, 22–31. [CrossRef]
19. Lim, K.O.; Ardekani, B.A.; Nierenberg, J.; Butler, P.D.; Javitt, D.C.; Hoptman, M.J. Voxelwise correlational analyses of white matter integrity in multiple cognitive domains in schizophrenia. *Am. J. Psychiatry* **2006**, *163*, 2008–2010. [CrossRef]
20. Fields, R.D. White matter in learning, cognition and psychiatric disorders. *Trends Neurosci.* **2008**, *31*, 361–370. [CrossRef]
21. Voineskos, A.N.; Felsky, D.; Kovacevic, N.; Tiwari, A.K.; Zai, C.; Chakravarty, M.M.; Lobaugh, N.J.; Shenton, M.E.; Rajji, T.K.; Miranda, D.; et al. Oligodendrocyte genes, white matter tract integrity, and cognition in schizophrenia. *Cereb Cortex* **2013**, *23*, 2044–2057. [CrossRef] [PubMed]
22. Kristensen, T.D.; Mandl, R.C.W.; Raghava, J.M.; Jessen, K.; Jepsen, J.R.M.; Fagerlund, B.; Glenthoj, L.B.; Wenneberg, C.; Krakauer, K.; Pantelis, C.; et al. Widespread higher fractional anisotropy associates to better cognitive functions in individuals at ultra-high risk for psychosis. *Hum. Brain Mapp.* **2019**, *40*, 5185–5201. [CrossRef] [PubMed]
23. Vostrikov, V.M.; Uranova, N.A.; Orlovskaya, D.D. Deficit of perineuronal oligodendrocytes in the prefrontal cortex in schizophrenia and mood disorders. *Schizophr Res.* **2007**, *94*, 273–280. [CrossRef] [PubMed]
24. Hof, P.R.; Haroutunian, V.; Friedrich, V.L., Jr.; Byne, W.; Buitron, C.; Perl, D.P.; Davis, K.L. Loss and altered spatial distribution of oligodendrocytes in the superior frontal gyrus in schizophrenia. *Biol. Psychiatry* **2003**, *53*, 1075–1085. [CrossRef]
25. Segal, D.; Schmitz, C.; Hof, P.R. Spatial distribution and density of oligodendrocytes in the cingulum bundle are unaltered in schizophrenia. *Acta Neuropathol.* **2009**, *117*, 385–394. [CrossRef] [PubMed]
26. Schmitt, A.; Steyskal, C.; Bernstein, H.G.; Schneider-Axmann, T.; Parlapani, E.; Schaeffer, E.L.; Gattaz, W.F.; Bogerts, B.; Schmitz, C.; Falkai, P. Stereologic investigation of the posterior part of the hippocampus in schizophrenia. *Acta Neuropathol.* **2009**, *117*, 395–407. [CrossRef]
27. Falkai, P.; Malchow, B.; Wetzestein, K.; Nowastowski, V.; Bernstein, H.G.; Steiner, J.; Schneider-Axmann, T.; Kraus, T.; Hasan, A.; Bogerts, B.; et al. Decreased Oligodendrocyte and Neuron Number in Anterior Hippocampal Areas and the Entire Hippocampus in Schizophrenia: A Stereological Postmortem Study. *Schizophr Bull.* **2016**, *42* Suppl. 1, S4–S12. [CrossRef]
28. Falkai, P.; Steiner, J.; Malchow, B.; Shariati, J.; Knaus, A.; Bernstein, H.G.; Schneider-Axmann, T.; Kraus, T.; Hasan, A.; Bogerts, B.; et al. Oligodendrocyte and Interneuron Density in Hippocampal Subfields in Schizophrenia and Association of Oligodendrocyte Number with Cognitive Deficits. *Front. Cell. Neurosci.* **2016**, *10*, 78. [CrossRef]
29. Arnett, H.A.; Fancy, S.P.; Alberta, J.A.; Zhao, C.; Plant, S.R.; Kaing, S.; Raine, C.S.; Rowitch, D.H.; Franklin, R.J.; Stiles, C.D. bHLH transcription factor Olig1 is required to repair demyelinated lesions in the CNS. *Science* **2004**, *306*, 2111–2115. [CrossRef]
30. Falkai, P.; Rossner, M.J.; Schulze, T.G.; Hasan, A.; Brzozka, M.M.; Malchow, B.; Honer, W.G.; Schmitt, A. Kraepelin revisited: Schizophrenia from degeneration to failed regeneration. *Mol. Psychiatry* **2015**, *20*, 671–676. [CrossRef]
31. Lavenex, P. Functional anatomy, development, and pathology of the hippocampus. In *The Clinical Neurobiology of The Hippocampus: An Integrative View*; Bartsch, T., Ed.; Oxford University Press: Oxford, UK, 2012.
32. Falkai, P.; Bogerts, B. Cell loss in the hippocampus of schizophrenics. *Eur. Arch. Psychiatry Neurol. Sci.* **1986**, *236*, 154–161. [CrossRef] [PubMed]
33. Das, T.; Ivleva, E.I.; Wagner, A.D.; Stark, C.E.; Tamminga, C.A. Loss of pattern separation performance in schizophrenia suggests dentate gyrus dysfunction. *Schizophr Res.* **2014**, *159*, 193–197. [CrossRef] [PubMed]
34. Williams, R.W.; Rakic, P. Three-dimensional counting: An accurate and direct method to estimate numbers of cells in sectioned material. *J. Comp. Neurol.* **1988**, *278*, 344–352. [CrossRef] [PubMed]
35. Schmitz, C.; Hof, P.R. Design-based stereology in neuroscience. *Neuroscience* **2005**, *130*, 813–831. [CrossRef] [PubMed]

36. Cassoli, J.S.; Guest, P.C.; Malchow, B.; Schmitt, A.; Falkai, P.; Martins-de-Souza, D. Disturbed macro-connectivity in schizophrenia linked to oligodendrocyte dysfunction: From structural findings to molecules. *NPJ Schizophr.* **2015**, *1*, 15034. [CrossRef] [PubMed]
37. Saia-Cereda, V.M.; Cassoli, J.S.; Schmitt, A.; Falkai, P.; Nascimento, J.M.; Martins-de-Souza, D. Proteomics of the corpus callosum unravel pivotal players in the dysfunction of cell signaling, structure, and myelination in schizophrenia brains. *Eur. Arch. Psychiatry Clin. Neurosci.* **2015**, *265*, 601–612. [CrossRef]
38. Martins-de-Souza, D.; Gattaz, W.F.; Schmitt, A.; Maccarrone, G.; Hunyadi-Gulyás, E.; Eberlin, M.N.; Souza, G.H.; Marangoni, S.; Novello, J.C.; Turck, C.W.; et al. Proteomic analysis of dorsolateral prefrontal cortex indicates the involvement of cytoskeleton, oligodendrocyte, energy metabolism and new potential markers in schizophrenia. *J. Psychiatr. Res.* **2009**, *43*, 978–986. [CrossRef]
39. Parlapani, E.; Schmitt, A.; Erdmann, A.; Bernstein, H.G.; Breunig, B.; Gruber, O.; Petroianu, G.; von Wilmsdorff, M.; Schneider-Axmann, T.; Honer, W.; et al. Association between myelin basic protein expression and left entorhinal cortex pre-alpha cell layer disorganization in schizophrenia. *Brain Res.* **2009**, *1301*, 126–134. [CrossRef]
40. Habib, N.; Li, Y.; Heidenreich, M.; Swiech, L.; Avraham-Davidi, I.; Trombetta, J.J.; Hession, C.; Zhang, F.; Regev, A. Div-Seq: Single-nucleus RNA-Seq reveals dynamics of rare adult newborn neurons. *Science* **2016**, *353*, 925–928. [CrossRef]
41. Miron, V.E.; Kuhlmann, T.; Antel, J.P. Cells of the oligodendroglial lineage, myelination, and remyelination. *Biochim. Biophys. Acta* **2011**, *1812*, 184–193. [CrossRef]
42. Jakel, S.; Agirre, E.; Mendanha Falcao, A.; van Bruggen, D.; Lee, K.W.; Knuesel, I.; Malhotra, D.; Ffrench-Constant, C.; Williams, A.; Castelo-Branco, G. Altered human oligodendrocyte heterogeneity in multiple sclerosis. *Nature* **2019**, *566*, 543–547. [CrossRef] [PubMed]
43. Cui, Q.L.; Kuhlmann, T.; Miron, V.E.; Leong, S.Y.; Fang, J.; Gris, P.; Kennedy, T.E.; Almazan, G.; Antel, J. Oligodendrocyte progenitor cell susceptibility to injury in multiple sclerosis. *Am. J. Pathol.* **2013**, *183*, 516–525. [CrossRef] [PubMed]
44. Mauney, S.A.; Pietersen, C.Y.; Sonntag, K.C.; Woo, T.W. Differentiation of oligodendrocyte precursors is impaired in the prefrontal cortex in schizophrenia. *Schizophr. Res.* **2015**, *169*, 374–380. [CrossRef] [PubMed]
45. Kuhlmann, T.; Remington, L.; Maruschak, B.; Owens, T.; Bruck, W. Nogo-A is a reliable oligodendroglial marker in adult human and mouse CNS and in demyelinated lesions. *J. Neuropathol. Exp. Neurol.* **2007**, *66*, 238–246. [CrossRef]
46. Kuhlmann, T.; Miron, V.; Cui, Q.; Wegner, C.; Antel, J.; Bruck, W. Differentiation block of oligodendroglial progenitor cells as a cause for remyelination failure in chronic multiple sclerosis. *Brain* **2008**, *131*, 1749–1758. [CrossRef]
47. van Kesteren, C.F.; Gremmels, H.; de Witte, L.D.; Hol, E.M.; Van Gool, A.R.; Falkai, P.G.; Kahn, R.S.; Sommer, I.E. Immune involvement in the pathogenesis of schizophrenia: A meta-analysis on postmortem brain studies. *Transl. Psychiatry* **2017**, *7*, e1075. [CrossRef]
48. Najjar, S.; Pearlman, D.M. Neuroinflammation and white matter pathology in schizophrenia: Systematic review. *Schizophr. Res.* **2015**, *161*, 102–112. [CrossRef]
49. Uranova, N.A.; Vostrikov, V.M.; Vikhreva, O.V.; Zimina, I.S.; Kolomeets, N.S.; Orlovskaya, D.D. The role of oligodendrocyte pathology in schizophrenia. *Int. J. Neuropsychoph.* **2007**, *10*, 537–545. [CrossRef]
50. Vikhreva, O.V.; Rakhmanova, V.I.; Orlovskaya, D.D.; Uranova, N.A. Ultrastructural alterations of oligodendrocytes in prefrontal white matter in schizophrenia: A post-mortem morphometric study. *Schizophr. Res.* **2016**, *177*, 28–36. [CrossRef]
51. Guest, P.C.; Iwata, K.; Kato, T.A.; Steiner, J.; Schmitt, A.; Turck, C.W.; Martins-de-Souza, D. MK-801 treatment affects glycolysis in oligodendrocytes more than in astrocytes and neuronal cells: Insights for schizophrenia. *Front. Cell. Neurosci.* **2015**, *9*, 180. [CrossRef]
52. Falkai, P.; Schmitt, A.; Cannon, T.D. Pathophysiology of Schizophrenia. In *Schizophrenia*; Herrman, H., Gaebel, W., Eds.; Wiley-Blackwell: Singapore, 2011; pp. 31–65.
53. Schmitt, A.; Malchow, B.; Keeser, D.; Falkai, P.; Hasan, A. Neurobiology of schizophrenia: New findings from the structure to the molecules. *Nervenarzt* **2015**, *86*, 324–326, 328–331. [CrossRef] [PubMed]
54. Lewis, D.A.; Curley, A.A.; Glausier, J.R.; Volk, D.W. Cortical parvalbumin interneurons and cognitive dysfunction in schizophrenia. *Trends Neurosci.* **2012**, *35*, 57–67. [CrossRef] [PubMed]

55. Stedehouder, J.; Kushner, S.A. Myelination of parvalbumin interneurons: A parsimonious locus of pathophysiological convergence in schizophrenia. *Mol. Psychiatry* **2017**, *22*, 4–12. [CrossRef] [PubMed]
56. Micheva, K.D.; Wolman, D.; Mensh, B.D.; Pax, E.; Buchanan, J.; Smith, S.J.; Bock, D.D. A large fraction of neocortical myelin ensheathes axons of local inhibitory neurons. *Elife* **2016**, *5*. [CrossRef]
57. Lin, S.C.; Bergles, D.E. Synaptic signaling between GABAergic interneurons and oligodendrocyte precursor cells in the hippocampus. *Nat. Neurosci.* **2004**, *7*, 24–32. [CrossRef]
58. Cardin, J.A.; Carlen, M.; Meletis, K.; Knoblich, U.; Zhang, F.; Deisseroth, K.; Tsai, L.H.; Moore, C.I. Driving fast-spiking cells induces gamma rhythm and controls sensory responses. *Nature* **2009**, *459*, 663–667. [CrossRef]
59. Sohal, V.S.; Zhang, F.; Yizhar, O.; Deisseroth, K. Parvalbumin neurons and gamma rhythms enhance cortical circuit performance. *Nature* **2009**, *459*, 698–702. [CrossRef]
60. Hormuzdi, S.G.; Pais, I.; LeBeau, F.E.N.; Towers, S.K.; Rozov, A.; Buhl, E.H.; Whittington, M.A.; Monyer, H. Impaired Electrical Signaling Disrupts Gamma Frequency Oscillations in Connexin 36-Deficient Mice. *Neuron* **2001**, *31*, 487–495. [CrossRef]
61. Traub, R.D.; Kopell, N.; Bibbig, A.; Buhl, E.H.; LeBeau, F.E.N.; Whittington, M.A. Gap Junctions between Interneuron Dendrites Can Enhance Synchrony of Gamma Oscillations in Distributed Networks. *J. Neurosci.* **2001**, *21*, 9478–9486. [CrossRef]
62. Hu, H.; Gan, J.; Jonas, P. Interneurons. Fast-spiking, parvalbumin(+) GABAergic interneurons: From cellular design to microcircuit function. *Science* **2014**, *345*, 1255263. [CrossRef]
63. Senkowski, D.; Gallinat, J. Dysfunctional prefrontal gamma-band oscillations reflect working memory and other cognitive deficits in schizophrenia. *Biol. Psychiatry* **2015**, *77*, 1010–1019. [CrossRef] [PubMed]
64. Gonzalez-Burgos, G.; Cho, R.Y.; Lewis, D.A. Alterations in cortical network oscillations and parvalbumin neurons in schizophrenia. *Biol. Psychiatry* **2015**, *77*, 1031–1040. [CrossRef] [PubMed]
65. Hall, M.H.; Chen, C.Y.; Cohen, B.M.; Spencer, K.M.; Levy, D.L.; Ongur, D.; Smoller, J.W. Genomewide association analyses of electrophysiological endophenotypes for schizophrenia and psychotic bipolar disorders: A preliminary report. *Am. J. Med. Genet. B Neuropsychiatr. Genet.* **2015**, *168B*, 151–161. [CrossRef] [PubMed]
66. Dricks, S. Effects of neonatal stress on gamma oscillations in hippocampus. *Sci. Rep.* **2016**, *6*, 29007. [CrossRef] [PubMed]
67. Schmitt, A.; Simons, M.; Cantuti-Castelvetri, L.; Falkai, P. A new role for oligodendrocytes and myelination in schizophrenia and affective disorders? *Eur. Arch. Psychiatry Clin. Neurosci.* **2019**, *269*, 371–372. [CrossRef] [PubMed]
68. Stedehouder, J.; Couey, J.J.; Brizee, D.; Hosseini, B.; Slotman, J.A.; Dirven, C.M.F.; Shpak, G.; Houtsmuller, A.B.; Kushner, S.A. Fast-spiking Parvalbumin Interneurons are Frequently Myelinated in the Cerebral Cortex of Mice and Humans. *Cereb Cortex* **2017**, *27*, 5001–5013. [CrossRef] [PubMed]
69. Battefeld, A.; Klooster, J.; Kole, M.H. Myelinating satellite oligodendrocytes are integrated in a glial syncytium constraining neuronal high-frequency activity. *Nat. Commun.* **2016**, *7*, 11298. [CrossRef]
70. Snaidero, N.; Simons, M. The logistics of myelin biogenesis in the central nervous system. *Glia* **2017**, *65*, 1021–1031. [CrossRef]
71. Funfschilling, U.; Supplie, L.M.; Mahad, D.; Boretius, S.; Saab, A.S.; Edgar, J.; Brinkmann, B.G.; Kassmann, C.M.; Tzvetanova, I.D.; Mobius, W.; et al. Glycolytic oligodendrocytes maintain myelin and long-term axonal integrity. *Nature* **2012**, *485*, 517–521. [CrossRef]
72. Lee, Y.; Morrison, B.M.; Li, Y.; Lengacher, S.; Farah, M.H.; Hoffman, P.N.; Liu, Y.; Tsingalia, A.; Jin, L.; Zhang, P.W.; et al. Oligodendroglia metabolically support axons and contribute to neurodegeneration. *Nature* **2012**, *487*, 443–448. [CrossRef]
73. Lee, S.H.; Kwan, A.C.; Zhang, S.; Phoumthipphavong, V.; Flannery, J.G.; Masmanidis, S.C.; Taniguchi, H.; Huang, Z.J.; Zhang, F.; Boyden, E.S.; et al. Activation of specific interneurons improves V1 feature selectivity and visual perception. *Nature* **2012**, *488*, 379–383. [CrossRef] [PubMed]
74. Nave, K.A. Myelination and support of axonal integrity by glia. *Nature* **2010**, *468*, 244–252. [CrossRef] [PubMed]
75. Yamazaki, Y.; Hozumi, Y.; Kaneko, K.; Fujii, S. Modulatory Effects of Perineuronal Oligodendrocytes on Neuronal Activity in the Rat Hippocampus. *Neurochem Res.* **2018**, *43*, 27–40. [CrossRef]

76. Toritsuka, M.; Makinodan, M.; Kishimoto, T. Social Experience-Dependent Myelination: An Implication for Psychiatric Disorders. *Neural Plast.* **2015**, *2015*, 465345. [CrossRef] [PubMed]
77. Varty, G.B.; Powell, S.B.; Lehmann-Masten, V.; Buell, M.R.; Geyer, M.A. Isolation rearing of mice induces deficits in prepulse inhibition of the startle response. *Behav. Brain Res.* **2006**, *169*, 162–167. [CrossRef] [PubMed]
78. Makinodan, M.; Rosen, K.M.; Ito, S.; Corfas, G. A critical period for social experience-dependent oligodendrocyte maturation and myelination. *Science* **2012**, *337*, 1357–1360. [CrossRef]
79. Liu, J.; Dupree, J.L.; Gacias, M.; Frawley, R.; Sikder, T.; Naik, P.; Casaccia, P. Clemastine Enhances Myelination in the Prefrontal Cortex and Rescues Behavioral Changes in Socially Isolated Mice. *J. Neurosci.* **2016**, *36*, 957–962. [CrossRef]
80. Varese, F.; Barkus, E.; Bentall, R.P. Dissociation mediates the relationship between childhood trauma and hallucination-proneness. *Psychol. Med.* **2012**, *42*, 1025–1036. [CrossRef]
81. Bonoldi, I.; Simeone, E.; Rocchetti, M.; Codjoe, L.; Rossi, G.; Gambi, F.; Balottin, U.; Caverzasi, E.; Politi, P.; Fusar-Poli, P. Prevalence of self-reported childhood abuse in psychosis: A meta-analysis of retrospective studies. *Psychiatry Res.* **2013**, *210*, 8–15. [CrossRef]
82. Najm, F.J.; Madhavan, M.; Zaremba, A.; Shick, E.; Karl, R.T.; Factor, D.C.; Miller, T.E.; Nevin, Z.S.; Kantor, C.; Sargent, A.; et al. Drug-based modulation of endogenous stem cells promotes functional remyelination in vivo. *Nature* **2015**, *522*, 216–220. [CrossRef]
83. Pardinas, A.F.; Holmans, P.; Pocklington, A.J.; Escott-Price, V.; Ripke, S.; Carrera, N.; Legge, S.E.; Bishop, S.; Cameron, D.; Hamshere, M.L.; et al. Common schizophrenia alleles are enriched in mutation-intolerant genes and in regions under strong background selection. *Nat. Genet.* **2018**. [CrossRef]
84. Gottesman, I.I.; Shields, J. A polygenic theory of schizophrenia. *Proc. Natl. Acad. Sci. USA* **1967**, *58*, 199–205. [CrossRef]
85. Tansey, K.E.; Hill, M.J. Enrichment of schizophrenia heritability in both neuronal and glia cell regulatory elements. *Transl. Psychiatry* **2018**, *8*, 7. [CrossRef] [PubMed]
86. Duncan, L.E.; Holmans, P.A.; Lee, P.H.; O'Dushlaine, C.T.; Kirby, A.W.; Smoller, J.W.; Ongur, D.; Cohen, B.M. Pathway analyses implicate glial cells in schizophrenia. *PLoS ONE* **2014**, *9*, e89441. [CrossRef] [PubMed]
87. Skene, N.G.; Bryois, J.; Bakken, T.E.; Breen, G.; Crowley, J.J.; Gaspar, H.A.; Giusti-Rodriguez, P.; Hodge, R.D.; Miller, J.A.; Munoz-Manchado, A.B.; et al. Genetic identification of brain cell types underlying schizophrenia. *Nat. Genet.* **2018**, *50*, 825–833. [CrossRef] [PubMed]
88. Pajonk, F.G.; Wobrock, T.; Gruber, O.; Scherk, H.; Berner, D.; Kaizl, I.; Kierer, A.; Muller, S.; Oest, M.; Meyer, T.; et al. Hippocampal plasticity in response to exercise in schizophrenia. *Arch. Gen. Psychiatry* **2010**, *67*, 133–143. [CrossRef]
89. Papiol, S.; Popovic, D.; Keeser, D.; Hasan, A.; Schneider-Axmann, T.; Degenhardt, F.; Rossner, M.J.; Bickeboller, H.; Schmitt, A.; Falkai, P.; et al. Polygenic risk has an impact on the structural plasticity of hippocampal subfields during aerobic exercise combined with cognitive remediation in multi-episode schizophrenia. *Transl. Psychiatry* **2017**, *7*, e1159. [CrossRef]
90. Firth, J.; Stubbs, B.; Rosenbaum, S.; Vancampfort, D.; Malchow, B.; Schuch, F.; Elliott, R.; Nuechterlein, K.H.; Yung, A.R. Aerobic Exercise Improves Cognitive Functioning in People with Schizophrenia: A Systematic Review and Meta-Analysis. *Schizophr Bull.* **2017**, *43*, 546–556. [CrossRef]
91. Papiol, S.; Keeser, D.; Hasan, A.; Schneider-Axmann, T.; Raabe, F.; Degenhardt, F.; Rossner, M.J.; Bickeböller, H.; Cantuti-Castelvetri, L.; Simons, M.; et al. Polygenic burden associated to oligodendrocyte precursor cells and radial glia influences the hippocampal volume changes induced by aerobic exercise in schizophrenia patients. *Transl. Psychiatry* **2019**, *9*. [CrossRef]
92. Soliman, M.A.; Aboharb, F.; Zeltner, N.; Studer, L. Pluripotent stem cells in neuropsychiatric disorders. *Mol. Psychiatry* **2017**, *22*, 1241–1249. [CrossRef]
93. Raabe, F.J.; Galinski, S.; Papiol, S.; Falkai, P.G.; Schmitt, A.; Rossner, M.J. Studying and modulating schizophrenia-associated dysfunctions of oligodendrocytes with patient-specific cell systems. *NPJ Schizophr.* **2018**, *4*, 23. [CrossRef]
94. Brennand, K.J.; Simone, A.; Jou, J.; Gelboin-Burkhart, C.; Tran, N.; Sangar, S.; Li, Y.; Mu, Y.; Chen, G.; Yu, D.; et al. Modelling schizophrenia using human induced pluripotent stem cells. *Nature* **2011**, *473*, 221–225. [CrossRef]

95. Prytkova, I.; Brennand, K.J. Prospects for Modeling Abnormal Neuronal Function in Schizophrenia Using Human Induced Pluripotent Stem Cells. *Front. Cell. Neurosci.* **2017**, *11*, 360. [CrossRef] [PubMed]
96. Gottesman, I.I.; Gould, T.D. The endophenotype concept in psychiatry: Etymology and strategic intentions. *Am. J. Psychiatry* **2003**, *160*, 636–645. [CrossRef] [PubMed]
97. Schmitt, A.; Hasan, A.; Gruber, O.; Falkai, P. Schizophrenia as a disorder of disconnectivity. *Eur. Arch. Psychiatry Clin. Neurosci.* **2011**, *261* (Suppl. 2), S150–S154. [CrossRef]
98. Insel, T.R. Rethinking schizophrenia. *Nature* **2010**, *468*, 187–193. [CrossRef] [PubMed]
99. Chen, X.; Ku, L.; Mei, R.; Liu, G.; Xu, C.; Wen, Z.; Zhao, X.; Wang, F.; Xiao, L.; Feng, Y. Novel schizophrenia risk factor pathways regulate FEZ1 to advance oligodendroglia development. *Transl. Psychiatry* **2017**, *7*, 1293. [CrossRef]
100. de Vrij, F.M.; Bouwkamp, C.G.; Gunhanlar, N.; Shpak, G.; Lendemeijer, B.; Baghdadi, M.; Gopalakrishna, S.; Ghazvini, M.; Li, T.M.; Quadri, M.; et al. Candidate CSPG4 mutations and induced pluripotent stem cell modeling implicate oligodendrocyte progenitor cell dysfunction in familial schizophrenia. *Mol. Psychiatry* **2018**. [CrossRef] [PubMed]
101. Windrem, M.S.; Osipovitch, M.; Liu, Z.; Bates, J.; Chandler-Militello, D.; Zou, L.; Munir, J.; Schanz, S.; McCoy, K.; Miller, R.H.; et al. Human iPSC Glial Mouse Chimeras Reveal Glial Contributions to Schizophrenia. *Cell Stem Cell* **2017**, *21*, 195–208. [CrossRef] [PubMed]
102. McPhie, D.L.; Nehme, R.; Ravichandran, C.; Babb, S.M.; Ghosh, S.D.; Staskus, A.; Kalinowski, A.; Kaur, R.; Douvaras, P.; Du, F.; et al. Oligodendrocyte differentiation of induced pluripotent stem cells derived from subjects with schizophrenias implicate abnormalities in development. *Transl. Psychiatry* **2018**, *8*, 230. [CrossRef]
103. Goldman, S.A.; Kuypers, N.J. How to make an oligodendrocyte. *Development* **2015**, *142*, 3983–3995. [CrossRef] [PubMed]
104. Chanoumidou, K.; Mozafari, S.; Baron-Van Evercooren, A.; Kuhlmann, T. Stem cell derived oligodendrocytes to study myelin diseases. *Glia* **2019**. [CrossRef] [PubMed]
105. Ehrlich, M.; Mozafari, S.; Glatza, M.; Starost, L.; Velychko, S.; Hallmann, A.L.; Cui, Q.L.; Schambach, A.; Kim, K.P.; Bachelin, C.; et al. Rapid and efficient generation of oligodendrocytes from human induced pluripotent stem cells using transcription factors. *Proc. Natl. Acad. Sci. USA* **2017**, *114*, E2243–E2252. [CrossRef] [PubMed]
106. Garcia-Leon, J.A.; Kumar, M.; Boon, R.; Chau, D.; One, J.; Wolfs, E.; Eggermont, K.; Berckmans, P.; Gunhanlar, N.; de Vrij, F.; et al. SOX10 Single Transcription Factor-Based Fast and Efficient Generation of Oligodendrocytes from Human Pluripotent Stem Cells. *Stem Cell Rep.* **2018**, *10*, 655–672. [CrossRef] [PubMed]
107. Spitzer, S.O.; Sitnikov, S.; Kamen, Y.; Evans, K.A.; Kronenberg-Versteeg, D.; Dietmann, S.; de Faria, O., Jr.; Agathou, S.; Karadottir, R.T. Oligodendrocyte Progenitor Cells Become Regionally Diverse and Heterogeneous with Age. *Neuron* **2019**. [CrossRef]
108. Li, T.; Wang, Q.; Zhang, J.; Rolls, E.T.; Yang, W.; Palaniyappan, L.; Zhang, L.; Cheng, W.; Yao, Y.; Liu, Z.; et al. Brain-Wide Analysis of Functional Connectivity in First-Episode and Chronic Stages of Schizophrenia. *Schizophr Bull.* **2017**, *43*, 436–448. [CrossRef]
109. Hakak, Y.; Walker, J.R.; Li, C.; Wong, W.H.; Davis, K.L.; Buxbaum, J.D.; Haroutunian, V.; Fienberg, A.A. Genome-wide expression analysis reveals dysregulation of myelination-related genes in chronic schizophrenia. *Proc. Natl. Acad. Sci. USA* **2001**, *98*, 4746–4751. [CrossRef]
110. Haroutunian, V.; Katsel, P.; Dracheva, S.; Stewart, D.G.; Davis, K.L. Variations in oligodendrocyte-related gene expression across multiple cortical regions: Implications for the pathophysiology of schizophrenia. *Int. J. Neuropsychoph.* **2007**, *10*, 565–573. [CrossRef]
111. Raabe, F.J.; Spengler, D. Epigenetic Risk Factors in PTSD and Depression. *Front. Psychiatry* **2013**, *4*, 80. [CrossRef]

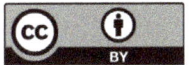

© 2019 by the authors. Licensee MDPI, Basel, Switzerland. This article is an open access article distributed under the terms and conditions of the Creative Commons Attribution (CC BY) license (http://creativecommons.org/licenses/by/4.0/).

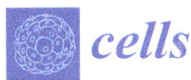

Article

Conditional Deletion of LRP1 Leads to Progressive Loss of Recombined NG2-Expressing Oligodendrocyte Precursor Cells in a Novel Mouse Model

Ina Schäfer [1], Johannes Kaisler [2], Anja Scheller [3], Frank Kirchhoff [3], Aiden Haghikia [2] and Andreas Faissner [1,*]

1. Department of Cell Morphology and Molecular Neurobiology, Ruhr University Bochum, Universitätsstr. 150, 44801 Bochum, Germany; Ina.Schaefer@rub.de
2. Research Center Neuroimmunology, Department of Neurology, Ruhr-University Bochum, Universitätsstr. 150, 44801 Bochum, Germany; Johannes.Kaisler@ruhr-uni-bochum.de (J.K.); Aiden.Haghikia@ruhr-uni-bochum.de (A.H.)
3. Department of Molecular Physiology, Center for Integrative Physiology and Molecular Medicine (CIPMM), University of Saarland, Building 48, 66421 Homburg, Germany; Anja.Scheller@uks.eu (A.S.); Frank.Kirchhoff@uks.eu (F.K.)
* Correspondence: andreas.faissner@rub.de; Tel.: +49-(0)234-32-28851

Received: 24 September 2019; Accepted: 27 November 2019; Published: 30 November 2019

Abstract: The low-density lipoprotein receptor-related protein 1 (LRP1) is a transmembrane receptor, mediating endocytosis and activating intracellular signaling cascades. LRP1 is highly expressed in the central nervous system (CNS), especially in oligodendrocyte precursor cells (OPCs). Previous studies have suggested LRP1 as a regulator in early oligodendrocyte development, repair of chemically induced white matter lesions, and cholesterol homeostasis. To circumvent embryonic lethality observed in the case of global LRP1 deletion, we generated a new inducible conditional knockout (KO) mouse model, which enabled an NG2-restricted LRP1 deficiency (NG2-CreERT2$^{ct2/wt}$xR26eGFP$^{flox/flox}$xLRP1$^{flox/flox}$). When characterizing our triple transgenic mouse model, we noticed a substantial and progressive loss of recombined LRP1-deficient cells in the oligodendrocyte lineage. On the other hand, we found comparable distributions and fractions of oligodendroglia within the Corpus callosum of the KO and control animals, indicating a compensation of these deficits. An initial study on experimental autoimmune encephalomyelitis (EAE) was performed in triple transgenic and control mice and the cell biology of oligodendrocytes obtained from the animals was studied in an in vitro myelination assay. Differences could be observed in these assays, which, however, did not achieve statistical significance, presumably because the majority of recombined LRP1-deficient cells has been replaced by non-recombined cells. Thus, the analysis of the role of LRP1 in EAE will require the induction of acute recombination in the context of the disease process. As LRP1 is necessary for the survival of OPCs in vivo, we assume that it will play an important role in myelin repair.

Keywords: cre-recombinase; demyelination; experimental autoimmune encephalomyelitis (EAE); glial progenitor cells; myelin; tamoxifen

---

1. Introduction

The low-density lipoprotein receptor-related protein 1 (LRP1) is a type-I transmembrane receptor. It consists of two covalently bound subunits, an 85 kDa intracellular α-chain and 515 kDa extracellular β-chain [1]. As a multifunctional receptor, LRP1 can bind a variety of up to 40 different ligands such as apolipoproteins (Apo), extracellular matrix molecules, and growth factors and is involved in their endocytosis [1,2]. Apolipoproteins, especially ApoE, mediate cholesterol transport in various cell types [3]. Beyond its endocytotic function, LRP1 is involved in intracellular signaling and can activate, for example, the ERK and AKT pathways [4–6].

The LRP1 receptor is widely expressed in the body (liver, lung, blood vessels) and particularly in the CNS [1,7,8]. Radial glia, neuroblasts, astrocytes, neurons, and especially oligodendrocyte precursor cells (OPCs) serve as main sources for LRP1 [9–12]. In the past, many studies have focused on LRP1 and demonstrated that a global deletion of the receptor leads to embryonic lethality [13]. Therefore, conditional *Lrp1*-knockout (KO) models have been developed. Previous studies have concentrated on LRP1 function in oligodendrocytes, the myelinating macroglia in the CNS. Originating from highly migratory and proliferative OPCs, which populate the forebrain, oligodendrocytes differentiate into mature cells in their target compartment. Due to cytoskeletal rearrangements, myelin membrane expansion of mature oligodendrocytes enables myelination, and thereby the electrical isolation of nerve fibers [14–16].

It has been shown that neural stem cells, which lack LRP1, have a significantly reduced potential to differentiate into OPCs, immature or mature oligodendrocytes, indicating a crucial role of LRP1 in oligodendrogenesis [10,11]. Accordingly, LRP1 has been found highly expressed in OPCs, whereas it is downregulated in mature, myelinating oligodendrocytes on both the mRNA and protein level [9,12,17]. This suggests a link between LRP1 and early oligodendrocyte development. Moreover, oligodendrocyte functions are affected by LRP1. Thus, LRP1 deletion in chemically induced white matter lesions revealed attenuated remyelination and compromised repair of white matter. Furthermore, cholesterol homeostasis is regulated by LRP1, which plays a key role in oligodendrocyte differentiation [16].

According to the preliminary data, we generated a new inducible, conditional KO mouse model with OPC-restricted LRP1-deficiency: NG2-CreERT2$^{ct2/wt}$xR26eGFP$^{flox/flox}$xLRP1$^{flox/flox}$. NG2, together with PDGFRα, serves as a marker for OPCs [18,19], which enabled us to delete LRP1 in early oligodendrocyte development and analyze the ensuing effects of LRP1-deficiency on the whole oligodendrocyte lineage. The characterization of our novel model revealed similar distributions and fractions of oligodendroglia in the Corpus callosum. However, substantial and progressive loss of recombined LRP1-deficient oligodendrocytes was observed over time. Moreover, when experimental autoimmune encephalomyelitis (EAE) was elicited by immunization with a MOG peptide, the LRP1 KO animals were more strongly affected, with greater functional deficits in comparison to the control. On the cellular level, the in vitro myelination assay revealed elongated internodes in the LRP1 KO condition. Considering our findings, we propose that LRP1 is a critical long-term regulator of oligodendrocyte survival in vivo and suggest a crucial role of LRP1 for myelin quality.

2. Materials and Methods

2.1. Ethics Statement

This study was carried out at the Ruhr-University Bochum with conformity to the recommendations of local guidelines in experimental animal handling. The animal experiments were approved by the "Landesamt für Natur, Umwelt, und Verbraucherschutz" (LANUV) in Recklinghausen, North Rhine-Westphalia with the reference number 84-02.04.2015.A149. The study referred to the 3Rs (Replacement, Reduction, Refinement) and tried to reduce animal numbers and refine experimental conditions.

2.2. Generation of the New Mouse Model and Housing

The new mouse model was generated by cross-breeding previously described mouse lines. LRP1$^{flox/flox}$ mice (B6;129S7-*Lrp1*^{tm2Her}/J), which were obtained from the Jackson Laboratory, and the transgenic constructs have been previously published by Rohlmann et al. [20]. In NG2-CreERT2$_{NGCE}$ mice, the inducible Cre DNA recombinase CreERT2 was knocked into the NG2 locus. Only heterozygous mice were used [21]. By crossbreeding the mice to homozygous floxed reporter mice [22], recombined cells could be identified by the genetically encoded GCaMP3 reporter expression that can be detected by anti-GFP antibodies. Since we did not take advantage of the Ca^{2+} indicating property of GCaMP3, we termed this reporter mouse line R26eGFP$^{flox/flox}$. By crossbreeding the two different mouse lines, NG2-CreERT2$^{ct2/wt}$xR26eGFP$^{flox/flox}$xLRP1$^{flox/flox}$ (KO) and NG2-CreERT2$^{wt/wt}$xR26eGFP$^{flox/flox}$xLRP1$^{flox/flox}$ (control) animals were generated in one litter. Both received tamoxifen via the lactating mother.

For in vivo analysis, postnatal day (P)7, P14, P21, P28, P42, P56, and P56–70 littermates were analyzed. An in vitro myelination assay (Figure S1) required P6 to P9 animals.

Animals were housed in an open cage system with 12 h-day/night-cycles and 25 °C room temperature. Water and diet were accessible ad libitum.

2.3. Genotyping

To genotype the littermates, genomic DNA from tail biopsies was used. All primers (Sigma, St. Louis, MO, USA), amplified product sizes, and sources are listed in Table 1 (base pairs: bp, for: forward, rev: reverse, WT: wildtype).

Table 1. Genotyping primers and amplified product sizes.

Gene	Primer Sequence	Product Size	Source
LRP1	for 5′-CATACCCTCTTCAAACCCCTTCCTG rev 5′-GCAAGCTCTCCTGCTCAGACCTGGA	WT: 291 bp KO: 350 bp	Jackson Laboratory
NG2-Cre (NGCE)	for 5′-GGCAAACCCAGAGCCCTGCC wt rev 5′-GCTGGAGCTGACAGCGGGTG Cre-ERT2 rev 5′-GCCCGGACCGACGATGAAGC	WT: 557 bp KO: 829 bP	[21]
Rosa26-GCaMP3	for wt 5′-CTCTGCTGCCTCCTGGCTTCT wt rev 5′-CGAGGCGGATCACAAGCAATA for KI 5′-CACGTGATGACAAACCTTGG rev KI 5′-GGCATTAAAGCAGCGTATCC	WT: 327 bp KO: 245 bp	[22]

2.4. Injection of Tamoxifen to Animals

The KO was induced via administration of tamoxifen. Therefore, feeding mothers were intraperitoneally injected with 100 mg/kg tamoxifen (Sigma) dissolved in corn oil (Sigma), on two consecutive days (Figure 1A). Maternal tamoxifen metabolites reached the pups via milk at postnatal days (p)3 and 4 (referring to [21]). Animals were monitored and weighed every 2–3 days and evaluated with a clinical score.

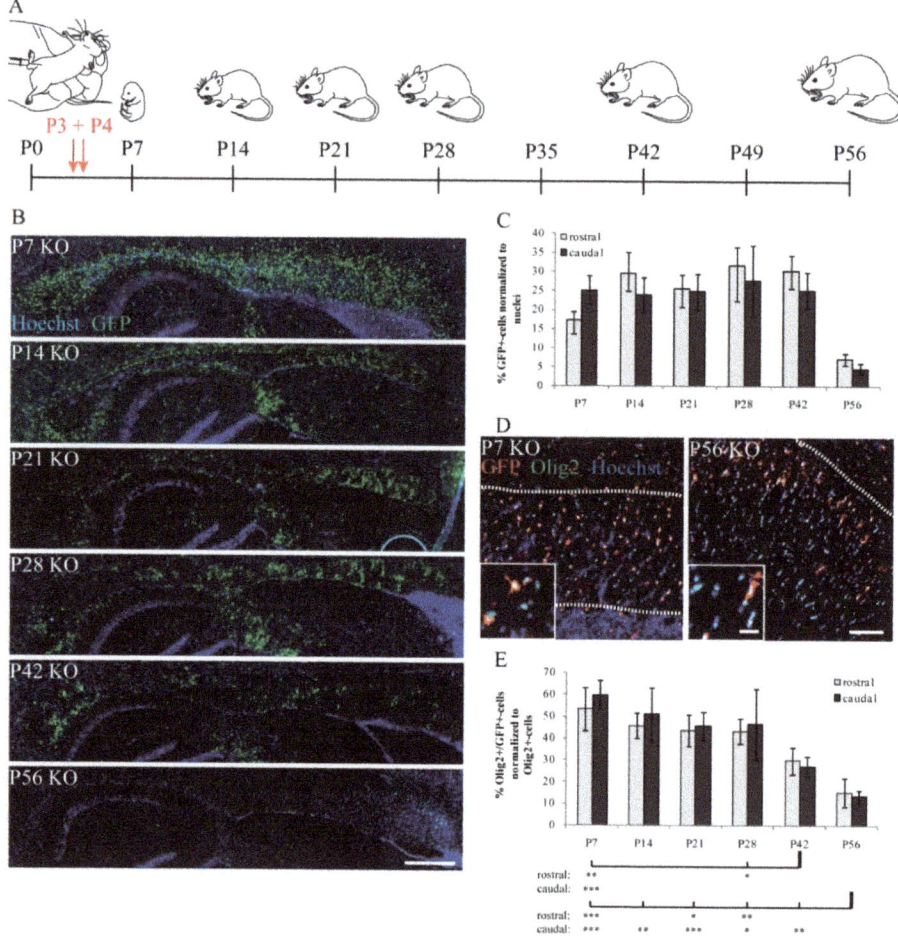

Figure 1. Recombination efficiency and portion of recombined cells over time. (**A**) Scheme of tamoxifen administration and analyzed ages of experimental animals. (**B**) Immunohistochemical stains against green fluorescent protein (GFP) indicating recombined cells within postnatal day (P) P7-P42 KO tissue (scale bars: 100 μm). (**C**) Quantification of GFP-expressing recombined cell fractions in the Corpus callosum of various analyzed stages. (**D**) Representative immunohistochemical staining against GFP and Olig2 (scale bars: 100 μm, 20 μm). (**E**) Quantification of double-positive cells for GFP and Olig2, defined as recombination efficiency, indicated an initial efficiency of more than 50%, before a significant and progressive loss of double-positive recombined LRP1 KO oligodendrocytes was observed over time. At P56, the loss of double-positive cells compared to earlier time points reached statistical significance, whereas this effect was not that prominent at P42 ($p \leq 0.05$ for *, $p \leq 0.01$ for **, and $p < 0.001$ for ***). Data are expressed as the mean ± SEM. N = 3–4, n = 9–12 per rostral and caudal part. At least 200–1200 cells per section were counted. Depending on normally or not normally distributed data, the Student's t-test or Mann–Whitney U test was used for evaluation within the individual ages.

2.5. Decapitation, Perfusion, and Dissection

For the experiments, P7 animals were decapitated, whereas P14, P21, P28, P42, P56, and P56–70 animals were anesthetized (100 mg/kg ketamine (CP-Pharma, Burgdorf, Germany), 10 mg/kg Xylazin (CP-Pharma)), and perfused with PBS/heparin (Ratiopharm, Ulm, Germany). Therefore, a constant pressure of 0.7 mL/min was generated with a peristaltic pump. After perfusion for 10–15 min, the animals were dissected. For all ages, the brains were removed from the skull and separated into hemispheres for cryosections, PCR, and western blot analysis.

2.6. Cryosections

For cryosections, the dissected tissue was postfixed in 4% paraformaldehyde (PFA; Carl Roth GmbH and Co. KG, Karlsruhe, Germany) overnight and afterward drained with 20% sucrose (Fisher Chemical by Thermo Fisher Scientific, Bedford, MA, USA), again overnight. The tissue was embedded in tissue freezing medium (Leica Biosystems, Mount Waverly, Australia) to prepare sagittal cryosections (14 μm). Cryosections were stored at −20 °C until further use.

2.7. Immunohistochemistry (IHC)

Intranuclear immunohistochemical staining started with incubation for 1 h in citrate buffer (solution A: 0.1 M citric acid-1-hydrate, solution B: 0.1 M Na-citrate-dihydrate; 1 mM of solution A and 4 mM of solution B in Aqua dest) at 70 °C. After three washes with PBS (10 × PBS: 137 mM NaCl, 3 mM KCl, 6.5 mM $Na_2HPO_4 \bullet 2H_2O$, 1.5 mM KH_2PO_4 in Aqua dest; 1 × PBS: 10 × PBS in Aqua dest, pH 7.4), blocking buffer (PBS, 0.1% Triton X-100, 1% bovine serum albumin (BSA, Sigma), 3% serum (Dianova GmbH, Hamburg, Germany)) was added to the slices for 1 h. The primary antibody was dissolved in blocking buffer and incubated on the sections overnight at 4 °C. Next, three washing steps with PBS followed and secondary antibody, dissolved in blocking buffer, was added for 2 h at room temperature. Finally, three washing steps in PBS and mounting with ImmuMount (Thermo Fisher Scientific) and coverslips were performed. Extranuclear immunohistochemical staining started with three PBS washes and followed the same protocol as described above. Antibodies: APC (clone CC1, 1:100, ab16794, Lot: GR322482-3, Abcam; Cambridge, UK), GFP (1:200, AB3080; Lot 2929345, Millipore by Merck, Darmstadt, Germany; 1:500, 600-101-215, Lot: 33301, Rockland Immunochemicals Inc., Limerick, PA, USA), LRP1 (1:500, ab92544, Lot: 6R259330-27, Abcam), Olig2 (1:400, AB9610, Lot: 3071572, Millipore), PDGFRα (1:300, sc-338, Lot: E2015, Santa Cruz Biotechnologies Inc., Dallas, TX, USA), Donkey α rabbit AF488 (1:250, 711-545-152, Lot: 127498, Jackson ImmunoResearch Laboratories Inc., West Grove, PA, USA), Donkey α rabbit Cy3 (1:500, 711-165-152, Lot: 130990, Jackson ImmunoResearch Laboratories Inc.), Donkey α mouse Cy5 (1:150, 715-175-150, Lot: 129945, Jackson ImmunoResearch Laboratories Inc.), rabbit α mouse Cy3 (1:500, 315-165-044, Lot: 131676, Jackson ImmunoResearch Laboratories Inc.), Donkey α goat AF488 (1:250, 705-545-147, Lot: 136089, Jackson ImmunoResearch Laboratories Inc.), and Donkey α goat Cy3 (1:500, 705-165-147, Lot: 139052, Jackson ImmunoResearch Laboratories Inc.).

2.8. Preparation of Tissue for Reverse Transcriptase-Polymerase Chain Reaction(RT-PCR) and Western Blot Analysis

For the PCR and western blot analysis, brain hemispheres were shortly thawed and Corpora callosa were dissected from the tissue with disposable scalpels (B. Braun, Melsungen, Germany). Afterward, the tissue was lysed with mRNA lysis buffer (Sigma: GenElute Mammalian Total RNA Miniprep Kit) or protein lysis buffer (50 mM Tris, 150 mM NaCl, 5 mM EDTA, 5 mM EGTA, 1% Triton X-100, 0.1% SDS, 0.1% Na-deoxycholate).

2.9. RT-PCR Analysis

To investigate mRNA expression in the tissue samples, mRNA was isolated from lysates and cDNA was synthesized following the manufacturer's instructions (Sigma: GenElute Mammalian Total RNA Miniprep Kit, Thermo Fisher Scientific: First Strand cDNA Synthesis Kit). Via RT-PCR *β-actin* (for: TAT GCC AAC ACA GTG CTG TCT GGT GG, rev: TAG AAG CAT TTG CGG TGG ACA ATG G), ***Mbp*** (for: TCT CAG CCC TGA CTT GTT CC, rev: ATC AAC CAT CAC CTG CCT TC) and ***Pdgfrα*** (for: GCA CCA AGT CAG GTC CCA TT, rev: CTT CAC TGG TGG CAT GGT CA) were amplified. All primers were from Sigma.

2.10. Western Blot Analysis

Proteins were separated by weight in 12% polyacrylamide-SDS-gels and transferred after to PVDF-membranes (Carl Roth) using a semi-dry transblot system (Carl Roth). Membranes were blocked with 5% skimmed milk powder (Heirler, Radolfzell, Germany) in tris-buffered saline with Tween TBST (0.05% Tween-20, 1 × TBS; 10 × TBS: 250 mM Tris/HCl pH 7.4, 1.5 M NaCl) (blocking solution) for 1 h. Membranes were incubated in primary antibody, dissolved in blocking solution at 4 °C overnight, followed by three washing steps in TBST. Next, a one-hour incubation with the secondary antibody, which was dissolved in blocking solution, and finally, three washing steps with TBST and one wash with 1 × TBS were carried out. Western blots were developed after incubation with the substrate solution (ECL Substrate, BioRad Lab. Inc., Hercules, CA, USA) for 5 min. Antibodies: LRP1 (1:10,000, ab92544, Lot: 6R259330-27, Abcam), MBP (1:1000, MCA409S, Lot: 161031A, BioRad), PDGFRα (1:10,000, sc-338, Lot: E2015, Santa Cruz), α-tubulin (1:10,000, T9026, Lot: 078M4796 V, Sigma), Goat α rabbit HRP (1:5000, 111-035-144, Lot: 132409, Jackson ImmunoResearch Laboratories Inc.), Goat α mouse HRP (1:10,000, 115-035-068, Lot: 132223, Jackson ImmunoResearch Laboratories Inc.), and Goat α rat (1:5000, 112-035-062, Lot: 90553, Jackson ImmunoResearch Laboratories Inc.).

2.11. Experimental Autoimmune Encephalomyelitis (EAE)

For the analysis of the functional effects of LRP1 on oligodendrocytes, experimental allergic encephalomyelitis (EAE) was induced. Tamoxifen-treated animals were generated and immunized with MOG_{35-55} peptide (synthesized at Charité Berlin, Germany) in complete Freund's adjuvant (incomplete Freund-adjuvant, M. tuberculosis H37 Ra, Difco Laboratories, Detroit, MI, USA) at the age of 8–10 weeks (P56–P70). Additionally, the animals received 250 ng/100 µL pertussis toxin (EMD Millipore Corporation by Merck) on the day of and two days after immunization. Clinical symptoms were evaluated using a 10-point-score scale (0 = normal, 1 = reduced tail tonus, 2 = complete tail palsy, 3 = lack of reflexive compensatory movements while walking, 4 = ataxia, 5 = slight paralysis of the hind legs, 6 = plegia of one leg or moderate paralysis of both legs, 7 = paraplegia with complete paralysis of both hind legs, 8 = tetraparesis with (slight) paralysis of front extremities, 9 = moribund, and 10 = death) and score and weight were documented on a daily basis. After 28 days of monitoring the course of disease, the experiment was stopped and the animals were sacrificed.

2.12. Imaging

Immunohistochemical stains were documented with AxioZoom V16, AxioCam 506mono, and Zen 2009 software by Zeiss (Oberkochen, Germany). Three caudal and three rostral images of each Corpus callosum were taken. RT-PCR results were kept by a documentation system from LTF Labortechnik (Wasserburg, Germany) with BioCaptw software. Protein gels and western blots were imaged with the documentation system MicroChemi and Gel Capture 6.6 software by DNR bio imaging systems (Jerusalem, Israel).

2.13. Quantification

Immunohistochemical stains were quantified by single cell counting in ImageJ/FIJI. Single cells were defined by nuclear stain with Hoechst dye, binding to nucleic acids. Immuno-positive cells were identified by expression of stage- or lineage-specific markers, depending on their expected localization (intranuclear, intracellular, extracellular). Three caudal and rostral sections of the Corpus callosum in the sagittal orientation were taken and at least 200–1200 cells per section were counted.

mRNA and protein expression were measured by intensity measurements in ImageJ/FIJI.

In some cases, significant reductions between two conditions were additionally calculated and mentioned in the text. Therefore, the higher value served as 100%.

2.14. Statistics

Statistics were depicted as mean ± SEM. Normal distribution of values was checked with the Shapiro–Wilk test. Depending on normally or not normally distributed values, the Student's *t*-test or Mann–Whitney U test was performed. Biological replicates were stated as "N" and technical replicates as "n". Immunohistochemical stains: N = 3–4, n = 9–12; PCR analysis: N = 4, n = 4; western blot analysis: N = 3, n = 3; EAE pilot study: N = 5, n = 5. Significant data were declared with a *p*-value (*p*) of 0.05. $p \leq 0.05$ for *, $p \leq 0.01$ for ** and $p < 0.001$ for ***. All statistical tests were performed with Microsoft Excel (Redmond, WA, USA).

3. Results

3.1. Induction of the NG2-Restricted LRP1-Deficient KO in the New Mouse Model

In order to investigate the role of LRP1 in the NG2-cell lineage, we generated the novel conditional knockout mouse model: NG2-CreERT2$^{ct2/wt}$xR26eGFP$^{flox/flox}$xLRP1$^{flox/flox}$ (KO) and NG2-CreERT2$^{wt/wt}$xR26eGFP$^{flox/flox}$xLRP1$^{flox/flox}$ (control). To induce the deletion, tamoxifen was applied to lactating mothers three and four days after the birth of the litters. For the analysis, we focused on six different age stages to evaluate different experimental aspects (Figure 1A).

First, we focused on the number of cells that recombined upon tamoxifen treatment by monitoring the expression of the reporter GCaMP3 detectable by anti-GFP antibodies. For the sake of simplicity, we refer to GCamP3-expressing cells as GFP- or reporter-expressing cells. Cells were counted in the Corpus callosum because this brain region represents a strongly myelinated fiber tract. Overall cell numbers were visualized using a nuclear marker (Hoechst dye) and the proportion of immunostained cells was recorded. Postnatally from P7 to P42, an increase in the number of GFP-expressing cells could be observed, before the fraction of immunopositive cells dropped rapidly at P56 (Figure 1B,C). For the rostral Corpus callosum, a range of maximally 31% ± 4.9% standard error of the mean (SEM) and minimally 7% ± 1.6% SEM was found over time. Similar to this finding, a maximum of 27% ± 9% SEM and a minimum of 4.7% ± 1.4% GFP-positive cells was present in the caudal region of the Corpus callosum (Figure 1C). These results suggest that initially from P7 to P42, about one third of the cells in the Corpus callosum showed Cre-mediated recombination, which represents the percentage of oligodendrocyte lineage cells generated by NG2 cells present at P3 to P5 at the time of tamoxifen injection.

To further assess the number of recombined cells that could be attributed to the oligodendrocyte lineage, we employed the lineage-specific marker Olig2 and analyzed the number of cells double-positive for GFP and Olig2. At P7, half of all oligodendrocytic Olig2-positive cells expressed GFP and revealed a recombination efficiency of 50% recombined LRP1-deficient oligodendrocytes. Surprisingly, we saw a significant reduction in the number of recombined oligodendrocytes over time (Figure 1D,E). Focusing at the maximum at P7, fractions of 53% ± 9.9% SEM rostrally and 59% ± 6.7% SEM caudally of GFP-expressing Olig2-positive cells were identified for the Corpus callosum. Reflecting a loss of recombined oligodendrocytes, a minimum of only 15% ± 6.6% SEM (rostral) and 13% ± 2.8% SEM (caudal) of GFP-expressing Olig2-positive cells was left at P56. Setting these fractions in relation to the starting point at P7, this signifies a rostral and caudal reduction of recombined oligodendrocyte lineage cells by 71.1% (53% ± 9.9% SEM reduced to 15% ± 6.6% SEM) and 77.3% (59% ± 6.7% SEM reduced to 13% ± 2.8% SEM), respectively. This strong effect illustrated a clear linkage between LRP1 expression and oligodendrocyte lineage cell survival. The most straightforward explanation for the progressive loss of recombined cells in the Olig2-lineage is presumably cell death as a consequence of LRP1 elimination.

3.2. LRP1 Expression in Oligodendrocyte Development

The new mouse model aims at LRP1-deficiency in OPCs and differentiating oligodendrocytes. Therefore, the analysis of LRP1-expressing cells was vitally important for the characterization of the model and the impact of LRP1 on oligodendrocytes. So, we performed immunohistochemical staining against LRP1 in relation to all cells assessed by nuclear stain (Figure 2 and Figure S2). Previous studies have demonstrated a decrease in LRP1-expression on the mRNA and protein level in the oligodendrocyte lineage during development [9,12], which was verified in our model during development with LRP1-expressing cells. LRP1-positive cells declined from P7 (Con maximum: 9.0% ± 1.9% SEM) to P56 (Con maximum: 0.2% ± 0.3% SEM) (Figure 2A,B). To assess the success of LRP1 deletion on protein level immunohistochemical staining against LRP1 were performed. Here, comparable fractions of LRP1-positive cells were observed in the KO when compared to the control at P7 (Con maximum: 9.0% ± 1.9%; KO maximum: 7.6 ± 2.0%). This indicates an incomplete recombination, or rather incomplete degradation of LRP1, at this time point shortly after tamoxifen-mediated induction. Notable differences were observed at P14 and P21, with significantly reduced fractions of LRP1-expressing cells in the KO when compared to the control. This demonstrated a successful recombination in terms of LRP1 deletion and the degradation of LRP1. In detail, we found a significant reduction by 72% (2.8% ± 1.4% SEM reduced to 0.8% ± 0.5% SEM) of LRP1-expressing cells from the control to KO condition at P14 in the caudal Corpus callosum ($p \leq 0.05$, *). One week later, highly significant reductions by 85% (2.1% ± 0.2% SEM reduced to 0.3% ± 0.3% SEM) rostrally and 73% (1.9% ± 0.5% SEM reduced to 0.5% ± 0.4% SEM) caudally in comparison with the control were shown for the KO at P21 ($p \leq 0.01$ **; $p \leq 0.001$ ***). Thus, a KO-dependent decrease in the LRP1-expressing cells was observed that confirmed the success of the inducible KO strategy. Accordingly, the loss of LRP1 in these cells might account for the previously detected reduced proportion of recombined cells (see above).

Strikingly, a significant difference between the control and KO was observed at P56. Whereas no LRP1-positive cells were found in the caudal Corpus callosum of the control, 0.5% of the cells expressed LRP1 in the KO (* $p \leq 0.05$).

In a complementary approach, we analyzed the time-dependent change of the cell fraction still double-positive for GFP and LRP1. This fraction represents the surviving cells of the oligodendrocyte lineage due to still incomplete protein degradation [23]. Immunohistochemical staining against LRP1 and GFP revealed a maximum at P7 with 2.4% ± 0.5% SEM (rostral) and 3.5% ± 0.7% SEM (caudal) of LRP1- and GFP-double-expressing cells. Within the next seven days, the fraction of double-positive cells dropped rapidly to 0.5% and less, and at P56, a minimum of 0.02% ± 0.03% SEM (rostral) and 0% (caudal) remained (Figure 2A,C). In conclusion, more than 95% of cells with recombined, and therefore activated reporter were devoid of LRP1 protein.

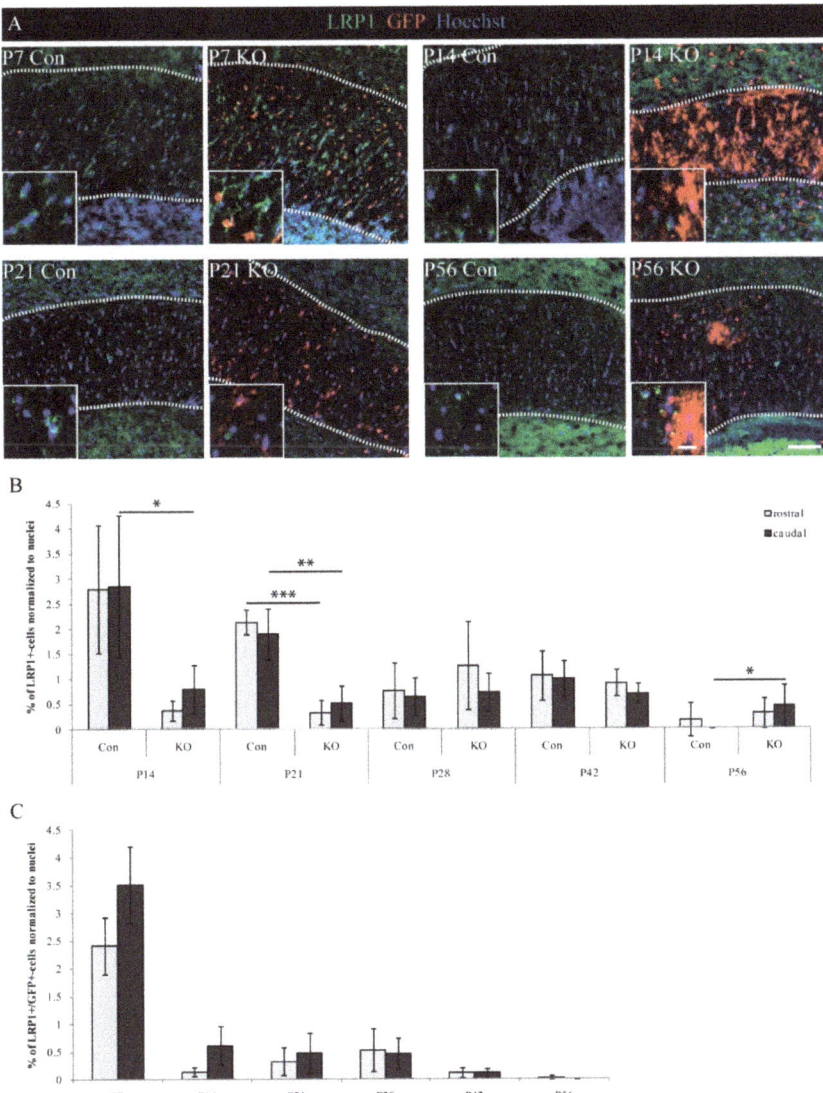

Figure 2. LRP1-expressing cells decreased over time. (**A**) Immunohistochemical staining against LRP1 and GFP to identify LRP1-expressing cells and double-positive cells, indicating reporter-positive cells that still expressed non-degraded LRP1 (scale bars: 100 µm, 20 µm). (**B**) Quantification of LRP1+-cells indicated a time-dependent reduction and proved the success of the inducible KO strategy with significantly reduced numbers of LRP1-expressing cells in the KO at P14 and P21 (* $p \leq 0.05$; ** $p \leq 0.01$; *** $p \leq 0.001$). (**C**) Time course of cell loss with LRP1 expression. Depicted is the remaining fraction of cells that were still double-positive for LRP1 and GFP. Please note that different experimental age stages are shown in diagrams (**B,C**). Data are expressed as the mean ± SEM. N = 3–4, n = 9–12 per rostral and caudal part. At least 200–1200 cells per section were counted. Depending on normally or not normally distributed data, the Student's *t*-test or Mann–Whitney U test was used for evaluation within the individual ages.

3.3. Proportion and Distribution of Control and KO Cells

In order to investigate the LRP1 KO-dependent effects specifically in the oligodendrocyte lineage, we analyzed the proportion and distribution of immature and mature oligodendrocytes in vivo. To this end, we prepared triple immunostainings to define different subpopulations of oligodendrocytes (Figure 3).

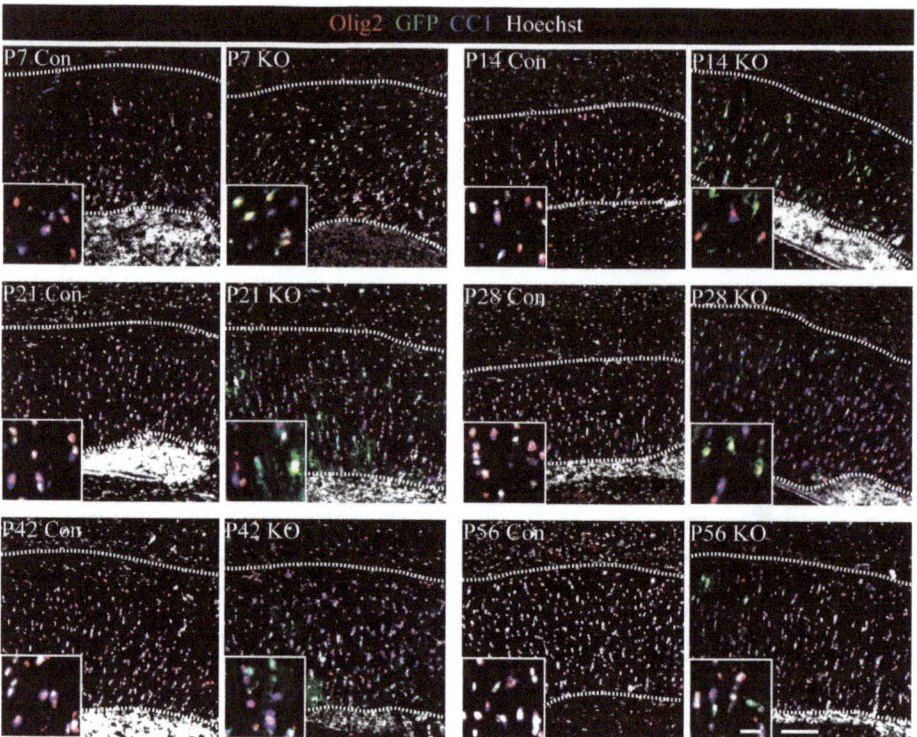

Figure 3. Triple immunohistochemical stainings showing mature and immature proportions within oligodendrocyte lineage in the Corpus callosum by Olig2, CC1, and GFP. Immunohistochemical stainings of P7–P56 control and KO tissue against Olig2, GFP, and CC1 (mature con cells defined as: Olig2+/CC1+/GFP−; mature KO cells: Olig2+/CC1+/GFP+; immature con cells defined as: Olig2+/CC1−/GFP−; immature KO cells: Olig2+/CC1−/GFP+) (scale bars: 100 µm, 20 µm).

Olig2 was used to label all oligodendrocytic cells. CC1-expressing cells were defined as mature oligodendrocytes, whereas CC1-negative cells were considered as immature cells. Based on the expression of GFP, KO cells (recombined) could be discriminated from non-recombined cells within the KO tissue. In this approach, mature oligodendrocytes were visualized by the marker combinations Olig2+/CC1+/GFP− (control; non-recombined in control tissue) and Olig2+/CC1+/GFP+ (KO; recombined in KO tissue). Immature oligodendrocytes were identified as Olig2+/CC1−/GFP− (control; non-recombined in control tissue) and Olig2+/CC1−/GFP+ (KO; recombined in KO tissue) (Figures 3–5).

First, the total numbers of Olig2-expressing cells served as references (100% value for the control and KO) for the analysis of mature and immature oligodendrocyte proportions in the control and KO tissue (Figures 4 and 5). For mature oligodendrocytes, an increase from P7 to P56 was observed in the control animals (rostral: 23.0% ± 3.9% to 67.8% ± 6.4%; caudal: 25.4% ± 1.7% to 66.6% ±

12.0%). However, the KO fraction supported our previously found progressive loss of LRP1-deficient oligodendrocytes with decreasing proportions in mature cells during development (rostral: 15.5% ± 3.2% to 5.7 ± 1.9%; caudal: 14.6% ± 3.3% to 8.6% ± 3.2%). For this comparison a highly significant impairment of the KO condition was observed when compared to the control (* $p \leq 0.05$; ** $p \leq 0.01$; *** $p \leq 0.001$).

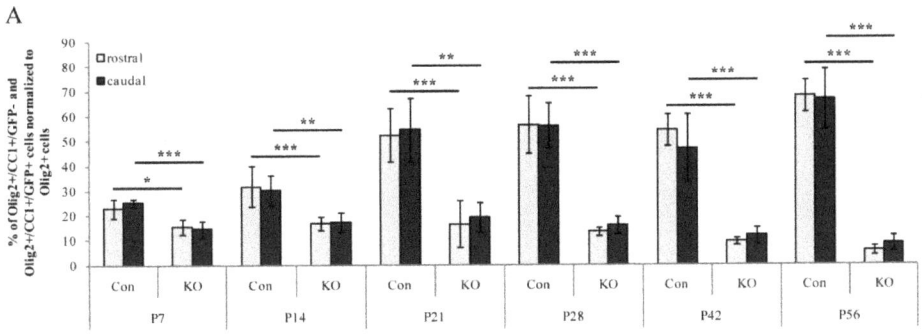

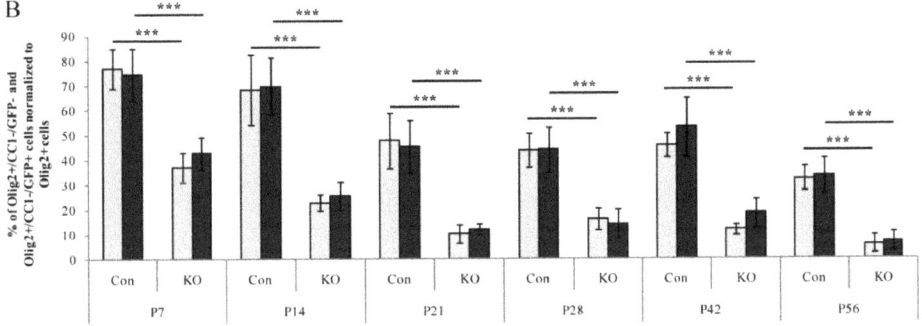

Figure 4. Comparison of mature and immature oligodendrocytes revealed significantly decreased fractions in the KO when compared to the control, indicating a progressive cell loss. (**A**) Quantification of mature proportions of recombined (Olig2+/CC1+/GFP+) and non-recombined oligodendrocytes (Olig2+/CC1+/GFP−), normalized to Olig2-positive cells indicated a significantly impaired KO fraction compared to the control (* $p \leq 0.05$; ** $p \leq 0.01$; *** $p \leq 0.001$). This observation demonstrated a progressive loss of LRP1-deficient oligodendrocytes during development. (**B**) Quantification of immature proportions of recombined (Olig2+/CC1−/GFP+) and non-recombined oligodendrocytes (Olig2+/CC1−/GFP−), normalized to Olig2-positive cells showed comparable results to the mature proportions. A significantly reduced fraction of LRP1-deficient oligodendrocytes developed over time (*** $p \leq 0.001$). Data are expressed as mean ± SEM. N = 3–4, n = 9–12 per rostral and caudal part. At least 200–1200 cells per section were counted. Depending on normally or not normally distributed data, the Student's *t*-test or Mann–Whitney U test was used for evaluation within the individual ages.

Furthermore, immature oligodendrocytes were investigated from P7 to P56 and revealed decreasing cell proportions for the control condition (rostral: 77.0% ± 8.0% to 32.2% ± 4.9%; caudal: 74.6% ± 10.5% to 33.4% ± 7.4%). Similar to mature LRP1-deficient KO oligodendrocytes, the proportion of immature KO cells also decreased over time (rostral: 37.2% ± 6.1% to 6.0% ± 3.7%; caudal: 42.8% ± 6.5% to 6.9% ± 3.9%). Again, a highly significant difference was seen between the control and the KO condition (*** $p \leq 0.001$). In summary, these findings support our previously shown data (Figure 1) regarding the progressive loss of LRP1-deficient oligodendrocytes compared to the control condition and the LRP1-dependent survival of oligodendrocytes.

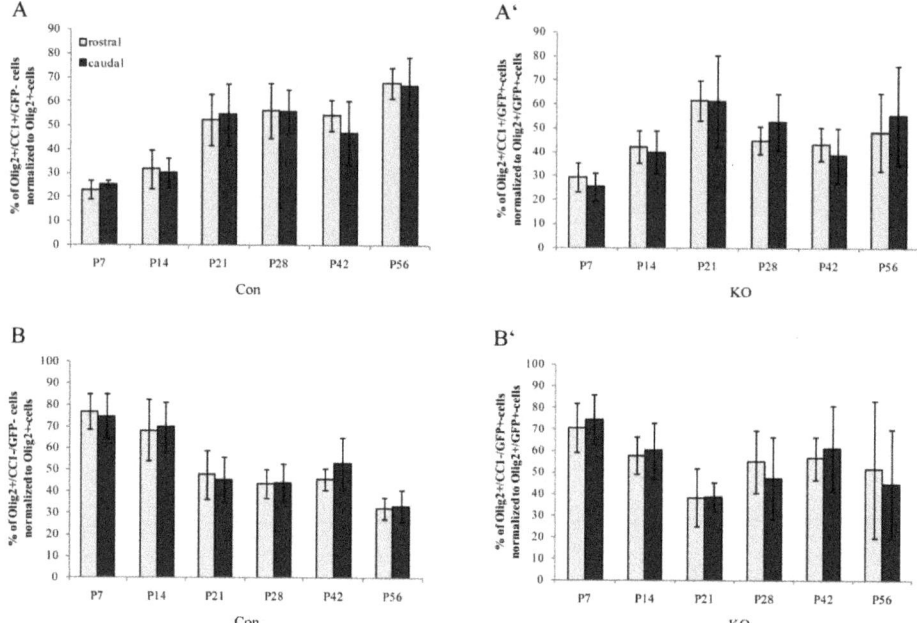

Figure 5. Proportions of persisting mature and immature oligodendrocyte lineage cells revealed similar differentiation and distribution in the KO condition when compared to the control. (A) Quantification of mature control oligodendrocyte proportions (Olig2+/CC1+/GFP− cells) normalized to Olig2+-cells revealed an increase from 20% to 65% over time. (A′) Quantification of mature KO oligodendrocyte proportions (Olig2+/CC1+/GFP+-cells) normalized to recombined Olig2+/GFP+-cells demonstrated an increase from P7 to P21 and comparable cell proportions afterwards. (B) Quantification of immature control oligodendrocyte proportions (Olig2+/CC1−/GFP-cells) normalized to Olig2+-cells exhibited decreasing proportions from 80% to 30% during development. (B′) Quantification of immature KO oligodendrocyte proportions (Olig2+/CC1−/GFP+-cells) normalized to Olig2+/GFP+-cells indicated a slight decrease over time. Please note that the presented proportions of mature and immature KO cells refer to the progressively decreasing recombined KO fraction (see Figure 1E). The minority of surviving LRP1-negative oligodendrocytes behaved similarly to the control. No statistically significant differences were observed between the KO and control conditions. Data are expressed as the mean ± SEM. N = 3–4, n = 9–12 per rostral and caudal part. At least 200–1200 cells per section were counted. Depending on normally or not normally distributed data, the Student's *t*-test or Mann–Whitney U test were used for evaluation within the individual ages.

In a further step, Olig2- (in the control tissue) as well as Olig2- and GFP-double expression (recombined cells in the KO tissue) were used to label the whole oligodendrocyte lineage fractions (100% reference values for the control and KO, respectively) (Figures 3 and 5). For this aspect, it is important to note that the following data showed relative proportions of mature/immature cells within the recombined LRP1-free cell fraction compared to the control. As shown in Figures 1 and 4, this recombined cell fraction was strongly reduced over time (compare Figure 1 reduction rostral: 71.1%, value: 53% ± 9.9% SEM reduced to 15% ± 6.6% SEM; reduction caudal: 77.3%, value: 59% ± 6.7% SEM reduced to 13% ± 2.8% SEM; see also Figure 4 and description above). This means that the absolute numbers of such KO cells found in the Corpus callosum were much lower than the control.

Focusing on the proportion of mature cells, a non-linear increase over time was observed (minimum: 23.0% ± 3.9% SEM, maximum: 67.8% ± 6.4% SEM) (Figure 5A,A'). At P21, the first peak was reached and the maximum of KO oligodendrocytes (67.8% ± 6.4% SEM) was detected, which slightly decreased until P56 (minimum 48.5% ± 16.4% SEM) (Figure 5A'). In contrast, the control condition revealed the opposite effect with a maximum at P56 (P21: 52.3% ± 10.6% SEM; P56: 67.8% ± 6.4% SEM) (Figure 5A).

The proportion of immature cells tended to decrease (Figure 5B,B'). From P7 to P21, a clear reduction in the fraction of immature cells was observed (maximum: 77.0% ± 8.0% SEM, minimum: 38.3% ± 13.3% SEM), which was comparable in both genotypes. Thereafter, the control cell fraction remained stable until P42 and finally decreased until P56 (minimum: 32.2% ± 4.9% SEM) (Figure 5B). Focusing on the KO, an increase to P42 (maximum: 61.3% ± 19.7% SEM) was determined, followed by a slight decrease until P56 (minimum: 44.7% ± 25.1% SEM) (Figure 5B').

Overall, the distribution of mature and immature oligodendrocytes in both genotypes was comparable at the individual postnatal age stages. However, the proportion of immature KO cells increased after P21, whereas the relating ratio of mature cells decreased in this LRP1-deficient fraction. In fact, our data suggest that although progressive elimination of Olig2-positive cells without LRP1 expression was observed via the loss of Olig2/GFP-double positive cells (Figures 1 and 4), the remaining fractions of oligodendrocyte lineage cells within the Corpus callosum revealed comparable characteristics. We assumed a compensatory effect by regenerative healthy cells at regions of progressive cell loss. The smaller proportion of remaining, recombined KO cells behaved similarly with regard to distribution and differentiation in the Corpus callosum compared to the control cells.

3.4. Cellular Characterization of Oligodendrocyte Lineage-Specific Cells

After the evaluation of the KO and successful recombination, we wanted to exclude side-effects on the oligodendrocyte population due to the tamoxifen-induced recombination. We aimed to compare oligodendrocyte lineage cell fractions in the Corpus callosum in a genotype-independent manner (including GFP+ and GFP− cells in the tissue) to validate potential gross differences in tissue composition between the control and KO animals. Therefore, subpopulations of oligodendrocytes of various differentiation stages (e.g., precursors and mature cells) were investigated. To this end, immunohistochemical stainings, using the lineage marker Olig2 (including OPCs and mature oligodendrocytes), the OPC marker PDGFRα (only OPCs), and the mature marker CC1 (mature oligodendrocytes only) were performed (Figure 6). Proportions of labeled cells were determined in relation to the overall cell number as revealed by staining the cell nuclei (Figure 6; see alternative analysis in Figure S3).

Focusing on the total number of Olig2-positive cells, we found slightly increasing numbers over time in both genotypes, starting with a minimum of 28.6% ± 3.8% SEM in the rostral KO Corpus callosum at P7, and reaching a maximum fraction of 65.9% ± 19.1% SEM in the rostral part at P56 (Figure 6A,B). Furthermore at P7 and P21, the KO conditions showed significantly different distributions of Olig2-positive cells within the Corpus callosum (* $p \leq 0.05$; ** $p \leq 0.01$). These can be explained with rostro-caudal differences due to differentiation, myelination, and development, which were the reason for the region-specific analysis in the present study [24–28]. As expected, the number of oligodendrocyte lineage cells in the Corpus callosum augmented with time.

Proceeding more specifically with progenitor and mature oligodendrocyte fractions, we noted inverse effects (Figure 6C,D). PDGFRα-positive OPCs decreased over time in the control and KO, starting with 17.8% ± 1.9% SEM (maximum, caudal, control) at P7, whereas only 0.9% ± 0.3% SEM (minimum, caudal, control) immunopositive cells remained in the adult stage at P56 (Figure 6C). In addition, a significantly increased OPC-fraction was observed at P56 for the KO in the rostral Corpus callosum compared to the control (** $p \leq 0.01$). In contrast, CC1-positive mature oligodendrocytes tended to increase within the first four weeks (until P28) (increase: 15%; value: 23.1% ± 2.7% SEM up to 44.3% ± 10.4% SEM) and surprisingly decreased afterward (reduction: 28%; value: 44.3 % ± 10.4% SEM reduced to 15.9% ± 3.8% SEM) (Figure 6D). Thus, the OPC population progressively matured, losing the PDGFRα marker, and expressing CC1. These data support the interpretation that the progressive loss of recombined LRP1-deleted oligodendrocytes is compensated by non-affected cells.

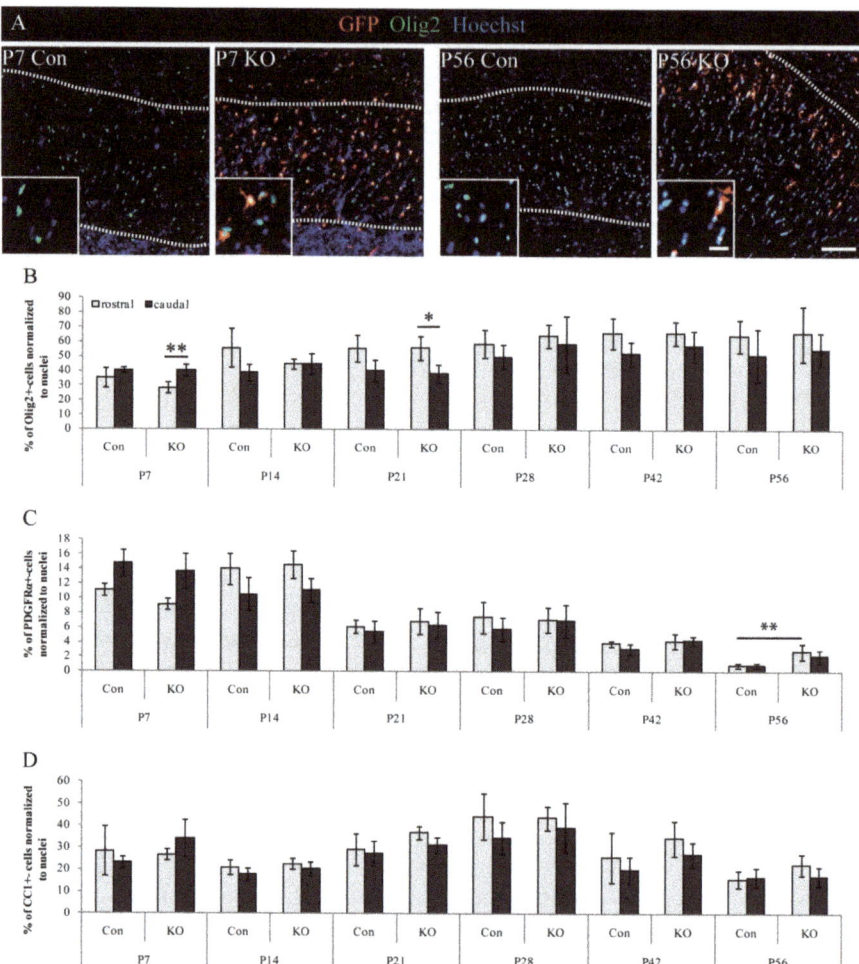

Figure 6. Analysis of stage-specific oligodendrocyte markers. (**A**) Representative immunohistochemical stainings against Olig2 and GFP for the control and KO animals at P7 and P56 (scale bars: 100 µm, 20 µm). (**B**) Quantification of Olig2+-cells indicated a slight increase over time with similar results for both genotypes. Significant caudo-rostral differences were observed in the KO at P7 and P21 (* $p \leq 0.05$; ** $p \leq 0.01$). (**C**) Quantification of PDGFRα+-OPCs from P7 to P56, demonstrating globally decreasing cell numbers and a significantly higher proportion of precursors in the KO when compared to the control at P56 (** $p \leq 0.01$). (**D**) Quantification of CC1-expressing mature oligodendrocytes revealed increasing numbers up to P28, followed by a decrease afterward. No difference was detectable between the control and KO. Data are expressed as mean ± SEM. N = 3–4, n = 9–12 per rostral and caudal part. At least 200–1200 cells per section were counted. Depending on normally or not normally distributed data, the Student's *t*-test or Mann–Whitney U test were used for evaluation within the individual ages (see supplementary analysis in Figure S3).

3.5. Molecular Characterization of Oligodendrocyte Lineage-Specific Cells

The above-mentioned results of the cellular characterization of oligodendrocytic cells by immunohistology were complemented by RT-PCR and western blot analysis referring to PDGFRα and MBP (myelin basic protein, a mature myelin marker) expression on the mRNA and protein level. Corpora callosa of the control and KO animals were prepared (Figure 7). In agreement with the results of immunohistochemistry, the RT-PCR and western blot results demonstrated increasing levels of the mature marker MBP and decreasing levels of the OPC marker PDGFRα over time (Figure 7A–E). Overall PCR and western blot analysis generally confirmed the previous findings obtained by immunohistochemistry, where a comparable outcome of oligodendrocyte maturation in both genotypes was observed. However, as an exception, we saw a significantly upregulated relative *Mbp* mRNA expression in the KO when compared to the control at P14 (** $p \leq 0.01$).

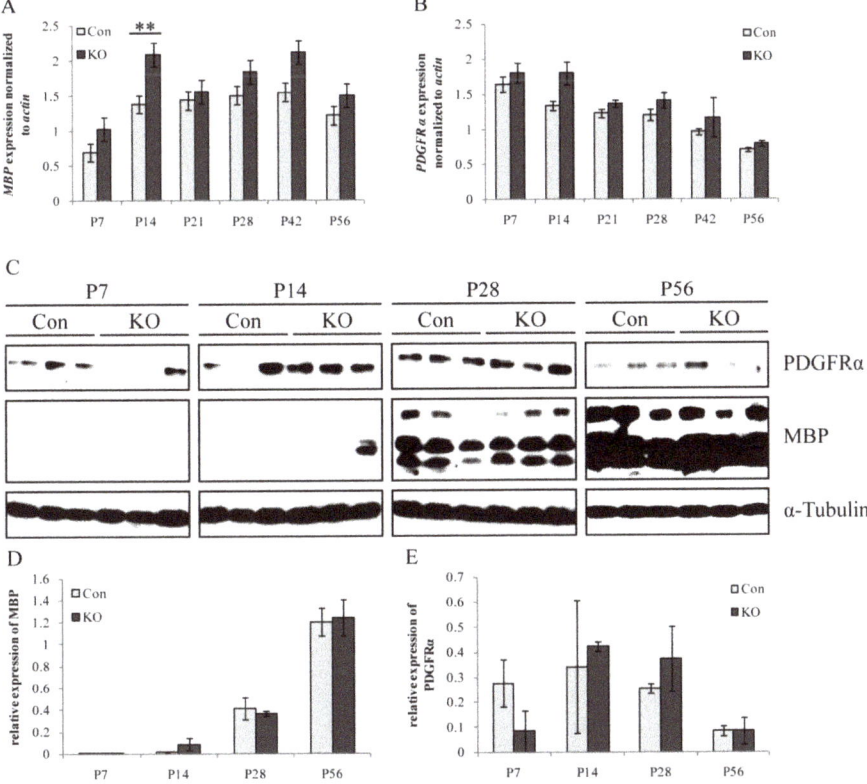

Figure 7. mRNA and protein levels of oligodendrocyte-specific markers were not impaired due to loss of LRP1. (**A**) Quantification of the relative expression of *Mbp* mRNA revealed a time-dependent upregulation with a significantly higher expression in the KO at P14 (** $p \leq 0.01$). (**B**) Quantification of the relative expression of *Pdgfra* mRNA showed a downregulation from P7 to P56 in the control and KO. (**C**) Western blot analysis of protein levels of PDGFRα and MBP. α-tubulin served as the loading control. (**D**) Quantification of the relative expression of MBP on protein level demonstrated a strong time-dependent upregulation of about 100% from P7 to P56. (**E**) Quantification of the relative expression of PDGFRα protein level illustrated a tendential downregulation from P14 to P56. Data are expressed as the mean ± SEM. PCR: N = 4, n = 4, western blot: N = 3, n = 3. Depending on normally or not normally distributed data, the Student's *t*-test or Mann–Whitney U test was used for evaluation within the individual ages.

In summary, the immunohistochemistry, RT-PCR, and western blot results suggested comparable rates of oligodendrocyte differentiation in response to the tamoxifen treatment excluding strong unspecific recombination-induced side-effects in our experimental approach, which could interfere with our analysis of cell-autonomous effects.

3.6. Experimental Autoimmune Encephalomyelitis (EAE)

Oligodendrocytes form myelin sheaths indispensable for integral CNS function and that are damaged in neuroinflammatory diseases. We wanted to examine whether LRP1 deletion compromises the myelination by oligodendrocytes. From this perspective, we induced EAE in tamoxifen-treated animals of both genotypes and sexes at the age of 8 to 10 weeks (P56–P70) and monitored and scored the animals for four weeks (Figure 8). The two parameters investigated in this study were the body weight and the clinical score of the animals over four weeks of the disease course (Figure 8B,C). Focusing on weight first, KO animals started with a slightly higher weight of 19.4 g ± 0.8 g SEM when compared to the control with 18 g ± 1.8 g SEM.

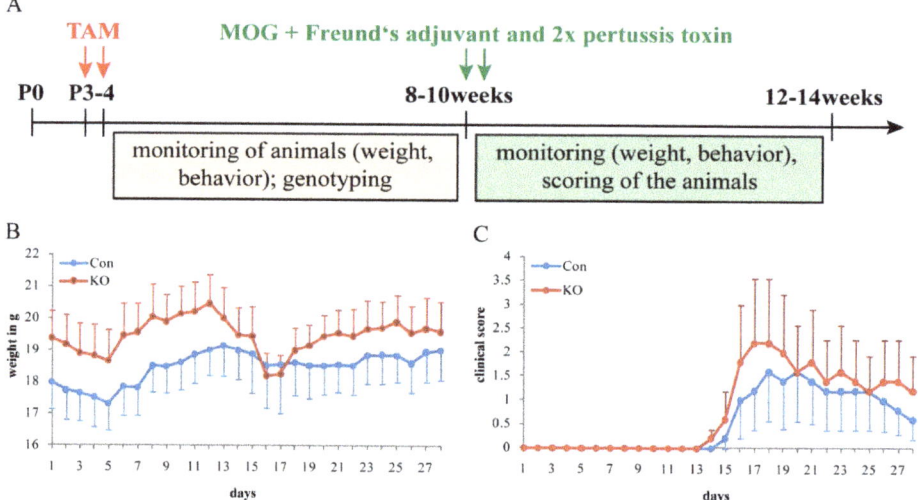

Figure 8. Experimental allergic encephalomyelitis (EAE) immunization reveals first hints toward more strongly affected KO animals, with greater deficits when compared to the control in the proof of concept experiment. (**A**) Timeline of experimental procedure. (**B**) Diagram of documented weights (g) during the course of disease over four weeks of control and KO animals. (**C**) Diagram of relating clinical scores of the control and KO animals over four weeks of EAE. Data are expressed as the mean ± SEM. N = 5, n = 5. Depending on normally or not normally distributed data, the Student's *t*-test or Mann–Whitney U test was used for evaluation within the individual ages. Score: 0 = normal; 1 = reduced tail tonus; 2 = complete tail palsy; 3 = lack of reflexive compensatory movements while walking; 4 = ataxia.

Within the first five days post immunization (dpi), a slight decrease of body weight was observed in both genotypes (control: 17.3 g ± 1.8 g SEM; KO: 18.7 g ± 0.8 g SEM), followed by an increase until 12 or rather 13 dpi, respectively (control: 19.1 g ± 2.1 g SEM; KO: 20.4 g ± 0.8 g SEM) (Figure 8B). While animals of the control condition remained constant in body weight until the end of the study (around 18.5–19 g), the KO animals demonstrated a notable reduction in body weight after 12 dpi with a minimum of 18.2 g ± 1.32 g SEM at 16 and 17 dpi.

The individual KO animals in our study appeared to be clearly affected by the EAE immunization, as indicated by the diminution in body weight. Following this reduction, the body weight of the

KO animals increased again (up to 22 dpi), transiting into a stable phase until the end of the study (Figure 8C).

According to the clinical score, as an indicator for the severity of symptoms due to EAE immunization (Figure 8C), both genotypes responded equally at the beginning of the experiment. A score of 0 revealed a lack of symptoms up to 13 dpi. Afterward, animals of both genotypes developed symptoms, reflected by an increased score of 1.6 in the control and 2.2 in the KO (control: 18 and 20 dpi, KO: 17 and 18 dpi). This score reflected a combination of a reduced tail tonus and complete tail palsy in control animals versus complete tail palsy in conjunction with a lack of reflexive compensatory movements while walking in KO animals. The proceeding disease course demonstrated a remitting phase in both genotypes with decreased scoring until the end of the experiment. In the control, a score of 0.6 indicated an intermediate stage between normal behavior and reduced tail tonus, whereas the KO condition was still more strongly affected with a score of 1.2 (Figure 8C). It has to be noted that our study comprised small collectives revealing mild differences in body weight and clinical score that did not, however, achieve statistical significance. This may be due to the fact that the majority of LRP1-deleted OPCs has been eliminated from the CNS of triple transgenic mice, as described above. Future studies will have to be performed to verify the asserted involvement of LRP1 in the recovery from EAE.

4. Discussion

In order to study LRP1 in the oligodendrocyte lineage, we decided to generate a tamoxifen-inducible conditional mouse line as it enables the selection of defined induction time points for the deletion of the gene. With our induction protocol, we benefited from the NG2-CreERT2 mouse, which was used to generate our novel model [21]. Depending on the reporter genes eYFP and tdTomato, recombination efficiencies of 50–95% respectively were observed by Huang et al. [21] and corresponded to our data at P7.

In our study, we present a new triple transgenic mouse model with LRP1-deficiency induced in postnatal OPCs: NG2-CreERT2$^{ct2/wt}$xR26eGFP$^{flox/flox}$xLRP1$^{flox/flox}$ (KO). Deletion of LRP1 in postnatal OPCs and their progeny resulted in the progressive loss of KO oligodendrocytes during development. Furthermore, EAE immunization hints at a clear response in LRP1 KO animals. On the cellular level, an in vitro myelination assay provided initial evidence for modified myelination behavior of recombined oligodendrocytes, as indicated by elongated internodes in the LRP1 KO condition (Figure S1). Focusing on the oligodendrocyte lineage, we were able to uncover a new role of LRP1 in oligodendrocyte survival during development in vivo and potentially also myelin formation in vitro.

In order to target the oligodendrocyte lineage, we induced the KO at P3 and P4 by injection of tamoxifen to lactating mothers, which metabolized tamoxifen to 4-hydroxy-tamoxifen in the liver [29] and fed the metabolites to the pups by milk. Early oligodendrocyte development is characterized by three independent OPC waves, which populate the forebrain at embryonic day (E) 11.5, E15.5, and P0, and are derived from different sources or structures of the early brain [15,30,31]. Based on the induction of the KO in young postnatal animals, we wanted to guarantee the deletion of LRP1 from a huge proportion of OPCs in their target compartment and aimed to analyze the effect of the lineage-restricted LRP1-deficiency in oligodendrocytes over time.

Additional to our focus on the oligodendrocyte lineage, the new mouse model also allowed us to investigate LRP1-deletion from NG2-glia with an adapted injection protocol (the tamoxifen treatment can be adjusted depending on the experimental question). The proteoglycan NG2 is not only expressed in OPCs [18,19], but also in pericytes, which are associated with blood vessels [32]. Pericytes are known to express LRP1 and therefore could have been affected in our conditional knockout mouse model. However, our experimental focus was on oligodendrocytes and myelination. Therefore, we used lineage-specific markers such as PDGFRα, CC1, MBP, and Olig2 to address this aspect in immunohistochemical stainings. PCR and western blot analysis were used to confirm the effects of LRP1 deletion on cells of the oligodendrocyte lineage. Additionally, for the in vitro myelination assay pure OPC cultures were used to compare LRP1-deficient OPCs with control cells. At present, we cannot exclude a potential intervention of LRP1-deficient pericytes in the EAE experiment.

OPCs not only exist in the young brain where they differentiate to oligodendrocytes, but proliferate and can be found throughout the brain into adulthood and were recently termed NG2 glia [33]. These macroglia-like cells in the CNS can generate oligodendrocytes and astrocytes during development [31,34]. In addition, NG2 glia has been suggested as an immature, progenitor-like cell type that can differentiate into mature cells with neural properties depending on specific environmental stimuli [35]. They are present in white and grey matter, but have also been found in stem cell niches such as the subventricular zone (SVZ) [33,36,37]. So far, nothing is known about LRP1 protein expression in NG2 glia, but the precursor properties of NG2 glia for oligodendrocyte lineage suggest an upregulation of LRP1 in NG2 glia. Our triple transgenic mouse model offers new possibilities to investigate LRP1-deletion in NG2 glia at different deliberately chosen time points. LRP1 deficiency from neural cell types results in multiple cellular or functional disorders (e.g., apoptosis in neurons [4], synapse loss and neurodegeneration in aging mice [38], and deficits in chemically induced white matter lesion repair [16]). Based on the knowledge concerning NG2 glia and LRP1, we propose potential effects of LRP1 on NG2 glia and their functions.

Deletion of LRP1 in postnatal OPCs in the new mouse model demonstrated a significant reduction of recombined cells during development. This indicated a progressive loss of LRP1-deficient oligodendrocytes in the Corpus callosum, the structure with the highest density of oligodendrocytes [39,40]. From this, we concluded a vulnerable phenotype of LRP1-deficient oligodendrocytes when compared to the control cells. To examine a potential global reduction of oligodendrocyte numbers during development due to the progressive loss of KO oligodendrocytes, we visualized the total fraction of oligodendrocytes with the help of Olig2, a specific lineage marker [41,42]. Increasing numbers of oligodendrocytes in the Corpus callosum over time support our interpretation that the progressively lost LRP1-deficient oligodendrocytes are replaced by GFP-negative non-recombined control cells in the KO over time.

Nevertheless, what happens to the disappearing, presumably weak and vulnerable LRP1 KO oligodendrocytes? We have previously shown that LRP1-deficient neural stem cells exhibited higher apoptosis rates when compared to the control conditions [11]. Pro-apoptotic effects in the absence of LRP1 have also been reported in neurons [4]. From this, we can conclude that the loss of LRP1-deficient oligodendrocytes could be explained by cell death, presumably apoptosis.

In order to study potential roles in myelination-related diseases, MOG_{35-55} EAE was induced in the control and KO animals. EAE is a model that mimics multiple sclerosis pathophysiology with focal inflammatory, demyelinating lesions, and axonal damage [43,44]. Furthermore, MOG_{35-55} EAE immunization is expected to generate a monophasic disease course [45], as also confirmed with our clinical score data. Defects preferentially appear in the spinal cord, but might also occur in the cerebellum and optic nerve, whereas symptoms are absent from the forebrain (including cortex and Corpus callosum) [43–45]. In explaining our preliminary findings in affected KO animals, the influences regarding the immune system should also be considered as the EAE model mimics autoimmune disease. Previously, anti-inflammatory effects of LRP1 in lipopolysaccharide, tumor necrosis factor α, and growth factor signaling as well as in phagocytosis have been observed [46]. These reports suggest an important role of LRP1 in the immune system. On the other hand, the LRP1 deletion in our model is restricted to the NG2-dependent lineage, and therefore it is questionable whether the immune system is modified in the EAE study. Furthermore, our observation of vulnerability in LRP1-deficient KO cells provides the first evidence for impairment in oligodendrocytes and potentially in myelin in our novel triple transgenic mouse model. Although these data refer to findings in the brain (Corpus callosum) and not the spinal cord, we expect similar conditions regarding cell fractions and recombination efficiency in the caudal sections of the CNS. We assumed that the affected KO animals might point to a late effect of progressive loss of LRP1-deficient oligodendrocytes. It is imaginable that the regenerative capacity of healthy LRP1-expressing oligodendrocytes is impaired at regions of progressive loss of LRP1 KO cells. As a consequence, vulnerable myelin might be formed around those axons exposed from myelin sheaths of perished oligodendrocytes, which might appear under EAE disease conditions. This concept will have to be validated by studies designed to eliminate LRP1 from non-recombined cells in parallel to EAE initiation. Our triple transgenic mouse model offers the option of timed elimination of LRP1 from OPCs recruited for myelin regeneration.

Based on our assumptions of altered myelin in the KO condition, we performed an in vitro myelination assay. Here, differentiated OPCs were placed on artificial fibers to investigate potential myelin impairment (Figure S1). This method allows the lengths of myelin sheaths, or rather internodes, to be measured [47]. Thereby it enables—and already has been used—to identify alterations in different conditions (e.g., due to genetically modified OPCs [48]). This myelination assay, performed with cortex-derived OPCs, revealed seemingly elongated internodes in the KO condition when compared to the control. Correlated with our findings of EAE, this in vitro study might point to myelin impairment in NG2-restricted LRP1-deficient mice in vivo. Again, one has to keep in mind that OPCs were derived from brain structures, and not from spinal cord, although this impaired myelination might represent a confident target of EAE inflammation. The elongated internodes might also display myelin dysregulation, referring to impaired thickness and/or wrapping of myelin, which could be addressed by electron microscopy.

The myelination assay suffered from strongly reduced numbers of surviving recombined KO cells in the immunopanning procedure and cultivation of cells on fibers. This underlined the weak and vulnerable KO cell phenotype in vitro and is in agreement with our previous observations. To circumvent the problems of OPC cultivation, in a future perspective, cells from another mouse model could be used that shows a higher proportion of recombined (KO) cells.

In addition to our observations regarding LRP1 loss and its marked consequences in the oligodendrocyte lineage, we also analyzed parameters that revealed a rather mild outcome. Namely, we concentrated on immature and mature oligodendrocytes in a global (control tissue vs. KO tissue including recombined and non-recombined cells) and cell-specific manner (control cells in control tissue vs. recombined cells in KO tissue). Decreasing proportions of precursors and increasing proportions of mature cells indicated oligodendrocyte differentiation and maturation over time [15,49,50]. mRNA and protein levels of PDGFRα (precursor marker) and MBP (mature marker) confirmed findings obtained by immunohistochemistry. Moreover, we found normally behaving and developing KO animals when compared to the control litter.

Despite the normal appearance of the mice, we found an important role of LRP1 in oligodendrocyte survival and vulnerability, which suggests a mechanism of compensation in our new model. The first plausible mechanism relies on the observed replacement of weak and apoptotic cells by healthy control cells, which might provide an immediate, but not optimum, compensation of cell loss. A second potential mechanism refers to LRP1 as a member of the low-density lipoprotein (LDL)-receptor gene family that shares structural elements and multiple functions and might account for compensatory effects [51]. In addition to LRP1, LRP3, LRP4, and LRP6 are highly expressed in OPCs [9]. LRP2 has been suggested to mediate OPC proliferation and migration in connection with sonic hedgehog [52]. These properties identify the LRPs as promising candidates for the substitution of specific LRP1 functions after deletion in our new mouse model. To name one function, LDL-receptor family members, especially LRP1, serve as the main receptors for cholesterol uptake into oligodendrocytes with the help of apolipoproteins such as ApoE [53]. Cholesterol itself is critically involved in the maturation of oligodendrocytes and induces myelin-specific gene expression, transports myelin proteins, and participates in internode formation [54–56].

5. Conclusions

In summary, our novel triple transgenic mouse model provides new insights into the field of LRP1 and its functions in oligodendrocytes. We found that LRP1-deficiency induced postnatally in NG2-expressing OPCs led to progressive loss of recombined LRP1 KO oligodendrocytes over time.

We conclude that LRP1-deficient OPCs are vulnerable and hardly survive. We propose a mechanism of cell death due to a phenotype susceptible to damage when LRP1 is deleted in the oligodendrocytic lineage. This was supported by observations in OPC cultures from cortical tissue, where only a few KO cells could be cultivated that hinted at a modified myelination behavior. In a further step, we found in an initial study that EAE can be elicited in the triple transgenic mouse line, where individual KO animals seemed to be clearly affected, yet without statistical significance. This presumably reflects the fact that most LRP1-deficient OPCs had been eliminated by the time the assay was carried out. Our model offers the perspective to test the roles of LRP1 by inducing recombination close to the commencement of inflammatory diseases. This experimental design might help to establish the role of LRP1 in myelin pathology in future studies.

Supplementary Materials: The following are available online at http://www.mdpi.com/2073-4409/8/12/1550/s1, Figure S1: Myelinated artificial fibers were examined for the length and the number of myelin sheaths in LRP1-deficient and in control oligodendrocytes, Figure S2: Immunohistochemical stainings to detect LRP1 and GFP and to verify the staining specificity by secondary antibody controls, Figure S3: Exemplary analysis of cell numbers per area to characterize oligodendrocyte-specific lineage markers alternatively.

Author Contributions: Conceptualization, I.S., J.K., A.H., and A.F.; Data curation, I.S.; Funding acquisition, A.F.; Investigation, I.S., J.K., and A.H.; Methodology, I.S., J.K., A.S., F.K., and A.H.; Project administration, A.F.; Resources, A.S., F.K., A.H., and A.F.; Supervision, A.F.; Validation, I.S.; Visualization, I.S.; Writing—original draft, I.S. and A.F.; Writing—review & editing, I.S., J.K., A.S., F.K., A.H., and A.F.

Funding: This research was funded by the German Research Foundation, grant number DFG SPP 1757/1,2, Fa 159/20-1,2 to A.F. and DFG FOR2289 to A.S. and F.K.

Acknowledgments: Special thanks go to Annika Ulc, who taught the immunopanning procedure and the artificial fiber assay to the researcher and to Lars Roll for helpful discussions. We acknowledge support from the DFG Open Access Publication Funds of the Ruhr-Universität Bochum.

Conflicts of Interest: The authors declare no conflicts of interest.

References

1. Boucher, P.; Herz, J. Signaling through LRP1: Protection from atherosclerosis and beyond. *Biochem. Pharmacol.* **2011**, *81*, 1–5. [CrossRef]
2. Bres, E.E.; Faissner, A. Low Density Receptor-Related Protein 1 Interactions with the Extracellular Matrix: More Than Meets the Eye. *Front. Cell Dev. Biol.* **2019**, *7*, 31. [CrossRef] [PubMed]
3. Mahley, R.W. Apolipoprotein E: Cholesterol transport protein with expanding role in cell biology. *Science* **1988**, *240*, 622–630. [CrossRef] [PubMed]
4. Fuentealba, R.A.; Liu, Q.; Kanekiyo, T.; Zhang, J.; Bu, G. Low density lipoprotein receptor-related protein 1 promotes anti-apoptotic signaling in neurons by activating Akt survival pathway. *J. Biol. Chem.* **2009**, *284*, 34045–34053. [CrossRef] [PubMed]
5. Martin, A.M.; Kuhlmann, C.; Trossbach, S.; Jaeger, S.; Waldron, E.; Roebroek, A.; Luhmann, H.J.; Laatsch, A.; Weggen, S.; Lessmann, V.; et al. The functional role of the second NPXY motif of the LRP1 beta-chain in tissue-type plasminogen activator-mediated activation of N-methyl-D-aspartate receptors. *J. Biol. Chem.* **2008**, *283*, 12004–12013. [CrossRef] [PubMed]
6. Muratoglu, S.C.; Mikhailenko, I.; Newton, C.; Migliorini, M.; Strickland, D.K. Low density lipoprotein receptor-related protein 1 (LRP1) forms a signaling complex with platelet-derived growth factor receptor-beta in endosomes and regulates activation of the MAPK pathway. *J. Biol. Chem.* **2010**, *285*, 14308–14317. [CrossRef]
7. Hussain, M.M.; Strickland, D.K.; Bakillah, A. The mammalian low-density lipoprotein receptor family. *Annu. Rev. Nutr.* **1999**, *19*, 141–172. [CrossRef]
8. Lorent, K.; Overbergh, L.; Delabie, J.; Van Leuven, F.; Van den Berghe, H. Distribution of mRNA coding for alpha-2-macroglobulin, the murinoglobulins, the alpha-2-macroglobulin receptor and the alpha-2-macroglobulin receptor associated protein during mouse embryogenesis and in adult tissues. *Differentiation* **1994**, *55*, 213–223. [CrossRef]

9. Zhang, Y.; Chen, K.; Sloan, S.A.; Bennett, M.L.; Scholze, A.R.; O'Keeffe, S.; Phatnani, H.P.; Guarnieri, P.; Caneda, C.; Ruderisch, N.; et al. An RNA-sequencing transcriptome and splicing database of glia, neurons, and vascular cells of the cerebral cortex. *J. Neurosci.* **2014**, *34*, 11929–11947. [CrossRef]
10. Hennen, E.; Safina, D.; Haussmann, U.; Wörsdörfer, P.; Edenhofer, F.; Poetsch, A.; Faissner, A. A LewisX glycoprotein screen identifies the low density lipoprotein receptor-related protein. 1 (LRP1) as a modulator of oligodendrogenesis in mice. *J. Biol. Chem.* **2013**, *288*, 16538–16545. [CrossRef]
11. Safina, D.; Schlitt, F.; Romeo, R.; Pflanzner, T.; Pietrzik, C.U.; Narayanaswami, V.; Edenhofer, F.; Faissner, A. Low-density lipoprotein receptor-related protein 1 is a novel modulator of radial glia stem cell proliferation, survival, and differentiation. *Glia* **2016**, *64*, 1363–1380. [CrossRef] [PubMed]
12. Auderset, L.; Cullen, C.L.; Young, K.M. Low Density Lipoprotein-Receptor Related Protein 1 is Differentially Expressed by Neuronal and Glial Populations in the Developing and Mature Mouse Central Nervous System. *PLoS ONE* **2016**, *11*, e0155878. [CrossRef] [PubMed]
13. Herz, J.; Clouthier, D.E.; Hammer, R.E. LDL receptor-related protein internalizes and degrades uPA-PAI-1 complexes and is essential for embryo implantation. *Cell* **1992**, *71*, 411–421. [CrossRef]
14. Simpson, P.B.; Armstrong, R.C. Intracellular signals and cytoskeletal elements involved in oligodendrocyte progenitor migration. *Glia* **1999**, *26*, 22–35. [CrossRef]
15. Rowitch, D.H.; Kriegstein, A.R. Developmental genetics of vertebrate glial-cell specification. *Nature* **2010**, *468*, 214–222. [CrossRef]
16. Lin, J.-P.; Mironova, Y.A.; Shrager, P.; Giger, R.J. LRP1 regulates peroxisome biogenesis and cholesterol homeostasis in oligodendrocytes and is required for proper CNS myelin development and repair. *eLife* **2017**, *6*, e30498. [CrossRef]
17. Cahoy, J.D.; Emery, B.; Kaushal, A.; Foo, L.C.; Zamanian, J.L.; Christopherson, K.S.; Xing, Y.; Lubischer, J.L.; Krieg, P.A.; Krupenko, S.A.; et al. A transcriptome database for astrocytes, neurons, and oligodendrocytes: A new resource for understanding brain development and function. *J. Neurosci.* **2008**, *28*, 264–278. [CrossRef]
18. Pringle, N.P.; Richardson, W.D. A singularity of PDGF alpha-receptor expression in the dorsoventral axis of the neural tube may define the origin of the oligodendrocyte lineage. *Development* **1993**, *117*, 525–533.
19. Horner, P.J.; Thallmair, M.; Gage, F.H. Defining the NG2-expressing cell of the adult CNS. *J. Neurocytol.* **2002**, *31*, 469–480. [CrossRef]
20. Rohlmann, A.; Gotthardt, M.; Willnow, T.E.; Hammer, R.E.; Herz, J. Sustained somatic gene inactivation by viral transfer of Cre recombinase. *Nat. Biotechnol.* **1996**, *14*, 1562–1565. [CrossRef]
21. Huang, W.; Zhao, N.; Bai, X.; Karram, K.; Trotter, J.; Goebbels, S.; Scheller, A.; Kirchhoff, F. Novel NG2-CreERT2 knock-in mice demonstrate heterogeneous differentiation potential of NG2 glia during development. *Glia* **2014**, *62*, 896–913. [CrossRef] [PubMed]
22. Paukert, M.; Agarwal, A.; Cha, J.; Doze, V.A.; Kang, J.U.; Bergles, D.E. Norepinephrine controls astroglial responsiveness to local circuit activity. *Neuron* **2014**, *82*, 1263–1270. [CrossRef] [PubMed]
23. Liu, J.; Willet, S.G.; Bankaitis, E.D.; Xu, Y.; Wright, C.V.; Gu, G. Non-parallel recombination limits Cre-LoxP-based reporters as precise indicators of conditional genetic manipulation. *Genesis* **2013**, *51*, 436–442. [CrossRef] [PubMed]
24. Xie, M.; Tobin, J.E.; Budde, M.D.; Chen, C.I.; Trinkaus, K.; Cross, A.H.; McDaniel, D.P.; Song, S.K.; Armstrong, R.C. Rostrocaudal analysis of corpus callosum demyelination and axon damage across disease stages refines diffusion tensor imaging correlations with pathological features. *J. Neuropathol. Exp. Neurol.* **2010**, *69*, 704–716. [CrossRef] [PubMed]
25. Reyes-Haro, D.; Mora-Loyola, E.; Soria-Ortiz, B.; Garcia-Colunga, J. Regional density of glial cells in the rat corpus callosum. *Biol. Res.* **2013**, *46*, 27–32. [CrossRef] [PubMed]
26. Van Tilborg, E.; de Theije Caroline, G.M.; van Hal, M.; Wagenaar, N.; de Vries, L.S.; Benders, M.J.; Rowitch, D.H.; Nijboer, C.H. Origin and dynamics of oligodendrocytes in the developing brain: Implications for perinatal white matter injury. *Glia* **2018**, *66*, 221–238. [CrossRef] [PubMed]
27. Steelman, A.J.; Thompson, J.P.; Li, J. Demyelination and remyelination in anatomically distinct regions of the corpus callosum following cuprizone intoxication. *Neurosci. Res.* **2012**, *72*, 32–42. [CrossRef]
28. Wu, Q.-Z.; Yang, Q.; Cate, H.S.; Kemper, D.; Binder, M.; Wang, H.X.; Fang, K.; Quick, M.J.; Marriott, M.; Kilpatrick, T.J.; et al. MRI identification of the rostral-caudal pattern of pathology within the corpus callosum in the cuprizone mouse model. *J. Magn. Reson. Imaging* **2008**, *27*, 446–453. [CrossRef]

29. Jahn, H.M.; Kasakow, C.V.; Helfer, A.; Michely, J.; Verkhratsky, A.; Maurer, H.H.; Scheller, A.; Kirchhoff, F. Refined protocols of tamoxifen injection for inducible DNA recombination in mouse astroglia. *Sci. Rep.* **2018**, *8*, 5913. [CrossRef]
30. Kessaris, N.; Fogarty, M.; Iannarelli, P.; Grist, M.; Wegner, M.; Richardson, W.D. Competing waves of oligodendrocytes in the forebrain and postnatal elimination of an embryonic lineage. *Nat. Neurosci.* **2006**, *9*, 173–179. [CrossRef]
31. Huang, W.; Guo, Q.; Bai, X.; Scheller, A.; Kirchhoff, F. Early embryonic NG2 glia are exclusively gliogenic and do not generate neurons in the brain. *Glia* **2019**, *67*, 1094–1103. [CrossRef] [PubMed]
32. Ozerdem, U.; Grako, K.A.; Dahlin-Huppe, K.; Monosov, E.; Stallcup, W.B. NG2 proteoglycan is expressed exclusively by mural cells during vascular morphogenesis. *Dev. Dyn.* **2001**, *222*, 218–227. [CrossRef] [PubMed]
33. Nishiyama, A.; Komitova, M.; Suzuki, R.; Zhu, X. Polydendrocytes (NG2 cells): Multifunctional cells with lineage plasticity. *Nat. Rev. Neurosci.* **2009**, *10*, 9–22. [CrossRef] [PubMed]
34. Dimou, L.; Gallo, V. NG2-glia and their functions in the central nervous system. *Glia* **2015**, *63*, 1429–1451. [CrossRef]
35. Richardson, W.D.; Young, K.M.; Tripathi, R.B.; McKenzie, I. NG2-glia as multipotent neural stem cells: Fact or fantasy? *Neuron* **2011**, *70*, 661–673. [CrossRef]
36. Aguirre, A.; Gallo, V. Postnatal neurogenesis and gliogenesis in the olfactory bulb from NG2-expressing progenitors of the subventricular zone. *J. Neurosci.* **2004**, *24*, 10530–10541. [CrossRef]
37. Aguirre, A.A.; Chittajallu, R.; Belachew, S.; Gallo, V. NG2-expressing cells in the subventricular zone are type C-like cells and contribute to interneuron generation in the postnatal hippocampus. *J. Cell Biol.* **2004**, *165*, 575–589. [CrossRef]
38. Liu, Q.; Trotter, J.; Zhang, J.; Peters, M.M.; Cheng, H.; Bao, J.; Han, X.; Weeber, E.J.; Bu, G. Neuronal LRP1 knockout in adult mice leads to impaired brain lipid metabolism and progressive, age-dependent synapse loss and neurodegeneration. *J. Neurosci.* **2010**, *30*, 17068–17078. [CrossRef]
39. Del Rio-Hortega, P. Studies on neuroglia: Glia with very few processes (oligodendroglia) by PÃo del RÃo-Hortega. 1921. *Clin. Neuropathol.* **2012**, *31*, 440–459.
40. Pérez-Cerdá, F.; Sánchez-Gómez, M.V.; Matute, C. Pío del Río Hortega and the discovery of the oligodendrocytes. *Front. Neuroanat.* **2015**, *9*, 92. [CrossRef]
41. Zhou, Q.; Wang, S.; Anderson, D.J. Identification of a novel family of oligodendrocyte lineage-specific basic helix-loop-helix transcription factors. *Neuron* **2000**, *25*, 331–343. [CrossRef]
42. Zhang, S.C. Defining glial cells during CNS development. *Nat. Rev. Neurosci.* **2001**, *2*, 840–843. [CrossRef] [PubMed]
43. Nikić, I.; Merkler, D.; Sorbara, C.; Brinkoetter, M.; Kreutzfeldt, M.; Bareyre, F.M.; Brück, W.; Bishop, D.; Misgeld, T.; Kerschensteiner, M. A reversible form of axon damage in experimental autoimmune encephalomyelitis and multiple sclerosis. *Nat. Med.* **2011**, *17*, 495–499. [CrossRef]
44. Kipp, M.; Nyamoya, S.; Hochstrasser, T.; Amor, S. Multiple sclerosis animal models: A clinical and histopathological perspective. *Brain Pathol.* **2017**, *27*, 123–137. [CrossRef]
45. Constantinescu, C.S.; Farooqi, N.; O'Brien, K.; Gran, B. Experimental autoimmune encephalomyelitis (EAE) as a model for multiple sclerosis (MS). *Br. J. Pharmacol.* **2011**, *164*, 1079–1106. [CrossRef]
46. May, P. The low-density lipoprotein receptor-related protein 1 in inflammation. *Curr. Opin. Lipidol.* **2013**, *24*, 134–137. [CrossRef]
47. Bechler, M.E.; Byrne, L.; Ffrench-Constant, C. CNS Myelin Sheath Lengths Are an Intrinsic Property of Oligodendrocytes. *Curr. Biol.* **2015**, *25*, 2411–2416. [CrossRef]
48. Ulc, A.; Zeug, A.; Bauch, J.; van Leeuwen, S.; Kuhlmann, T.; ffrench-Constant, C.; Ponimaskin, E.; Faissner, A. The guanine nucleotide exchange factor Vav3 modulates oligodendrocyte precursor differentiation and supports remyelination in white matter lesions. *Glia* **2019**, *67*, 376–392. [CrossRef]
49. Zuchero, J.B.; Barres, B.A. Intrinsic and extrinsic control of oligodendrocyte development. *Curr. Opin. Neurobiol.* **2013**, *23*, 914–920. [CrossRef]
50. Elbaz, B.; Popko, B. Molecular Control of Oligodendrocyte Development. *Trends Neurosci.* **2019**. [CrossRef]
51. Herz, J.; Strickland, D.K. LRP: A multifunctional scavenger and signaling receptor. *J. Clin. Investig.* **2001**, *108*, 779–784. [CrossRef] [PubMed]

52. Auderset, L.; Landowski, L.M.; Foa, L.; Young, K.M. Low Density Lipoprotein Receptor Related Proteins as Regulators of Neural Stem and Progenitor Cell Function. *Stem Cells Int.* **2016**, *2016*, 2108495. [CrossRef] [PubMed]
53. Van de Sluis Bart Wijers, M.; Herz, J. News on the molecular regulation and function of hepatic low-density lipoprotein receptor and LDLR-related protein 1. *Curr. Opin. Lipidol.* **2017**, *28*, 241–247. [CrossRef] [PubMed]
54. Krämer-Albers, E.-M.; Gehrig-Burger, K.; Thiele, C.; Trotter, J.; Nave, K.A. Perturbed interactions of mutant proteolipid protein/DM20 with cholesterol and lipid rafts in oligodendroglia: Implications for dysmyelination in spastic paraplegia. *J. Neurosci.* **2006**, *26*, 11743–11752. [CrossRef] [PubMed]
55. Mathews, E.S.; Mawdsley, D.J.; Walker, M.; Hines, J.H.; Pozzoli, M.; Appel, B. Mutation of 3-hydroxy-3-methylglutaryl CoA synthase I reveals requirements for isoprenoid and cholesterol synthesis in oligodendrocyte migration arrest, axon wrapping, and myelin gene expression. *J. Neurosci.* **2014**, *34*, 3402–3412. [CrossRef] [PubMed]
56. Saher, G.; Brügger, B.; Lappe-Siefke, C.; Mobius, W.; Tozawa, R.; Wehr, M.C.; Wieland, F.; Ishibashi, S.; Nave, K.A. High cholesterol level is essential for myelin membrane growth. *Nat. Neurosci.* **2005**, *8*, 468–475. [CrossRef] [PubMed]

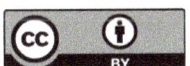 © 2019 by the authors. Licensee MDPI, Basel, Switzerland. This article is an open access article distributed under the terms and conditions of the Creative Commons Attribution (CC BY) license (http://creativecommons.org/licenses/by/4.0/).

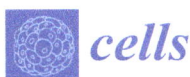

Review

Aberrant Oligodendrogenesis in Down Syndrome: Shift in Gliogenesis?

Laura Reiche, Patrick Küry [†] and Peter Göttle *,[†]

Department of Neurology, Medical Faculty, Heinrich-Heine-University, 40225 Düsseldorf, Germany; Laura.Reiche@hhu.de (L.R.); Patrick.kuery@uni-duesseldorf.de (P.K.)
* Correspondence: Peter.Goettle@uni-duesseldorf.de; Tel.: +49-211/81-08071; Fax: +49-(0211)-81-18469
† These authors contributed equally to this work.

Received: 31 October 2019; Accepted: 4 December 2019; Published: 7 December 2019

Abstract: Down syndrome (DS), or trisomy 21, is the most prevalent chromosomal anomaly accounting for cognitive impairment and intellectual disability (ID). Neuropathological changes of DS brains are characterized by a reduction in the number of neurons and oligodendrocytes, accompanied by hypomyelination and astrogliosis. Recent studies mainly focused on neuronal development in DS, but underestimated the role of glial cells as pathogenic players. Aberrant or impaired differentiation within the oligodendroglial lineage and altered white matter functionality are thought to contribute to central nervous system (CNS) malformations. Given that white matter, comprised of oligodendrocytes and their myelin sheaths, is vital for higher brain function, gathering knowledge about pathways and modulators challenging oligodendrogenesis and cell lineages within DS is essential. This review article discusses to what degree DS-related effects on oligodendroglial cells have been described and presents collected evidence regarding induced cell-fate switches, thereby resulting in an enhanced generation of astrocytes. Moreover, alterations in white matter formation observed in mouse and human post-mortem brains are described. Finally, the rationale for a better understanding of pathways and modulators responsible for the glial cell imbalance as a possible source for future therapeutic interventions is given based on current experience on pro-oligodendroglial treatment approaches developed for demyelinating diseases, such as multiple sclerosis.

Keywords: down syndrome; white matter; glial fate

1. Introduction

The majority of central nervous system (CNS) diseases are characterized by neuronal damage and white matter malfunctions, which can lead to detrimental motor and sensory effects. Trisomy 21, as an aneuploidy disorder, is characterized by an additional copy of human chromosome 21 (Hsa21) and causes Down syndrome (DS). DS is the most abundant human trisomy, affecting around 1 in 1100 neonates annually [1], making it the most common genetic cause for intellectual disability (ID) [2]. DS patients suffer from several cognitive impairments, accompanied by a low intelligence quotient (IQ) ranging from 30 to 70 [2], which can be attributed to brain abnormalities. In accordance with the neurocentric paradigm, brain research in DS has followed the concept that neuronal dysfunctions primarily lead to neurological diseases [3]. Therefore, much of the DS research aimed at identifying the underlying genetic interventions of altered neurogenesis. This information is essential for unraveling pharmacological approaches to ameliorate cognitive function (summarized in recent reviews [1,4–8]). Nevertheless, over the last few years consideration has been given to the re-evaluation of the role of astroglial and oligodendroglial lineage cells in CNS pathologies characterized by neurodegeneration [3,9]. Interestingly, several studies in DS indicated a neuro- to gliogenic shift, mainly focusing on the observed bias toward astrocytes [3,4,6,10]. Even though oligodendroglial cells—as a source of CNS myelin sheaths—are essential for higher brain functions by assuring long-term axonal integrity, metabolic and trophic support, and accelerated electrical signal propagation, this crucial cell population has not attracted much attention in DS. The notion that aberrant oligodendrogenesis may contribute to cognitive impairments and ID in DS is supported by a recent developmental transcriptome analysis of post-mortem human DS brains [11]. Of note, the analysis of this study revealed a dysregulated gene cluster associated with oligodendroglial cell differentiation and myelination, showing that hypomyelination in DS is caused by a cell-autonomous phenomenon in oligodendrocyte development. To further highlight the importance of the oligodendroglial lineage in DS development, this review article summarizes the current knowledge regarding altered oligodendrogenesis and white matter malformations in human and rodent DS research. We show that signaling pathways assumed to lead to defective neurogenesis and to a neuro-to astrogenic shift also affect oligodendrogenesis. Such knowledge may help to devise new treatments that aim to improve brain development and ID by stabilization of the oligodendroglial lineage.

2. Down Syndrome: A Brief Neurological Profile

Associated with more than 80 clinical features affecting many organs, both the occurrence (penetrance) and severity (expressivity) of phenotypes vary across the DS population [4]. Nonetheless, certain characteristics, such as facial dysmorphology, reduced brain volume accompanied by ID, and an early-onset Alzheimer's disease (AD)-like pathology are common in all DS individuals. This neurological profile is distinctly marked by hypocellularity in the cerebral hemispheres, frontal lobe, temporal cortex, hippocampus, and cerebellum, most likely explained by a complex spatiotemporal perturbation in neurogenesis, resulting in a reduced neuronal cell population and a subsequently altered neuronal connectivity [1,4,6].

Moreover, aberrant astrogliogenesis and changes in several astrocytic marker expression patterns have been demonstrated in DS (reviewed in [3]). Notably, an over-population of astroglial cells in the frontal lobe of DS fetuses [12], as well as in the frontal cortex, calcarine cortex, and mainly hippocampus of infant and adult DS brains [13], has been observed. At an advanced age, astrogliosis in the amygdala [14], related to the occurrence of senile plaques and neurofibrillary tangles [13] and in areas of basal ganglia calcification [15], was shown to be implicated in DS.

Furthermore, DS brains of old adults are marked by reduced numbers of oligodendrocytes when compared to age-matched individuals [16]. More devastating is the observed hypomyelination in DS, pointing to an impaired myelination process which proceeds until adulthood, as demonstrated by myelin protein expression [11], histological [17,18], or magnetic resonance imaging (MRI) [19] examinations. Assessed by diffusion tensor imaging (DTI) fractional anisotropy (FA) analysis, white matter in DS patients showed lower fiber density, smaller axonal diameters, and a reduced myelination degree compared to healthy controls [20]. Decreased FA and early white matter damage were particularly observed in the region of the anterior thalamic radiation, the inferior fronto-occipital fasciculus, the inferior longitudinal fasciculus and the corticospinal tract, bilaterally, the corpus callosum (CC), and the anterior limb of the internal capsule [21–23]. Of note, diminished white matter integrity in DS was associated with poorer performance at neuropsychological assessments [20,23]. In this context, recent evidence in animal models suggests that ongoing myelin remodeling is important for behavior, cognition, and learning throughout adulthood [24,25]. Notably, the onset of cognitive deficits in DS is thought to occur in late infancy, becoming more obvious in adolescence [11,26–33]. This time course indeed correlates with the peak of myelination during the first years of life, continuing into young adulthood [34]. Moreover, immunohistochemical analysis for myelin basic protein (MBP) revealed a decreased density of myelinated axons and a generally delayed myelin formation in DS compared to age-matched controls [18], indicating that the oligodendroglial lineage was directly affected upon gene-dosage effects of Hsa21. Accordingly, a recent multi-region transcriptome analysis of DS and healthy brains spanning from fetal development to adulthood revealed that genes associated with oligodendroglial cell differentiation and myelination are dysregulated in trisomy 21 during late fetal development and the first years of postnatal life [11]. Weighted-gene co-expression network analysis (WGCNA) within this study identified several modules of co-expressed genes, including the module number 43 (M43) which is related to oligodendrocyte development and myelination including, for example, 2′,3′-cyclic nucleotide-3′-phosphodiesterase (CNPase), proteolipid protein (PLP), Sox10, and G protein coupled receptor 17 (GPR17). This module exhibited a distinct downregulation throughout the DS neocortex and hippocampus during development [11]. Of note, GPR17, a modulator of oligodendroglial cell maturation [35], is linked to a significantly reduced expression of sorting nexin family member 27 (SNX27) in DS [36], which was demonstrated to impair oligodendroglial precursor cell (OPC) maturation, resulting in myelination deficits in Ts65Dn mice, a mouse model for DS [37]. However, there is much evidence on aberrant oligodendrogenesis correlating with or contributing to DS-related cognitive impairments, but the underlying mechanisms have so far not been investigated in detail.

3. Gliogenesis and Cell Types in Healthy CNS

The mammalian central nervous system (CNS) consists of neurons and glial cells, the latter of which make up at least 50% of human brain cells. Glial cell function is essential for the evolutionary increase in complexity of neurological function in mammals [38] and can be divided in macroglial cells deriving from the neuroepithelium and microglia with a hematopoietic (mesodermal) origin [38]. Despite their crucial importance for various physiological processes [39,40], these cells are not further addressed in this review article. Macroglial cells are generally categorized into astrocytes and oligodendrocytes. Due to upcoming knowledge about the functions of proteoglycan nerve-glial antigen 2 (NG2) expressing glial cells, NG2 glia are considered a further category of macroglia [41].

Approximately 40% of the human brain is considered to be white matter. It consists of (i) axons, the functional unit of neurons providing the basis for signal transduction and information, (ii) astrocytes, which are essential for structural and metabolic support to neurons, and (iii) myelin. In the CNS, myelin is imperative for the stabilization, protection, and electrical insulation of axons, enabling accelerated electrical signal propagation [34–36]. Myelin sheaths are generated by oligodendrocytes. These specialized glial cells either derive from oligodendroglial precursor cells (OPCs) or niche-located neural stem cells (NSCs) [37]. The structural integrity of myelin is of crucial importance for CNS function and restoration [38]. Unfortunately, pathological degeneration and inflammation [35] or genetic intervention [39] can result in myelin loss, which may lead to impaired neuronal signaling, functional deficits, and a shortened lifetime [40]. Hence, white matter deficits and myelin dysfunctions are considered to be a main contributing factor for neurodegenerative diseases and malfunctions of the CNS [41].

The major cell types of the CNS are produced by several spatiotemporal, partially overlapping generation and division waves of progenitor cells, which are guided by extrinsic and intrinsic cues [38,42], resulting in a well-defined brain anatomy and cytoarchitecture. In the oligodendrogenic context, it is important to briefly introduce OPCs/NG2 glia and their differentiation potency (Figure 1). These cells derive from radial glia, the primary progenitor cells at embryonic stages, and are produced in three waves following a ventral-dorsal temporal progression in the developing forebrain [38]. They populate the brain and spinal cord to generate oligodendrocytes that myelinate the entire CNS during postnatal life [34]. A small fraction of OPCs is maintained as an immature, slowly proliferative, or quiescent cell population in the adult CNS [43]. Noteworthy, accumulating evidence indicates that beyond generating oligodendrocytes, OPCs exhibit the potential to also give rise to astroglial cells in vitro [44] and in vivo [45–47]. As mentioned above, OPCs can additionally be generated postnatally and in the adult brain from transient amplifying cells (TAPs or C cells) derived from NSCs located in the subventricular zone (SVZ) [48], mainly from the dorsal part (facing the corpus callosum) [49]. For OPC differentiation and subsequent myelination to occur, various signals are necessary in order to stabilize oligodendroglial fate and to regulate extensive changes in cell shape and membrane architecture. Pro-oligodendroglial extracellular signals comprise several pathways, such as those elicited by sonic hedgehog (SHH), Wnt/β-catenin, bone morphogenic protein (BMP), cytokines (LIF, Cxcl1), neurotransmitters (glutamate, ATP, adenosine), hormones (thyroid hormone T3, insulin), extracellular matrix molecules (fibronectin, laminin), metabolic signals (hypoxia), or in response to physical cues (spatial constrain, rigid substrate), and axonal receptors (Lingo-1, PSA-Ncam) [9,50,51]. Additionally, intrinsic regulators, such as the transcription factors basic helix-loop-helix oligodendrocyte lineage transcription factor 2 (Olig2) and sex determining region Y-Box 10 (Sox10), have also been implicated in OPC differentiation [52] in that, for example, exposure to SHH, expressed by the ventral telencephalon, instructs early progenitor cells to become OPCs, possibly via upregulation of Olig2 [53]. This induction is antagonized by the dorsally expressed Wnt/β-catenin and BMP pathways [54]. BMP4, on the other hand, has been shown to promote the expression of a family of inhibitor of DNA-binding (Id) proteins Id2 and Id4, which form complexes with Olig2. This interaction prevents Olig2 from binding to DNA, blocking its ability to act as a transcription factor and therefore inhibiting the differentiation along the oligodendroglial lineage but promoting astrogliogenesis [55]. Furthermore, post-translation processes, such as the regulation of the JAK/STAT3 activity by modulating STAT3's acetylation state, mediated by the histone deacetylase Hdac3, which has been shown to control Olig2 expression, are also needed to suppress astrogliogenesis [56].

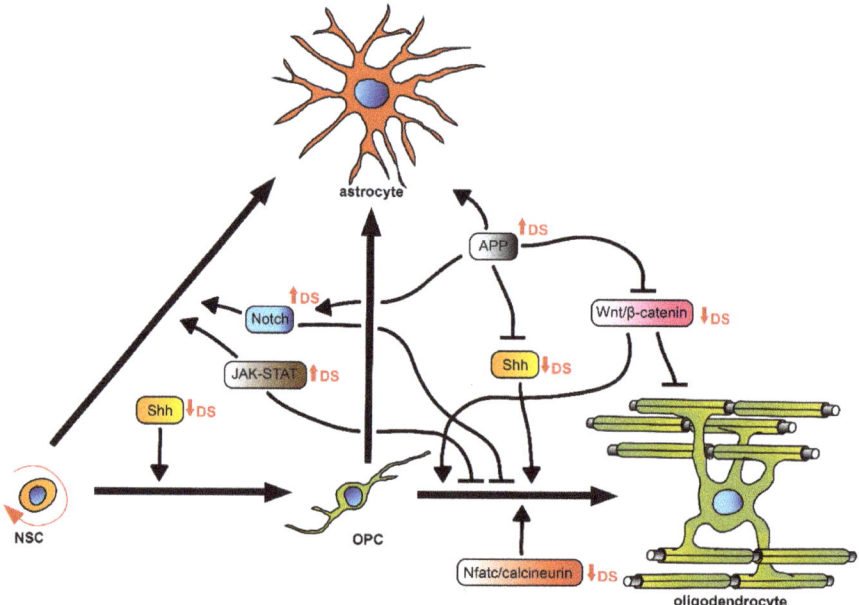

Figure 1. Representation of key signaling pathways involved in oligodendrogenesis. Neural stem cells (NSCs) exhibit astrogenic and oligodendrogenic potential. For oligodendroglial precursor cells (OPCs) derived from NSCs to successfully differentiate into myelinating oligodendrocytes, OPCs follow a highly regulated differentiation process that is affected by a fine-tuned network of signaling pathways. Within Down syndrome (DS) (red arrows), signaling pathways reveal aberrant dynamics.

Hence, based on this fine-tuned regulation of cell fate and differentiation mediators, it is likely that neurogenesis and gliogenesis are misguided in their responses to gene-dosage abnormalities caused by aneuploidy disorders. This holds true for DS brain development, where not only altered progenitor cell proliferation and apoptosis but also potential signaling pathways responsible for a neuro- to astrogenic shift are assumed to be responsible for observed neuronal hypocellularity and concurrent over-population of astroglial cells. However, so far, an oligodendrogenic to astrogenic shift has not been taken into account, although the number of oligodendrocytes and myelination rate are decreased in DS [11,16,18]. Furthermore, the differentiation of OPCs to mature oligodendrocytes was shown to be negatively affected in the DS mouse model Ts65Dn [11].

4. Defective OPC Differentiation in DS—Possible Interfering Regulators

Overall brain volume reduction and hypocellularity are already present in fetuses and children with DS [57–60]. This fact indicates that defective neuro- and gliogenesis during early phases of brain development may be a major causal factor of DS-associated brain abnormalities, which might be a consequence of early apoptosis and impaired proliferation in DS [6,61]. Also, the comparison of hippocampal regions of DS fetuses between 17 and 21 weeks of gestation to age-matched controls showed a higher percentage of cells with astrocytic phenotypes, but a smaller percentage of cells with neuronal phenotypes [62]. A few studies demonstrated elevated numbers of Olig2 expressing cells (thus declared as OPCs) in DS fetal brains at 14 and 18 weeks of gestation [63], even up to 34 weeks [10], suggesting a cell-fate shift from neurogenesis to gliogenesis at early developmental stages. Of note, the number of Olig2 expressing cells in the DS mouse model Ts65Dn is increased at embryonic day 13.5 and 14 [64], but decreases thereafter [11] when compared to age-matched controls. Intriguingly, the percentage of mature oligodendrocytes was drastically diminished from postnatal days 15–60 [11], whereas a massive increase of astrocyte numbers and reactivity was shown at the age of 48 weeks in the same DS mouse model [65]. Considering the capacity of OPCs to generate astroglial cells instead of oligodendrocytes, a shift within the glial cell commitment in DS accompanied with a generally defective differentiation capacity of oligodendroglial progenitors might be suggested.

Several authors have already discussed the involvement of pathways essential for cell fate and differentiation within neurogenesis in DS, thereby giving strong evidence that therapeutic approaches targeting these pathways could improve aberrant brain cytoarchitecture, in particular the neuro- to astrogliogenic shift [4–7,61]. Hereinafter, we focus on pathways relevant for oligodendrogenesis (Figure 1) instead and highlight to what extent they might constitute new therapeutic avenues.

4.1. JAK-STAT Signaling

One of the most important signaling pathways for the gliogenic cascade in NSCs is the Janus kinase-signal transducer and activator of transcription (JAK-STAT) pathway, mediated by ligands such as interleukins (ILs), interferons (INFs), the glycoprotein (gp) 130 family, and the γ-chain (gC) family [6,66]. Common downstream targets, such as GFAP and S100β which specify glial cell fate, are transcriptionally activated by STATs [6,67]. STAT3 in particular plays an essential role in regulating astrogliogenesis during brain development [66]. In vivo studies showed that overexpression of STAT3 in the neocortex of DS mice (Ts1Cje) enhanced astrogliogenesis [68], whereas its knockout inhibited the astroglial fate in mouse NSCs [69]. Additionally, it was reported that IL-6 in DS children and IFN-γ in embryonic trisomy 16 mouse brains (Ts16, a model used for human trisomy 21 (DS)), were increased respectively [70,71], both of which are capable of activating the STAT3 pathway [72]. Indeed, neonate DS mice (Ts65Dn) exhibited hyperactivation of STAT3 in the hippocampus [73]. More importantly, four IFN receptors, IFN-α receptor 1 and 2 (IFNAR1, IFNAR2), IFN-γ R2 (IFNGR2), and interleukin 10 receptor β (IL10RB), are located on Hsa21 and overexpressed in DS with a mean ratio of ~1.5 proportional to the gene-dosage effect of trisomy 21 [74–76]. This disposition leads to a generally increased INF sensitivity in DS [74].

Overstimulation of the JAK-STAT signaling pathway can also be linked to dual-specificity tyrosine-(Y)-phosphorylation-regulated kinase 1A (DYRK1A), which is also overexpressed in DS due to the location on Hsa21 [77]. Overexpression of this protein was shown to result in elevated STAT3 activity, which promoted the astrocytic differentiation of neocortical progenitors in Ts1Cje mice [68].

Interestingly, the STAT3 pathway was also shown to be a crucial regulator of OPC differentiation by means of shifting oligodendroglia toward an astrocytic fate, thereby causing astrogliosis and insufficient remyelination in Theiler's murine encephalomyelitis [78]. Given that STAT3 pathway can be activated by IFN-γ, the expression of which is increased in DS mice, it needs to be pointed out that IFN-γ was demonstrated to decrease rat OPC differentiation into oligodendrocytes [47]. Moreover, this study also indicated that IFN-γ might shift cell commitment toward the astrocytic lineage. Accordingly, transgenic mice overexpressing IFN-γ under control of the MBP promotor exhibited hypomyelination accompanied by an increase of astrocyte numbers, as well as reactive gliosis in white matter tracts [79]—a shift in brain cytoarchitecture that is strikingly similar to DS neuropathology. Therefore, overstimulation of JAK-STAT signaling caused by overexpressed levels of INFRs, ligands, and subsequent overactivation of the STAT3 pathway may promote an NSC/OPC fate toward an astrogliogenic pathway in the DS brain.

4.2. SHH Signaling

The spatiotemporal activity of Sonic Hedgehog (SHH) controls cell proliferation, migration, fate and differentiation of progenitor cell waves during brain development [80]. SHH is a well-known regulator that promotes oligodendroglial fate, OPC generation, differentiation, and myelin production in the spinal cord and forebrain during embryonic development [81,82], as well as OPC production and recruitment throughout adulthood [83] and in demyelination [84]. In the canonical SHH pathway, in the absence of SHH, the inhibitory transmembrane receptor Patched1 (Ptch1) suppresses the activity of the SHH signaling activator Smoothened (Smo) [85]. SHH binding to Ptch1 interrupts its inhibition on Smo, which triggers a complex intracellular signaling cascade including the transcription factors of the Glioma-associated oncogene (Gli) family to mediate downstream gene transcription, such as Mammalian achaetescute homolog-1 (Ascl1/Mash1), Olig2, or Nk2 homeobox 2 (Nkx2.2) [86–88]. Ptch1 was shown to be overexpressed in 17–21 week old fetuses and the DS mouse Ts65Dn [89], leading to the assumption that the SHH pathway is repressed in DS. Indeed, Gli 1 and 2, as well as Mash1, are downregulated in trisomic neuronal precursor cells (NPCs) of Ts65Dn mice, which could be restored by the maintenance of SHH signaling activity by Smoothened Agonist (SAG) treatment [73].

Of note, inhibition of Gli1 activity was previously shown to be important for NSC-dependent remyelination [90]. Furthermore, OPC differentiation was shown to be defective and diminished in SHH$^{-/-}$ mutants [87,91] and rat OPCs treated with the steroidal alkaloid cyclopamine, which inhibits SHH signaling by targeting Smo [92]. Thus, the increased inhibition of Smo due to elevated Ptch1 levels in DS, subsequently leading to repressed SHH activity, may contribute to the observed downregulation of a whole cluster of genes associated with OPC differentiation and myelination [11] and the delayed differentiation of OPCs, subsequently leading to hypomyelination in DS brains [18].

4.3. Notch Signaling

Notch signaling was shown to cross-talk with JAK-STAT [72] and SHH signaling pathways [93], thereby inducing gliogenic shift during brain development. Mediated by binding of ligands such as delta-like protein 1 (Dll1), cleavage of the transmembrane receptor Notch by γ-secretase is initiated. This liberates the Notch intracellular domain (NICD), which translocates to the nucleus to transcriptionally activate Notch effector proteins, such as hairy/enhancer of split 1 and 5 (Hes1, Hes5) [94], which are proteins that were shown to promote the activation of STAT3 [95]. Notch1, Notch2, and Dll1 expression were demonstrated to be significantly upregulated in adult DS fibroblasts and cortices [94]. This process may increase Hes protein activity, thus contributing to the activation of STAT3 and enhancing astroglial differentiation. Notably, Wu and colleagues demonstrated, independently of DS studies, that Notch1 overexpression in glial restricted precursor cells (GRPs) upregulated *Hes1* mRNA levels and that overexpression of Hes1 promoted astrocyte generation at the expense of oligodendrocytes [96]. Taken together, the upregulation of JAK-STAT and Notch signaling may synergistically contribute to astrogliogenesis, thereby suppressing neurogenesis [6] and oligodendrogenesis in the DS brain.

4.4. Wnt/β-Catenin Signaling

The wingless and integration site (Wnt) signaling pathway is another fundamental mechanism that directs cell proliferation, polarity, and fate determination during embryonic development and tissue homeostasis [97,98]. Activation of the canonical Wnt pathway is dependent on the nuclear translocation of β-catenin, which drives the expression of several target genes [99]. The canonical Wnt signaling consists of extracellular Wnt proteins/ligands, surface membrane frizzled receptors (Fzd), low density lipoprotein (LDL) receptor related protein-5 and 6 (LRP-5/6), cytoplasmic β-catenin, and intranuclear transcription factors of the T cell factor/lymphoid enhancer factor (TCF/LEF) family. Binding of a Wnt ligand to Fzd and Lrp5/6 causes the degradation of the β-catenin destruction complex, which consists of adenomatous polyposis coli (APC), axin, glycogen synthase kinase 3 β (Gsk3β), and casein kinase 1 (CK1). This leads to the accumulation of β-catenin in the cytoplasm, which then translocates to the nucleus where it induces the expression of downstream target genes, including cyclin Dl, which is mediated by binding to TCF4 [99]. Signaling via the Wnt/β-catenin pathway is also a key regulator of oligodendrocyte development, as it is transiently activated in OPCs concurrent with the initiation of terminal differentiation [100]. β-catenin activity is down-regulated in mature oligodendrocytes, which is necessary for accurate oligodendrocyte differentiation [100], as mutant mice with elevated Wnt/β-catenin signaling in the oligodendrocyte lineage display blocked differentiation and hypomyelination [101]. Paradoxically, however, deletion of the Wnt effector TCF4 does not cause precocious oligodendrocyte differentiation as may be expected, but rather blocks oligodendrocyte differentiation [100,102,103]. Interestingly, loss of β-catenin in NPCs was demonstrated to cause precocious specification and differentiation to astrocytes [104].

In the context of DS, general downregulation of the Wnt/β-catenin signaling pathway was demonstrated in human DS and the DS mouse Tc1 hippocampus [99]. In particular, free, and thus activated, β-catenin levels were dramatically diminished. Contrary to this finding, Li and colleagues observed elevated β-catenin signaling in gene perturbation studies targeting a specific Hsa21-endcoded gene that they suggested was implicated in DS pathogenesis, which nevertheless resulted in defective neurogenesis [105]. Taken together, the aberrant Wnt/β-catenin signaling observed in DS may also contribute to defective oligodendrogenesis and lead to a gliogenic cell-fate shift during early brain development and homeostasis.

4.5. Nfatc/Calcineurin Signaling

The nuclear factor of activated T cell (Nfat) pathway is an essential regulator of vertebrate development, which is necessary for the regulation of proliferation and differentiation of NPCs from the SVZ [106]. Activated by calcineurin, a calcium and calmodulin-dependent serine/threonine protein phosphatase, cytoplasmic Nfatc is dephosphorylated and subsequently translocated into the nucleus, where it regulates protein expression such as IL-2 [6]. Regulator of calcineurin 1 (RCAN1), formerly known as DS critical region 1 (DSCR1), inhibits the calcineurin-mediated activation of Nfatc. Interestingly, RCAN1 is located on Hsa21 and was shown to be overexpressed in the DS fetal brain and in Ts1Cje and Ts65Dn mice [107,108]. Accordingly, Nfatc4 was reported to be hyperphosphorylated in the human fetal DS brain at gestation week 20 [109]. In this context, it needs to be mentioned that DYRK1A and RCAN1 were shown to act synergistically to control phosphorylation levels of Nfatc [109,110]. DYRK1A increases RCAN1 inhibitory activity by phosphorylating it and is capable of reducing Nfatc transcriptional activity by directly phosphorylating Nfatc proteins.

Notably, Nfat/calcineurin signaling was shown to be required for oligodendroglial differentiation and myelination by transcription factor network tuning [111]. When Nfatc activation was inhibited by preventing calcineurin binding to Nfats, OPC maturation and differentiation was strongly reduced. This pathway may therefore contribute to aberrant oligodendrogenesis and hypomyelination in DS, as inhibition of Nfatc/calcineurin signaling is mediated by elevated RCAN1 and DYRK1A activities.

4.6. APP-Mediated Signaling

The Hsa21-encoded *Amyloid precursor protein (APP)* gene is involved in cell migration and cell-cycle progression in brain development [112], specifically influencing NPC proliferation, cell-fate specification, and maturation [113]. Depending on the APP processing pathway (non-/amyloidogenic), APP is cleaved by α-, β-, and γ-secretases, resulting in N-terminal soluble secreted APP (sAPP) and C-terminal fragments, such as Aβ and the APP intracellular domain (AICD). The dysregulation of APP due to triplication was suggested to result in early-onset AD-like pathology in DS. Indeed, APP protein levels were shown to be increased in homogenates from the temporal cortex of fetuses with DS [6,114], and neuritic Aβ plaque formation is present in the hippocampus and enthorinal cortex of almost all adults with DS and in some DS children [115–117]. Furthermore, the triplication of APP in Ts65Dn mice was demonstrated to impair NPC proliferation, differentiation and maturation due to increased levels of AICD [73,89,118].

Notably, elevated levels of AICD increased the Ptch1 expression in trisomic NPCs [89], hence the APP/AICD system may at least contribute to the derangement of SHH signaling, as outlined above. Moreover, increased AICD levels can promote Gsk3β activity, thereby reducing the translocation of β-catenin to the nucleus, which may contribute to the suppression of the Wnt/β-catenin pathway [118]. Interestingly, a study in the field of intraventricular hemorrhage (IVH), a common neurological complication of prematurity causing cognitive deficits and ID [119], which is accompanied by inhibited proliferation/maturation of OPCs and hypomyelination [120], demonstrated that Gsk3β activity interfered with OPC differentiation and myelination [121]. Furthermore, a cross-talk of Gsk3β and Notch signaling was shown, as inhibition of Gsk3β downregulated Notch signaling. Accordingly, it can be suggested that increased Gsk3β activity due to APP overexpression may contribute to increased Notch signaling, thus enhancing astrogliogenesis at the expense of oligodendrogenesis. Indeed, exposure to soluble APP was demonstrated to regulate human NPC differentiation through activation of JAK-STAT and Notch signaling and to induce astrocytic differentiation [122]. As Aβ itself was reported to increase apoptosis in oligodendroglia in vitro [123], a more widespread implication of this protein is suggested to lead to aberrant oligodendrogenesis in DS.

5. Regulators of Glia Cell Fate: Avenues to Adjust Aberrant White Matter?

Adjusting glia cell-fate imbalance, hence overcoming intrinsic defects in oligodendroglial cell maturation and subsequently developmental dysmyelination, will be a major target in order to improve white matter structures in DS. To this end, repurposing pre-existing modulators or compounds developed for the promotion of endogenous oligodendroglial cell maturation in demyelinating diseases such as multiple sclerosis (MS) [9,124–126] represents a possible strategy. In this context, currently evaluated drugs related to the development of myelin-repair therapies are discussed here.

Modulating the Wnt/β-catenin pathway by means of indometacin, a non-steroidal anti-inflammatory drug (NSAID) [127], or Gsk3β inhibitors, such as CHIR99021 or LY-294002, exhibited the potential to promote oligodendrogenesis in healthy and demyelinated paradigms [86,87]. Furthermore, the antifungal agent miconazole, which interferes with ergosterol synthesis, as well as corticosteroid betamethasone clobetasol, which suppresses inflammatory responses, were demonstrated as therapeutic compounds for enhancing (re)myelination in vivo and in human OPCs in vitro [128]. Moreover, modulation of histamine receptor signaling by means of GSK239512, a histamine H3 receptor antagonist, was demonstrated to boost oligodendroglial differentiation as indicated by phenotypic screening and genetic association of human demyelination lesion samples of patients with MS [129]. In this regard, magnetization transfer ratio (MTR)-based post-hoc analyses indicated a small mean improvement in myelin content in treated patients with relapsing remitting (RR) MS relative to placebo [130]. On the other hand, the first-generation histamine H1 receptor blocker clemastine was initially identified as a remyelinating drug in a high-throughput screening [131] and was further investigated in a RRMS clinical study demonstrating a reduction in P100 latency delay in visual evoked potentials (VEPs) [132]. This readout could be used to monitor myelination dependent signal propagation in the visual system. In addition to these OPC-directed drugs, several experimental compounds have been described to trigger signaling pathways modulating oligodendrogenesis. The endothelin (ET) receptor antagonist BQ788 was demonstrated to block endothelin-B receptor activation on astrocytes, thereby rescuing oligodendrogenesis and promoting remyelination [133]. The flavonoid molecule quercetin leads to enhanced oligodendrogenesis and remyelination in several ways, as it suppresses Notch signaling by inhibiting γ-secretase activity and disrupts the binding of β-catenin to TCF4 [134]. In a recent study by Granno and colleagues, a major role of Wnt/β-catenin signaling in DS was implicated. They combined bioinformatics with RNA and protein analyses using post-mortem tissue from adult DS individuals. Among other molecules, they identified axin2 to be significantly decreased in DS [99]. As the small molecule XAV939 was previously shown to stabilize axin2 by inhibiting the poly-ADP-ribosylating enzymes tankyrase 1 and 2 in hypoxic and demyelinating injuries, thereby accelerating OPC differentiation and myelination [135], it might also constitute a possible treatment approach for white matter deficits in DS.

Moreover, small molecule approaches addressing transcriptional/epigenetic regulators affecting oligodendrogenesis could also provide additional therapeutic perspectives. In this regard, GANT61, a blocker of the transcription factor Gli1, was demonstrated to promote the generation of oligodendrocytes from adult NSCs [90]. In accordance, specific inactivation of SIRT1 by means of the small molecule inhibitor EX-527, a protein deacetylase implicated in energy metabolism, increased the production of new NSC-derived OPCs in the adult mouse brain [136]. Likewise, a similar promoting effect could also be attributed to this molecule in the OPC context [137]. Furthermore, activation of the fibroblast growth factor receptor-3 (FGFR3) signaling was recently shown to redirect the differentiation of SVZ-derived NSCs from neuronal to oligodendroglial lineage, hence, promoting remyelination [138]. In this context, the membrane-bound and the cleaved ectodomains of the klotho protein were observed to be associated with FGFR3 signaling. This protein acts as a co-receptor and was found to modulate the Wnt and IGF pathways, thereby enhancing remyelination in demyelinating animal models [139,140].

However, promoting oligodendroglial maturation and axonal ensheathment might not be sufficient for successful white matter restoration or rescue. Reprogramming or reconverting astroglial to oligodendroglial cells, as well as a preservation of the oligodendroglial lineage by means of genetic or pharmacological approaches, are most likely mandatory for white matter stabilization in DS [9,141]. In 2014, information on FDA-approved drugs/small molecules, suitable for rescuing cognitive impairment due to neurodevelopmental alterations, neurotransmitter imbalances, and neurodegeneration in the Ts65Dn DS mouse, was compiled [5]. Of note, the preclinical evaluations that emerged from this study need to be considered critically, as this mouse model did not reflect all trisomic orthologues in individuals with DS, hence an effective translation to human clinical trials is still unclear. However, beside neurogenic effects, some identified drugs are also likely to foster oligodendrogenesis, thus representing potential therapeutics for enhanced myelin development and stabilization. Among these listed drugs, the selective generic estrogen receptor (ER) β agonist diarylpropionitrile (DPN) could be of interest based on the observation that it confers functional neuroprotection in a chronic experimental autoimmune encephalomyelitis (EAE) mouse model of MS by stimulating endogenous remyelination [142]. The stimulation of glial progenitor cells (GPCs) derived from both the SVZ and white matter with memantine, a low-affinity antagonist of NMDA receptors used to treat AD, was found to promote oligodendrogenesis, and therefore myelin repair, upon ischemic periventricular leukomalacia (PVL) [143]. Moreover, fluoxetine, an antidepressant based on selective serotonin reuptake inhibition, also known as Prozac, was demonstrated to boost oligodendrocyte-related gene transcripts such as *CNPase*, *OLIG1*, and *MOG* when applied to rhesus monkeys with major depressive disorders [144]. Lithium chloride (LiCl), which was established for the treatment of bipolar disorder (BD), can stimulate oligodendrocyte morphological maturation and promote remyelination after toxin-induced demyelination of organotypic slice cultures [145]. In addition, melatonin, a sleep/wake-cycle regulating hormone, was shown to increase oligodendrocyte generation from NSCs [146]. Further to this, the vitamin E derivate TFA-12 was found to reduce astrogliosis and to accelerate remyelination of toxin-induced demyelinated lesions [147]. Given the impact of SHH signaling in oligodendrogenesis, a recent study demonstrated that the small molecule Smo agonist SAG could alter SHH signaling in DS [148]. Notably, SAG modulates oligodendroglial differentiation and additionally steers commitment of NSCs to the oligodendroglial lineage [92]. Interestingly, the γ-secretase inhibitor DAPT (N-[N-(3,5-difluorophenacetyl)-1-alanyl]-S-phenyl-glycinet-butylester) is an effective inhibitor of the Notch signaling pathway and might also confer benefits to white matter, as it was found to promote differentiation of NSCs/NPCs into oligodendrocytes, astrocytes, and neurons in vitro [149]. Nevertheless, to what degree the balance between these two glial cell types is affected remains to be shown. In this context, such a preferred shift toward oligodendroglia could be mediated via the acetylcholine esterase inhibitor donepezil, an FDA-approved drug for Alzheimer's disease and dementia. Donepezil was shown to promote the differentiation of primary NSCs into mature oligodendrocytes at the expense of astrocytes [150], and it was also found to enhance myelin sheath generation in neuron/glia co-cultures [151]. The FDA-approved anti-seizure drug ethosuximide was described to be capable of inducing trans-differentiation of muscle-derived stem cells into Olig2-positive oligodendroglial cells [152]. Whether ethosuximide activity could also be used to re-establish the glial cell balance needs to be shown, keeping in mind that Olig2 expression itself is not restricted to oligodendroglial cells, but is also found in the cytoplasm of astroglia [153].

The histone deacetylase class I and II inhibitors trichostatin A and valproate (VPA) were previously demonstrated to promote the conversion of astrocytes to OPCs [154,155], and could thus be considered as potential regulators for the desired glial shift in DS. A similar mode of action was revealed in response to forced expression of the microRNA miR-302/367 cluster, thereby enhancing the generation of oligodendroglia from astrocytes [156]. Likewise, injection of Sox2 lentiviral particles into the corpus callosum following cuprizone-mediated demyelination in vivo as well as lentiviral transduction of astroglial cells in vitro resulted in a conversion of astrocytes to oligodendroglial cells [156]. Similarly, overexpression of pro-oligodendroglial transcription factors, such as Olig2 or Ascl1/Mash1, also resulted in reprogramming of NSCs toward an oligodendroglial fate [157–160]. Of note, *Olig2* is an Hsa21-encoded gene, which was shown to be overexpressed in DS and assumed to interfere with neurogenesis in DS [6]. However, we demonstrated here that oligodendrogenesis is negatively affected in DS.

Nevertheless, it appears that the drugs and transcriptional/epigenetic regulators described here could indeed provide new avenues for the experimental and clinical rescue of white matter deficits in DS. To what degree some of these candidates are applicable in the context of DS in terms of application and opportunity windows certainly needs additional experimental and pre-clinical research efforts.

6. Concluding Remarks

Given the importance of myelinating glial cells for axonal support, trophism, maintenance, and electrical insulation, an overall increase in the number of functional oligodendrocytes would likely confer an overall benefit on neuronal cell numbers and functionality, which in turn could ameliorate ID, even in light of known neurogenic deficits in DS. Strikingly, DS research has so far mainly focused on aberrant neurogenesis and the underlying signaling pathways leading to defective neuronal cell proliferation, differentiation, and progenitor cell fate in DS. In this review, the collected evidence suggests that many of these dysregulated signaling pathways may also be involved in defective DS-related NSC/OPC proliferation, differentiation, and fate commitment. Furthermore, we demonstrated that several drugs and molecules identified to restore brain developmental deficits in rodent DS models based on neurogenesis criteria [5] might also mediate beneficial effects on the oligodendroglial lineage.

Hsa21 is the smallest human chromosome, currently known to encode more than 400 genes. This number might increase over time due to the recognition of non-coding RNAs [161,162]. Nevertheless, the description of dosage-sensitive Hsa21 genes resulting in a specific phenotype by gene-copy number variations is currently limited to only a few. This may be due to the fact that over 20 proteins encoded by Hsa21 are involved in signal transduction and more than 30 proteins are considered to belong to transcription factors, both of which most likely influence the expression of other genes in the genomes of DS patients [7]. By implication, this inevitably results in a genome-wide dysregulation of several networks at the same time, which could be demonstrated, for example, in the case of the gene cluster M43, which is related to oligodendroglial differentiation and myelination [11].

Interestingly, pharmacological approaches addressing neurogenic deficits were found to be successful in a broad age range (prenatal, perinatal, and adult) of treated Ts65Dn mice, suggesting that the prevention or amelioration of cognitive deficits in DS may indeed be possible. This paves the way toward clinical trials, some of which (donepezil, folate or memantine) are still in progress, but no differences in outcome between treated and placebo have occurred as yet [5]. In humans, however, prenatal treatments will be challenging due to specific safety requirements. Nevertheless, the window of opportunity to improve differentiation and homeostasis in the oligodendroglial lineage might stretch over several developmental phases, as myelination is mainly a postnatal event. In this regard, it is worth mentioning that dysregulation of the M43 gene cluster, which is related to oligodendroglial lineage, appears during late neonate's development and during the first years of postnatal life in DS [11], a period that coincides with massive upregulation of oligodendroglial and myelination genes [163], as well as oligodendrocyte expansion in the human brain [164].

A number of mouse models with DS-related features were generated and used to study Hsa21 dosage-sensitive genes and to understand their roles leading to cognitive impairment (reviewed in [5,165,166]). Although well-established mouse models such as Ts65Dn, Ts1Cje, and Ts16 recapitulate the human neuropathological phenotype to a certain extent, modeling of DS in rodent system remains challenging because Hsa21 genes are distributed throughout mouse chromosomes 16, 17, and 10 (Mmu16/17/10). Therefore, mouse models may provide different outcomes, hence negatively affecting translation to humans.

Author Contributions: Conceptualization, L.R. and P.G.; writing—original draft preparation, L.R., P.K., and P.G.; writing—review and editing, L.R., P.K., and P.G.; supervision, P.G.

Funding: This study was supported by the Jürgen Manchot foundation, Düsseldorf. Research on white matter deficits, myelin repair, and neuroregeneration in the laboratory of P.K. was additionally funded by the Deutsche Forschungsgemeinschaft (DFG; grants KU1934/2-1, KU1934/5-1), Christiane and Claudia Hempel Foundation for clinical stem cell research, DMSG Ortsvereinigung Düsseldorf und Umgebung e.V., iBrain, Stifterverband/Novartisstiftung, and the James and Elisabeth Cloppenburg, Peek and Cloppenburg Düsseldorf Stiftung. The MS Center at the Department of Neurology is supported in part by the Walter and Ilse Rose Foundation.

Conflicts of Interest: The authors declare no conflict of interest.

References

1. Baburamani, A.A.; Patkee, P.A.; Arichi, T.; Rutherford, M.A. New approaches to studying early brain development in Down syndrome. *Dev. Med. Child Neurol.* **2019**, *61*, 867–879. [CrossRef] [PubMed]
2. Chapman, R.S.; Hesketh, L.J. Behavioral phenotype of individuals with Down syndrome. *Ment. Retard. Dev. Disabil. Res. Rev.* **2000**, *6*, 84–95. [CrossRef]
3. Dossi, E.; Vasile, F.; Rouach, N. Human astrocytes in the diseased brain. *Brain Res. Bull.* **2017**. [CrossRef] [PubMed]
4. Haydar, T.F.; Reeves, R.H. Trisomy 21 and early brain development. *Trends Neurosci.* **2012**, *35*, 81–91. [CrossRef]
5. Gardiner, K.J. Pharmacological approaches to improving cognitive function in Down syndrome: Current status and considerations. *Drug Des. Dev. Ther.* **2015**, *9*, 103–125. [CrossRef]
6. Stagni, F.; Giacomini, A.; Emili, M.; Guidi, S.; Bartesaghi, R. Neurogenesis impairment: An early developmental defect in Down syndrome. *Free Radic. Biol. Med.* **2017**. [CrossRef]
7. Antonarakis, S.E. Down syndrome and the complexity of genome dosage imbalance. *Nat. Rev. Genet.* **2017**, *18*, 147–163. [CrossRef]

8. Xu, R.; Brawner, A.T.; Li, S.; Liu, J.J.; Kim, H.; Xue, H.; Pang, Z.P.; Kim, W.Y.; Hart, R.P.; Liu, Y.; et al. OLIG2 Drives Abnormal Neurodevelopmental Phenotypes in Human iPSC-Based Organoid and Chimeric Mouse Models of Down Syndrome. *Cell Stem Cell* **2019**, *24*, 908–926.e908. [CrossRef]
9. Kremer, D.; Göttle, P.; Hartung, H.-P.; Küry, P. Pushing Forward: Remyelination as the New Frontier in CNS Diseases. *Trends Neurosci.* **2016**, *39*, 246–263. [CrossRef]
10. Kanaumi, T.; Milenkovic, I.; Adle-Biassette, H.; Aronica, E.; Kovacs, G.G. Non-neuronal cell responses differ between normal and Down syndrome developing brains. *Int. J. Dev. Neurosci.* **2013**, *31*, 796–803. [CrossRef]
11. Olmos-Serrano, J.L.; Kang, H.J.; Tyler, W.A.; Silbereis, J.C.; Cheng, F.; Zhu, Y.; Pletikos, M.; Jankovic-Rapan, L.; Cramer, N.P.; Galdzicki, Z.; et al. Down Syndrome Developmental Brain Transcriptome Reveals Defective Oligodendrocyte Differentiation and Myelination. *Neuron* **2016**, *89*, 1208–1222. [CrossRef]
12. Zdaniuk, G.; Wierzba-Bobrowicz, T.; Szpak, G.M.; Stepien, T. Astroglia disturbances during development of the central nervous system in fetuses with Down's syndrome. *Folia Neuropathol.* **2011**, *49*, 109–114.
13. Mito, T.; Becker, L.E. Developmental changes of S-100 protein and glial fibrillary acidic protein in the brain in Down syndrome. *Exp. Neurol.* **1993**, *120*, 170–176. [CrossRef]
14. Murphy, G.M., Jr.; Ellis, W.G.; Lee, Y.L.; Stultz, K.E.; Shrivastava, R.; Tinklenberg, J.R.; Eng, L.F. Astrocytic gliosis in the amygdala in Down's syndrome and Alzheimer's disease. *Prog. Brain Res.* **1992**, *94*, 475–483.
15. Takashima, S.; Becker, L.E. Basal ganglia calcification in Down's syndrome. *J. Neurol. Neurosurg. Psychiatry* **1985**, *48*, 61–64. [CrossRef]
16. Karlsen, A.S.; Pakkenberg, B. Total numbers of neurons and glial cells in cortex and basal ganglia of aged brains with Down syndrome—A stereological study. *Cereb. Cortex* **2011**, *21*, 2519–2524. [CrossRef]
17. Wisniewski, K.E.; Schmidt-Sidor, B. Postnatal delay of myelin formation in brains from Down syndrome infants and children. *Clin. Neuropathol.* **1989**, *8*, 55–62.
18. Abraham, H.; Vincze, A.; Veszpremi, B.; Kravjak, A.; Gomori, E.; Kovacs, G.G.; Seress, L. Impaired myelination of the human hippocampal formation in Down syndrome. *Int. J. Dev. Neurosci.* **2012**, *30*, 147–158. [CrossRef]
19. Koo, B.K.; Blaser, S.; Harwood-Nash, D.; Becker, L.E.; Murphy, E.G. Magnetic resonance imaging evaluation of delayed myelination in Down syndrome: A case report and review of the literature. *J. Child Neurol.* **1992**, *7*, 417–421. [CrossRef]
20. Fenoll, R.; Pujol, J.; Esteba-Castillo, S.; de Sola, S.; Ribas-Vidal, N.; Garcia-Alba, J.; Sanchez-Benavides, G.; Martinez-Vilavella, G.; Deus, J.; Dierssen, M.; et al. Anomalous White Matter Structure and the Effect of Age in Down Syndrome Patients. *J. Alzheimers Dis.* **2017**, *57*, 61–70. [CrossRef]
21. Romano, A.; Moraschi, M.; Cornia, R.; Bozzao, A.; Rossi-Espagnet, M.C.; Giove, F.; Albertini, G.; Pierallini, A. White matter involvement in young non-demented Down's syndrome subjects: A tract-based spatial statistic analysis. *Neuroradiology* **2018**, *60*, 1335–1341. [CrossRef]
22. Gunbey, H.P.; Bilgici, M.C.; Aslan, K.; Has, A.C.; Ogur, M.G.; Alhan, A.; Incesu, L. Structural brain alterations of Down's syndrome in early childhood evaluation by DTI and volumetric analyses. *Eur. Radiol.* **2017**, *27*, 3013–3021. [CrossRef]
23. Powell, D.; Caban-Holt, A.; Jicha, G.; Robertson, W.; Davis, R.; Gold, B.T.; Schmitt, F.A.; Head, E. Frontal white matter integrity in adults with Down syndrome with and without dementia. *Neurobiol. Aging* **2014**, *35*, 1562–1569. [CrossRef]
24. McKenzie, I.A.; Ohayon, D.; Li, H.; de Faria, J.P.; Emery, B.; Tohyama, K.; Richardson, W.D. Motor skill learning requires active central myelination. *Science* **2014**, *346*, 318–322. [CrossRef]
25. Liu, J.; Dietz, K.; DeLoyht, J.M.; Pedre, X.; Kelkar, D.; Kaur, J.; Vialou, V.; Lobo, M.K.; Dietz, D.M.; Nestler, E.J.; et al. Impaired adult myelination in the prefrontal cortex of socially isolated mice. *Nat. Neurosci.* **2012**, *15*, 1621–1623. [CrossRef]
26. Lanfranchi, S.; Jerman, O.; Dal Pont, E.; Alberti, A.; Vianello, R. Executive function in adolescents with Down Syndrome. *J. Intellect. Disabil. Res.* **2010**, *54*, 308–319. [CrossRef]
27. Baddeley, A.; Jarrold, C. Working memory and Down syndrome. *J. Intellect. Disabil. Res.* **2007**, *51*, 925–931. [CrossRef]
28. Rowe, J.; Lavender, A.; Turk, V. Cognitive executive function in Down's syndrome. *Br. J. Clin. Psychol.* **2006**, *45*, 5–17. [CrossRef]
29. Nelson, L.; Johnson, J.K.; Freedman, M.; Lott, I.; Groot, J.; Chang, M.; Milgram, N.W.; Head, E. Learning and memory as a function of age in Down syndrome: A study using animal-based tasks. *Prog. Neuro-Psychopharmacol. Biol. Psychiatry* **2005**, *29*, 443–453. [CrossRef]

30. Pennington, B.F.; Moon, J.; Edgin, J.; Stedron, J.; Nadel, L. The neuropsychology of Down syndrome: Evidence for hippocampal dysfunction. *Child Dev.* **2003**, *74*, 75–93. [CrossRef]
31. Lanfranchi, S.; Carretti, B.; Spano, G.; Cornoldi, C. A specific deficit in visuospatial simultaneous working memory in Down syndrome. *J. Intellect. Disabil. Res.* **2009**, *53*, 474–483. [CrossRef] [PubMed]
32. Lanfranchi, S.; Cornoldi, C.; Vianello, R. Verbal and Visuospatial Working Memory Deficits in Children With Down Syndrome. *Am. J. Ment. Retard.* **2004**, *109*, 456–466. [CrossRef]
33. Lanfranchi, S.; Jerman, O.; Vianello, R. Working Memory and Cognitive Skills in Individuals with Down Syndrome. *Child Neuropsychol.* **2009**, *15*, 397–416. [CrossRef] [PubMed]
34. Fields, R.D. White matter in learning, cognition and psychiatric disorders. *Trends Neurosci.* **2008**, *31*, 361–370. [CrossRef]
35. Simon, K.; Hennen, S.; Merten, N.; Blattermann, S.; Gillard, M.; Kostenis, E.; Gomeza, J. The Orphan G Protein-coupled Receptor GPR17 Negatively Regulates Oligodendrocyte Differentiation via Galphai/o and Its Downstream Effector Molecules. *J. Biol. Chem.* **2016**, *291*, 705–718. [CrossRef]
36. Wang, X.; Zhao, Y.; Zhang, X.; Badie, H.; Zhou, Y.; Mu, Y.; Loo, L.S.; Cai, L.; Thompson, R.C.; Yang, B.; et al. Loss of sorting nexin 27 contributes to excitatory synaptic dysfunction by modulating glutamate receptor recycling in Down's syndrome. *Nat. Med.* **2013**, *19*, 473–480. [CrossRef]
37. Meraviglia, V.; Ulivi, A.F.; Boccazzi, M.; Valenza, F.; Fratangeli, A.; Passafaro, M.; Lecca, D.; Stagni, F.; Giacomini, A.; Bartesaghi, R.; et al. SNX27, a protein involved in down syndrome, regulates GPR17 trafficking and oligodendrocyte differentiation. *Glia* **2016**, *64*, 1437–1460. [CrossRef]
38. Rowitch, D.H.; Kriegstein, A.R. Developmental genetics of vertebrate glial-cell specification. *Nature* **2010**, *468*, 214–222. [CrossRef]
39. Casano, A.M.; Peri, F. Microglia: Multitasking specialists of the brain. *Dev. Cell.* **2015**, *32*, 469–477. [CrossRef]
40. Michell-Robinson, M.A.; Touil, H.; Healy, L.M.; Owen, D.R.; Durafourt, B.A.; Bar-Or, A.; Antel, J.P.; Moore, C.S. Roles of microglia in brain development, tissue maintenance and repair. *Brain* **2015**, *138*, 1138–1159. [CrossRef]
41. Peters, A. A fourth type of neuroglial cell in the adult central nervous system. *J. Neurocytol.* **2004**, *33*, 345–357. [CrossRef] [PubMed]
42. Kriegstein, A.; Alvarez-Buylla, A. The glial nature of embryonic and adult neural stem cells. *Annu. Rev. Neurosci.* **2009**, *32*, 149–184. [CrossRef] [PubMed]
43. Dawson, M.R.; Polito, A.; Levine, J.M.; Reynolds, R. NG2-expressing glial progenitor cells: An abundant and widespread population of cycling cells in the adult rat CNS. *Mol. Cell. Neurosci.* **2003**, *24*, 476–488. [CrossRef]
44. Raff, M.C.; Miller, R.H.; Noble, M. A glial progenitor cell that develops in vitro into an astrocyte or an oligodendrocyte depending on culture medium. *Nature* **1983**, *303*, 390–396. [CrossRef] [PubMed]
45. Dimou, L.; Gotz, M. Glial cells as progenitors and stem cells: New roles in the healthy and diseased brain. *Physiol. Rev.* **2014**, *94*, 709–737. [CrossRef]
46. Nishiyama, A.; Boshans, L.; Goncalves, C.M.; Wegrzyn, J.; Patel, K.D. Lineage, fate, and fate potential of NG2-glia. *Brain Res.* **2016**, *1638*, 116–128. [CrossRef]
47. Tanner, D.C.; Cherry, J.D.; Mayer-Pröschel, M. Oligodendrocyte Progenitors Reversibly Exit the Cell Cycle and Give Rise to Astrocytes in Response to Interferon-γ. *J. Neurosci.* **2011**, *31*, 6235. [CrossRef]
48. Menn, B.; Garcia-Verdugo, J.M.; Yaschine, C.; Gonzalez-Perez, O.; Rowitch, D.; Alvarez-Buylla, A. Origin of oligodendrocytes in the subventricular zone of the adult brain. *J. Neurosci.* **2006**, *26*, 7907–7918. [CrossRef]
49. Ortega, F.; Gascon, S.; Masserdotti, G.; Deshpande, A.; Simon, C.; Fischer, J.; Dimou, L.; Chichung Lie, D.; Schroeder, T.; Berninger, B. Oligodendrogliogenic and neurogenic adult subependymal zone neural stem cells constitute distinct lineages and exhibit differential responsiveness to Wnt signalling. *Nat. Cell Biol.* **2013**, *15*, 602–613. [CrossRef]
50. Snaidero, N.; Simons, M. Myelination at a glance. *J. Cell Sci.* **2014**, *127*, 2999–3004. [CrossRef]
51. Snaidero, N.; Simons, M. The logistics of myelin biogenesis in the central nervous system. *Glia* **2017**, *65*, 1021–1031. [CrossRef] [PubMed]
52. Miron, V.E.; Kuhlmann, T.; Antel, J.P. Cells of the oligodendroglial lineage, myelination, and remyelination. *Biochim. Biophys. Acta* **2011**, *1812*, 184–193. [CrossRef] [PubMed]
53. Lu, Q.R.; Sun, T.; Zhu, Z.; Ma, N.; Garcia, M.; Stiles, C.D.; Rowitch, D.H. Common developmental requirement for Olig function indicates a motor neuron/oligodendrocyte connection. *Cell* **2002**, *109*, 75–86. [CrossRef]
54. El Waly, B.; Macchi, M.; Cayre, M.; Durbec, P. Oligodendrogenesis in the normal and pathological central nervous system. *Front. Neurosci.* **2014**, *8*, 145. [CrossRef]

55. Samanta, J.; Kessler, J.A. Interactions between ID and OLIG proteins mediate the inhibitory effects of BMP4 on oligodendroglial differentiation. *Development* **2004**, *131*, 4131–4142. [CrossRef]
56. Zhang, L.; He, X.; Liu, L.; Jiang, M.; Zhao, C.; Wang, H.; He, D.; Zheng, T.; Zhou, X.; Hassan, A.; et al. Hdac3 Interaction with p300 Histone Acetyltransferase Regulates the Oligodendrocyte and Astrocyte Lineage Fate Switch. *Dev. Cell* **2016**, *37*, 582. [CrossRef]
57. Golden, J.A.; Hyman, B.T. Development of the superior temporal neocortex is anomalous in trisomy 21. *J. Neuropathol. Exp. Neurol.* **1994**, *53*, 513–520. [CrossRef]
58. Winter, T.C.; Ostrovsky, A.A.; Komarniski, C.A.; Uhrich, S.B. Cerebellar and frontal lobe hypoplasia in fetuses with trisomy 21: Usefulness as combined US markers. *Radiology* **2000**, *214*, 533–538. [CrossRef]
59. Pinter, J.D.; Eliez, S.; Schmitt, J.E.; Capone, G.T.; Reiss, A.L. Neuroanatomy of Down's syndrome: A high-resolution MRI study. *Am. J. Psychiatry* **2001**, *158*, 1659–1665. [CrossRef]
60. Schmidt-Sidor, B.; Wisniewski, K.E.; Shepard, T.H.; Sersen, E.A. Brain growth in Down syndrome subjects 15 to 22 weeks of gestational age and birth to 60 months. *Clin. Neuropathol.* **1990**, *9*, 181–190.
61. Liu, B.; Filippi, S.; Roy, A.; Roberts, I. Stem and progenitor cell dysfunction in human trisomies. *EMBO Rep.* **2015**, *16*, 44–62. [CrossRef] [PubMed]
62. Guidi, S.; Bonasoni, P.; Ceccarelli, C.; Santini, D.; Gualtieri, F.; Ciani, E.; Bartesaghi, R. Neurogenesis impairment and increased cell death reduce total neuron number in the hippocampal region of fetuses with Down syndrome. *Brain Pathol.* **2008**, *18*, 180–197. [CrossRef] [PubMed]
63. Lu, J.; Lian, G.; Zhou, H.; Esposito, G.; Steardo, L.; Delli-Bovi, L.C.; Hecht, J.L.; Lu, Q.R.; Sheen, V. OLIG2 over-expression impairs proliferation of human Down syndrome neural progenitors. *Hum. Mol. Genet.* **2012**, *21*, 2330–2340. [CrossRef] [PubMed]
64. Chakrabarti, L.; Best, T.K.; Cramer, N.P.; Carney, R.S.; Isaac, J.T.; Galdzicki, Z.; Haydar, T.F. Olig1 and Olig2 triplication causes developmental brain defects in Down syndrome. *Nat. Neurosci.* **2010**, *13*, 927–934. [CrossRef] [PubMed]
65. Lockrow, J.; Fortress, A.; Granholm, A.-C. Age-Related Neurodegeneration and Memory Loss in Down Syndrome. *Curr. Gerontol. Geriatr. Res.* **2012**, *2012*, 463909. [CrossRef]
66. Bonni, A.; Sun, Y.; Nadal-Vicens, M.; Bhatt, A.; Frank, D.A.; Rozovsky, I.; Stahl, N.; Yancopoulos, G.D.; Greenberg, M.E. Regulation of gliogenesis in the central nervous system by the JAK-STAT signaling pathway. *Science* **1997**, *278*, 477–483. [CrossRef]
67. Hong, S.; Song, M.-R. STAT3 but not STAT1 is required for astrocyte differentiation. *PLoS ONE* **2014**, *9*, e86851. [CrossRef]
68. Kurabayashi, N.; Nguyen, M.D.; Sanada, K. DYRK1A overexpression enhances STAT activity and astrogliogenesis in a Down syndrome mouse model. *EMBO Rep.* **2015**, *16*, 1548–1562. [CrossRef]
69. Cao, F.; Hata, R.; Zhu, P.; Nakashiro, K.; Sakanaka, M. Conditional deletion of Stat3 promotes neurogenesis and inhibits astrogliogenesis in neural stem cells. *Biochem. Biophys. Res. Commun.* **2010**, *394*, 843–847. [CrossRef]
70. Corsi, M.M.; Dogliotti, G.; Pedroni, F.; Palazzi, E.; Magni, P.; Chiappelli, M.; Licastro, F. Plasma nerve growth factor (NGF) and inflammatory cytokines (IL-6 and MCP-1) in young and adult subjects with Down syndrome: An interesting pathway. *Neuro Endocrinol. Lett.* **2006**, *27*, 773–778.
71. Hallam, D.M.; Capps, N.L.; Travelstead, A.L.; Brewer, G.J.; Maroun, L.E. Evidence for an interferon-related inflammatory reaction in the trisomy 16 mouse brain leading to caspase-1-mediated neuronal apoptosis. *J. Neuroimmunol.* **2000**, *110*, 66–75. [CrossRef]
72. Lee, H.C.; Tan, K.L.; Cheah, P.S.; Ling, K.H. Potential Role of JAK-STAT Signaling Pathway in the Neurogenic-to-Gliogenic Shift in Down Syndrome Brain. *Neural Plasticity* **2016**, *2016*, 7434191. [CrossRef] [PubMed]
73. Trazzi, S.; Fuchs, C.; Valli, E.; Perini, G.; Bartesaghi, R.; Ciani, E. The amyloid precursor protein (APP) triplicated gene impairs neuronal precursor differentiation and neurite development through two different domains in the Ts65Dn mouse model for Down syndrome. *J. Biol. Chem.* **2013**, *288*, 20817–20829. [CrossRef] [PubMed]
74. Sullivan, K.D.; Lewis, H.C.; Hill, A.A.; Pandey, A.; Jackson, L.P.; Cabral, J.M.; Smith, K.P.; Liggett, L.A.; Gomez, E.B.; Galbraith, M.D.; et al. Trisomy 21 consistently activates the interferon response. *Elife* **2016**, *5*. [CrossRef]

75. Wilcock, D.M. Neuroinflammation in the aging down syndrome brain; lessons from Alzheimer's disease. *Curr. Gerontol. Geriatr. Res.* **2012**, *2012*, 170276. [CrossRef]
76. Ferrando-Miguel, R.; Shim, K.S.; Cheon, M.S.; Gimona, M.; Furuse, M.; Lubec, G. Overexpression of Interferon α/β Receptor β Chain in Fetal Down Syndrome Brain. *Neuroembryol. Aging* **2003**, *2*, 147–155. [CrossRef]
77. Guimera, J.; Casas, C.; Estivill, X.; Pritchard, M. Human minibrain homologue (MNBH/DYRK1): Characterization, alternative splicing, differential tissue expression, and overexpression in Down syndrome. *Genomics* **1999**, *57*, 407–418. [CrossRef]
78. Sun, Y.; Lehmbecker, A.; Kalkuhl, A.; Deschl, U.; Sun, W.; Rohn, K.; Tzvetanova, I.D.; Nave, K.A.; Baumgartner, W.; Ulrich, R. STAT3 represents a molecular switch possibly inducing astroglial instead of oligodendroglial differentiation of oligodendroglial progenitor cells in Theiler's murine encephalomyelitis. *Neuropathol. Appl. Neurobiol.* **2015**, *41*, 347–370. [CrossRef]
79. Corbin, J.G.; Kelly, D.; Rath, E.M.; Baerwald, K.D.; Suzuki, K.; Popko, B. Targeted CNS expression of interferon-gamma in transgenic mice leads to hypomyelination, reactive gliosis, and abnormal cerebellar development. *Mol. Cell. Neurosci.* **1996**, *7*, 354–370. [CrossRef]
80. Martí, E.; Bovolenta, P. Sonic hedgehog in CNS development: One signal, multiple outputs. *Trends Neurosci.* **2002**, *25*, 89–96. [CrossRef]
81. Alberta, J.A.; Park, S.-K.; Mora, J.; Yuk, D.-i.; Pawlitzky, I.; Iannarelli, P.; Vartanian, T.; Stiles, C.D.; Rowitch, D.H. Sonic Hedgehog Is Required during an Early Phase of Oligodendrocyte Development in Mammalian Brain. *Mol. Cell. Neurosci.* **2001**, *18*, 434–441. [CrossRef] [PubMed]
82. Danesin, C.; Agius, E.; Escalas, N.; Ai, X.; Emerson, C.; Cochard, P.; Soula, C. Ventral Neural Progenitors Switch toward an Oligodendroglial Fate in Response to Increased Sonic Hedgehog (Shh) Activity: Involvement of Sulfatase 1 in Modulating Shh Signaling in the Ventral Spinal Cord. *J. Neurosci.* **2006**, *26*, 5037. [CrossRef] [PubMed]
83. Loulier, K.; Ruat, M.; Traiffort, E. Increase of proliferating oligodendroglial progenitors in the adult mouse brain upon Sonic hedgehog delivery in the lateral ventricle. *J. Neurochem.* **2006**, *98*, 530–542. [CrossRef] [PubMed]
84. Ferent, J.; Zimmer, C.; Durbec, P.; Ruat, M.; Traiffort, E. Sonic Hedgehog Signaling Is a Positive Oligodendrocyte Regulator during Demyelination. *J. Neurosci.* **2013**, *33*, 1759. [CrossRef] [PubMed]
85. Taipale, J.; Cooper, M.K.; Maiti, T.; Beachy, P.A. Patched acts catalytically to suppress the activity of Smoothened. *Nature* **2002**, *418*, 892–896. [CrossRef] [PubMed]
86. Laouarem, Y.; Traiffort, E. Developmental and Repairing Production of Myelin: The Role of Hedgehog Signaling. *Front. Cell. Neurosci.* **2018**, *12*. [CrossRef] [PubMed]
87. Oh, S.; Huang, X.; Chiang, C. Specific requirements of sonic hedgehog signaling during oligodendrocyte development. *Dev. Dyn.* **2005**, *234*, 489–496. [CrossRef]
88. Yu, K.; McGlynn, S.; Matise, M.P. Floor plate-derived sonic hedgehog regulates glial and ependymal cell fates in the developing spinal cord. *Development* **2013**, *140*, 1594–1604. [CrossRef]
89. Trazzi, S.; Mitrugno, V.M.; Valli, E.; Fuchs, C.; Rizzi, S.; Guidi, S.; Perini, G.; Bartesaghi, R.; Ciani, E. APP-dependent up-regulation of Ptch1 underlies proliferation impairment of neural precursors in Down syndrome. *Hum. Mol. Genet.* **2011**, *20*, 1560–1573. [CrossRef]
90. Samanta, J.; Grund, E.M.; Silva, H.M.; Lafaille, J.J.; Fishell, G.; Salzer, J.L. Inhibition of Gli1 mobilizes endogenous neural stem cells for remyelination. *Nature* **2015**, *526*, 448–452. [CrossRef]
91. Tan, M.; Hu, X.; Qi, Y.; Park, J.; Cai, J.; Qiu, M. Gli3 mutation rescues the generation, but not the differentiation, of oligodendrocytes in Shh mutants. *Brain Res.* **2006**, *1067*, 158–163. [CrossRef] [PubMed]
92. Wang, L.C.; Almazan, G. Role of Sonic Hedgehog Signaling in Oligodendrocyte Differentiation. *Neurochem. Res.* **2016**, *41*, 3289–3299. [CrossRef] [PubMed]
93. Ravanelli, A.M.; Kearns, C.A.; Powers, R.K.; Wang, Y.; Hines, J.H.; Donaldson, M.J.; Appel, B. Sequential specification of oligodendrocyte lineage cells by distinct levels of Hedgehog and Notch signaling. *Dev. Biol.* **2018**, *444*, 93–106. [CrossRef] [PubMed]
94. Fischer, D.F.; van Dijk, R.; Sluijs, J.A.; Nair, S.M.; Racchi, M.; Levelt, C.N.; van Leeuwen, F.W.; Hol, E.M. Activation of the Notch pathway in Down syndrome: Cross-talk of Notch and APP. *FASEB J.* **2005**, *19*, 1451–1458. [CrossRef] [PubMed]
95. Kamakura, S.; Oishi, K.; Yoshimatsu, T.; Nakafuku, M.; Masuyama, N.; Gotoh, Y. Hes binding to STAT3 mediates crosstalk between Notch and JAK-STAT signalling. *Nat. Cell Biol.* **2004**, *6*, 547–554. [CrossRef]

96. Wu, Y.; Liu, Y.; Levine, E.M.; Rao, M.S. Hes1 but not Hes5 regulates an astrocyte versus oligodendrocyte fate choice in glial restricted precursors. *Dev. Dyn.* **2003**, *226*, 675–689. [CrossRef]
97. Logan, C.Y.; Nusse, R. The Wnt signaling pathway in development and disease. *Annu. Rev. Cell Dev. Biol.* **2004**, *20*, 781–810. [CrossRef]
98. Soomro, S.; Jie, J.; Fu, H. Oligodendrocytes Development and Wnt Signaling Pathway. *Int. J. Hum. Anat.* **2018**, *1*, 17–35. [CrossRef]
99. Granno, S.; Nixon-Abell, J.; Berwick, D.C.; Tosh, J.; Heaton, G.; Almudimeegh, S.; Nagda, Z.; Rain, J.C.; Zanda, M.; Plagnol, V.; et al. Downregulated Wnt/beta-catenin signalling in the Down syndrome hippocampus. *Sci. Rep.* **2019**, *9*, 7322. [CrossRef]
100. Emery, B. Regulation of oligodendrocyte differentiation and myelination. *Science* **2010**, *330*, 779–782. [CrossRef]
101. Fancy, S.P.; Baranzini, S.E.; Zhao, C.; Yuk, D.I.; Irvine, K.A.; Kaing, S.; Sanai, N.; Franklin, R.J.; Rowitch, D.H. Dysregulation of the Wnt pathway inhibits timely myelination and remyelination in the mammalian CNS. *Genes Dev.* **2009**, *23*, 1571–1585. [CrossRef] [PubMed]
102. Ye, F.; Chen, Y.; Hoang, T.; Montgomery, R.L.; Zhao, X.H.; Bu, H.; Hu, T.; Taketo, M.M.; van Es, J.H.; Clevers, H.; et al. HDAC1 and HDAC2 regulate oligodendrocyte differentiation by disrupting the beta-catenin-TCF interaction. *Nat. Neurosci.* **2009**, *12*, 829–838. [CrossRef] [PubMed]
103. Fu, H.; Qi, Y.; Tan, M.; Cai, J.; Takebayashi, H.; Nakafuku, M.; Richardson, W.; Qiu, M. Dual origin of spinal oligodendrocyte progenitors and evidence for the cooperative role of Olig2 and Nkx2.2 in the control of oligodendrocyte differentiation. *Development* **2002**, *129*, 681–693. [PubMed]
104. Sun, S.; Zhu, X.-J.; Huang, H.; Guo, W.; Tang, T.; Xie, B.; Xu, X.; Zhang, Z.; Shen, Y.; Dai, Z.-M.; et al. WNT signaling represses astrogliogenesis via Ngn2-dependent direct suppression of astrocyte gene expression. *Glia* **2019**, *67*, 1333–1343. [CrossRef] [PubMed]
105. Li, S.S.; Qu, Z.D.; Haas, M.; Ngo, L.; Heo, Y.J.; Kang, H.J.; Britto, J.M.; Cullen, H.D.; Vanyai, H.K.; Tan, S.S.; et al. The HSA21 gene EURL/C21ORF91 controls neurogenesis within the cerebral cortex and is implicated in the pathogenesis of Down Syndrome. *Sci. Rep.* **2016**, *6*, 14. [CrossRef] [PubMed]
106. Serrano-Pérez, M.C.; Fernández, M.; Neria, F.; Berjón-Otero, M.; Doncel-Pérez, E.; Cano, E.; Tranque, P. NFAT transcription factors regulate survival, proliferation, migration, and differentiation of neural precursor cells. *Glia* **2015**, *63*, 987–1004. [CrossRef] [PubMed]
107. Kurabayashi, N.; Sanada, K. Increased dosage of DYRK1A and DSCR1 delays neuronal differentiation in neocortical progenitor cells. *Genes Dev.* **2013**, *27*, 2708–2721. [CrossRef]
108. Baek, K.H.; Zaslavsky, A.; Lynch, R.C.; Britt, C.; Okada, Y.; Siarey, R.J.; Lensch, M.W.; Park, I.H.; Yoon, S.S.; Minami, T.; et al. Down's syndrome suppression of tumour growth and the role of the calcineurin inhibitor DSCR1. *Nature* **2009**, *459*, 1126–1130. [CrossRef]
109. Arron, J.R.; Winslow, M.M.; Polleri, A.; Chang, C.P.; Wu, H.; Gao, X.; Neilson, J.R.; Chen, L.; Heit, J.J.; Kim, S.K.; et al. NFAT dysregulation by increased dosage of DSCR1 and DYRK1A on chromosome 21. *Nature* **2006**, *441*, 595–600. [CrossRef]
110. Jung, M.S.; Park, J.H.; Ryu, Y.S.; Choi, S.H.; Yoon, S.H.; Kwen, M.Y.; Oh, J.Y.; Song, W.J.; Chung, S.H. Regulation of RCAN1 protein activity by Dyrk1A protein-mediated phosphorylation. *J. Biol. Chem.* **2011**, *286*, 40401–40412. [CrossRef]
111. Weider, M.; Starost, L.J.; Groll, K.; Kuspert, M.; Sock, E.; Wedel, M.; Frob, F.; Schmitt, C.; Baroti, T.; Hartwig, A.C.; et al. Nfat/calcineurin signaling promotes oligodendrocyte differentiation and myelination by transcription factor network tuning. *Nat. Commun.* **2018**, *9*, 899. [CrossRef] [PubMed]
112. Nalivaeva, N.N.; Turner, A.J. The amyloid precursor protein: A biochemical enigma in brain development, function and disease. *FEBS Lett.* **2013**, *587*, 2046–2054. [CrossRef] [PubMed]
113. Zhou, Z.D.; Chan, C.H.; Ma, Q.H.; Xu, X.H.; Xiao, Z.C.; Tan, E.K. The roles of amyloid precursor protein (APP) in neurogenesis: Implications to pathogenesis and therapy of Alzheimer disease. *Cell Adhes. Migr.* **2011**, *5*, 280–292. [CrossRef] [PubMed]
114. Guidi, S.; Emili, M.; Giacomini, A.; Stagni, F.; Bartesaghi, R. Neuroanatomical alterations in the temporal cortex of human fetuses with Down syndrome. In Proceedings of the 2nd International Conference of the Trisomy 21 Research Society, Chicago, IL, USA, 7–11 June 2017; p. 79.

115. Hof, P.R.; Bouras, C.; Perl, D.P.; Sparks, D.L.; Mehta, N.; Morrison, J.H. Age-related distribution of neuropathologic changes in the cerebral cortex of patients with Down's syndrome. Quantitative regional analysis and comparison with Alzheimer's disease. *Arch. Neurol.* **1995**, *52*, 379–391. [CrossRef] [PubMed]
116. Hyman, B.T.; West, H.L.; Rebeck, G.W.; Lai, F.; Mann, D.M. Neuropathological changes in Down's syndrome hippocampal formation. Effect of age and apolipoprotein E genotype. *Arch. Neurol.* **1995**, *52*, 373–378. [CrossRef] [PubMed]
117. Leverenz, J.B.; Raskind, M.A. Early amyloid deposition in the medial temporal lobe of young Down syndrome patients: A regional quantitative analysis. *Exp. Neurol.* **1998**, *150*, 296–304. [CrossRef] [PubMed]
118. Trazzi, S.; Fuchs, C.; De Franceschi, M.; Mitrugno, V.M.; Bartesaghi, R.; Ciani, E. APP-dependent alteration of GSK3β activity impairs neurogenesis in the Ts65Dn mouse model of Down syndrome. *Neurobiol. Dis.* **2014**, *67*, 24–36. [CrossRef]
119. Ballabh, P. Intraventricular hemorrhage in premature infants: Mechanism of disease. *Pediatr. Res.* **2010**, *67*, 1–8. [CrossRef]
120. Dummula, K.; Vinukonda, G.; Chu, P.; Xing, Y.; Hu, F.; Mailk, S.; Csiszar, A.; Chua, C.; Mouton, P.; Kayton, R.J.; et al. Bone morphogenetic protein inhibition promotes neurological recovery after intraventricular hemorrhage. *J. Neurosci.* **2011**, *31*, 12068–12082. [CrossRef]
121. Dohare, P.; Cheng, B.; Ahmed, E.; Yadala, V.; Singla, P.; Thomas, S.; Kayton, R.; Ungvari, Z.; Ballabh, P. Glycogen synthase kinase-3β inhibition enhances myelination in preterm newborns with intraventricular hemorrhage, but not recombinant Wnt3A. *Neurobiol. Dis.* **2018**, *118*, 22–39. [CrossRef]
122. Sugaya, K. Mechanism of glial differentiation of neural progenitor cells by amyloid precursor protein. *Neurodegener. Dis.* **2008**, *5*, 170–172. [CrossRef]
123. Roth, A.D.; Ramirez, G.; Alarcon, R.; Von Bernhardi, R. Oligodendrocytes damage in Alzheimer's disease: Beta amyloid toxicity and inflammation. *Biol. Res.* **2005**, *38*, 381–387. [CrossRef]
124. Kremer, D.; Akkermann, R.; Küry, P.; Dutta, R. Current advancements in promoting remyelination in multiple sclerosis. *Mult. Scler.* **2019**, *25*, 7–14. [CrossRef] [PubMed]
125. Küry, P.; Kremer, D.; Göttle, P. Drug repurposing for neuroregeneration in multiple sclerosis. *Neural Regen. Res.* **2018**, *13*, 1366–1367. [CrossRef] [PubMed]
126. Azim, K.; Angonin, D.; Marcy, G.; Pieropan, F.; Rivera, A.; Donega, V.; Cantu, C.; Williams, G.; Berninger, B.; Butt, A.M.; et al. Pharmacogenomic identification of small molecules for lineage specific manipulation of subventricular zone germinal activity. *PLoS Biol.* **2017**, *15*, e2000698. [CrossRef] [PubMed]
127. Preisner, A.; Albrecht, S.; Cui, Q.L.; Hucke, S.; Ghelman, J.; Hartmann, C.; Taketo, M.M.; Antel, J.; Klotz, L.; Kuhlmann, T. Non-steroidal anti-inflammatory drug indometacin enhances endogenous remyelination. *Acta Neuropathol.* **2015**, *130*, 247–261. [CrossRef]
128. Najm, F.J.; Madhavan, M.; Zaremba, A.; Shick, E.; Karl, R.T.; Factor, D.C.; Miller, T.E.; Nevin, Z.S.; Kantor, C.; Sargent, A.; et al. Drug-based modulation of endogenous stem cells promotes functional remyelination in vivo. *Nature* **2015**, *522*, 216–220. [CrossRef]
129. Chen, Y.; Zhen, W.; Guo, T.; Zhao, Y.; Liu, A.; Rubio, J.P.; Krull, D.; Richardson, J.C.; Lu, H.; Wang, R. Histamine Receptor 3 negatively regulates oligodendrocyte differentiation and remyelination. *PLoS ONE* **2017**, *12*, e0189380. [CrossRef]
130. Schwartzbach, C.J.; Grove, R.A.; Brown, R.; Tompson, D.; Then Bergh, F.; Arnold, D.L. Lesion remyelinating activity of GSK239512 versus placebo in patients with relapsing-remitting multiple sclerosis: A randomised, single-blind, phase II study. *J. Neurol.* **2017**, *264*, 304–315. [CrossRef]
131. Mei, F.; Fancy, S.P.J.; Shen, Y.A.; Niu, J.; Zhao, C.; Presley, B.; Miao, E.; Lee, S.; Mayoral, S.R.; Redmond, S.A.; et al. Micropillar arrays as a high-throughput screening platform for therapeutics in multiple sclerosis. *Nature Med.* **2014**, *20*, 954–960. [CrossRef]
132. Green, A.J.; Gelfand, J.M.; Cree, B.A.; Bevan, C.; Boscardin, W.J.; Mei, F.; Inman, J.; Arnow, S.; Devereux, M.; Abounasr, A.; et al. Clemastine fumarate as a remyelinating therapy for multiple sclerosis (ReBUILD): A randomised, controlled, double-blind, crossover trial. *Lancet* **2017**, *390*, 2481–2489. [CrossRef]
133. Hammond, T.R.; McEllin, B.; Morton, P.D.; Raymond, M.; Dupree, J.; Gallo, V. Endothelin-B Receptor Activation in Astrocytes Regulates the Rate of Oligodendrocyte Regeneration during Remyelination. *Cell Rep.* **2015**, *13*, 2090–2097. [CrossRef] [PubMed]

134. Wu, X.; Qu, X.; Zhang, Q.; Dong, F.; Yu, H.; Yan, C.; Qi, D.; Wang, M.; Liu, X.; Yao, R. Quercetin promotes proliferation and differentiation of oligodendrocyte precursor cells after oxygen/glucose deprivation-induced injury. *Cell Mol. Neurobiol.* **2014**, *34*, 463–471. [CrossRef] [PubMed]
135. Fancy, S.P.; Harrington, E.P.; Yuen, T.J.; Silbereis, J.C.; Zhao, C.; Baranzini, S.E.; Bruce, C.C.; Otero, J.J.; Huang, E.J.; Nusse, R.; et al. Axin2 as regulatory and therapeutic target in newborn brain injury and remyelination. *Nat. Neurosci.* **2011**, *14*, 1009–1016. [CrossRef] [PubMed]
136. Rafalski, V.A.; Ho, P.P.; Brett, J.O.; Ucar, D.; Dugas, J.C.; Pollina, E.A.; Chow, L.M.; Ibrahim, A.; Baker, S.J.; Barres, B.A.; et al. Expansion of oligodendrocyte progenitor cells following SIRT1 inactivation in the adult brain. *Nat. Cell Biol.* **2013**, *15*, 614–624. [CrossRef] [PubMed]
137. Prozorovski, T.; Ingwersen, J.; Lukas, D.; Göttle, P.; Koop, B.; Graf, J.; Schneider, R.; Franke, K.; Schumacher, S.; Britsch, S.; et al. Regulation of sirtuin expression in autoimmune neuroinflammation: Induction of SIRT1 in oligodendrocyte progenitor cells. *Neurosci. Lett.* **2019**, *704*, 116–125. [CrossRef]
138. Kang, W.; Nguyen, K.C.Q.; Hebert, J.M. Transient Redirection of SVZ Stem Cells to Oligodendrogenesis by FGFR3 Activation Promotes Remyelination. *Stem Cell Rep.* **2019**, *12*, 1223–1231. [CrossRef]
139. Kuro-o, M. Klotho. *Pflug. Arch.* **2010**, *459*, 333–343. [CrossRef]
140. Torbus-Paluszczak, M.; Bartman, W.; Adamczyk-Sowa, M. Klotho protein in neurodegenerative disorders. *Neurol. Sci.* **2018**, *39*, 1677–1682. [CrossRef]
141. Zare, L.; Baharvand, H.; Javan, M. In vivo conversion of astrocytes to oligodendrocyte lineage cells using chemicals: Targeting gliosis for myelin repair. *Regen. Med.* **2018**, *13*, 803–819. [CrossRef]
142. Khalaj, A.J.; Hasselmann, J.; Augello, C.; Moore, S.; Tiwari-Woodruff, S.K. Nudging oligodendrocyte intrinsic signaling to remyelinate and repair: Estrogen receptor ligand effects. *J. Steroid Biochem. Mol. Biol.* **2016**, *160*, 43–52. [CrossRef] [PubMed]
143. Li, W.J.; Mao, F.X.; Chen, H.J.; Qian, L.H.; Buzby, J.S. Treatment with UDP-glucose, GDNF, and memantine promotes SVZ and white matter self-repair by endogenous glial progenitor cells in neonatal rats with ischemic PVL. *Neuroscience* **2015**, *284*, 444–458. [CrossRef] [PubMed]
144. Rajkowska, G.; Mahajan, G.; Maciag, D.; Sathyanesan, M.; Iyo, A.H.; Moulana, M.; Kyle, P.B.; Woolverton, W.L.; Miguel-Hidalgo, J.J.; Stockmeier, C.A.; et al. Oligodendrocyte morphometry and expression of myelin—Related mRNA in ventral prefrontal white matter in major depressive disorder. *J. Psychiatr. Res.* **2015**, *65*, 53–62. [CrossRef] [PubMed]
145. Meffre, D.; Massaad, C.; Grenier, J. Lithium chloride stimulates PLP and MBP expression in oligodendrocytes via Wnt/beta-catenin and Akt/CREB pathways. *Neuroscience* **2015**, *284*, 962–971. [CrossRef] [PubMed]
146. Ghareghani, M.; Sadeghi, H.; Zibara, K.; Danaei, N.; Azari, H.; Ghanbari, A. Melatonin Increases Oligodendrocyte Differentiation in Cultured Neural Stem Cells. *Cell. Mol. Neurobiol.* **2017**, *37*, 1319–1324. [CrossRef]
147. Blanchard, B.; Heurtaux, T.; Garcia, C.; Moll, N.M.; Caillava, C.; Grandbarbe, L.; Klopstein, A.; Kerninon, C.; Frah, M.; Coowar, D.; et al. Tocopherol derivative TFA-12 promotes myelin repair in experimental models of multiple sclerosis. *J. Neurosci.* **2013**, *33*, 11633–11642. [CrossRef]
148. Das, I.; Park, J.-M.; Shin, J.H.; Jeon, S.K.; Lorenzi, H.; Linden, D.J.; Worley, P.F.; Reeves, R.H. Hedgehog agonist therapy corrects structural and cognitive deficits in a Down syndrome mouse model. *Sci. Transl. Med.* **2013**, *5*, 201ra120. [CrossRef]
149. Wang, J.; Ye, Z.; Zheng, S.; Chen, L.; Wan, Y.; Deng, Y.; Yang, R. Lingo-1 shRNA and Notch signaling inhibitor DAPT promote differentiation of neural stem/progenitor cells into neurons. *Brain Res.* **2016**, *1634*, 34–44. [CrossRef]
150. Imamura, O.; Arai, M.; Dateki, M.; Takishima, K. Donepezil promotes differentiation of neural stem cells into mature oligodendrocytes at the expense of astrogenesis. *J. Neurochem.* **2017**, *140*, 231–244. [CrossRef]
151. Cui, X.; Guo, Y.E.; Fang, J.H.; Shi, C.J.; Suo, N.; Zhang, R.; Xie, X. Donepezil, a drug for Alzheimer's disease, promotes oligodendrocyte generation and remyelination. *Acta Pharmacol. Sin* **2019**. [CrossRef]
152. Kang, M.L.; Kwon, J.S.; Kim, M.S. Induction of neuronal differentiation of rat muscle-derived stem cells in vitro using basic fibroblast growth factor and ethosuximide. *Int. J. Mol. Sci.* **2013**, *14*, 6614–6623. [CrossRef] [PubMed]
153. Setoguchi, T.; Kondo, T. Nuclear export of OLIG2 in neural stem cells is essential for ciliary neurotrophic factor-induced astrocyte differentiation. *J. Cell Biol.* **2004**, *166*, 963–968. [CrossRef] [PubMed]

154. Zare, L.; Baharvand, H.; Javan, M. Trichostatin A Promotes the Conversion of Astrocytes to Oligodendrocyte Progenitors in a Defined Culture Medium. *Iran J. Pharm. Res.* **2019**, *18*, 286–295. [PubMed]
155. Ghasemi-Kasman, M.; Zare, L.; Baharvand, H.; Javan, M. In vivo conversion of astrocytes to myelinating cells by miR-302/367 and valproate to enhance myelin repair. *J. Tissue Eng. Regen. Med.* **2018**, *12*, e462–e472. [CrossRef] [PubMed]
156. Farhangi, S.; Dehghan, S.; Totonchi, M.; Javan, M. In vivo conversion of astrocytes to oligodendrocyte lineage cells in adult mice demyelinated brains by Sox2. *Mult. Scler. Relat. Disord.* **2019**, *28*, 263–272. [CrossRef] [PubMed]
157. Hack, M.A.; Saghatelyan, A.; de Chevigny, A.; Pfeifer, A.; Ashery-Padan, R.; Lledo, P.M.; Gotz, M. Neuronal fate determinants of adult olfactory bulb neurogenesis. *Nat. Neurosci.* **2005**, *8*, 865–872. [CrossRef]
158. Maire, C.L.; Wegener, A.; Kerninon, C.; Nait Oumesmar, B. Gain-of-function of Olig transcription factors enhances oligodendrogenesis and myelination. *Stem Cells* **2010**, *28*, 1611–1622. [CrossRef]
159. Jessberger, S.; Toni, N.; Clemenson, G.D., Jr.; Ray, J.; Gage, F.H. Directed differentiation of hippocampal stem/progenitor cells in the adult brain. *Nat. Neurosci.* **2008**, *11*, 888–893. [CrossRef]
160. Braun, S.M.; Pilz, G.A.; Machado, R.A.; Moss, J.; Becher, B.; Toni, N.; Jessberger, S. Programming Hippocampal Neural Stem/Progenitor Cells into Oligodendrocytes Enhances Remyelination in the Adult Brain after Injury. *Cell Rep.* **2015**, *11*, 1679–1685. [CrossRef]
161. Gardiner, K.; Costa, A.C. The proteins of human chromosome 21. *Am. J. Med. Genet C Semin Med. Genet.* **2006**, *142C*, 196–205. [CrossRef]
162. Wiseman, F.K.; Alford, K.A.; Tybulewicz, V.L.J.; Fisher, E.M.C. Down syndrome-recent progress and future prospects. *Hum. Mol. Genet.* **2009**, *18*, R75–R83. [CrossRef] [PubMed]
163. Kang, H.J.; Kawasawa, Y.I.; Cheng, F.; Zhu, Y.; Xu, X.; Li, M.; Sousa, A.M.; Pletikos, M.; Meyer, K.A.; Sedmak, G.; et al. Spatio-temporal transcriptome of the human brain. *Nature* **2011**, *478*, 483–489. [CrossRef] [PubMed]
164. Yeung, M.S.; Zdunek, S.; Bergmann, O.; Bernard, S.; Salehpour, M.; Alkass, K.; Perl, S.; Tisdale, J.; Possnert, G.; Brundin, L.; et al. Dynamics of oligodendrocyte generation and myelination in the human brain. *Cell* **2014**, *159*, 766–774. [CrossRef] [PubMed]
165. Herault, Y.; Delabar, J.M.; Fisher, E.M.C.; Tybulewicz, V.L.J.; Yu, E.; Brault, V. Rodent models in Down syndrome research: Impact and future opportunities. *Dis. Model. Mech.* **2017**, *10*, 1165–1186. [CrossRef] [PubMed]
166. Gupta, M.; Dhanasekaran, A.R.; Gardiner, K.J. Mouse models of Down syndrome: Gene content and consequences. *Mamm. Genome* **2016**, *27*, 538–555. [CrossRef] [PubMed]

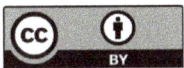

© 2019 by the authors. Licensee MDPI, Basel, Switzerland. This article is an open access article distributed under the terms and conditions of the Creative Commons Attribution (CC BY) license (http://creativecommons.org/licenses/by/4.0/).

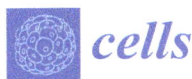

Article

Investigation of Cuprizone-Induced Demyelination in mGFAP-Driven Conditional Transient Receptor Potential Ankyrin 1 (TRPA1) Receptor Knockout Mice

Gábor Kriszta [1,2,3], Balázs Nemes [1], Zoltán Sándor [1], Péter Ács [4], Sámuel Komoly [4], Zoltán Berente [3,5], Kata Bölcskei [1,2,†] and Erika Pintér [1,2,*,†]

1. Department of Pharmacology and Pharmacotherapy, University of Pécs Medical School, Pécs H-7624, Hungary; gabor.kriszta@aok.pte.hu (G.K.); balazs.nemes@aok.pte.hu (B.N.); zoltan.sandor@aok.pte.hu (Z.S.); kata.bolcskei@aok.pte.hu (K.B.)
2. Molecular Pharmacology Research Group and Center for Neuroscience, János Szentágothai Research Center, University of Pécs, Pécs H-7624, Hungary
3. Research Group for Experimental Diagnostic Imaging, University of Pécs Medical School, Pécs H-7624, Hungary; zoltan.berente@aok.pte.hu
4. Department of Neurology, University of Pécs Medical School, Pécs H-7623, Hungary; acs.peter@pte.hu (P.Á.); komoly.samuel@pte.hu (S.K.)
5. Department of Biochemistry and Medical Chemistry, University of Pécs Medical School, Pécs H-7624, Hungary
* Correspondence: erika.pinter@aok.pte.hu
† These authors contributed equally to this work.

Received: 7 November 2019; Accepted: 20 December 2019; Published: 28 December 2019

Abstract: Transient receptor potential ankyrin 1 (TRPA1) receptors are non-selective cation channels responsive to a variety of exogenous irritants and endogenous stimuli including products of oxidative stress. It is mainly expressed by primary sensory neurons; however, expression of TRPA1 by astrocytes and oligodendrocytes has recently been detected in the mouse brain. Genetic deletion of TRPA1 was shown to attenuate cuprizone-induced oligodendrocyte apoptosis and myelin loss in mice. In the present study we aimed at investigating mGFAP-Cre conditional TRPA1 knockout mice in the cuprizone model. These animals were generated by crossbreeding GFAP-Cre$^{+/-}$ and floxed TRPA1 (TRPA1$^{Fl/Fl}$) mice. Cuprizone was administered for 6 weeks and demyelination was followed by magnetic resonance imaging (MRI). At the end of the treatment, demyelination and glial activation was also investigated by histological methods. The results of the MRI showed that demyelination was milder at weeks 3 and 4 in both homozygous (GFAP-Cre$^{+/-}$ TRPA1$^{Fl/Fl}$) and heterozygous (GFAP-Cre$^{+/-}$ TRPA1$^{Fl/-}$) conditional knockout animals compared to Cre$^{-/-}$ control mice. However, by week 6 of the treatment the difference was not detectable by either MRI or histological methods. In conclusion, TRPA1 receptors on astrocytes may transiently contribute to the demyelination induced by cuprizone, however, expression and function of TRPA1 receptors by other cells in the brain (oligodendrocytes, microglia, neurons) warrant further investigation.

Keywords: transient receptor potential ankyrin 1; cuprizone; demyelination; astrocyte; conditional knockout; magnetic resonance imaging

1. Introduction

Transient receptor potential ankyrin 1 (TRPA1) receptors are non-selective cation channels which are responsive to a variety of exogenous and endogenous stimuli including mustard oil, cinnamaldehyde, irritant chemicals such as formalin or acrolein, as well as reactive oxygen species and oxidized lipid molecules [1–3]. Apart from being a nocisensor for exogenous irritant compounds, it has been suggested to work as a sensor for oxidative stress [4]. Originally described to be localized on a subgroup of nociceptive primary afferent neurons [5,6], it was later revealed that TRPA1 is also expressed at lower levels by various non-neuronal cells including keratinocytes, endothelial cells and cells of the gastrointestinal mucosa [1–3,7]. More importantly, several studies have supported the presence of TRPA1 receptors in the brain on astrocytes [8–10], as well as oligodendrocytes [11]. A recent cell-specific transcriptome analysis of the mouse cortex revealed low level expression of TRPA1 on neurons, astrocytes, oligodendrocytes and microglia, as well [12].

In astrocytes, TRPA1 receptors were implicated in both physiological and pathophysiological processes. Astrocyte TRPA1 receptors were shown to regulate resting Ca^{2+} levels and modulate GABA-ergic inhibitory transmission by reducing GABA transport [8]. TRPA1 receptors on astrocytes were also suggested to play a role in long-term potentiation in the mouse hippocampus [9]. Since reactive astrocytes can contribute to the progression of neuroinflammation in neurodegenerative diseases [13,14], several workgroups, including ours, had started to investigate the role of TRPA1 in animal models of neurodegenerative diseases. Our previous study aimed at examining the role of TRPA1 in the cuprizone-induced demyelination model in mice. Cuprizone treatment constitutes an accepted non-immune animal model of multiple sclerosis [15,16] which produces lesions resembling type III lesions seen in patients [17]. Feeding mice with cuprizone leads to a well-reproducible demyelination of the corpus callosum as well as other subcortical and cortical brain areas by inducing oligodendrocyte apoptosis and a secondary activation of astrocytes and microglia [15,16,18–21]. We have revealed that demyelination of the corpus callosum was significantly reduced in TRPA1 receptor gene-deleted mice [22,23]. Based on our data we have assumed that TRPA1 receptors localized on astrocytes may influence the astrocyte-oligodendrocyte crosstalk. Activation of these receptors on the astrocytes increases the intracellular Ca^{2+} concentration and subsequent release of mediators. Astrocyte-derived signaling molecules may contribute to the apoptosis of oligodendrocytes by promoting the proapoptotic p38-MAPK pathway resulting in c-Jun activation [22]. We have also shown that TRPA1 deficiency did not affect the number of oligodendrocyte precursor cells (OPCs) during cuprizone treatment. In TRPA1 KO mice, there was no increase or a less pronounced increase of growth factors promoting OPC proliferation (FGF-2, IGF-1). The level of Bak mRNA, a marker of apoptosis and levels of pro-apoptotic signalling proteins were significantly lower in cuprizone-treated TRPA1 KO animals. All these data suggest that TRPA1 deficiency did not affect oligodendrocyte development but reduced the apoptosis of mature oligodendrocytes [22]. In contrast with our theory, Hamilton and coworkers assumed a direct action of TRPA1 activation on myelination. They detected the functional expression of TRPA1 on oligodendrocytes and showed that ischemia-induced demyelination was diminished in the lack of TRPA1 receptors [11]. Likewise, another group showed that in TRPA1 receptor gene-deleted mice behavioral deficits and neuroinflammation were less severe in a transgenic mouse model of Alzheimer's disease [24]. The same group also later demonstrated that the loss of TRPA1 is associated with decreased anxiety-like behavior and improved performance in spatial memory and social discrimination tests [25].

Based on these prior data we focused on further elucidating the role of TRPA1 receptors in the cuprizone model. In the present study, the effects of cuprizone in the corpus callosum were studied in mGFAP-driven conditional TRPA1 knockout mice.

2. Materials and Methods

2.1. Ethics

The study was designed and conducted according to European legislation (Directive 2010/63/EU) and Hungarian Government regulation (40/2013., II. 14.) on the protection of animals used for scientific purposes. The project was approved by the Animal Welfare Committee of the University of Pécs and the National Scientific Ethical Committee on Animal Experimentation of Hungary and licensed by the Government Office of Baranya County (license No. BA02/2000-82/2017).

2.2. Animals

Animals were bred in the Animal House of the Department of Pharmacology and Pharmacotherapy of the University of Pécs and kept in the Animal House of the Szentágothai Research Center during the experiments. Mice were housed in groups of 3–7 in standard polycarbonate cages on wood shavings bedding. Food and water were provided *ad libitum*. The temperature was maintained at 24 °C and the lighting was set to a 12 h light-dark cycle (lights on from 6:00 a.m. to 6:00 p.m.).

The mGFAP-driven conditional TRPA1 receptor knockout mice were produced via crossbreeding floxed TRPA1 carrying mice (B6.129S-Trpa1tm2Kykw/J) by GFAP promoter directed Cre recombinase gene expressing mice (B6.Cg-Tg(Gfap-cre) 77.6Mvs/2J) both obtained from The Jackson Laboratory (Bar Harbor, ME, USA), stock numbers #008650 and #024098, respectively. Only female mice carrying the GFAP-Cre transgene were used to prevent non-specific Cre activation during spermatogenesis. The GFAP-Cre transgene was also maintained in heterozygote form, to minimize the chance of non-specific recombination. As the first step, GFAP-Cre heterozygote females were crossbred by floxed TRPA1 homozygote males. Next, female mice heterozygote for both genes were backcrossed by floxed TRPA1 homozygote males. The obtained male Cre$^{+/-}$ TRPA1$^{Fl/Fl}$ mice were the main subjects of the experiments, whereas their male siblings (Cre$^{+/-}$ TRPA1$^{Fl/-}$ and Cre$^{-/-}$ TRPA1$^{Fl/Fl}$) were used as hetero controls and Cre negative controls, respectively. Animals showing a global KO genotype by tail analysis were excluded from the experiments (approximately 10% of all genotyped Cre$^{+/-}$ animals).

Genotyping of floxed TRPA1 was done according to the protocol suggested by the provider, using forward primer oIMR9168 (AGC AGG AGC AGA AGT ATG AAA) and reverse primer oIMR9169 (GAA GGC CAT GGC ATC TTA AC) producing 359 bp (floxed) and/or 472 bp (wild type) PCR products.

Genotyping of GFAP-Cre was done by forward primer 15831 (TCC ATA AGC CTG ACA TC) and reverse primer 15832 (TGC GAA CCT CAT CAC TCG T) also using internal positive control forward primer oIMR8744 (CAA ATG TTG CTT GTC TGG TG) and reverse primer oIMR8745 (GTC AGT CGA GTG CAC AGT TT) which produced 200 bp (internal positive control) and ~400 bp (GFAP-Cre positive) PCR products. Genotyping of conditional TRPA1 receptor knockout was carried out by using forward primer exon 21 (TGT TCC TCA ACA TCC CAG CG), second forward primer oIMR9168 (AGC AGG AGC AGA AGT ATG AAA) and reverse primer oIMR9169 (GAA GGC CAT GGC ATC TTA AC) producing 609 bp (knockout), 359 bp (intact floxed) and/or 472 bp (intact wild type) PCR products, respectively. RT-PCR analysis of conditional TRPA1 receptor knockout messenger RNA was done by forward primer exon 21 (TGT TCC TCA ACA TCC CAG CG) and reverse primer exon 25 (CGT GCC TGG GTC TAT TTG GA) which produce 573 bp (intact) or 191 bp (knockout) RT-PCR products.

2.3. Mouse TRPA1 Quantitative RT-PCR

Total RNA was isolated from homogenized brain samples by using TRI Reagent (Molecular Research Centre Inc., Cincinnati, OH, USA) and Direct-Zol RNA isolation kit (Zymo Research, Irvine, CA, USA) according to the manufacturer's instructions. Purified RNA was quantified by a NanoDrop ND-1000 spectrophotometer and 1 µg total RNA was treated with DNAse I (Thermo Scientific, Waltham, MA, USA) to remove genomic DNA contamination from the samples. First strand cDNA synthesis was carried out with 0.5 µg of total RNA/sample using Maxima™ First Strand cDNA Synthesis Kit for RT-qPCR (Thermo Scientific, Waltham, MA, USA). In the PCR reaction we used SensiFast Probe Lo-ROX Kit (Bioline Inc., London, UK) and forward primer 5′ atgccttcagcaccccattg (binding site in exon 23), reverse primer 5′ gacctcagcaatgtccccaa (binding site in exon 24) and labeled probe 56FAM/tgggcagct/ZEN/tattgccttcacaat/3IABkFQ (binding site in exon 23), 1 µM each, all obtained from Integrated DNA Technologies (Coralville, IA, USA). The following PCR protocol was used on an Applied Biosystems (Foster City, CA, USA) Quantstudio5 quantitative PCR machine: 3 min 95 °C original denaturation, followed by 40 cycles of 30 s 95 °C denaturation, 30 s 62 °C annealing, 1 min 72 °C extension. The sites of the primers and probe are missing from the Cre-Lox recombined mRNA therefore this assay measures only the amount of intact TRPA1 mRNA. Mouse beta-actin mRNA was used as reference and the expression was determined by using Prime Time Std qPCR Assay

Mm.PT.58.33540333 obtained from Integrated DNA Technologies (Coralville, IA, USA) under the same PCR conditions. All qRT-PCR assays were done in duplicates in each sample and Ct values were determined. dCt values were obtained by subtracting the corresponding beta-actin Ct values from the TRPA1 Ct values. ddCt values were calculated for each sample by subtracting the average dCt value of the $Cre^{-/-}$ group (representing the 100% expression level) from each dCt value. Finally, for each sample the obtained ddCt were converted to relative expression level by the $100/(2^{ddCt})$ formula.

2.4. Cuprizone Treatment

Cuprizone was administered orally for 6 weeks as previously described [22,23]. Briefly, standard rodent chow was ground and 0.2% cuprizone was thoroughly mixed into ground chow which was placed into the cages in small ceramic bowls. Control mice were fed the milled chow without the addition of cuprizone. The chow was provided *ad libitum* to all groups and it was changed to a fresh batch each day. The general health status of animals was also monitored daily and body weights were measured every 2 days.

2.5. Magnetic Resonance Imaging (MRI)

The timeline of demyelination was monitored by T2-weighted MRI measurements on 4 mice from each group. Animals were scanned once before cuprizone administration and later once per week starting from week 2 of the treatment. The measurements were performed using a Bruker® PharmaScan® (4.7 T) small animal MRI instrument (Bruker, Billerica, MA, USA).

Anesthesia was induced by 3.5% *v/v* of isoflurane in a gas mixture of 33% O_2 and 66% N_2O via induction chamber and maintained with 1–2% isoflurane in a rodent face mask controlled by respiratory monitoring and gating system.

The imaging protocol was performed on the same day and same time each week. After B_0 mapping a multislice T2 Rapid Acquisition with Relaxation Enhancement (RARE) experiment was performed (TR/TE: 3000/50 ms, FOV: 16 × 16 mm, Thk: 0.8 mm, Gap: 0.2 mm, matrix: 160 × 160, 4 averages, RARE factor: 4) on seven coronal slices positioned to cover the whole corpus callosum. The total imaging time was roughly 12 min per animal.

Before the analysis, all imaging data were converted first into a Digital Imaging Communications in Medicines (DICOM) format and stored in an isolated hardware in a local system. Any further processing was performed via DICOM-handling software packages. (3D-Slicer v4.6 NA-MIC and Onis v2.5, Digitalcore, Tokyo, Japan) [26]. For the quantification of the damage, regions of interests (ROI) were manually circumscribed, fitted by anatomical structures in the medial corpus callosum and the signal intensities (as mean ± SEM) of ROIs have been recorded. Results were expressed in percentage of intensity ratio, compared to the pre-treatment intensity (considered as 100%) measured in the identical brain area of the same individual animal. The evaluation was performed in a blinded manner.

2.6. Histological Assessment of Cuprizone-Induced Changes in the Corpus Callosum

Animals were anesthetized with pentobarbital (70 mg/kg i.p.) at the end of the cuprizone treatment (week 6) and perfused transcardially in two steps, first with phosphate buffered saline (PBS, pH 7.4) and then with 4% paraformaldehyde in 0.1M phosphate buffer. Brains were postfixed over one night in the same fixative. 5 µm thin coronal sections from paraffin embedded brains were made and mounted onto a silane-coated slides.

2.6.1. Luxol Fast Blue-cresyl Violet (LFB/CV) Staining

LFB/CV staining was used to evaluate the severity of demyelination as described previously [20,22] on coronal sections obtained from different regions (0.14, −0.22,−1.06, and −1.94 mm) according to the mouse brain atlas of Paxinos and Franklin [27]. Brain sections on silane-coated slides were rehydrated in graded series of alcohol and incubated at 60 °C in LFB solution (0.01%), overnight. Thereafter, sections were differentiated in a solution of Li_2CO_3 (0.05%) and counterstained with CV. Four sections of each animal were scored by a semiquantitative four-tiered scoring system (0–3) in a blinded manner. Intact myelin was scored with 0 and the totally damaged myelin was labeled with score 3.

2.6.2. Immunohistochemical Detection of Myelin Basic Protein (MBP) and Astrocyte and Microglia Markers

In addition to the LFB/CV staining, immunohistochemical detection of myelin basic protein (MBP) was also performed to evaluate demyelination. Furthermore, astrocyte and microglia activation in the corpus callosum was detected with immunohistochemical staining of glial fibrillary acidic protein (GFAP) and ionized calcium-binding adaptor molecule 1 (Iba1), respectively. Briefly, 8 µm-thick paraffin sections were deparaffinized and heat-unmasked in citrate buffer. Sections were treated with 3% hydrogen peroxide to block endogenous peroxidase activity, treated with BSA and incubated for 1 h with the following primary antibodies: anti-MBP (1:100, mouse monoclonal antibody from Novocastra/Leica Biosystems (Nussloch, Germany, catalogue No. NCL-MBP; Antibody Registry No AB_563893), anti-GFAP (1:1000, rabbit polyclonal antibody from Dako, Glostrup, Denmark; catalogue No. Z0334; Antibody Registry No AB_10013382) to visualize astrocytes, anti-Iba1, (1:500, rabbit polyclonal antibody from Wako Chemicals, Neuss, Germany; catalogue No. 019-19741; Antibody Registry No AB_839504) as a marker for microglia/macrophages. Incubation was performed with the HISTO-Labeling System, the reaction was visualized using 3,3′-diaminobenzidine reaction. Sections were photographed with an Olympus DP50 camera attached to an Olympus BX51 microscope (Olympus, Tokyo, Japan) under 200x magnification. Quantification was performed by determining the mean density of equal-sized regions of interest of the medial corpus callosum with the Image-ProPlus software (Media Cybernetics, Rockville, MD, USA). The experimenter evaluating the slides was blinded to the group allocation.

2.7. Materials

Cuprizone and all other chemicals were purchased from Sigma-Aldrich (St. Louis, MO, USA), unless otherwise previously indicated. Pentobarbital (Euthanimal 20% injection ad us. vet.) was obtained from Alfasan Nederland B.V. (Woerden, The Netherlands) while isoflurane was purchased from Medicus Partner Ltd. (Biatorbágy, Hungary).

2.8. Statistics

In each group, means ± S.E.M. of parameters were calculated. Statistical analysis was carried out with the GraphPad Prism 8.0.1 software (GraphPad Software Inc., San Diego, CA, USA). For comparison of qPCR relative expression values and MRI relative intensity values, one-way ANOVA followed by Tukey's multiple comparisons test was used. Paired t-test was used to compare density values of LFB/CV and immunohistological staining, $*p < 0.05$ or $**p < 0.01$ was considered as statistically significant.

3. Results

3.1. Determination of TRPA1 mRNA Levels in the Mouse Brain

Intact TRPA1 mRNA levels were determined by quantitative RT-PCR in brain samples of GFAP-Cre$^{-/-}$ TRPA1$^{Fl/Fl}$ compared to GFAP-Cre$^{+/-}$ TRPA1$^{Fl/-}$ and GFAP-Cre$^{+/-}$ TRPA1$^{Fl/Fl}$ mice. The obtained relative expression levels, means and standard deviations are presented in Figure 1 for each group. Compared to GFAP-Cre$^{-/-}$ control mice where TRPA1 expression level was 102 ± 22%, both the GFAP-Cre$^{+/-}$ TRPA1$^{Fl/-}$ and GFAP-Cre$^{+/-}$ TRPA1$^{Fl/Fl}$ mouse groups had lower expression levels, 68 ± 28% and 77 ± 23%, respectively. These results indicate that some of the TRPA1 mRNA was lost due to Cre-LoxP recombination in both GFAP-Cre$^{+/-}$ groups. ANOVA statistical analysis showed that there was a significant difference between the groups (p=0.0017). The post hoc test demonstrated that the differences were significant when both the GFAP-Cre$^{+/-}$ TRPA1$^{Fl/-}$ and GFAP-Cre$^{+/-}$ TRPA1$^{Fl/Fl}$ group were compared to the GFAP-Cre$^{-/-}$ TRPA1$^{Fl/Fl}$ control group ($p < 0.01$ and $p < 0.05$ respectively), but there was no significant difference in TRPA1 mRNA expression between the GFAP-Cre$^{+/-}$ groups (Figure 1).

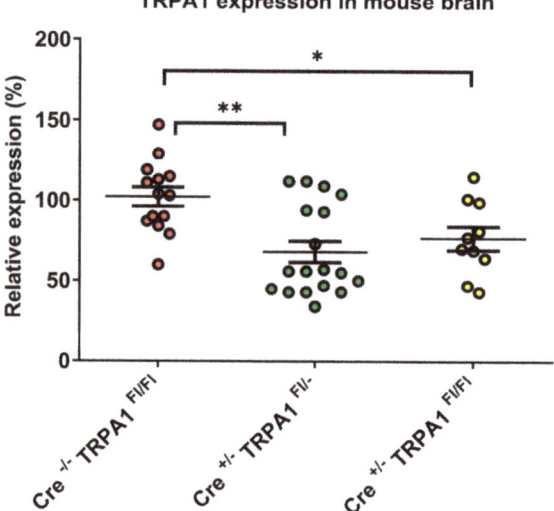

Figure 1. Relative expression levels of TRPA1 mRNA in the brain in GFAP-Cre$^{-/-}$ TRPA1$^{Fl/Fl}$ ($n = 7$), GFAP-Cre$^{+/-}$ TRPA1$^{Fl/-}$ ($n = 5$) and GFAP-Cre$^{+/-}$ TRPA1$^{Fl/Fl}$ mice ($n = 9$). Asterisks show statistically significant differences between the indicated groups (*$p < 0.05$, **$p < 0.01$).

3.2. Magnetic Resonance Imaging (MRI)

The timeline of damage was followed by the evaluation of signal intensity changes of T2 weighted MRI (Figure 2) in the medial part of the corpus callosum between week 2 and 6.

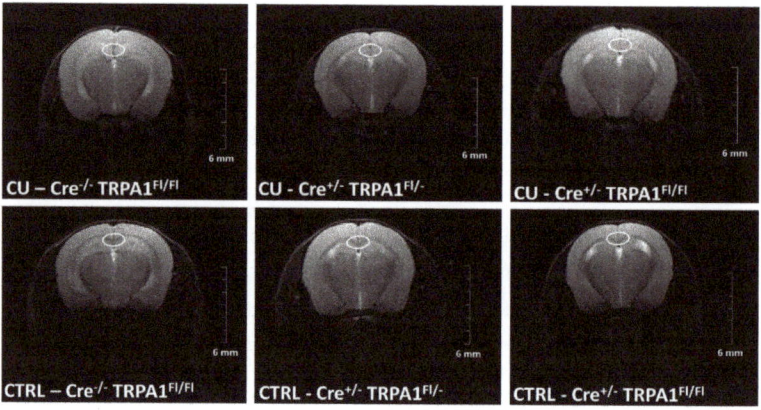

Figure 2. Representative MR images, constructed on fourth week. The medial corpus callosum is highlighted by a white ellipse.

The intensities in the untreated control groups were not significantly different and no changes were detected in any of the control animals throughout the whole experiment. (Figure 3a). In contrast, the signal intensity was significantly increased in cuprizone-treated GFAP-Cre$^{-/-}$ TRPA1$^{Fl/Fl}$ mice compared to GFAP-Cre$^{+/-}$ TRPA1$^{Fl/-}$ and GFAP-Cre$^{+/-}$ TRPA1$^{Fl/Fl}$ animals on week 3 and week 4 (*$p < $

0.05, **$p < 0.01$; Figure 3b). The most pronounced increase was detected on the fourth week, 179.75% in GFAP-Cre$^{-/-}$ TRPA1$^{Fl/Fl}$ group versus 134.25% (GFAP-Cre$^{+/-}$ TRPA1$^{Fl/-}$) and 134.75% (GFAP Cre$^{+/-}$ TRPA1$^{Fl/Fl}$). These results indicate that the myelin damage was less severe in the corpus callosum of both heterozygous and homozygous mGFAP-Cre conditional TRPA1 knockout mice on weeks 3 and 4. The difference between genotypes decreased at later time points. At the end of the treatment we did not detect significant differences between the cuprizone-treated GFAP-Cre$^{-/-}$ TRPA1$^{Fl/Fl}$, GFAP-Cre$^{+/-}$ TRPA1$^{Fl/-}$ and GFAP-Cre$^{+/-}$ TRPA1$^{Fl/Fl}$ animals. Each cuprizone-treated group showed a significantly elevated intensity from the third to sixth weeks compared to their respective control groups (Figure 3a,b; significance not shown).

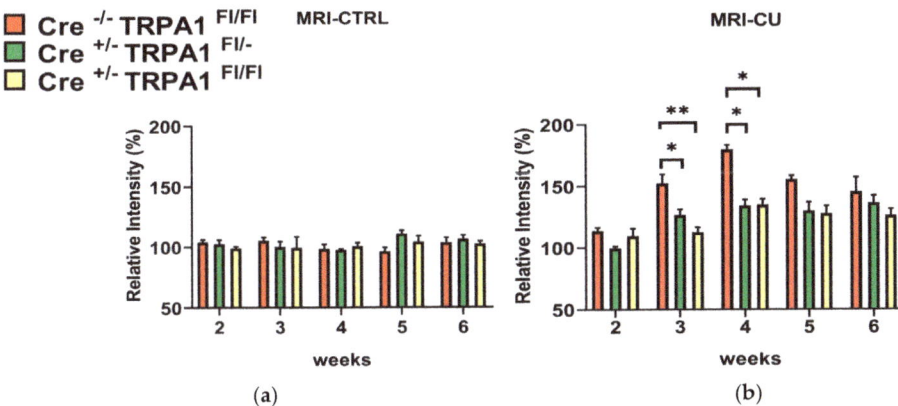

Figure 3. Changes of signal intensity in the medial corpus callosum measured by magnetic resonance imaging between week 2 and 6 of cuprizone treatment in (**a**) control (CTRL) and (**b**) cuprizone-treated (CU) groups of GFAP-Cre$^{-/-}$ TRPA1$^{Fl/Fl}$, GFAP-Cre$^{+/-}$ TRPA1$^{Fl/-}$ and GFAP-Cre$^{+/-}$ TRPA1$^{Fl/Fl}$ mice. Data are means ± S.E.M. of images obtained from animals (n = 4/group). The signal intensities were normalized to the baseline values (100%) for each animal and indicated by percentages of relative intensity. Asterisks show statistically significant differences between respective CU and CTRL groups (* $p < 0.05$, ** $p < 0.01$).

3.3. Cuprizone-Induced Demyelination Determined by LFB/CV Staining and MBP Immunohistochemistry

After the six weeks of the treatment, significant demyelination was detected in all three cuprizone-treated groups with the LFB/CV staining, compared to their respective control groups (Figure 4a,b). No statistically significant differences were found between the demyelination scores of the three genotypes. Likewise, immunohistochemical staining of MBP revealed a significant reduction in all cuprizone-fed animals compared to controls, but no difference was detected between the MBP content of GFAP-Cre$^{-/-}$ TRPA1$^{Fl/Fl}$, GFAP-Cre$^{+/-}$ TRPA1$^{Fl/-}$ and GFAP-Cre$^{+/-}$ TRPA1$^{Fl/Fl}$ mice (Figure 5a,b). The results show that the attenuating effect of mGFAP-driven conditional deletion of the TRPA1 receptor on the severity of cuprizone-induced demyelination was diminished by week 6 of treatment.

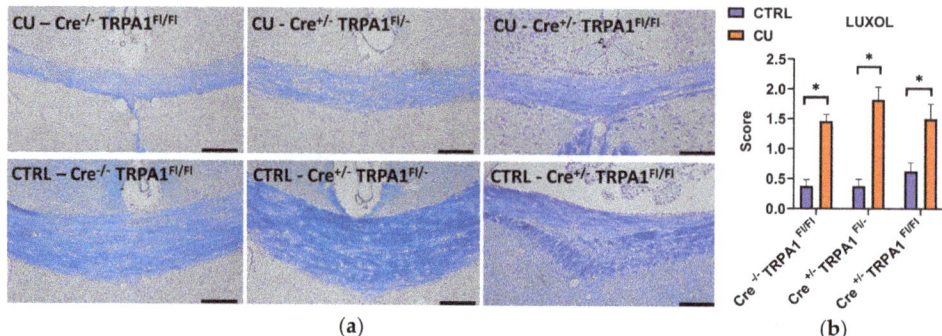

Figure 4. Evaluation of myelin content with Luxol Fast Blue/cresyl violet (LFB/CV) staining after 6 weeks of cuprizone treatment (**a**). Representative images of control (CTRL) and cuprizone-treated (CU) groups in GFAP-Cre$^{-/-}$ TRPA1$^{Fl/Fl}$, GFAP-Cre$^{+/-}$ TRPA1$^{Fl/-}$ and GFAP-Cre$^{+/-}$ TRPA1$^{Fl/Fl}$ mice.; (**b**) Semiquantitative demyelination scores of LFB/CV staining, *$p < 0.05$, n = 3–5/group, Scale bar = 100 µm.

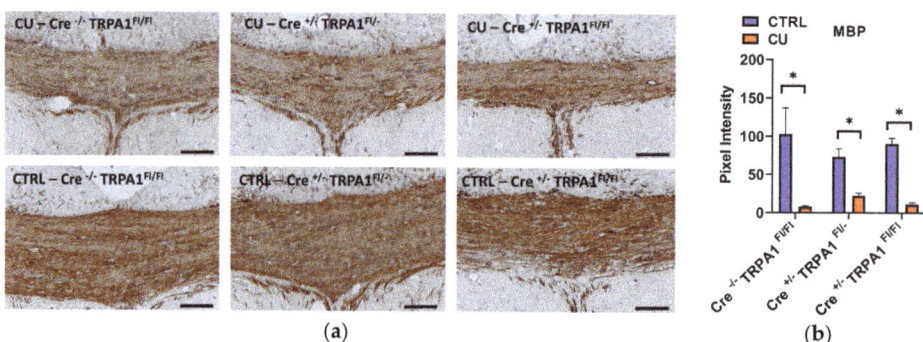

Figure 5. Evaluation of myelin content with myelin basic protein (MBP) immunohistochemistry after 6 weeks of cuprizone treatment (**a**). Representative images of control (CTRL) and cuprizone-treated (CU) groups in GFAP-Cre$^{-/-}$ TRPA1$^{Fl/Fl}$, GFAP-Cre$^{+/-}$ TRPA1$^{Fl/-}$ and GFAP-Cre$^{+/-}$ TRPA1$^{Fl/Fl}$ mice.; (**b**) Pixel intensities of diaminobenzidine staining in the middle part of the corpus callosum in each group, *$p < 0.05$, n = 3–5/group, Scale bar = 100 µm.

3.4. Cuprizone-Induced Astrocyte and Microglia Activation

At the end of the 6-week treatment, a significant increase of GFAP and Iba1 immunostaining was detected in all three cuprizone-treated groups, compared to their respective control groups (Figures 6a and 7a). Quantifying the intensity of the staining, no statistically significant differences were found in the DAB staining intensities between the three genotypes (Figures 6b and 7b). Therefore, by the end of the 6-week treatment the mGFAP-driven conditional deletion of the TRPA1 receptor had no effect on the astrocyte and microglia accumulation induced by cuprizone.

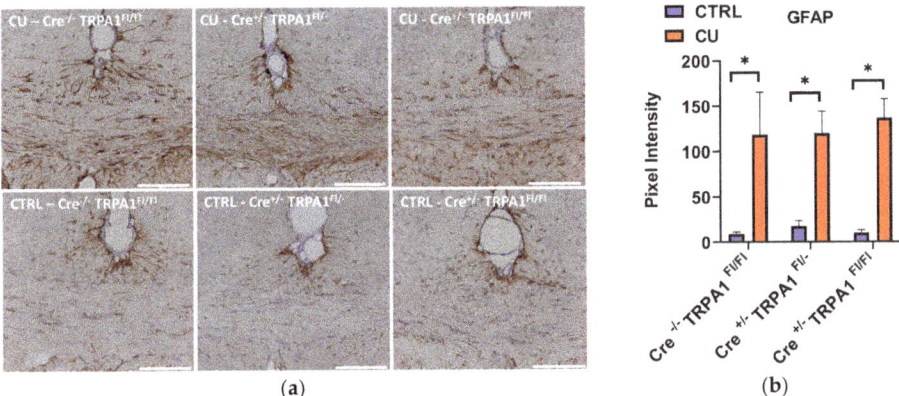

Figure 6. Evaluation of astrocyte activation by GFAP immunohistochemistry after 6 weeks of cuprizone treatment (**a**) Representative images of control (CTRL) and cuprizone-treated (CU) groups in GFAP-Cre$^{-/-}$ TRPA1$^{Fl/Fl}$, GFAP-Cre$^{+/-}$ TRPA1$^{Fl/-}$ and GFAP-Cre$^{+/-}$ TRPA1$^{Fl/Fl}$ mice.; (**b**) Pixel intensities of diaminobenzidine staining in the middle part of the corpus callosum in each group; *$p <$ 0.05, n = 3–5/group, Scale bar = 100 µm.

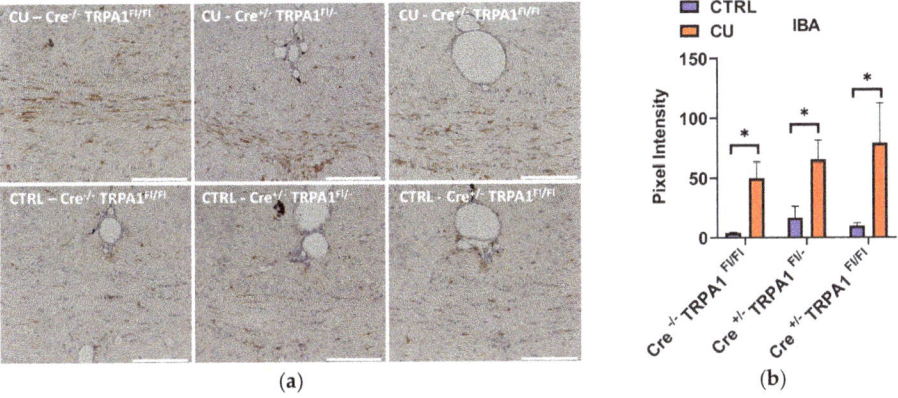

Figure 7. Evaluation of microglia activation by Iba1 immunohistochemistry after 6 weeks of cuprizone treatment (**a**) Representative images of control (CTRL) and cuprizone-treated (CU) groups in GFAP-Cre$^{-/-}$ TRPA1$^{Fl/Fl}$, GFAP-Cre$^{+/-}$ TRPA1$^{Fl/-}$ and GFAP-Cre$^{+/-}$ TRPA1$^{Fl/Fl}$ mice.; (**b**) Pixel intensities of diaminobenzidine staining in the middle part of the corpus callosum in each group *$p <$ 0.05, n = 3–5/group, Scale bar = 100 µm.

4. Discussion

In the present study we have investigated the modulatory role of TRPA1 receptors expressed by GFAP positive cells in the cuprizone-induced demyelination model using mGFAP-driven conditional TRPA1 receptor knockout mice. The glial fibrillary acidic protein (GFAP) is a generally accepted marker of astrocytes. Brain diseases are characterized by the active inflammatory state of astrocytes, which is usually manifested as up-regulation of GFAP [28].

Our results show that the genetic lack of TRPA1 receptors in GFAP positive cells influences the demyelination process induced by cuprizone feeding in mice. Reduced pathological changes were detected in the corpus callosum by MRI between the 3rd and 5th weeks of the treatment. In contrast, at the end of week 6, no significant differences were found in the demyelination evaluated either by MRI or histology.

In a previous study using embryonic global TRPA1 KO animals we demonstrated that TRPA1 receptor deficiency attenuated the cuprizone-induced demyelination by reduction of apoptosis of mature oligodendrocytes [22]. Additionally, it was recently published that oligodendrocytes express TRPA1 receptors [11]. Therefore, a direct effect of TRPA1 activation on oligodendrocyte apoptosis in the cuprizone model could be hypothesized. Since our investigations have not provided sufficient evidence for TRPA1 expression in oligodendrocytes, it was presumed that TRPA1 receptor deficiency might alleviate the cuprizone-induced loss of mature oligodendrocytes by altering the release of mediators by astrocytes. TRPA1 receptors localized on astrocytes may participate in the astrocyte-oligodendrocyte crosstalk. Since TRPA1 can be triggered by several noxious stimuli, including inflammation, tissue damage or oxidative stress on one hand, and astrocytes influence the extent of this toxin-induced demyelination on the other [29], we assumed that this receptor might modulate the demyelination process. Numerous earlier studies have provided substantial morphological and functional evidence that astrocytes express the TRPA1 receptor, functioning as a regulator of resting Ca^{2+} levels [8,9,24,30,31]. In a very recent study, Oh et al., using the cell-type-specific gene-silencing and ultrasensitive sniffer-patch techniques, identified astrocytes as the cellular target and TRPA1 as the molecular sensor for the low intensity, low frequency ultrasound (LILFU). They demonstrated that LILFU-induced neuromodulation was initiated by opening of TRPA1 channels in astrocytes. The Ca^{2+} entry through TRPA1 caused a release of gliotransmitters including glutamate from the astrocytes activating NMDA receptors in neighboring neurons [32]. In another newly-published paper, Xia et al. raised the involvement of TRPA1 in myelin damage and oxidative stress injury in a mouse intracerebral hemorrhage (ICH) model. They showed that TRPA1 was activated by the increased reactive oxygen species (ROS) after ICH, leading to an increase of Ca^{2+} influx. The increased Ca^{2+} further contributed to the rise in NOX1 and Calpain1, causing oxidative stress damage and myelin degradation. [33].

Since our previous data also supported the TRPA1 immunopositivity of astrocytes in the corpus callosum and astrocytic reactions were less prominent in cuprizone-treated TRPA1 receptor deficient mice compared to wild-type counterparts, we have supposed a pivotal role of TRPA1 receptors expressed by astrocytes [22]. For our further investigations, mGFAP-driven conditional TRPA1 knockout mice were bred by our laboratory in order to reveal the precise role of astrocytic TRPA1 receptors. These mice were created via crossbreeding floxed TRPA1 carrying mice (B6.129S-Trpa1tm2Kykw/J) by GFAP promoter-directed Cre recombinase gene expressing mice (B6.Cg-Tg(Gfap-cre) 77.6Mvs/2J. This technique allows the selective cutout of the Trpa1 gene only from the GFAP-positive cells and the examination of cuprizone-induced demyelination in the lack of astrocyte-specific TRPA1 receptors.

Cuprizone-treatment significantly increased T2-weighted MRI signal intensities measured on the 3rd and 4th weeks in all three animal groups compared to the baseline, proving the reliability of the model. Myelin loss with the concomitant water accumulation enhances the signal intensity on T2-weighted MR images [34]. The intensity of T2-weighted images of ROIs corresponding to the medial corpus callosum was reproducible. Remarkably, the MRI was sensitive enough to notice the milder severity of myelin loss in GFAP-Cre$^{+/-}$ TRPA1$^{Fl/-}$ and GFAP-Cre$^{+/-}$ TRPA1$^{Fl/Fl}$ animals compared to the GFAP-Cre$^{-/-}$ TRPA1$^{Fl/Fl}$ group. The most pronounced difference was detected on the 4th week, but the disparity decreased at later time points. In our previous study in the cuprizone model with embryonic global TRPA1 KO mice, we provided MRI-based evidence that the severity of myelin loss in the gene-deleted animals was significantly lower at all measurement points during the six-week experiment compared to the wild-type controls [23]. In accordance with the present results, the largest differences in signal intensities were detected on the 3rd and 4th weeks. Considering the data of the follow-up in vivo imaging, we conclude that genetic loss of the astrocyte-specific TRPA1 receptors attenuates the progress of demyelination in the corpus callosum, but these effects can be noticed only at the time of the most intensive pathological changes. The homozygote (Cre$^{+/-}$ TRPA1$^{Fl/Fl}$) and heterozygote (Cre$^{+/-}$ TRPA1$^{Fl/-}$) mice showed similar alterations which is explained by a similar reduction of mRNA levels in both genotypes. However, by the 6th week these disparities had disappeared, as we could not detect any differences with histological examinations at the end of the study. Neither the semiquantitative scoring of demyelination, based on Luxol fast blue staining technique, nor the MBP immunohistochemistry showed significant differences in the mGFAP-driven conditional TRPA1 knockout mice compared to the Cre$^{-/-}$ controls. Similarly to the demyelination, the cuprizone-induced accumulation of the astrocytes and microglial cells in the corpus callosum was not influenced by the genetic loss of TRPA1 in the GFAP positive cells. In contrast to the results obtained with embryonic global TRPA1 KO mice, these results suggest that deletion of the receptor in the astrocytes does not exert substantial inhibitory effect eventually on the six-week cuprizone treatment-induced demyelination of the corpus callosum.

5. Conclusions

According to the currently available data, we presume that TRPA1 receptors localized on astrocytes can be activated by electrophilic ligands, reactive oxygen species in response to cuprizone challenge and the consequent release of pro-inflammatory mediators contributes to the progression of oligodendrocyte apoptosis. However, since the global TRPA1 KO mice presented a more attenuated demyelination compared to the conditional KO mice, it can be concluded that TRPA1 receptors on astrocytes contribute to the demyelination induced by cuprizone only transiently and TRPA1 receptors expressed by other cell types in the brain (e. g. oligodendrocytes, microglia, neurons) may participate in the demyelination process [11,33]. The expression and function of TRPA1 receptors by other cells in the brain warrant further investigation.

Author Contributions: Conceptualization, E.P., Z.S., K.B., P.Á. S.K.; methodology, G.K., K.B., P.Á., Z.S., Z.B., E.P.; formal analysis, G.K., K.B., B.N., Z.S., P.Á., Z.B.; investigation, G.K., K.B., B.N., Z.S., P.Á.; writing—original draft preparation, G.K., K.B., B.N., Z.S., E.P.; writing—review and editing, G.K., K.B., B.N., Z.S., P.Á., S.K., Z.B., E.P.; supervision, E.P., Z.S., K.B., P.Á., Z.B.; funding acquisition, E.P. All authors have read and agreed to the published version of the manuscript.

Funding: This research was funded by grants "The role of neuro-inflammation in neurodegeneration: from molecules to clinics" (EFOP-3.6.2-16-2017-00008); EFOP-3.6.3-VEKOP-16-2017-00009; Hungarian Brain Research Program 2. 2017-1.2.1-NKP-2017-00002. and the University of Pécs is acknowledged for a support by the 17886-4/23018/FEKUTSTRAT excellence grant. G.K. was supported by Richter Gedeon Centenárium Foundation.

Acknowledgments: The authors wish to thank Krisztina Fülöp and Anikó Perkecz for expert technical assistance in the histological techniques. The authors also acknowledge Anett Vranesics for contributing to the development of the MRI protocol.

Conflicts of Interest: The authors declare no conflict of interest. The funders had no role in the design of the study; in the collection, analyses, or interpretation of data; in the writing of the manuscript, or in the decision to publish the results.

References

1. Nilius, B.; Appendino, G.; Owsianik, G. The transient receptor potential channel TRPA1: From gene to pathophysiology. *Pflug. Arch.* **2012**, *464*, 425–458. [CrossRef] [PubMed]
2. Chen, J.; Hackos, D.H. TRPA1 as a drug target—promise and challenges. *Naunyn-Schmiedeberg's Arch. Pharmacol.* **2015**, *388*, 451–463. [CrossRef] [PubMed]
3. Talavera, K.; Startek, J.B.; Alvarez-Collazo, J.; Boonen, B.; Alpizar, Y.A.; Sanchez, A.; Naert, R.; Nilius, B. Mammalian transient receptor potential TRPA1 channels: From structure to disease. *Physiol. Rev.* **2019**. [CrossRef] [PubMed]
4. Andersson, D.A.; Gentry, C.; Moss, S.; Bevan, S. Transient receptor potential A1 is a sensory receptor for multiple products of oxidative stress. *J. Neurosci.* **2008**, *28*, 2485–2494. [CrossRef]
5. Story, G.M.; Peier, A.M.; Reeve, A.J.; Eid, S.R.; Mosbacher, J.; Hricik, T.R.; Earley, T.J.; Hergarden, A.C.; Andersson, D.A.; Hwang, S.W.; et al. ANKTM1, a TRP-like channel expressed in nociceptive neurons, is activated by cold temperatures. *Cell* **2003**, *112*, 819–829. [CrossRef]
6. Kobayashi, K.; Fukuoka, T.; Obata, K.; Yamanaka, H.; Dai, Y.; Tokunaga, A.; Noguchi, K. Distinct expression of TRPM8, TRPA1, and TRPV1 mRNAs in rat primary afferent neurons with aδ/c-fibers and colocalization with trk receptors. *J. Comp. Neurol.* **2005**, *493*, 596–606. [CrossRef]

7. Fernandes, E.; Fernandes, M.; Keeble, J. The functions of TRPA1 and TRPV1: Moving away from sensory nerves. *Br. J. Pharm.* **2012**, *166*, 510–521. [CrossRef]
8. Shigetomi, E.; Tong, X.; Kwan, K.Y.; Corey, D.P.; Khakh, B.S. TRPA1 channels regulate astrocyte resting calcium and inhibitory synapse efficacy through GAT-3. *Nat. Neurosci.* **2012**, *15*, 70–80. [CrossRef]
9. Shigetomi, E.; Jackson-Weaver, O.; Huckstepp, R.T.; O'Dell, T.J.; Khakh, B.S. TRPA1 Channels Are Regulators of Astrocyte Basal Calcium Levels and Long-Term Potentiation via Constitutive D-Serine Release. *J. Neurosci.* **2013**, *33*, 10143–10153. [CrossRef]
10. Verkhratsky, A.; Reyes, R.C.; Parpura, V. TRP Channels Coordinate Ion Signalling in Astroglia. *Rev. Physiol Biochem Pharm.* **2014**, *166*, 1–22. [CrossRef]
11. Hamilton, N.B.; Kolodziejczyk, K.; Kougioumtzidou, E.; Attwell, D. Proton-gated Ca^{2+}-permeable TRP channels damage myelin in conditions mimicking ischaemia. *Nature* **2016**, *529*, 523–527. [CrossRef]
12. Zhang, Y.; Chen, K.; Sloan, S.A.; Bennett, M.L.; Scholze, A.R.; O'Keeffe, S.; Phatnani, H.P.; Guarnieri, P.; Caneda, C.; Ruderisch, N.; et al. An RNA-Sequencing Transcriptome and Splicing Database of Glia, Neurons, and Vascular Cells of the Cerebral Cortex. *J. Neurosci.* **2014**, *34*, 11929–11947. [CrossRef]
13. Ben Haim, L.; Carrillo-de Sauvage, M.-A.; Ceyzériat, K.; Escartin, C. Elusive roles for reactive astrocytes in neurodegenerative diseases. *Front. Cell. Neurosci.* **2015**, *9*. [CrossRef]
14. Li, K.; Li, J.; Zheng, J.; Qin, S. Reactive Astrocytes in Neurodegenerative Diseases. *Aging Dis* **2019**, *10*, 664–675. [CrossRef]
15. Kipp, M.; Clarner, T.; Dang, J.; Copray, S.; Beyer, C. The cuprizone animal model: New insights into an old story. *Acta Neuropathol.* **2009**, *118*, 723–736. [CrossRef]
16. Kipp, M.; Nyamoya, S.; Hochstrasser, T.; Amor, S. Multiple sclerosis animal models: A clinical and histopathological perspective. *Brain Pathol.* **2017**, *27*, 123–137. [CrossRef]
17. Lucchinetti, C.; Brück, W.; Parisi, J.; Scheithauer, B.; Rodriguez, M.; Lassmann, H. Heterogeneity of multiple sclerosis lesions: Implications for the pathogenesis of demyelination. *Ann. Neurol.* **2000**, *47*, 707–717. [CrossRef]
18. Matsushima, G.K.; Morell, P. The neurotoxicant, cuprizone, as a model to study demyelination and remyelination in the central nervous system. *Brain Pathol.* **2001**, *11*, 107–116. [CrossRef]
19. Praet, J.; Guglielmetti, C.; Berneman, Z.; Van der Linden, A.; Ponsaerts, P. Cellular and molecular neuropathology of the cuprizone mouse model: Clinical relevance for multiple sclerosis. *Neurosci. Biobehav. Rev.* **2014**, *47*, 485–505. [CrossRef]
20. Ács, P.; Kálmán, B. Pathogenesis of Multiple Sclerosis: What Can We Learn from the Cuprizone Model. In *Autoimmunity*; Perl, A., Ed.; Humana Press: Totowa, NJ, USA, 2012; Volume 900, pp. 403–431. ISBN 978-1-60761-719-8.
21. Gudi, V.; Gingele, S.; Skripuletz, T.; Stangel, M. Glial response during cuprizone-induced de- and remyelination in the CNS: Lessons learned. *Front. Cell Neurosci* **2014**, *8*, 73. [CrossRef]
22. Sághy, É.; Sipos, É.; Ács, P.; Bölcskei, K.; Pohóczky, K.; Kemény, Á.; Sándor, Z.; Szőke, É.; Sétáló, G.; Komoly, S.; et al. TRPA1 deficiency is protective in cuprizone-induced demyelination-A new target against oligodendrocyte apoptosis. *Glia* **2016**, *64*, 2166–2180. [CrossRef]
23. Bölcskei, K.; Kriszta, G.; Sághy, É.; Payrits, M.; Sipos, É.; Vranesics, A.; Berente, Z.; Ábrahám, H.; Ács, P.; Komoly, S.; et al. Behavioural alterations and morphological changes are attenuated by the lack of TRPA1 receptors in the cuprizone-induced demyelination model in mice. *J. Neuroimmunol.* **2018**, *320*, 1–10. [CrossRef] [PubMed]
24. Lee, K.-I.; Lee, H.-T.; Lin, H.-C.; Tsay, H.-J.; Tsai, F.-C.; Shyue, S.-K.; Lee, T.-S. Role of transient receptor potential ankyrin 1 channels in Alzheimer's disease. *J. Neuroinflammation* **2016**, *13*, 92. [CrossRef] [PubMed]
25. Lee, K.-I.; Lin, H.-C.; Lee, H.-T.; Tsai, F.-C.; Lee, T.-S. Loss of Transient Receptor Potential Ankyrin 1 Channel Deregulates Emotion, Learning and Memory, Cognition, and Social Behavior in Mice. *Mol Neurobiol* **2017**, *54*, 3606–3617. [CrossRef] [PubMed]
26. Fedorov, A.; Beichel, R.; Kalpathy-Cramer, J.; Finet, J.; Fillion-Robin, J.-C.; Pujol, S.; Bauer, C.; Jennings, D.; Fennessy, F.; Sonka, M.; et al. 3D Slicer as an image computing platform for the Quantitative Imaging Network. *Magn Reson Imaging* **2012**, *30*, 1323–1341. [CrossRef] [PubMed]
27. Paxinos, G.; Franklin, K.B.J. *The Mouse Brain in Stereotaxic Coordinates*, 2nd ed.; Academic Press: San Diego, CA, USA, 2001; ISBN 978-0-12-547636-2.

28. Siracusa, R.; Fusco, R.; Cuzzocrea, S. Astrocytes: Role and Functions in Brain Pathologies. *Front. Pharmacol.* **2019**, *10*. [CrossRef]
29. Skripuletz, T.; Hackstette, D.; Bauer, K.; Gudi, V.; Pul, R.; Voss, E.; Berger, K.; Kipp, M.; Baumgärtner, W.; Stangel, M. Astrocytes regulate myelin clearance through recruitment of microglia during cuprizone-induced demyelination. *Brain* **2013**, *136*, 147–167. [CrossRef]
30. Lee, S.M.; Cho, Y.S.; Kim, T.H.; Jin, M.U.; Ahn, D.K.; Noguchi, K.; Bae, Y.C. An ultrastructural evidence for the expression of transient receptor potential ankyrin 1 (TRPA1) in astrocytes in the rat trigeminal caudal nucleus. *J. Chem. Neuroanat.* **2012**, *45*, 45–49. [CrossRef]
31. Bosson, A.; Paumier, A.; Boisseau, S.; Jacquier-Sarlin, M.; Buisson, A.; Albrieux, M. TRPA1 channels promote astrocytic Ca2+ hyperactivity and synaptic dysfunction mediated by oligomeric forms of amyloid-β peptide. *Mol. Neurodegener.* **2017**, *12*, 53. [CrossRef]
32. Oh, S.-J.; Lee, J.M.; Kim, H.-B.; Lee, J.; Han, S.; Bae, J.Y.; Hong, G.-S.; Koh, W.; Kwon, J.; Hwang, E.-S.; et al. Ultrasonic Neuromodulation via Astrocytic TRPA1. *Curr. Biol.* **2019**, *29*, 3386–3401.e8. [CrossRef]
33. Xia, M.; Chen, W.; Wang, J.; Yin, Y.; Guo, C.; Li, C.; Li, M.; Tang, X.; Jia, Z.; Hu, R.; et al. TRPA1 Activation-Induced Myelin Degradation Plays a Key Role in Motor Dysfunction After Intracerebral Hemorrhage. *Front. Mol. Neurosci.* **2019**, *12*. [CrossRef]
34. Merkler, D.; Boretius, S.; Stadelmann, C.; Ernsting, T.; Michaelis, T.; Frahm, J.; Brück, W. Multicontrast MRI of remyelination in the central nervous system. *Nmr Biomed.* **2005**, *18*, 395–403. [CrossRef]

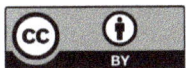 © 2019 by the authors. Licensee MDPI, Basel, Switzerland. This article is an open access article distributed under the terms and conditions of the Creative Commons Attribution (CC BY) license (http://creativecommons.org/licenses/by/4.0/).

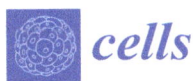

Review

Astrocyte and Oligodendrocyte Cross-Talk in the Central Nervous System

Erik Nutma [1], Démi van Gent [1], Sandra Amor [1,2,†] and Laura A. N. Peferoen [1,*,†]

1. Department of Pathology, Amsterdam UMC, Location VUmc, 1081 HV Amsterdam, The Netherlands
2. Centre for Neuroscience and Trauma, Blizard Institute, Barts and the London School of Medicine & Dentistry, Queen Mary University of London, London E1 2AT, UK
* Correspondence: l.peferoen@amsterdamumc.nl; Tel.: +31-6-5148-1284
† These authors have equally contributed to this work.

Received: 14 February 2020; Accepted: 28 February 2020; Published: 3 March 2020

Abstract: Over the last decade knowledge of the role of astrocytes in central nervous system (CNS) neuroinflammatory diseases has changed dramatically. Rather than playing a merely passive role in response to damage it is clear that astrocytes actively maintain CNS homeostasis by influencing pH, ion and water balance, the plasticity of neurotransmitters and synapses, cerebral blood flow, and are important immune cells. During disease astrocytes become reactive and hypertrophic, a response that was long considered to be pathogenic. However, recent studies reveal that astrocytes also have a strong tissue regenerative role. Whilst most astrocyte research focuses on modulating neuronal function and synaptic transmission little is known about the cross-talk between astrocytes and oligodendrocytes, the myelinating cells of the CNS. This communication occurs via direct cell-cell contact as well as via secreted cytokines, chemokines, exosomes, and signalling molecules. Additionally, this cross-talk is important for glial development, triggering disease onset and progression, as well as stimulating regeneration and repair. Its critical role in homeostasis is most evident when this communication fails. Here, we review emerging evidence of astrocyte-oligodendrocyte communication in health and disease. Understanding the pathways involved in this cross-talk will reveal important insights into the pathogenesis and treatment of CNS diseases.

Keywords: astrocytes; oligodendrocytes; white matter disease; cross-talk; CNS; glial cells

---

1. Introduction

Astrocytes, the most abundant glial cell type in the central nervous system (CNS), have long been considered to be cells that only respond to damage in CNS diseases. This view is gradually changing with the accumulating evidence that astrocytes fulfil many functions in health, during development and in response to damage [1]. Astrocytes regulate processes critical for cell-cell interactions and homeostasis such as ion and water transport, pH, neuroplasticity, synapse pruning and cerebral blood flow thus providing trophic and metabolic support to all cells in the CNS. Astrocytes also play a major role in maintaining the blood-brain barrier (BBB) and blood-cerebrospinal fluid barrier. During CNS injury, infection and inflammation astrocytes produce a wide range of pro-inflammatory factors including chemokines, cytokines, increased expression of innate immune receptors and molecules including MHC-II [2–5]. On the other hand, astrocytes produce anti-inflammatory cytokines, heat shock proteins and neuroprotective factors aiding in processes such as neuroregeneration and remyelination [2]. These different characteristics present the astrocyte as a versatile player in regulatory processes depending on context and time of injury and disease. While much of the knowledge of astrocytes relates to their interaction with neurons and neuronal functions astrocytes collaborate and impact on other cells within the CNS as well, such as endothelial cells and pericytes in BBB formation.

They also share their lineage with oligodendrocytes and interact with these myelin forming cells by sharing gap junctions allowing passage of small metabolites and molecules for communication [6].

Oligodendrocytes have the highest metabolic rate of cells in the CNS, producing myelin up to three times their weight per day for up to 50 axons each. The myelin sheaths are critical for action potentials and need to be maintained constantly [7]. Additionally, oligodendrocytes provide axons with trophic support and are crucial for neuronal functionality [2,7]. Due to their high turnover of myelin oligodendrocytes are sensitive to reactive oxygen species and oxidative stress [7,8]. They have been shown to participate intricately in immune mediated processes by producing immune regulatory factors and expressing receptors to communicate with microglia [9]. As it becomes more apparent that astrocytes participate in immune mediated processes as well, their cross-talk with oligodendrocytes might elucidate new mechanisms in neuroinflammatory diseases.

The importance of astrocytes in oligodendrocyte functioning is exemplified in primary astrocytopathies such as Alexander disease (AxD) and vanishing white matter (VWM) [10] where astrocyte damage leads to demyelination and oligodendrocyte death. In osmotic demyelination syndrome astrocyte death is observed due to loss of gap junctions and proteostasis defects in astrocytes prior to oligodendrocyte loss and demyelination [11–13]. In addition, astrocyte dysfunction has been associated with many other neurological diseases including epilepsy [14], amyotrophic lateral sclerosis (ALS) [15], Huntington's disease (HD) [16], and Alzheimer's disease (AD) [17]. In neuroinflammatory diseases, such as multiple sclerosis (MS) oligodendrocyte loss might be a consequence of aberrant immune responses. MS is characterized by inflammatory lesions with demyelination, neurodegeneration, and astrogliosis, in which astrocytes and oligodendrocytes are damaged [18,19]. Similarly, numerous other white matter disorders also show important cross-talk between astrocytes and oligodendrocytes (Table 1) [10].

Here we review the evidence for cross-talk between astrocytes and oligodendrocytes demonstrating an emerging role for astrocytes in oligodendrocyte damage, as well as contributing to tissue regeneration and remyelination. Understanding how astrocytes interact with oligodendrocytes will provide a deeper insight into the pathophysiology of neurological disorders that may elucidate new pathways to drug strategies for myelin damage in CNS diseases.

Table 1. Astrocyte involvement in white matter CNS diseases [1].

	Disease	Pathology	Detrimental Impact on Astrocytes	Beneficial Impact on Astrocytes	References
Inflammatory	MS	Inflammation, myelin loss, neurodegeneration, astrogliosis, astrocyte damage.	BBB damage, impaired signal transduction and glutamate clearance. Reduced OPC proliferation	Gliosis may aid remyelination and regenerate integrity of BBB, aid remyelination and provide trophic support	[5,20–23]
	NMO	Inflammation, myelin loss in optic nerve and spinal cord. Reduction in AQP4 and GFAP. Decreased EAAT2.	Impaired water and ion homeostasis, impaired glutamate clearance	Stimulation of remyelination, trophic support	[21,24–26]
	ADEM	Widespread CNS inflammation associated with infection.	Dependent on infectious agent	Infection may trigger protective response via TLR-dependent mechanism	[27]
	AHL	Perivascular demyelination, inflammation, oedema, haemorrhages. Hyper-reactive astrocytes.	Swelling of protoplasmic and fibrous astrocyte end-feet, beading consistent with degeneration.	Demyelination is secondary to astrocyte injury indicating a beneficial effect of astrocytes in early disease	[28]
Infectious	PML	Cytolytic JC virus induces oligodendrocytes death and focal myelin loss. Abnormal astrocytes with inclusion bodies.	Astrocytes aid the spread of JC virus to neighbouring oligodendrocytes	Unknown	[29–31]
	SSPE	Viral inclusion bodies in neurons, neuronal damage and loss. Virion inclusion in some astrocytes.	Infection of (perivascular) astrocytes may aid spread of virus	Reactive gliosis in longstanding disease may be beneficial	[32,33]
	Congenital CMV	Encephalitis, microglial activation.	CMV infection of astrocytes induces TGF-beta known to enhance productive infection. Infection of foetal astrocytes alters uptake and metabolism of glutamate	Unknown	[34,35]
Toxic-Metabolic	PNND	Depends on position and type of tumour.	Pathogenic antibodies and CD8+ T cells to astrocytic antigens expressed on tumour induces neurological damage	Unknown	[36,37]

Table 1. *Cont.*

	Disease	Pathology	Detrimental Impact on Astrocytes	Beneficial Impact on Astrocytes	References
Hypoxia-Ischemia	Binswanger disease	Chronic microvascular leukoencephalopathy, white matter lesions, axonal damage.	Damage to BBB leads to peri-infarct reactive astrocytes	Unknown	[38]
	Cerebral hypoxia and ischemia in new-borns	Diffuse white matter damage, gliosis, decrease in oligodendrocytes.	Reactive astrocytes form a glia scar and secret inflammatory molecules e.g., ROS	Astrocytes produce PDGF, IGF-1, elevated levels of EAAT2 aid glutamate removal in response to hypoxia. VEGF production mobilises stem cells. BDNF reduces apoptosis.	[39,40]
TBI	Diffuse axonal injury	Axonal damage, tau accumulation, secondary white matter damage, astrogliosis.	Glial scar inhibits remyelination and axonal regrowth	Glial scar prevents spread of toxic molecules	[2,41]
Lysosomal Storage	MLD	Accumulated sulfatides leads to demyelination, sparing of U-fibres. Eosinophilic granules in macrophages, metachromasia.	Sulfatide accumulates in astrocytes impairing differentiation	Unknown	[42]
Peroxisomal	X-linked ALD	Defective ABCD1 transport protein. Increased saturated VLCFA in serum. Progressive demyelination. VLCFA accumulate in glia.	Astrocyte stress prior to myelin damage due to accumulated VLCFA. Astrocytes produce ROS and have impaired oxidative ATP synthesis and decreased Ca^{2+} uptake capacity	Unknown	[43,44]
Mitochondrial	Leber's hereditary optic neuropathy	Loss of retinal ganglion cells, optic nerve degeneration.	Unknown	Unknown	
DNA Repair Defects	Cockayne syndrome	Patchy myelin loss, neuronal loss, astrocytic gliosis, microglia nodules.	Multinucleated astrocytes	Unknown	[45]

Table 1. Cont.

	Disease	Pathology	Detrimental Impact on Astrocytes	Beneficial Impact on Astrocytes	References
Defects in Myelin Genes	PMD	PLP1 duplication or gene alterations, dysmyelination, failure to form myelin.	Increased astrocytic activity, astrogliosis.	Unknown	[46]
AA/Organic Acid Metabolism Disorders	Canavan disease	Mutations of aspartoacylase gene diffuse spongiform white matter degeneration, dysmyelination and intramyelinic oedema. Hypertrophy and hyperplasia of astrocytes.	Metabolic disturbance of mitochondria in abnormal astrocyte	Unknown	[47,48]
Miscellaneous	Alexander disease	Myelin damage, Rosenthal fibres, non-neoplastic astrocytes	Mutations in GFAP lead to diminished glutamate transporter, accumulation of CD44, and loss of EAAT-2. Loss of Cx43 and Cx30	Unknown	[49]
	VWM	Progressive demyelination, blunted dysmorphic astrocytes.	Failure to reach maturity of astrocytes. Overexpression of nestin and GFAPδ	Unknown	[50]
	CADASIL	Diffuse white matter lesions, subcortical infarcts. Granular osmiophilic material in small vessels	Astrocytes undergo autophagy-like cell death. Glia-vascular unit damaged, BBB disturbed	Unknown	[51]
	PMLD	Lack of the gap junction protein Cx47 leads to splitting and decompaction of myelin sheaths and axonal spheroids.	Gap junctions between astrocytes and oligodendrocytes are disturbed compromising oligodendrocyte survival and myelination.	Unknown	[52]

Abbreviations: ADEM, acute disseminated encephalomyelitis; AHL, acute haemorrhagic leukoencephalopathy; AQP4, Aquaporin-4; BBB, blood brain barrier; BDNF, Brain-derived neurotrophic factor; CMV, cytomegalovirus; CNS, central nervous system; EAAT, Excitatory amino acid transporter; GFAP, Glial fibrillary acidic protein; IGF, insulin-like growth factor; MLD, Metachromatic leukodystrophy; MS, multiple sclerosis; NMO, neuromyelitis optica; OPC, oligodendrocyte precursor cell; PDGF, platelet derived growth factor; PMD, Pelizaeus-Merzbacher disease; PMLD, Pelizaeus-Merzbacher-like disease; PML, progressive multifocal leukoencephalopathy; PNND, paraneoplastic neurological disorders; ROS, Reactive oxygen species; SSPE, subacute sclerosing panencephalitis; TBI, traumatic brain injury; TGF, transforming growth factor; TLR, toll-like receptor; VEGF, vascular endothelial growth factor; VLCFA, very long chain fatty acid; VWM, vanishing white matter. [1] As classified by van der Knaap and Valk [53].

2. Astrocyte and Oligodendrocyte Cross-Talk during Brain Development

In neurogenesis, a "gliogenic switch" occurs and dividing neural stem cells develop into glial cells [54,55]. From these cells, both astrocyte precursor cells and oligodendrocyte progenitor cells (OPCs) arise [55,56]. Astrogenesis is mediated through cardiotrophin-1 (CT-1), a factor secreted by cortical neurons. CT-1 induces glial fibrillary acidic protein (GFAP) expression by immature astrocytes through activation of the janus kinase signal transducer and activator of transcription proteins (JAK-STAT). The importance of CT-1 is exemplified by the 50–80% decrease in GFAP expression in CT-1 knock-out mice [57]. Astrogenesis-related genes are silenced during the neurogenic period through epigenetic mechanisms [57–59]. Oligodendrogenesis, on the other hand, is subject to a morphogen gradient of Sonic hedgehog (Shh) and bone morphogenic protein (BMP) and OPCs arise on the ventral side of the neural tube [60,61]. Critical in proliferation and timing of oligodendrocyte maturation is secretion of platelet derived growth factor AA (PDGF-AA) by astrocytes [62]. Once generated, OPCs migrate due to chemokines and Shh signalling, all while being guided by astrocytes [63]. In the optic nerve, astrocytes transiently express high levels of the megalin receptor that regulates the availability of Shh in the microenvironment and thus guides OPC migration. Inhibition of the megalin receptor has been shown to result in impaired migration of OPCs to the optic nerve [64]. Furthermore, astrocytes tightly control release of BMPs and prevent maturation of OPCs into myelin-producing oligodendrocytes [65]. Clearly, cross-talk between astrocytes and oligodendrocytes during development is essential for migration and maturation of OPCs through the CNS.

Various areas in the brain give rise to different types of astrocytes. Fibrous astrocytes are located in the white matter while protoplasmic astrocytes are present in the grey matter. These phenotypes of astrocytes differ in morphology and expression patterns. One example is the expression of excitatory amino acid transporters (EAATs), which is higher in the white matter and results in extracellular glutamate levels being lower in white than in grey matter [3,5,66,67]. Additionally, the astrocytic syncytium formed by protoplasmic astrocytes is larger than that of fibrous astrocytes [67]. The differences observed in morphology and protein expression impact the way these cells interact with their environment and with other glia cells such as oligodendrocytes.

During development astrocytes provide critical metabolic support of oligodendrocytes by supplying e.g., sterol regulatory element-binding protein (SREBP) cleavage-activating protein, a protein essential in lipid production. Mice in which SREBP cleavage activating protein is conditionally knocked out in astrocytes, develop microcephaly and a decrease in white matter volume [68], indicating the importance of astrocyte-derived lipids in myelination. Astrocytes also provide cholesterol for myelin production, and since cholesterol cannot cross the BBB it has to be synthesized de novo in the CNS by astrocytes and oligodendrocytes [3,69,70]. However, inhibition of the oligodendrocyte cholesterol synthesis pathway in mice leads to a delay in myelination suggesting cholesterol production by oligodendrocytes and astrocytes is critical for early myelination [70]. This suggests that cholesterol availability is a rate-limiting factor in myelin production. In experimental autoimmune encephalomyelitis (EAE), an animal model of MS, the cholesterol synthesis pathway is downregulated in astrocytes of the cerebellum and spinal cord [69]. Determining whether this is a cause of limited remyelination requires more investigation. The metabolite exchange between oligodendrocytes and astrocytes may be key for astrocytic leukodystrophies, as disturbed astrocyte function in these disorders may limit lipid exchange from astrocytes to oligodendrocytes.

3. Astrocytic Communication with Oligodendrocytes

3.1. Blood-Brain Barrier Interactions

Astrocyte end-feet cover up to 90% of the brain vasculature and are exchange sites for nutrients, metabolites, and ions from the blood to the brain. BBB dysfunction is a key step in the pathogenesis of inflammatory and neurodegenerative CNS diseases [71].

Iron from the blood is provided by astrocytes to oligodendrocytes through endocytosis and transferred to the cells as protein-bound iron. Iron is essential for several enzymatic functions of oligodendrocytes, such as energy metabolism enzymes, including the mitochondrial respiratory chain protein complexes I-IV, which use it as a co-factor [4,72]. When oligodendrocytes are deprived of iron, proliferation and differentiation of OPCs is impaired as shown in vitro, leading to a delay in remyelination after injury in vivo [72,73]. The importance of iron in myelination is exemplified by prenatal iron deficiency in which abnormal oligodendrocyte distribution is observed [73]. Abnormalities in iron metabolism are also reported in MS [72] and HD [74] and restoration of normal metabolism is required for remyelination. Maintenance and development of the BBB is regulated by astrocytic Shh [75]. In MS, Shh acts as an anti-inflammatory molecule at the level of the neurovascular unit and is increased during neuroinflammation to promote BBB repair and integrity [75]. These examples underscore the critical role of astrocytes in BBB functioning in order to provide metabolic support to oligodendrocytes, essential in processes such as myelination.

While astrocytes are considered to be key players in maintaining BBB integrity, OPCs have also been shown to play a role in BBB integrity through TGF-β signalling [76]. Additionally, BBB integrity is enhanced by OPCs through PDGF-BB/PDGFRα signalling while oligodendrocytes control BBB integrity independent of this pathway [77]. Conversely, a recent study combining pathology, in vivo and in vitro cultures indicates that clusters of OPCs contribute to altered vascular permeability by impacting the astrocyte foot processes in MS [78]. OPCs require a vascular scaffold for migration throughout the CNS to repopulate demyelinated areas in MS but detachment of the vasculature fails which results in a disruption of the BBB integrity [78].

3.2. Gap Junctions Connect Astrocytes and Oligodendrocytes

Astrocytes are connected to other glial cells via gap junctions, allowing free flow of ions and small metabolites. Gap junctions between astrocytes are made up of connexin (Cx) 30 and/or 43 that forms either homotypic (Cx30:Cx30 or Cx43:Cx43) or heterotypic channels (Cx30:Cx43). Using these gap junctions, astrocytes form a syncytium with free flow of small molecules including gliotransmitters and lactate that aids buffering of K^+ [20,79]. Astrocytes express Cx30 and Cx43 that couples to adjacent oligodendrocytes expressing Cx32 and Cx47 by forming heterotypic gap junctions respectively Cx30:Cx32 and Cx43:Cx47 [6,79]. This physical contact is important in oligodendrocyte maturation and is often disrupted in demyelinating conditions. In EAE the reduction in Cx47 and Cx32 reduces oligodendrocyte-oligodendrocyte and astrocyte-oligodendrocyte interactions [20]. This reduction is also observed in active and chronic lesions in MS, neuromyelitis optica (NMO) and Baló's disease [80]. Absence of Cx47 or Cx32 in oligodendrocytes exacerbates clinical EAE in mice associated with increased myelin loss but does not affect Cx30 and Cx43 expression in astrocytes [81]. Pathogenic mutations in Cx32 also contribute to Charcot-Marie-Tooth disease characterized by peripheral demyelination and neuropathy [80]. In contrast, Cx43 is upregulated in remyelinating MS lesions, emphasizing the importance of communication via gap junctions in remyelination [80]. The detrimental effect of Cx loss on remyelination may be attributed to the necessity of trophic support of oligodendrocytes by astrocytes, although whether the loss of Cx in gap junctions is the cause or consequence of myelin damage is unclear [82].

4. Astrocytes and Oligodendrocytes Play Active Roles in Immune Responses

Emerging studies have changed the perception that astrocytes and oligodendrocytes are solely bystanders in inflammatory processes. In infectious and inflammatory CNS diseases oligodendrocytes have been reported to act as antigen presenting cells and produce immune molecules [9] (Table 2). In neuroinflammation oligodendrocytes express many factors known to activate astrocytes [83,84] (Figure 1). For example, in vitro astrocytes express receptors for e.g., CCL2 and CXCL10 which are mostly secreted to attract monocytes and macrophages [85–88]. In MS lesions oligodendrocyte and astrocyte expression of IL-17 suggests that glia, as well as T cells, promote the pro-inflammatory environment that attracts macrophages to the lesion [89]. In mice, administration of cuprizone, that damages and ablates oligodendrocytes, both oligodendrocytes and OPCs secrete IL-1β, a known pro-inflammatory cytokine [90–92]. CXCL1, CXCL2, CXCL3, CXCL5, and CXCL6 all bind the CXCR2 receptor, which is constitutively expressed on oligodendrocytes, but not present on astrocytes [88,93]. The CXCR2 receptor is upregulated in response to these cytokines that are secreted by oligodendrocytes, supporting autocrine regulation. Several CXCR2 ligands have previously been associated with OPC proliferation and differentiation [94], indicating that oligodendrocytes regulate their own proliferation. Granulocyte macrophage colony stimulating factor (GM-CSF) is upregulated in resting oligodendrocytes [93] which has been found to be anti-apoptotic for neurons and neuroprotective in models of stroke.

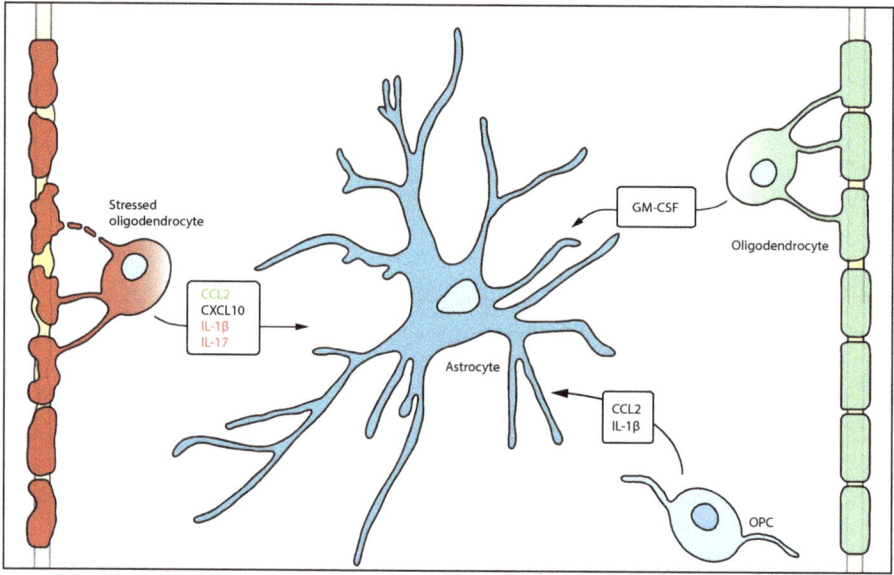

Figure 1. Oligodendrocytes secrete factors that impact on astrocytes. Stressed oligodendrocytes release factors that have beneficial effects (green) on astrocytes such as CCL2 to reduce inflammation. In contrast detrimental factors (red) such as IL-1β exacerbates inflammation. Healthy oligodendrocytes and OPCs also interact with astrocytes by secretion of GM-CSF and CCL2 as well as IL-1β.

Additionally, astrocytes secrete CXCL1 in spinal cord injury and in MS lesions, both in vivo and in vitro, which may act to recruit oligodendrocytes [88,95]. Gap junctions are also reported to play an immunoregulatory role for example Cx43 loss in astrocytes increases recruitment of immune cells in the brain as well as inducing an atypical reactive astrocyte phenotype that secretes both pro- and anti-inflammatory factors [82,96,97].

Many immune factors are secreted by both oligodendrocytes and astrocytes in vitro i.e., IL-1β, CXCL10 and IL17, underscoring a possible immune function of these cells [90]. In addition, astrocytes also secrete tumour necrosis factor-α (TNF-α), IL-1β, interferon-γ (IFN-γ), fibroblast growth factor-2 (FGF-2), PDGF, and BMPs, factors known to influence oligodendrocytes and OPCs [3,98] (Figure 2, Table 2). TNF-α is recognized by TNFR1 and induces pro-inflammatory effects, while binding to TNF-αR2 induces anti-inflammatory effects. Both TNFR1 and TNFR2 are expressed on oligodendrocytes [9], and both are upregulated during inflammation [8] indicating that oligodendrocytes could trigger both pro- and anti-inflammatory responses. Likewise, astrocytes express predominantly TNFR1 but are capable of upregulating TNFR2 after stimulation by TNF-α [3,99], suggesting an autocrine feedback loop. While inhibition of TNF-α is an effective therapy in autoimmune diseases such as rheumatoid arthritis, this approach has been less straightforward in MS [100], recent data shows that selective modulation of TNFRs by activating TNFR2 and/or silencing TNFR1 might have therapeutic potential [101]. IL-1β is expressed by astrocytes during ischemic stroke, as well as neuroinflammatory disease although the precise mechanisms of IL-1β remain unclear [102,103]. IL-1β was also found in active MS lesions in reactive astrocytes and in pre-active lesions where it might act on oligodendrocytes and astrocytes in lesion formation [104]. IFN-γ has both pro- and anti-inflammatory effects, as treatment with IFN-γ exacerbates MS pathology, but also induces neurotrophic factor production in astrocytes, which are also able to produce IFN-γ [105,106]. FGF-2 is secreted by astrocytes after focal demyelination in mice, and has been shown to promote OPC proliferation yet inhibit their differentiation to oligodendrocytes [4,21]. BMPs are upregulated in EAE, and direct OPC differentiation into the astrocyte lineage [21]. Lastly, insulin-like growth factor-1 (IGF-1) also induces OPC maturation [107].

Table 2. Immunologic interplay between astrocytes and oligodendrocytes.

	Detrimental	Beneficial	References
Astrocyte Mediator	**Impact on Oligodendrocytes**		
TNF-α	Induces demyelination and oligodendrocyte necrosis	Induces PDGF, and LIF on astrocytes which enhances OPC survival and differentiation	[3,108–112]
IL-1β	Induces oligodendrocyte apoptosis and hypomyelination		[102]
IFN-γ	Reversibly reduces OPC proliferation	Limits inflammation, limits Th17 activation, limits IL-1β signalling, protects oligodendrocytes from endoplasmic reticulum stress	[106,113–115]
FGF-2	Induces loss of myelin and myelin-producing oligodendrocytes	Induces proliferation of OPCs	[4,116]
BMP	BMPs induce OPC differentiation into the astrocyte lineage		[21,117]
CNTF		Induces proliferation and differentiation of OPCs	[21,105]
IGF-1		Induces OPC differentiation	[21,107,118]
Oligodendrocyte Mediator	**Impact on Astrocytes**		
CCL2		Reduces IL-6 expression in astrocytes, leading to a less inflammatory environment	[92,119,120]
CXCL10	Induces CXCR3 receptor expression		[119,121]
IL-17	Induces GFAP, IL-1β, and VEGF, reduces BBB integrity Induces astrogliosis		[89,122]
IL-1β	Induces IL-1β and NF-κB, and P2X$_7$ receptor.		[90,92,123,124]
GM-CSF		Inhibits glial scar formation. Induces proliferation, and migration of astrocytes	[93,125]

Abbreviations: BMP, bone morphogenic protein, CNTF, ciliary neurotrophic factor; FGF, Fibroblast growth factor; IFN, interferon; IGF, insulin-like growth factor; LIF, leukaemia inhibitory factor; OPC, oligodendrocyte precursor cell; PDGF, Platelet-derived growth factor; TNF, tumour necrosis factor.

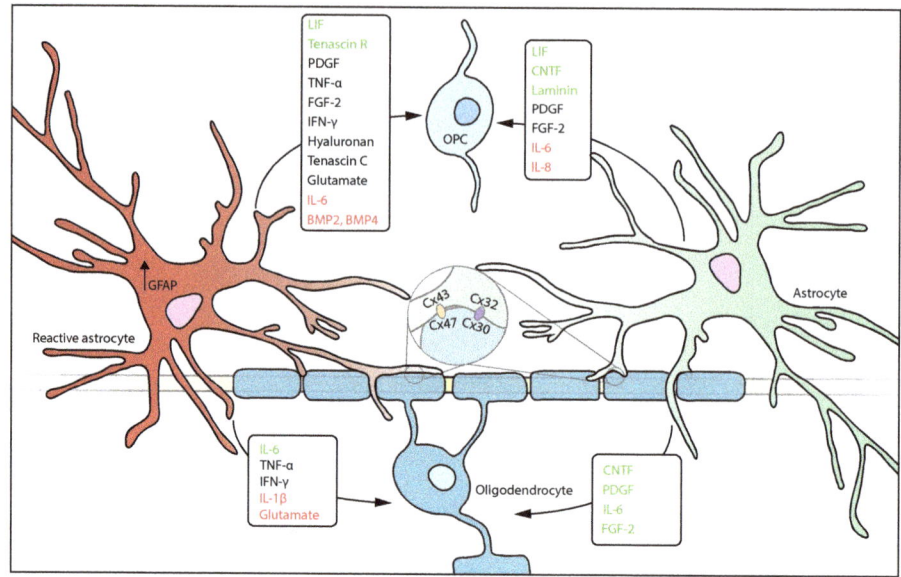

Figure 2. Astrocytes release a wide variety of molecules that impact oligodendrocyte functioning. Reactive and homeostatic astrocytes can release both beneficial (green) as well as detrimental (red) molecules. Most molecules that are secreted by astrocytes have a context dependent effect as well as a differential effect on oligodendrocytes and OPCs.

5. Astrocyte—Oligodendrocyte Interplay in Disease

5.1. Reactive Gliosis and Glial Scar Formation

Reactive astrocytes are a hallmark of many CNS diseases for example in MS lesions [3,22,25,126], around the injured site during spinal cord injury (SCI) [41], within Rosenthal fibres in AxD [127], after ischemic stroke [128], and near amyloid plaques in AD [129], indicating their importance in both classic white matter and grey matter disease. Reactive gliosis is a spectrum rather than an all-or-nothing reaction, and the severity may differ between diseases, patients, or even within a patient. Mildly reactive astrocytes are associated with milder CNS injury or inflammation, and do not proliferate, showing only moderate changes in gene expression. Severely reactive astrocytes are characterized by upregulation of GFAP, hypertrophy and proliferation, and are present in severe injury and infection, as well as in chronic neurodegenerative disease. The most severe reaction is the glial scar, where astrocytes proliferate and intertwine to form a physical barrier that surrounds injured CNS tissue and isolates it from healthy tissue. It is associated with severe necrosis or inflammation [130].

In the acute stages of CNS damage, glial scarring is essential to prevent more widespread inflammation and the spread of toxic factors, protecting neurons from secondary degeneration [131]. An astrocyte-specific STAT3 knock-out inhibits formation of the glial scar, and leads to increased inflammation and motor dysfunction in mice after SCI [2,4,98]. On the other hand, in an AD mouse model, inhibition of the JAK2-STAT3 pathway leads to reduced astrocyte reactivity and increased learning abilities [132]. Glial scars are also involved in restoration of BBB integrity in inflammatory CNS disorders [20,131]. However, in the chronic stages, the glial scars inhibit OPC migration and differentiation and is thus considered to be detrimental blocking tissue repair [3,4,66,103]. This is observed in ischemic stroke, where the glial scar secretes growth inhibiting factors that prevent axonal regrowth [128], and in MS, where OPC migration into demyelinated lesions is inhibited [22].

Astrocytes become reactive in response to both direct and indirect activation; indirect activation is mediated by cytokines secreted by microglia, while direct activation is mediated by damage or pathogen associated molecular patterns that are released by pathogens or during cell death, oxidative stress, or chemical stress [3,22]. This implies that oligodendrocyte injury induces astrocyte reactivity. Upon activation, astrocytes secrete factors e.g., TNF-α, IL-1β, IL-6, brain derived neurotrophic factor (BDNF), leukemia inhibitory factor (LIF), CCL2, and CXCL10 [3,22,98,103,133]. These factors play a critical role in generating the immune responses during infection or damage, but also lead to collateral damage of oligodendrocytes and OPCs. The glial scar is essential to keep these factors isolated in the acute phase of disease, and abolishing it is adverse to recovery, while modulation of the glial scar in the chronic phase of disease may stimulate remyelination in white matter disorders.

5.2. Astrocytes in Neuroinflammation

The NF-κB pathway is a major inflammatory pathway involved in activation of the innate and adaptive immune responses essential for e.g., generation of T-cell and B-cells. The pathway is constitutively active in many inflammatory disorders of the white matter [90,134]. In vitro, astrocytes upregulate NF-κB in response to pro-inflammatory cytokines such as IL-17, IL-1β, and TNF-α [90,135]. In vivo, overexpression of the NF-κB inhibitor IκBα in astrocytes results in protection of oligodendrocytes via reduced leukocyte infiltration and lower levels of chemokines during EAE [136]. NF-κB is also relevant in other CNS disorders that are not classically seen as white matter disorders, including AD, where amyloid-β plaques induce NF-κB activation in an astrocyte-specific manner [137]. In SOD1 mice, a mouse model of ALS, astrocytic NF-κB promotes degeneration of motor neurons and accelerates disease progression [138]. Subtle white matter changes are found in neurodegenerative diseases as early as pre-clinical AD where the NF-κB pathway could play a role in exacerbating inflammatory signaling [139]. Intervention in this pathway is effective, as demonstrated by the MS drug laquinimod, which inhibits astrocytic NF-κB expression [4,134]. NF-κB signalling represents an important inflammatory pathway in various neurological disorders that is frequently used by astrocytes to exacerbate inflammation. Alleviation of oligodendrocyte pathology via astrocytic NF-κB targeting may be relevant in more white matter disorders, and its use in MS treatment is proof of concept for the relevance of cross-talk in white matter disease therapy.

5.3. Excitotoxicity

Oligodendrocytes are sensitive to excitotoxic damage due to their expression of α-amino-3-hydroxy-5-methyl-4-isoxazolepropionic acid (AMPA) and kainate receptors. In EAE, treatment with AMPA and kainate antagonists significantly reduces oligodendrocyte death and disease severity, suggesting a role for excitotoxic cell death in MS [22,140]. Moreover, TNF-α triggers astrocytic upregulation of prostaglandin-E2 in vitro, which induces release of glutamate into the extracellular space [141], indicating that neuroinflammation exacerbates excitotoxic damage, leading to oligodendrocyte death. Excitotoxicity is further facilitated by downregulation of EAATs, which occurs in the senile plaques in AD, and in ALS [129,137]. Excitotoxicity in oligodendrocytes is not just glutamate-mediated, but also ATP-mediated, via overstimulation of the P2X purinoreceptor-7 (P2X7) ATP receptors. Similar to the AMPA and kainate receptors, the P2X7 receptor is Ca^{2+} permeable, and the intracellular Ca^{2+} damages oligodendrocytes.

Studies by Matute and colleagues show that in mice P2X7 antagonists prevent ATP toxicity in oligodendrocytes [7]. P2X7 receptors are significantly increased in oligodendrocytes in the optic nerves of people with MS compared to healthy controls, indicating that ATP toxicity might be a relevant pathogenic mechanism in disease [142]. ATP toxicity is also pathogenic after SCI, increasing demyelination and neuronal death after injury [143]. In support of this, treatment of rats with P2X7 antagonists increases neuronal survival and functional recovery after SCI [143]. Stimulation of the P2X7 receptor of neonatal rat-derived astrocytes results in glutamate release, supplying the environment with more excitotoxic molecules [142]. Astrocytic overexpression of P2X7 was also found in the white and grey matter in secondary progressive MS [144] as well as upon stimulation with IL-1β [123], suggesting that this signalling pathway is especially relevant during inflammation.

P2X7 is also of importance in epilepsy, since sufferers have higher P2X7 expression than healthy controls in the neocortical nerve terminals. P2X7 antagonist treatment decreases the severity and number of epileptic seizures in rats [145]. Excitotoxicity is a relevant mechanism of cell death in many disorders, and astrocyte-oligodendrocyte cross-talk plays an important role here, as astrocytes are able to create a hostile environment with glutamate and ATP which then damages oligodendrocytes. Inhibition of astrocytic glutamate release or increasing the activity of the EAAT receptors may thus be a relevant treatment mechanism in epilepsy or white matter diseases.

6. Astrocyte Control of Remyelination and the Extracellular Matrix

The white matter of the brain primarily consists of myelinated axons formed by oligodendrocytes, after differentiating from OPCs [4]. In demyelinating diseases such as MS and NMO, functional recovery requires remyelination. Although in these diseases astrocytes are known to be detrimental to oligodendrocytes and OPCs, they also promote and mediate remyelination [7,41]. For example, in vivo ablation of astrocytes results in impaired recovery from SCI [2]. In MS or SCI remyelination occurs but often fails despite the presence of significant numbers of OPCs suggesting the lack of remyelination is likely due to a failure in OPC differentiation rather than migration [20,146,147]. However, migration failure and clustering of OPCs at astrocyte endfeet indicates that astrocytes may also play a role in restricting migration of OPCs [78]. Recruitment of OPCs to the demyelinating area occurs through astrocyte chemokine signalling of IL-1β and CCL2, confirming the necessity of cellular cross-talk in remyelination [20,148]. After migration, OPCs exit the cell cycle and differentiate into oligodendrocytes through stimulation of PDGF and FGF-2 [147]. FGF-2 is highly upregulated by astrocytes in remyelinating spinal cord lesions where it acts on oligodendrocytes as well as in autocrine fashion on astrocytes [149]. Recently, a new study has found that OPCs might not be as important for remyelination as previously thought. Remyelination was found to be mainly dependent on the pool of surviving mature oligodendrocytes present in the lesions based on carbon dating of oligodendrocytes [150].

Astrocytes influence oligodendrocytes via modification of the extracellular matrix (ECM). A major ECM component secreted by astrocytes is hyaluronan, which acts on T-cells and OPCs, blocking OPC differentiation into oligodendrocytes and promoting astrocytic differentiation [41]. Hyaluronan is especially abundant in white matter lesions of MS patients [21], as well as patients with rare familial leukodystrophies VWM [50] and AxD [127]. Exaggerated hyaluronan secretion is a common feature of leukodystrophies, and likely has a role in neurological pathogenesis. Another astrocytic ECM factor is laminin that controls the differentiation and migration of OPCs, and promotes their survival by binding integrin and dystroglycan receptors. Mutations in laminin result in profound muscular and white matter abnormalities [151–153]. In inflammatory conditions, reactive astrocytes also produce tenascin C and R. Tenascin C is linked to inhibition of OPC migration, but tenascin R induces myelin gene expression and OPC differentiation. In chronic MS plaques, both tenascin C and R were shown to be upregulated in reactive astrocytes [153]. Lastly, astrocytes secrete proteoglycans that inhibit remyelination in high concentrations [154]. Proteoglycans also capture chemokines and growth factors, localizing them and targeting immune cells to the area of inflammation. This helps to prevent immune-mediated collateral damage [131]. These studies underscore the importance of the ECM in providing a healthy environment for remyelination. If disrupted, a remyelination promoting environment turns inhibitory, leading to impaired differentiation and proliferation of OPCs. Astrocytes are an important source of many ECM factors, and communicate with and influence OPCs and oligodendrocytes via secretion of ECM factors.

In inflammatory CNS conditions infiltration of immune cells is a hallmark of disease and heavily dependent on the breakdown of the ECM. MMP2 and 9 are important in degradation of the *Lamina basalis*, as well as infiltration of immune cells into the brain parenchyma. The activity of these proteins is regulated by tissue inhibitors of metalloproteinases (TIMPs). Although astrocytes express MMP2 and 9 both in vivo and in vitro, they also produce TIMP-1 [103]. Astrocytes promote oligodendrogenesis during and after injury through secretion of BDNF and TIMP-1 [155,156]. This is also shown in TIMP-1 deficient mice that exhibit defective myelin repair [20], indicating the importance of the ECM in remyelination. Another MMP that is active in remyelination is MMP7, which cleaves fibronectin aggregates present in demyelinating lesions in MS. These aggregates prevent OPC maturation and remyelination. Secreted proMMP7 is activated by astrocytic MMP3, indicating that astrocytes assist in this cleavage [157]. This shows that astrocytes are not only involved in the building of the ECM, but also in its breakdown and maintenance.

In summary, astrocytic dysfunction results in a toxic extracellular environment with high levels of excitotoxic molecules and pro-inflammatory cytokines such as IL-1β and TNF-α. On the other hand, their basal functions are essential in maintaining a healthy brain microenvironment where oligodendrocytes thrive and remyelinate the CNS. Although astrocytes can be detrimental in neurological disease they are also essential for the recovery from damage. Astrocytes are particularly important in early recovery by supporting oligodendrocyte migration and OPC differentiation. However, astrocytes become pathological in the chronic phase, exemplified by the glial scar formation in SCI or MS, in which hypertrophic astrocytes produce many factors that induce a harmful environment for mature oligodendrocytes and inhibit OPC differentiation [41,131].

7. Conclusions

Astrocyte and oligodendrocyte interactions in healthy conditions and disease are complex and multifaceted. The widely considered view that astrocytes only react to damage in neurological diseases is changing to embrace the emerging evidence that these cells are essential to the development of the healthy CNS. On the other hand, astrocytes are involved in the pathogenesis of several CNS diseases since loss of normal trophic functions of astrocytes results in damage to neurons and oligodendrocytes thereby exacerbating pathology.

Furthermore, astrocytes are important for the regenerative capacities of the brain aiding oligodendrocyte proliferation, maturation and migration—a key step in repair in diseases such as MS and other demyelinating diseases. There is also a growing awareness that astrocytes and oligodendrocytes are not only targets for autoimmune responses in the context of neuroinflammation. Astrocytes play an important role as innate immune cells, e.g., by secreting chemokines, and as such influence other glia cells.

Future studies into the communication between astrocytes and oligodendrocytes as well as their impact on other CNS cell types will provide new clues for controlling innate immunity and aiding repair in the CNS.

Author Contributions: Writing—original draft preparation, E.N., D.v.G., S.A.; writing—review and editing, L.A.N.P. and S.A. All authors have read and agreed to the published version of the manuscript.

Funding: This research received no external funding.

Acknowledgments: We thank the Multiple Sclerosis Society of Great Britain and Northern Ireland and the Stichting MS Research, The Netherlands for supporting studies discussed in this review.

Conflicts of Interest: The authors declare no conflict of interest.

References

1. Colombo, E.; Farina, C. Astrocytes: Key Regulators of Neuroinflammation. *Trends Immunol.* **2016**, *37*, 608–620. [CrossRef] [PubMed]
2. Gaudet, A.D.; Fonken, L.K. Glial Cells Shape Pathology and Repair After Spinal Cord Injury. *Neurotherapeutics* **2018**, *15*, 554–577. [CrossRef] [PubMed]
3. Kiray, H.; Lindsay, S.L.; Hosseinzadeh, S.; Barnett, S.C. The multifaceted role of astrocytes in regulating myelination. *Exp. Neurol.* **2016**, *283*, 541–549. [CrossRef] [PubMed]

4. Li, J.; Zhang, L.; Chu, Y.; Namaka, M.; Deng, B.; Kong, J.; Bi, X. Astrocytes in Oligodendrocyte Lineage Development and White Matter Pathology. *Front. Cell Neurosci.* **2016**, *10*, 119. [CrossRef] [PubMed]
5. Seth, P.; Koul, N. Astrocyte, the star avatar: Redefined. *J. Biosci.* **2008**, *33*, 405–421. [CrossRef]
6. Orthmann-Murphy, J.L.; Abrams, C.K.; Scherer, S.S. Gap junctions couple astrocytes and oligodendrocytes. *J. Mol. Neurosci.* **2008**, *35*, 101–116. [CrossRef]
7. McTigue, D.M.; Tripathi, R.B. The life, death, and replacement of oligodendrocytes in the adult CNS. *J. Neurochem.* **2008**, *107*, 1–19. [CrossRef]
8. Patel, J.; Balabanov, R. Molecular mechanisms of oligodendrocyte injury in multiple sclerosis and experimental autoimmune encephalomyelitis. *Int. J. Mol. Sci.* **2012**, *13*, 10647–10659. [CrossRef]
9. Peferoen, L.; Kipp, M.; van der Valk, P.; van Noort, J.M.; Amor, S. Oligodendrocyte-microglia cross-talk in the central nervous system. *Immunology* **2014**, *141*, 302–313. [CrossRef]
10. van der Knaap, M.S.; Bugiani, M. Leukodystrophies: A proposed classification system based on pathological changes and pathogenetic mechanisms. *Acta Neuropathol.* **2017**, *134*, 351–382. [CrossRef]
11. Bouchat, J.; Couturier, B.; Marneffe, C.; Gankam-Kengne, F.; Balau, B.; De Swert, K.; Brion, J.-P.; Poncelet, L.; Gilloteaux, J.; Nicaise, C. Regional oligodendrocytopathy and astrocytopathy precede myelin loss and blood–brain barrier disruption in a murine model of osmotic demyelination syndrome. *Glia* **2018**, *66*, 606–622. [CrossRef] [PubMed]
12. Gankam Kengne, F.; Nicaise, C.; Soupart, A.; Boom, A.; Schiettecatte, J.; Pochet, R.; Brion, J.P.; Decaux, G. Astrocytes are an early target in osmotic demyelination syndrome. *J. Am. Soc. Nephrol.* **2011**, *22*, 1834–1845. [CrossRef] [PubMed]
13. Gankam-Kengne, F.; Couturier, B.S.; Soupart, A.; Brion, J.P.; Decaux, G. Osmotic Stress-Induced Defective Glial Proteostasis Contributes to Brain Demyelination after Hyponatremia Treatment. *J. Am. Soc. Nephrol.* **2017**, *28*, 1802–1813. [CrossRef] [PubMed]
14. Coulter, D.A.; Eid, T. Astrocytic regulation of glutamate homeostasis in epilepsy. *Glia* **2012**, *60*, 1215–1226. [CrossRef] [PubMed]
15. Seifert, G.; Schilling, K.; Steinhauser, C. Astrocyte dysfunction in neurological disorders: A molecular perspective. *Nat. Rev. Neurosci.* **2006**, *7*, 194–206. [CrossRef] [PubMed]
16. Faideau, M.; Kim, J.; Cormier, K.; Gilmore, R.; Welch, M.; Auregan, G.; Dufour, N.; Guillermier, M.; Brouillet, E.; Hantraye, P.; et al. In vivo expression of polyglutamine-expanded huntingtin by mouse striatal astrocytes impairs glutamate transport: A correlation with Huntington's disease subjects. *Hum. Mol. Genet.* **2010**, *19*, 3053–3067. [CrossRef]
17. Simpson, J.E.; Ince, P.G.; Lace, G.; Forster, G.; Shaw, P.J.; Matthews, F.; Savva, G.; Brayne, C.; Wharton, S.B.; Function, M.R.C.C.; et al. Astrocyte phenotype in relation to Alzheimer-type pathology in the ageing brain. *Neurobiol. Aging* **2010**, *31*, 578–590. [CrossRef]
18. Reich, D.S.; Lucchinetti, C.F.; Calabresi, P.A. Multiple Sclerosis. *New Engl. J. Med.* **2018**, *378*, 169–180. [CrossRef]
19. Thompson, A.J.; Baranzini, S.E.; Geurts, J.; Hemmer, B.; Ciccarelli, O. Multiple sclerosis. *Lancet* **2018**, *391*, 1622–1636. [CrossRef]
20. Domingues, H.S.; Portugal, C.C.; Socodato, R.; Relvas, J.B. Oligodendrocyte, Astrocyte, and Microglia Crosstalk in Myelin Development, Damage, and Repair. *Front. Cell Dev. Biol.* **2016**, *4*, 71. [CrossRef]
21. Moore, C.S.; Abdullah, S.L.; Brown, A.; Arulpragasam, A.; Crocker, S.J. How factors secreted from astrocytes impact myelin repair. *Neurosci. Res.* **2011**, *89*, 13–21. [CrossRef] [PubMed]
22. Ponath, G.; Park, C.; Pitt, D. The Role of Astrocytes in Multiple Sclerosis. *Front. Immunol.* **2018**, *9*, 217. [CrossRef]
23. Torkildsen, O.; Myhr, K.M.; Bo, L. Disease-modifying treatments for multiple sclerosis - a review of approved medications. *Eur. J. Neurol.* **2016**, *23*, 18–27. [CrossRef]
24. Hostenbach, S.; Cambron, M.; D'Haeseleer, M.; Kooijman, R.; De Keyser, J. Astrocyte loss and astrogliosis in neuroinflammatory disorders. *Neurosci. Lett.* **2014**, *565*, 39–41. [CrossRef] [PubMed]
25. Popescu, B.F.; Lucchinetti, C.F. Pathology of demyelinating diseases. *Annu. Rev. Pathol.* **2012**, *7*, 185–217. [CrossRef] [PubMed]
26. Uzawa, A.; Mori, M.; Arai, K.; Sato, Y.; Hayakawa, S.; Masuda, S.; Taniguchi, J.; Kuwabara, S. Cytokine and chemokine profiles in neuromyelitis optica: Significance of interleukin-6. *Mult. Scler.* **2010**, *16*, 1443–1452. [CrossRef] [PubMed]

27. Vitturi, B.K.; Rosemberg, S.; Arita, F.N.; da Rocha, A.J.; Forte, W.C.N.; Tilbery, C.P. Multiphasic disseminated encephalomyelitis associated with herpes virus infection in a patient with TLR3 deficiency. *Mult. Scler. Relat. Disord.* **2019**, *36*, 101379. [CrossRef]
28. Robinson, C.A.; Adiele, R.C.; Tham, M.; Lucchinetti, C.F.; Popescu, B.F. Early and widespread injury of astrocytes in the absence of demyelination in acute haemorrhagic leukoencephalitis. *Acta Neuropathol. Commun.* **2014**, *2*, 52. [CrossRef]
29. Bauer, J.; Gold, R.; Adams, O.; Lassmann, H. Progressive multifocal leukoencephalopathy and immune reconstitution inflammatory syndrome (IRIS). *Acta Neuropathol.* **2015**, *130*, 751–764. [CrossRef]
30. Gheuens, S.; Wuthrich, C.; Koralnik, I.J. Progressive multifocal leukoencephalopathy: Why gray and white matter. *Annu. Rev. Pathol.* **2013**, *8*, 189–215. [CrossRef]
31. Langer-Gould, A.; Atlas, S.W.; Green, A.J.; Bollen, A.W.; Pelletier, D. Progressive multifocal leukoencephalopathy in a patient treated with natalizumab. *New Engl. J. Med.* **2005**, *353*, 375–381. [CrossRef] [PubMed]
32. Lewandowska, E.; Szpak, G.M.; Lechowicz, W.; Pasennik, E.; Sobczyk, W. Ultrastructural changes in neuronal and glial cells in subacute sclerosing panencephalitis: Correlation with disease duration. *Folia Neuropathol.* **2001**, *39*, 193–202. [PubMed]
33. Mesquita, R.; Castanos-Velez, E.; Biberfeld, P.; Troian, R.M.; de Siqueira, M.M. Measles virus antigen in macrophage/microglial cells and astrocytes of subacute sclerosing panencephalitis. *Apmis Acta Pathol. Microbiol. Et Immunol. Scand.* **1998**, *106*, 553–561. [CrossRef] [PubMed]
34. Kossmann, T.; Morganti-Kossmann, M.C.; Orenstein, J.M.; Britt, W.J.; Wahl, S.M.; Smith, P.D. Cytomegalovirus production by infected astrocytes correlates with transforming growth factor-beta release. *J. Infect. Dis.* **2003**, *187*, 534–541. [CrossRef]
35. Zhang, L.; Li, L.; Wang, B.; Qian, D.M.; Song, X.X.; Hu, M. HCMV induces dysregulation of glutamate uptake and transporter expression in human fetal astrocytes. *Neurochem. Res.* **2014**, *39*, 2407–2418. [CrossRef]
36. Banjara, M.; Ghosh, C.; Dadas, A.; Mazzone, P.; Janigro, D. Detection of brain-directed autoantibodies in the serum of non-small cell lung cancer patients. *PLoS ONE* **2017**, *12*, e0181409. [CrossRef]
37. Fang, B.; McKeon, A.; Hinson, S.R.; Kryzer, T.J.; Pittock, S.J.; Aksamit, A.J.; Lennon, V.A. Autoimmune Glial Fibrillary Acidic Protein Astrocytopathy: A Novel Meningoencephalomyelitis. *JAMA Neurol.* **2016**, *73*, 1297–1307. [CrossRef]
38. Rosenberg, G.A. Binswanger's disease: Biomarkers in the inflammatory form of vascular cognitive impairment and dementia. *J. Neurochem.* **2018**, *144*, 634–643. [CrossRef]
39. Pregnolato, S.; Chakkarapani, E.; Isles, A.R.; Luyt, K. Glutamate Transport and Preterm Brain Injury. *Front. Physiol.* **2019**, *10*, 417. [CrossRef]
40. Revuelta, M.; Elicegui, A.; Moreno-Cugnon, L.; Buhrer, C.; Matheu, A.; Schmitz, T. Ischemic stroke in neonatal and adult astrocytes. *Mech. Ageing Dev.* **2019**, *183*, 111147. [CrossRef]
41. Wang, H.F.; Liu, X.K.; Li, R.; Zhang, P.; Chu, Z.; Wang, C.L.; Liu, H.R.; Qi, J.; Lv, G.Y.; Wang, G.Y.; et al. Effect of glial cells on remyelination after spinal cord injury. *Neural. Regen Res.* **2017**, *12*, 1724–1732. [CrossRef] [PubMed]
42. Frati, G.; Luciani, M.; Meneghini, V.; De Cicco, S.; Stahlman, M.; Blomqvist, M.; Grossi, S.; Filocamo, M.; Morena, F.; Menegon, A.; et al. Human iPSC-based models highlight defective glial and neuronal differentiation from neural progenitor cells in metachromatic leukodystrophy. *Cell Death Dis.* **2018**, *9*, 698. [CrossRef] [PubMed]
43. Kruska, N.; Schonfeld, P.; Pujol, A.; Reiser, G. Astrocytes and mitochondria from adrenoleukodystrophy protein (ABCD1)-deficient mice reveal that the adrenoleukodystrophy-associated very long-chain fatty acids target several cellular energy-dependent functions. *Biochim. Et Biophys. Acta* **2015**, *1852*, 925–936. [CrossRef] [PubMed]
44. Gortz, A.L.; Peferoen, L.A.N.; Gerritsen, W.H.; van Noort, J.M.; Bugiani, M.; Amor, S. Heat shock protein expression in cerebral X-linked adrenoleukodystrophy reveals astrocyte stress prior to myelin loss. *Neuropathol. Appl. Neurobiol.* **2018**, *44*, 363–376. [CrossRef] [PubMed]
45. Weidenheim, K.M.; Dickson, D.W.; Rapin, I. Neuropathology of Cockayne syndrome: Evidence for impaired development, premature aging, and neurodegeneration. *Mech. Ageing Dev.* **2009**, *130*, 619–636. [CrossRef] [PubMed]

46. Takanashi, J.; Inoue, K.; Tomita, M.; Kurihara, A.; Morita, F.; Ikehira, H.; Tanada, S.; Yoshitome, E.; Kohno, Y. Brain N-acetylaspartate is elevated in Pelizaeus-Merzbacher disease with PLP1 duplication. *Neurology* **2002**, *58*, 237–241. [CrossRef]
47. Adachi, M.; Schneck, L.; Cara, J.; Volk, B.W. Spongy degeneration of the central nervous system (van Bogaert and Bertrand type; Canavan's disease). A review. *Hum. Pathol.* **1973**, *4*, 331–347. [CrossRef]
48. Baslow, M.H.; Guilfoyle, D.N. Are astrocytes the missing link between lack of brain aspartoacylase activity and the spongiform leukodystrophy in Canavan disease? *Neurochem. Res.* **2009**, *34*, 1523–1534. [CrossRef]
49. Borrett, D.; Becker, L.E. Alexander's disease. A disease of astrocytes. *Brain A J. Neurol.* **1985**, 367–385. [CrossRef]
50. Bugiani, M.; Vuong, C.; Breur, M.; van der Knaap, M.S. Vanishing white matter: A leukodystrophy due to astrocytic dysfunction. *Brain Pathol. (Zur. Switz.)* **2018**, *28*, 408–421. [CrossRef]
51. Hase, Y.; Chen, A.; Bates, L.L.; Craggs, L.J.L.; Yamamoto, Y.; Gemmell, E.; Oakley, A.E.; Korolchuk, V.I.; Kalaria, R.N. Severe white matter astrocytopathy in CADASIL. *Brain Pathol. (Zur. Switz.)* **2018**, *28*, 832–843. [CrossRef]
52. Orthmann-Murphy, J.L.; Enriquez, A.D.; Abrams, C.K.; Scherer, S.S. Loss-of-function GJA12/Connexin47 mutations cause Pelizaeus-Merzbacher-like disease. *Mol. Cell Neurosci.* **2007**, *34*, 629–641. [CrossRef] [PubMed]
53. van der Knaap, M.S.; Valk, J. *Magnetic Resonance of Myelination and Myelin Disorders*; Springer: Berlin/Heidelberg, Germany, 2005.
54. Sloan, S.A.; Barres, B.A. Mechanisms of astrocyte development and their contributions to neurodevelopmental disorders. *Curr. Opin. Neurobiol.* **2014**, *27*, 75–81. [CrossRef] [PubMed]
55. Zuchero, J.B.; Barres, B.A. Glia in mammalian development and disease. *Development* **2015**, *142*, 3805–3809. [CrossRef] [PubMed]
56. Noble, M.; Davies, J.E.; Mayer-Proschel, M.; Proschel, C.; Davies, S.J. Precursor cell biology and the development of astrocyte transplantation therapies: Lessons from spinal cord injury. *Neurotherapeutics* **2011**, *8*, 677–693. [CrossRef] [PubMed]
57. Molofsky, A.V.; Krencik, R.; Ullian, E.M.; Tsai, H.H.; Deneen, B.; Richardson, W.D.; Barres, B.A.; Rowitch, D.H. Astrocytes and disease: A neurodevelopmental perspective. *Genes Dev.* **2012**, *26*, 891–907. [CrossRef] [PubMed]
58. Miller, F.D.; Gauthier, A.S. Timing is everything: Making neurons versus glia in the developing cortex. *Neuron* **2007**, *54*, 357–369. [CrossRef] [PubMed]
59. Yang, Y.; Higashimori, H.; Morel, L. Developmental maturation of astrocytes and pathogenesis of neurodevelopmental disorders. *J. Neurodev. Disord.* **2013**, *5*, 22. [CrossRef]
60. Naruse, M.; Ishizaki, Y.; Ikenaka, K.; Tanaka, A.; Hitoshi, S. Origin of oligodendrocytes in mammalian forebrains: A revised perspective. *J. Physiol. Sci.* **2017**, *67*, 63–70. [CrossRef]
61. Rowitch, D.H.; Kriegstein, A.R. Developmental genetics of vertebrate glial-cell specification. *Nature* **2010**, *468*, 214–222. [CrossRef]
62. Durand, B.; Raff, M. A cell-intrinsic timer that operates during oligodendrocyte development. *Bioessays* **2000**, *22*, 64–71. [CrossRef]
63. Ortega, M.C.; Cases, O.; Merchan, P.; Kozyraki, R.; Clemente, D.; de Castro, F. Megalin mediates the influence of sonic hedgehog on oligodendrocyte precursor cell migration and proliferation during development. *Glia* **2012**, *60*, 851–866. [CrossRef] [PubMed]
64. Clemente, D.; Ortega, M.C.; Melero-Jerez, C.; de Castro, F. The effect of glia-glia interactions on oligodendrocyte precursor cell biology during development and in demyelinating diseases. *Front. Cell Neurosci.* **2013**, *7*, 268. [CrossRef] [PubMed]
65. See, J.; Zhang, X.; Eraydin, N.; Mun, S.B.; Mamontov, P.; Golden, J.A.; Grinspan, J.B. Oligodendrocyte maturation is inhibited by bone morphogenetic protein. *Mol. Cell Neurosci.* **2004**, *26*, 481–492. [CrossRef]
66. Lanciotti, A.; Brignone, M.S.; Bertini, E.; Petrucci, T.C.; Aloisi, F.; Ambrosini, E. Astrocytes: Emerging Stars in Leukodystrophy Pathogenesis. *Transl. Neurosci.* **2013**, *4*. [CrossRef]
67. Lundgaard, I.; Osorio, M.J.; Kress, B.T.; Sanggaard, S.; Nedergaard, M. White matter astrocytes in health and disease. *Neuroscience* **2014**, *276*, 161–173. [CrossRef]

68. Camargo, N.; Goudriaan, A.; van Deijk, A.F.; Otte, W.M.; Brouwers, J.F.; Lodder, H.; Gutmann, D.H.; Nave, K.A.; Dijkhuizen, R.M.; Mansvelder, H.D.; et al. Oligodendroglial myelination requires astrocyte-derived lipids. *PLoS Biol.* **2017**, *15*, e1002605. [CrossRef]
69. Itoh, N.; Itoh, Y.; Tassoni, A.; Ren, E.; Kaito, M.; Ohno, A.; Ao, Y.; Farkhondeh, V.; Johnsonbaugh, H.; Burda, J.; et al. Cell-specific and region-specific transcriptomics in the multiple sclerosis model: Focus on astrocytes. *Proc. Natl. Acad. Sci. USA* **2018**, *115*, E302–E309. [CrossRef]
70. Liu, J.P.; Tang, Y.; Zhou, S.; Toh, B.H.; McLean, C.; Li, H. Cholesterol involvement in the pathogenesis of neurodegenerative diseases. *Mol. Cell Neurosci.* **2010**, *43*, 33–42. [CrossRef]
71. Sweeney, M.D.; Kisler, K.; Montagne, A.; Toga, A.W.; Zlokovic, B.V. The role of brain vasculature in neurodegenerative disorders. *Nat. Neurosci..* **2018**, *21*, 1318–1331. [CrossRef]
72. Stephenson, E.; Nathoo, N.; Mahjoub, Y.; Dunn, J.F.; Yong, V.W. Iron in multiple sclerosis: Roles in neurodegeneration and repair. *Nat. Rev. Neurol.* **2014**, *10*, 459–468. [CrossRef] [PubMed]
73. Morath, D.J.; Mayer-Proschel, M. Iron deficiency during embryogenesis and consequences for oligodendrocyte generation in vivo. *Dev. Neurosci.* **2002**, *24*, 197–207. [CrossRef] [PubMed]
74. Heneka, M.T.; Kummer, M.P.; Latz, E. Innate immune activation in neurodegenerative disease. *Nat. Rev. Immunol.* **2014**, *14*, 463–477. [CrossRef] [PubMed]
75. Alvarez, J.I.; Dodelet-Devillers, A.; Kebir, H.; Ifergan, I.; Fabre, P.J.; Terouz, S.; Sabbagh, M.; Wosik, K.; Bourbonnière, L.; Bernard, M.; et al. The Hedgehog pathway promotes blood-brain barrier integrity and CNS immune quiescence. *Sci. (New Yorkn.Y.)* **2011**, *334*, 1727–1731. [CrossRef]
76. Seo, J.H.; Maki, T.; Maeda, M.; Miyamoto, N.; Liang, A.C.; Hayakawa, K.; Pham, L.D.; Suwa, F.; Taguchi, A.; Matsuyama, T.; et al. Oligodendrocyte precursor cells support blood-brain barrier integrity via TGF-beta signaling. *PLoS ONE* **2014**, *9*, e103174. [CrossRef]
77. Kimura, I.; Dohgu, S.; Takata, F.; Matsumoto, J.; Watanabe, T.; Iwao, T.; Yamauchi, A.; Kataoka, Y. Oligodendrocytes upregulate blood-brain barrier function through mechanisms other than the PDGF-BB/PDGFRalpha pathway in the barrier-tightening effect of oligodendrocyte progenitor cells. *Neurosci. Lett.* **2020**, *715*, 134594. [CrossRef]
78. Niu, J.; Tsai, H.H.; Hoi, K.K.; Huang, N.; Yu, G.; Kim, K.; Baranzini, S.E.; Xiao, L.; Chan, J.R.; Fancy, S.P.J. Aberrant oligodendroglial-vascular interactions disrupt the blood-brain barrier, triggering CNS inflammation. *Nat. Neurosci.* **2019**, *22*, 709–718. [CrossRef]
79. Giaume, C.; Naus, C.C. Connexins, gap junctions, and glia. *Wiley Interdiscip. Rev. Membr. Transport. Signal.* **2013**, *2013*, 133–142. [CrossRef]
80. Masaki, K. Early disruption of glial communication via connexin gap junction in multiple sclerosis, Balo's disease and neuromyelitis optica. *Neuropathology* **2015**, *35*, 469–480. [CrossRef]
81. Papaneophytou, C.P.; Georgiou, E.; Karaiskos, C.; Sargianidou, I.; Markoullis, K.; Freidin, M.M.; Abrams, C.K.; Kleopa, K.A. Regulatory role of oligodendrocyte gap junctions in inflammatory demyelination. *Glia* **2018**, *66*, 2589–2603. [CrossRef]
82. Boulay, A.-C.; Mazeraud, A.; Cisternino, S.; Saubaméa, B.; Mailly, P.; Jourdren, L.; Blugeon, C.; Mignon, V.; Smirnova, M.; Cavallo, A.; et al. Immune quiescence of the brain is set by astroglial connexin 43. *J. Neurosci.* **2015**, *35*, 4427–4439. [CrossRef] [PubMed]
83. Darbinyan, A.; Kaminski, R.; White, M.K.; Darbinian-Sarkissian, N.; Khalili, K. Polyomavirus JC infection inhibits differentiation of oligodendrocyte progenitor cells. *Neurosci. Res.* **2013**, *91*, 116–127. [CrossRef] [PubMed]
84. Ramesh, G.; Benge, S.; Pahar, B.; Philipp, M.T. A possible role for inflammation in mediating apoptosis of oligodendrocytes as induced by the Lyme disease spirochete Borrelia burgdorferi. *J. Neuroinflammation* **2012**, *9*, 72. [CrossRef] [PubMed]
85. Andjelkovic, A.V.; Song, L.; Dzenko, K.A.; Cong, H.; Pachter, J.S. Functional expression of CCR2 by human fetal astrocytes. *Neurosci. Res.* **2002**, *70*, 219–231. [CrossRef] [PubMed]
86. Ashutosh; Kou, W.; Cotter, R.; Borgmann, K.; Wu, L.; Persidsky, R.; Sakhuja, N.; Ghorpade, A. CXCL8 protects human neurons from amyloid-beta-induced neurotoxicity: Relevance to Alzheimer's disease. *Biochem. Biophys. Res. Commun.* **2011**, *412*, 565–571. [CrossRef] [PubMed]
87. Hsu, M.P.; Frausto, R.; Rose-John, S.; Campbell, I.L. Analysis of IL-6/gp130 family receptor expression reveals that in contrast to astroglia, microglia lack the oncostatin M receptor and functional responses to oncostatin M. *Glia* **2015**, *63*, 132–141. [CrossRef] [PubMed]

88. Omari, K.M.; John, G.; Lango, R.; Raine, C.S. Role for CXCR2 and CXCL1 on glia in multiple sclerosis. *Glia* **2006**, *53*, 24–31. [CrossRef]
89. Tzartos, J.S.; Friese, M.A.; Craner, M.J.; Palace, J.; Newcombe, J.; Esiri, M.M.; Fugger, L. Interleukin-17 production in central nervous system-infiltrating T cells and glial cells is associated with active disease in multiple sclerosis. *Am. J. Pathol.* **2008**, *172*, 146–155. [CrossRef]
90. Choi, S.S.; Lee, H.J.; Lim, I.; Satoh, J.; Kim, S.U. Human astrocytes: Secretome profiles of cytokines and chemokines. *PLoS ONE* **2014**, *9*, e92325. [CrossRef]
91. Moynagh, P.N. The interleukin-1 signalling pathway in astrocytes: A key contributor to inflammation in the brain. *J. Anat* **2005**, *207*, 265–269. [CrossRef]
92. Moyon, S.; Dubessy, A.L.; Aigrot, M.S.; Trotter, M.; Huang, J.K.; Dauphinot, L.; Potier, M.C.; Kerninon, C.; Melik Parsadaniantz, S.; Franklin, R.J.; et al. Demyelination causes adult CNS progenitors to revert to an immature state and express immune cues that support their migration. *J. Neurosci.* **2015**, *35*, 4–20. [CrossRef] [PubMed]
93. Kim, W.K.; Kim, D.; Cui, J.; Jang, H.H.; Kim, K.S.; Lee, H.J.; Kim, S.U.; Ahn, S.M. Secretome analysis of human oligodendrocytes derived from neural stem cells. *PLoS ONE* **2014**, *9*, e84292. [CrossRef]
94. Kadi, L.; Selvaraju, R.; de Lys, P.; Proudfoot, A.E.; Wells, T.N.; Boschert, U. Differential effects of chemokines on oligodendrocyte precursor proliferation and myelin formation in vitro. *J. Neuroimmunol.* **2006**, *174*, 133–146. [CrossRef] [PubMed]
95. Zhang, Z.J.; Cao, D.L.; Zhang, X.; Ji, R.R.; Gao, Y.J. Chemokine contribution to neuropathic pain: Respective induction of CXCL1 and CXCR2 in spinal cord astrocytes and neurons. *Pain* **2013**, *154*, 2185–2197. [CrossRef] [PubMed]
96. Boulay, A.-C.; Cisternino, S.; Cohen-Salmon, M. Immunoregulation at the gliovascular unit in the healthy brain: A focus on Connexin 43. *Brain Behaviour Immunol.* **2016**, *56*, 1–9. [CrossRef] [PubMed]
97. Boulay, A.-C.; Gilbert, A.; Oliveira Moreira, V.; Blugeon, C.; Perrin, S.; Pouch, J.; Le Crom, S.; Ducos, B.; Cohen-Salmon, M. Connexin 43 Controls the Astrocyte Immunoregulatory Phenotype. *Brain Sci.* **2018**, *8*, 50. [CrossRef]
98. Allaman, I.; Belanger, M.; Magistretti, P.J. Astrocyte-neuron metabolic relationships: For better and for worse. *Trends Neurosci.* **2011**, *34*, 76–87. [CrossRef]
99. Choi, S.J.; Lee, K.H.; Park, H.S.; Kim, S.K.; Koh, C.M.; Park, J.Y. Differential expression, shedding, cytokine regulation and function of TNFR1 and TNFR2 in human fetal astrocytes. *Yonsei Med. J.* **2005**, *46*, 818–826. [CrossRef]
100. Kemanetzoglou, E.; Andreadou, E. CNS Demyelination with TNF-alpha Blockers. *Curr. Neurol. Neurosci. Rep.* **2017**, *17*, 36. [CrossRef]
101. Pegoretti, V.; Baron, W.; Laman, J.D.; Eisel, U.L.M. Selective Modulation of TNF-TNFRs Signaling: Insights for Multiple Sclerosis Treatment. *Front. Immunol.* **2018**, *9*, 925. [CrossRef]
102. Deng, Y.; Xie, D.; Fang, M.; Zhu, G.; Chen, C.; Zeng, H.; Lu, J.; Charanjit, K. Astrocyte-derived proinflammatory cytokines induce hypomyelination in the periventricular white matter in the hypoxic neonatal brain. *PLoS ONE* **2014**, *9*, e87420. [CrossRef]
103. Miljkovic, D.; Timotijevic, G.; Mostarica Stojkovic, M. Astrocytes in the tempest of multiple sclerosis. *FEBS Lett.* **2011**, *585*, 3781–3788. [CrossRef]
104. Burm, S.M.; Peferoen, L.A.; Zuiderwijk-Sick, E.A.; Haanstra, K.G.; t Hart, B.A.; van der Valk, P.; Amor, S.; Bauer, J.; Bajramovic, J.J. Expression of IL-1beta in rhesus EAE and MS lesions is mainly induced in the CNS itself. *J. Neuroinflammation.* **2016**, *13*, 138. [CrossRef] [PubMed]
105. Hesp, Z.C.; Goldstein, E.Z.; Miranda, C.J.; Kaspar, B.K.; McTigue, D.M. Chronic oligodendrogenesis and remyelination after spinal cord injury in mice and rats. *J. Neurosci.* **2015**, *35*, 1274–1290. [CrossRef] [PubMed]
106. Panitch, H.S.; Hirsch, R.L.; Schindler, J.; Johnson, K.P. Treatment of multiple sclerosis with gamma interferon: Exacerbations associated with activation of the immune system. *Neurology* **1987**, *37*, 1097–1102. [CrossRef] [PubMed]
107. McMorris, F.A.; Smith, T.M.; DeSalvo, S.; Furlanetto, R.W. Insulin-like growth factor I/somatomedin C: A potent inducer of oligodendrocyte development. *Proc. Natl. Acad. Sci. USA* **1986**, *83*, 822–826. [CrossRef]
108. Chang, R.; Yee, K.L.; Sumbria, R.K. Tumor necrosis factor alpha Inhibition for Alzheimer's Disease. *J. Cent. Nerv. Syst. Dis.* **2017**, *9*, 1179573517709278. [CrossRef]

109. Fischer, R.; Wajant, H.; Kontermann, R.; Pfizenmaier, K.; Maier, O. Astrocyte-specific activation of TNFR2 promotes oligodendrocyte maturation by secretion of leukemia inhibitory factor. *Glia* **2014**, *62*, 272–283. [CrossRef]
110. Hofman, F.M.; Hinton, D.R.; Johnson, K.; Merrill, J.E. Tumor necrosis factor identified in multiple sclerosis brain. *J. Exp. Med.* **1989**, *170*, 607–612. [CrossRef]
111. Selmaj, K.; Raine, C.S.; Farooq, M.; Norton, W.T.; Brosnan, C.F. Cytokine cytotoxicity against oligodendrocytes. Apoptosis induced by lymphotoxin. *J. Immunol.* **1991**, *147*, 1522–1529.
112. Selmaj, K.; Raine, C.S. Tumor necrosis factor mediates myelin damage in organotypic cultures of nervous tissue. *Ann. N. Y. Acad. Sci.* **1988**, *540*, 568–570. [CrossRef] [PubMed]
113. Agresti, C.; D'Urso, D.; Levi, G. Reversible inhibitory effects of interferon-gamma and tumour necrosis factor-alpha on oligodendroglial lineage cell proliferation and differentiation in vitro. *Eur. J. Neurosci.* **1996**, *8*, 1106–1116. [CrossRef] [PubMed]
114. Hindinger, C.; Bergmann, C.C.; Hinton, D.R.; Phares, T.W.; Parra, G.I.; Hussain, S.; Savarin, C.; Atkinson, R.D.; Stohlman, S.A. IFN-gamma signaling to astrocytes protects from autoimmune mediated neurological disability. *PLoS ONE* **2012**, *7*, e42088. [CrossRef] [PubMed]
115. LaFerla, F.M.; Sugarman, M.C.; Lane, T.E.; Leissring, M.A. Regional hypomyelination and dysplasia in transgenic mice with astrocyte-directed expression of interferon-gamma. *J. Mol. Neurosci.* **2000**, *15*, 45–59. [CrossRef]
116. Butt, A.M.; Dinsdale, J. Fibroblast growth factor 2 induces loss of adult oligodendrocytes and myelin in vivo. *Exp. Neurol.* **2005**, *192*, 125–133. [CrossRef]
117. Gross, R.E.; Mehler, M.F.; Mabie, P.C.; Zang, Z.; Santschi, L.; Kessler, J.A. Bone morphogenetic proteins promote astroglial lineage commitment by mammalian subventricular zone progenitor cells. *Neuron* **1996**, *17*, 595–606. [CrossRef]
118. Clarner, T.; Parabucki, A.; Beyer, C.; Kipp, M. Corticosteroids impair remyelination in the corpus callosum of cuprizone-treated mice. *J. Neuroendocr.* **2011**, *23*, 601–611. [CrossRef]
119. Balabanov, R.; Strand, K.; Goswami, R.; McMahon, E.; Begolka, W.; Miller, S.D.; Popko, B. Interferon-gamma-oligodendrocyte interactions in the regulation of experimental autoimmune encephalomyelitis. *J. Neurosci.* **2007**, *27*, 2013–2024. [CrossRef]
120. Semple, B.D.; Frugier, T.; Morganti-Kossmann, M.C. CCL2 modulates cytokine production in cultured mouse astrocytes. *J. Neuroinflammation* **2010**, *7*, 67. [CrossRef]
121. Goldberg, S.H.; van der Meer, P.; Hesselgesser, J.; Jaffer, S.; Kolson, D.L.; Albright, A.V.; Gonzalez-Scarano, F.; Lavi, E. CXCR3 expression in human central nervous system diseases. *Neuropathol. Appl. Neurobiol.* **2001**, *27*, 127–138. [CrossRef]
122. You, T.; Bi, Y.; Li, J.; Zhang, M.; Chen, X.; Zhang, K.; Li, J. IL-17 induces reactive astrocytes and up-regulation of vascular endothelial growth factor (VEGF) through JAK/STAT signaling. *Sci. Rep.* **2017**, *7*, 41779. [CrossRef] [PubMed]
123. Narcisse, L.; Scemes, E.; Zhao, Y.; Lee, S.C.; Brosnan, C.F. The cytokine IL-1beta transiently enhances P2X7 receptor expression and function in human astrocytes. *Glia* **2005**, *49*, 245–258. [CrossRef] [PubMed]
124. Zeis, T.; Enz, L.; Schaeren-Wiemers, N. The immunomodulatory oligodendrocyte. *Brain Res.* **2016**, *1641*, 139–148. [CrossRef] [PubMed]
125. Choi, J.K.; Park, S.Y.; Kim, K.H.; Park, S.R.; Lee, S.G.; Choi, B.H. GM-CSF reduces expression of chondroitin sulfate proteoglycan (CSPG) core proteins in TGF-beta-treated primary astrocytes. *BMB Rep.* **2014**, *47*, 679–684. [CrossRef] [PubMed]
126. Prins, M.; Schul, E.; Geurts, J.; van der Valk, P.; Drukarch, B.; van Dam, A.M. Pathological differences between white and grey matter multiple sclerosis lesions. *Ann. N. Y. Acad. Sci.* **2015**, *1351*, 99–113. [CrossRef] [PubMed]
127. Sosunov, A.; Olabarria, M.; Goldman, J.E. Alexander disease: An astrocytopathy that produces a leukodystrophy. *Brain Pathol. (Zur. Switz.)* **2018**, *28*, 388–398. [CrossRef]
128. Huang, L.; Wu, Z.B.; Zhuge, Q.; Zheng, W.; Shao, B.; Wang, B.; Sun, F.; Jin, K. Glial scar formation occurs in the human brain after ischemic stroke. *Int. J. Med. Sci.* **2014**, *11*, 344–348. [CrossRef]
129. Verkhratsky, A.; Parpura, V.; Pekna, M.; Pekny, M.; Sofroniew, M. Glia in the pathogenesis of neurodegenerative diseases. *Biochem. Soc. Trans.* **2014**, *42*, 1291–1301. [CrossRef]

130. Anderson, M.A.; Ao, Y.; Sofroniew, M.V. Heterogeneity of reactive astrocytes. *Neurosci. Lett.* **2014**, *565*, 23–29. [CrossRef]
131. Rolls, A.; Shechter, R.; Schwartz, M. The bright side of the glial scar in CNS repair. *Nat. Rev. Neurosci.* **2009**, *10*, 235–241. [CrossRef]
132. Ceyzériat, K.; Ben Haim, L.; Denizot, A.; Pommier, D.; Matos, M.; Guillemaud, O.; Palomares, M.-A.; Abjean, L.; Petit, F.; Gipchtein, P.; et al. Modulation of astrocyte reactivity improves functional deficits in mouse models of Alzheimer's disease. *Acta Neuropathol. Commun.* **2018**, *6*, 104. [CrossRef] [PubMed]
133. Ludwin, S.K.; Rao, V.; Moore, C.S.; Antel, J.P. Astrocytes in multiple sclerosis. *Mult. Scler.* **2016**, *22*, 1114–1124. [CrossRef] [PubMed]
134. Leibowitz, S.M.; Yan, J. NF-kappaB Pathways in the Pathogenesis of Multiple Sclerosis and the Therapeutic Implications. *Front. Mol. Neurosci.* **2016**, *9*, 84. [CrossRef] [PubMed]
135. Yi, H.; Bai, Y.; Zhu, X.; Lin, L.; Zhao, L.; Wu, X.; Buch, S.; Wang, L.; Chao, J.; Yao, H. IL-17A induces MIP-1alpha expression in primary astrocytes via Src/MAPK/PI3K/NF-kB pathways: Implications for multiple sclerosis. *J. Neuroimmune Pharm.* **2014**, *9*, 629–641. [CrossRef] [PubMed]
136. Brambilla, R.; Persaud, T.; Hu, X.; Karmally, S.; Shestopalov, V.I.; Dvoriantchikova, G.; Ivanov, D.; Nathanson, L.; Barnum, S.R.; Bethea, J.R. Transgenic inhibition of astroglial NF-kappa B improves functional outcome in experimental autoimmune encephalomyelitis by suppressing chronic central nervous system inflammation. *J. Immunol.* **2009**, *182*, 2628–2640. [CrossRef]
137. Gonzalez-Reyes, R.E.; Nava-Mesa, M.O.; Vargas-Sanchez, K.; Ariza-Salamanca, D.; Mora-Munoz, L. Involvement of Astrocytes in Alzheimer's Disease from a Neuroinflammatory and Oxidative Stress Perspective. *Front. Mol. Neurosci.* **2017**, *10*, 427. [CrossRef]
138. Ouali Alami, N.; Schurr, C.; Olde Heuvel, F.; Tang, L.; Li, Q.; Tasdogan, A.; Kimbara, A.; Nettekoven, M.; Ottaviani, G.; Raposo, C.; et al. NF-kappaB activation in astrocytes drives a stage-specific beneficial neuroimmunological response in ALS. *EMBO J.* **2018**, *37*, e98697. [CrossRef]
139. Butt, A.M.; De La Rocha, I.C.; Rivera, A. Oligodendroglial Cells in Alzheimer's Disease. *Adv. Exp. Med. Biol.* **2019**, *1175*, 325–333. [CrossRef]
140. Matute, C.; Torre, I.; Perez-Cerda, F.; Perez-Samartin, A.; Alberdi, E.; Etxebarria, E.; Arranz, A.M.; Ravid, R.; Rodriguez-Antiguedad, A.; Sanchez-Gomez, M.; et al. P2X(7) receptor blockade prevents ATP excitotoxicity in oligodendrocytes and ameliorates experimental autoimmune encephalomyelitis. *J. Neurosci.* **2007**, *27*, 9525–9533. [CrossRef]
141. Bezzi, P.; Domercq, M.; Brambilla, L.; Galli, R.; Schols, D.; De Clercq, E.; Vescovi, A.; Bagetta, G.; Kollias, G.; Meldolesi, J.; et al. CXCR4-activated astrocyte glutamate release via TNFalpha: Amplification by microglia triggers neurotoxicity. *Nat. Neurosci.* **2001**, *4*, 702–710. [CrossRef]
142. Jeremic, A.; Jeftinija, K.; Stevanovic, J.; Glavaski, A.; Jeftinija, S. ATP stimulates calcium-dependent glutamate release from cultured astrocytes. *J. Neurochem.* **2001**, *77*, 664–675. [CrossRef] [PubMed]
143. Wang, X.; Arcuino, G.; Takano, T.; Lin, J.; Peng, W.G.; Wan, P.; Li, P.; Xu, Q.; Liu, Q.S.; Goldman, S.A.; et al. P2X7 receptor inhibition improves recovery after spinal cord injury. *Nat. Med.* **2004**, *10*, 821–827. [CrossRef] [PubMed]
144. Amadio, S.; Parisi, C.; Piras, E.; Fabbrizio, P.; Apolloni, S.; Montilli, C.; Luchetti, S.; Ruggieri, S.; Gasperini, C.; Laghi-Pasini, F.; et al. Modulation of P2X7 Receptor during Inflammation in Multiple Sclerosis. *Front. Immunol.* **2017**, *8*, 1529. [CrossRef] [PubMed]
145. Beamer, E.; Fischer, W.; Engel, T. The ATP-Gated P2X7 Receptor As a Target for the Treatment of Drug-Resistant Epilepsy. *Front. Neurosci.* **2017**, *11*, 21. [CrossRef]
146. Olsen, J.A.; Akirav, E.M. Remyelination in multiple sclerosis: Cellular mechanisms and novel therapeutic approaches. *Neurosci. Res.* **2015**, *93*, 687–696. [CrossRef]
147. Van Strien, M.E.; Baron, W.; Bakker, E.N.; Bauer, J.; Bol, J.G.; Breve, J.J.; Binnekade, R.; Van Der Laarse, W.J.; Drukarch, B.; Van Dam, A.M. Tissue transglutaminase activity is involved in the differentiation of oligodendrocyte precursor cells into myelin-forming oligodendrocytes during CNS remyelination. *Glia* **2011**, *59*, 1622–1634. [CrossRef]
148. Franklin, R.J.M.; Ffrench-Constant, C. Regenerating CNS myelin - from mechanisms to experimental medicines. *Nat. Rev. Neurosci.* **2017**, *18*, 753–769. [CrossRef]

149. Albrecht, P.J.; Murtie, J.C.; Ness, J.K.; Redwine, J.M.; Enterline, J.R.; Armstrong, R.C.; Levison, S.W. Astrocytes produce CNTF during the remyelination phase of viral-induced spinal cord demyelination to stimulate FGF-2 production. *Neurobiol. Dis.* **2003**, *13*, 89–101. [CrossRef]
150. Yeung, M.S.Y.; Djelloul, M.; Steiner, E.; Bernard, S.; Salehpour, M.; Possnert, G.; Brundin, L.; Frisen, J. Dynamics of oligodendrocyte generation in multiple sclerosis. *Nature* **2019**, *566*, 538–542. [CrossRef]
151. Lau, L.W.; Cua, R.; Keough, M.B.; Haylock-Jacobs, S.; Yong, V.W. Pathophysiology of the brain extracellular matrix: A new target for remyelination. *Nat. Rev. Neurosci.* **2013**, *14*, 722–729. [CrossRef]
152. Mohassel, P.; Foley, A.R.; Bonnemann, C.G. Extracellular matrix-driven congenital muscular dystrophies. *Matrix Biol.* **2018**, *71–72*, 188–204. [CrossRef] [PubMed]
153. van Horssen, J.; Dijkstra, C.D.; de Vries, H.E. The extracellular matrix in multiple sclerosis pathology. *J. Neurochem.* **2007**, *103*, 1293–1301. [CrossRef] [PubMed]
154. Lau, L.W.; Keough, M.B.; Haylock-Jacobs, S.; Cua, R.; Döring, A.; Sloka, S.; Stirling, D.P.; Rivest, S.; Yong, V.W. Chondroitin sulfate proteoglycans in demyelinated lesions impair remyelination. *Ann. Neurol.* **2012**, *72*, 419–432. [CrossRef] [PubMed]
155. Jiang, P.; Chen, C.; Liu, X.B.; Pleasure, D.E.; Liu, Y.; Deng, W. Human iPSC-Derived Immature Astroglia Promote Oligodendrogenesis by Increasing TIMP-1 Secretion. *Cell Rep.* **2016**, *15*, 1303–1315. [CrossRef] [PubMed]
156. Miyamoto, N.; Maki, T.; Shindo, A.; Liang, A.C.; Maeda, M.; Egawa, N.; Itoh, K.; Lo, E.K.; Lok, J.; Ihara, M.; et al. Astrocytes Promote Oligodendrogenesis after White Matter Damage via Brain-Derived Neurotrophic Factor. *J. Neurosci.* **2015**, *35*, 14002–14008. [CrossRef] [PubMed]
157. Wang, P.; Gorter, R.P.; de Jonge, J.C.; Nazmuddin, M.; Zhao, C.; Amor, S.; Hoekstra, D.; Baron, W. MMP7 cleaves remyelination-impairing fibronectin aggregates and its expression is reduced in chronic multiple sclerosis lesions. *Glia* **2018**, *66*, 1625–1643. [CrossRef] [PubMed]

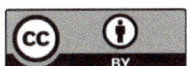 © 2020 by the authors. Licensee MDPI, Basel, Switzerland. This article is an open access article distributed under the terms and conditions of the Creative Commons Attribution (CC BY) license (http://creativecommons.org/licenses/by/4.0/).

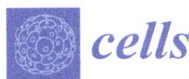

Article

Delayed Demyelination and Impaired Remyelination in Aged Mice in the Cuprizone Model

Stefan Gingele [†], Florian Henkel [†], Sandra Heckers, Thiemo M. Moellenkamp, Martin W. Hümmert, Thomas Skripuletz, Martin Stangel [†] and Viktoria Gudi [*,†]

Department of Neurology, Hannover Medical School, D-30625 Hannover, Germany; gingele.stefan@mh-hannover.de (S.G.); Florian.Henkel@stud.mh-hannover.de (F.H.); sandra.heckers@gmx.de (S.H.); thiemo.m.moellenkamp@stud.mh-hannover.de (T.M.M.); huemmert.martin@mh-hannover.de (M.W.H.); skripuletz.thomas@mh-hannover.de (T.S.); stangel.martin@mh-hannover.de (M.S.)
* Correspondence: gudi.viktoria@mh-hannover.de; Tel.: +49-511-532-3816; Fax: +49-511-532-3115
† These authors contributed equally to this work.

Received: 10 March 2020; Accepted: 7 April 2020; Published: 11 April 2020

Abstract: To unravel the failure of remyelination in multiple sclerosis (MS) and to test promising remyelinating treatments, suitable animal models like the well-established cuprizone model are required. However, this model is only standardized in young mice. This does not represent the typical age of MS patients. Furthermore, remyelination is very fast in young mice, hindering the examination of effects of remyelination-promoting agents. Thus, there is the need for a better animal model to study remyelination. We therefore aimed to establish the cuprizone model in aged mice. 6-month-old C57BL6 mice were fed with different concentrations of cuprizone (0.2–0.6%) for 5–6.5 weeks. De- and remyelination in the medial and lateral parts of the corpus callosum were analyzed by immunohistochemistry. Feeding aged mice 0.4% cuprizone for 6.5 weeks resulted in the best and most reliable administration scheme with virtually complete demyelination of the corpus callosum. This was accompanied by a strong accumulation of microglia and near absolute loss of mature oligodendrocytes. Subsequent remyelination was initially robust but remained incomplete. The remyelination process in mature adult mice better represents the age of MS patients and offers a better model for the examination of regenerative therapies.

Keywords: multiple sclerosis; cuprizone; age; oligodendrocyte; myelin; demyelination; remyelination; microglia; astrocyte

1. Introduction

Multiple sclerosis (MS) is a chronic inflammatory disease of the central nervous system (CNS). Destruction and loss of oligodendrocytes resulting in demyelination represent the pathological core characteristics of MS [1]. Remyelination is a naturally occurring and highly effective repair mechanism after demyelination that can restore rapid axonal conduction velocity [2] and lead to functional recovery and neuroprotection [3–5]. It was suggested that remyelination might prevent axonal injury and chronic clinical disability [6,7]. However, remyelination varies considerably between individual patients and lesion location and is often incomplete or fails, particularly in chronic MS lesions [8,9]. To decipher the pathophysiology of remyelination and the reasons for its failure as well as to investigate remyelination-supporting agents, toxic demyelination animal models such as the cuprizone mouse model are needed. In the cuprizone model, usually young mice are fed with the copper chelator cuprizone (bis-cyclohexanone oxaldihydrazone) which leads to highly reproducible oligodendrocyte apoptosis followed by demyelination. Typically, C57BL6 mice aged 8–10 weeks are fed a diet containing 0.2% cuprizone for 5 weeks to induce complete demyelination of the midline of the corpus callosum

(CC). After withdrawal of cuprizone, robust remyelination occurs within days [10–12]. However, this standard protocol of cuprizone intoxication does not reflect the complex situation in MS lesions with limited remyelination capacity. Furthermore, myelin repair occurs rapidly, which causes difficulties for the investigation of remyelination-promoting therapeutic approaches. In addition, the age of 8–10 weeks in mice is equivalent to a human age below 18 years, rather representing the situation in pediatric MS [13–15]. In contrast, an age of 6 months in C57BL6 mice represents a mature adult phenotype and corresponds better to the mean age of MS disease onset in humans of approximately 30 years [13–15]. Additionally, remyelination efficiency shows an age related decline in different toxic demyelination models and thus investigation of this regenerative process in aged animals represents a promising approach to gain insights into impediments of remyelination [16–20]. Although the cuprizone model has previously been used in aged mice, the protocols differed considerably regarding the age, the concentration, and duration of cuprizone treatment [21–24]. However, it is crucial to exactly determine the cuprizone dose and feeding period to achieve complete and reproducible demyelination of the region of interest to investigate subsequent remyelination [12,25,26]. Thus, we established a protocol to induce complete demyelination of the corpus callosum in 6-month-old male C57BL6 mice and characterized the de- and remyelination processes in detail.

2. Materials and Methods

2.1. Animals

Male C57BL6/J mice were purchased from Charles River Laboratories (Sulzfeld, Germany). Animals underwent routine cage maintenance once a week and were microbiologically monitored according to the Federation of European Laboratory Animal Science Associations recommendations [27]. Food and water were available ad libitum. All research procedures were approved by the Review Board for the Care of Animal Subjects of the district government (LAVES, Lower Saxony, Germany; ethic approval number: 15/1762) and performed according to international guidelines on the use of laboratory animals.

2.2. Induction of De- and Remyelination

In order to establish the cuprizone treatment protocol for aged mice representing a mature adult phenotype [13] and resulting in complete demyelination of the midline of the corpus callosum, 6-month-old male C57BL6/J mice were fed with different concentrations (0.2%, 0.3%, 0.4%, 0.5%, or 0.6%) of cuprizone (bis-cyclohexanone oxaldihydrazone, Sigma-Aldrich, St. Louis, MO, USA) mixed into a milled standard rodent chow (maintenance diet, rats/mice, Altromin, Lage, Germany). For induction of experimental demyelination, cuprizone was administered for up to 6.5 weeks. In total, demyelination in aged mice was studied in 12 different treatment groups. After cuprizone feeding, mice were changed to standard rodent chow and subsequent remyelination was assessed at different time points (up to 3.5 weeks after the end of cuprizone feeding) (see Figure S1 for experimental setup). Age-matched male C57BL6/J control mice received standard rodent chow without cuprizone. Toxic demyelination in young mice was induced as previously described [28] by feeding 2-month-old male C57BL6/J mice a diet containing 0.2% cuprizone for 5 weeks. After 5 weeks, cuprizone was removed from the diet and remyelination was assessed after another 1.5 weeks (Figure S1). Five to six animals were analyzed for each cuprizone concentration and every time point during de- and remyelination in young and aged mice.

2.3. Tissue Processing

Mice were perfused at different time points with 4% paraformaldehyde in phosphate buffer through the left cardiac ventricle as previously described [29,30]. The brains were removed, post-fixed in 4% paraformaldehyde and embedded in paraffin. For light microscopy, 7 μm serial coronal paraffin sections between bregma −0.82 mm and bregma −1.94 mm according to the mouse atlas by

Paxinos and Franklin [31] were cut with a rotary microtome (RM2245, Leica, Wetzlar, Germany) and evaluated microscopically.

2.4. Immunohistochemistry

Paraffin-embedded sections were dewaxed and heat-unmasked in 10 mM citrate buffer (pH 6.0). The following primary antibodies were used for immunostaining: for myelin, anti-myelin basic protein (MBP, mouse monoclonal IgG2a, 1:500, BioLegend, San Diego, CA, USA) and anti-proteolipid protein (PLP, mouse monoclonal IgG2a, 1:500, BIO-RAD); for microglia, anti-ionized calcium-binding adaptor molecule 1 (Iba-1, rabbit polyclonal IgG, 1:200, Wako, Osaka, Japan) and for activated microglia Ricinus communis antigen 1 (RCA-1, 1:1000, Vector); for mature oligodendrocytes anti-adenomatous polyposis coli (APC, mouse IgG2b, 1:200, Calbiochem) and anti-myelin-associated neurite outgrowth inhibitor (NOGO-A, rabbit polyclonal IgG, 1:750, Millipore, Burlington, MA, USA); for astrocytes, anti-glial fibrillary acidic protein (GFAP, polyclonal rabbit IgG, 1:200, Dako, Santa Clara, CA, USA); for axonal damage anti-amyloid precursor protein (APP, rabbit polyclonal IgG, 1:200, Serotec, Hercules, CA, USA) and anti-Synaptophysin (mouse monoclonal IgG1, 1:200, BIO-RAD, Hercules, CA, USA). All antibodies were diluted in PBS containing 0.3% Triton-X100. Sections were further incubated with biotinylated secondary antibodies, followed by peroxidase-coupled avidin-biotin complex (ABC Kit, Vector Laboratories, Burlingame, CA, USA). For immunofluorescence double staining, sections were incubated with secondary antibodies Alexa Fluor 555 goat anti-rabbit IgG (H + L) and Alexa Fluor 488 goat anti-mouse IgG (H + L) (all 1:500, Invitrogen, Carlsbad, CA, USA). Brain slices were counterstained either with Mayer's hemalum solution (Merck, Darmstadt, Germany) for DAB-based cell analysis or with 4′,6-diamidino-2-phenylindole (DAPI, Invitrogen, Carlsbad, CA, USA) for immunofluorescence staining.

2.5. Determination of Demyelination and Quantification of Glial Reaction

The extent of cuprizone-induced demyelination was assessed as previously described [32,33]. Sections immunostained for myelin proteins were scored by three independent observers using a magnification of 200× in the midline of the corpus callosum and in the lateral parts directly adjacent to the midline using a light microscope (Olympus BX61, Olympus, Hamburg, Germany). On a scale from 0 (complete loss of myelin staining), to 3 (normal, fully myelinated corpus callosum) the different grades of demyelination were assessed (see [34] for representative images of the respective grades). In this grading system, a score of 1 is equivalent to one third myelinated area and a score of 2 corresponds to two thirds myelinated area of the investigated region of the corpus callosum, respectively [35]. Control tissues did not display any abnormalities. To quantify the reactions of different glial cell populations, immunopositive cells were counted at a magnification of 400× (Olympus BX61, Olympus cellSens Software) in the midline and in the flanking lateral parts of the corpus callosum. Results of cell counting refer to the number of cells per mm^2. Synaptophysin/APP double positive spheroids in the size >2 µm were counted in the central corpus callosum using a magnification of 400× (Olympus BX61, Olympus cellSens Software). The results are presented as mean with standard error of the mean (SEM) of spheroid numbers per mm^2.

2.6. Statistical Analysis

Normal distribution was evaluated by using Kolmogorov-Smirnov test and statistical analysis was performed using analysis of variance one-way ANOVA followed by Bonferroni´s multiple comparison test or Kruskal-Wallis test followed by Dunn's multiple comparison test when appropriate.

All data are given as arithmetic means ± standard error of the mean (SEM). Significant effects are indicated by asterisks (compared to the prior time point) or hash marks (compared to controls) (*/# $p < 0.05$; **/## $p < 0.01$; ***/### $p < 0.001$) and are shown in the respective figures.

3. Results

3.1. The Standard 0.2% Cuprizone Treatment is Not Sufficient to Induce Demyelination of the Corpus Callosum in Aged Mice

To establish a cuprizone treatment protocol in mature adult mice, we first followed the feeding protocols in young mice and fed 6-month-old male C57BL6/J mice a ground standard rodent chow containing 0.2% cuprizone for 5 or 6 weeks. To determine demyelination in aged mice, the midline and lateral parts of the corpus callosum in MBP and PLP-stained sections were investigated. The commonly established feeding protocol for young mice (5 weeks, 0.2% cuprizone) was not sufficient to induce significant loss of MBP or PLP myelin protein in both the medial and lateral parts of the corpus callosum of aged mice (Figure 1 and Figure S2). Moreover, a prolonged treatment period of 6 weeks 0.2% cuprizone did not lead to significant demyelination (Figure 1 and Figure S2).

3.2. Feeding of 0.4% Cuprizone for 6.5 Weeks Results in Complete Demyelination of the Corpus Callosum in Aged Mice

An increase of cuprizone dose to 0.3–0.6% for 5 weeks resulted in a significant but nonetheless incomplete reduction of MBP and PLP in the midline of the corpus callosum (Figure 1 and Figure S2). After an extended feeding period of cuprizone for 6 weeks, nearly complete loss of MBP protein in the medial and lateral parts of the corpus callosum was evident (Figure S2), whereas PLP immunoreactivity was only partially reduced in the midline and adjacent lateral sections of the corpus callosum (Figure 1). Since demyelination in the midline of the corpus callosum was most pronounced after treatment with 0.3% and 0.4% cuprizone for 6 weeks with no dose-dependent advancement of demyelination by feeding higher concentrations of cuprizone, we prolonged the cuprizone treatment with 0.3% and 0.4% for an additional 3 days to 6.5 weeks in total to achieve complete demyelination. As expected, 0.4% cuprizone feeding for 6.5 weeks resulted in virtually complete demyelination of the midline and adjacent parts of the corpus callosum as judged by distinct loss of MBP and PLP immunoreactivity (Figure 1 and Figure S2). In contrast, after treatment with 0.3% cuprizone for 6.5 weeks, demyelination was insufficient (Figure 1 and Figure S2) and re-expression of myelin proteins, especially of MBP, was already evident in the corpus callosum (Figure S2). Interestingly, demyelination in the lateral segments of the corpus callosum generally preceded demyelination of the medial part of the corpus callosum (Figure S2).

3.3. Cuprizone Treatment Leads to Significant Oligodendrocyte Loss Independent of Cuprizone Concentration

To evaluate how mature oligodendrocytes were affected by different cuprizone feeding protocols, the oligodendrocyte markers APC and Nogo-A were examined in the corpus callosum. Each cuprizone concentration and feeding duration was sufficient to significantly deplete oligodendrocytes as compared to controls (Figure 2 and Figure S3). However, the reduction of APC and Nogo-A-positive cells in the corpus callosum of aged mice was less pronounced after feeding 0.2% cuprizone, as used as standard protocol for young mice compared to higher concentrations of 0.3–0.6%. This result is of particular interest as it demonstrates that treatment with 0.2% cuprizone is sufficient to significantly damage mature oligodendrocytes in aged mice without inducing relevant demyelination, as mentioned before. Feeding higher doses of 0.3–0.6% cuprizone resulted in more distinctive depletion of mature oligodendrocytes with the most extensive loss of adult oligodendrocytes in the midline of the corpus callosum being observed after feeding 0.4% cuprizone for 6.5 weeks (Figure 2 and Figure S3). Again, in line with the findings from the myelin stainings, a dose-dependent effect on oligodendrocyte loss appeared to exist up to a concentration of 0.4% and higher concentrations of cuprizone did not result in faster or more pronounced oligodendrocyte damage. Rather, a duration-dependent effect was observed with feeding durations of 6 and 6.5 weeks being more effective than 5 weeks for concentrations between 0.3% and 0.5% cuprizone (Figure 2). Similar to the medial part, pronounced oligodendrocyte depletion was detected in the lateral segments of the corpus callosum as well (Figure S5).

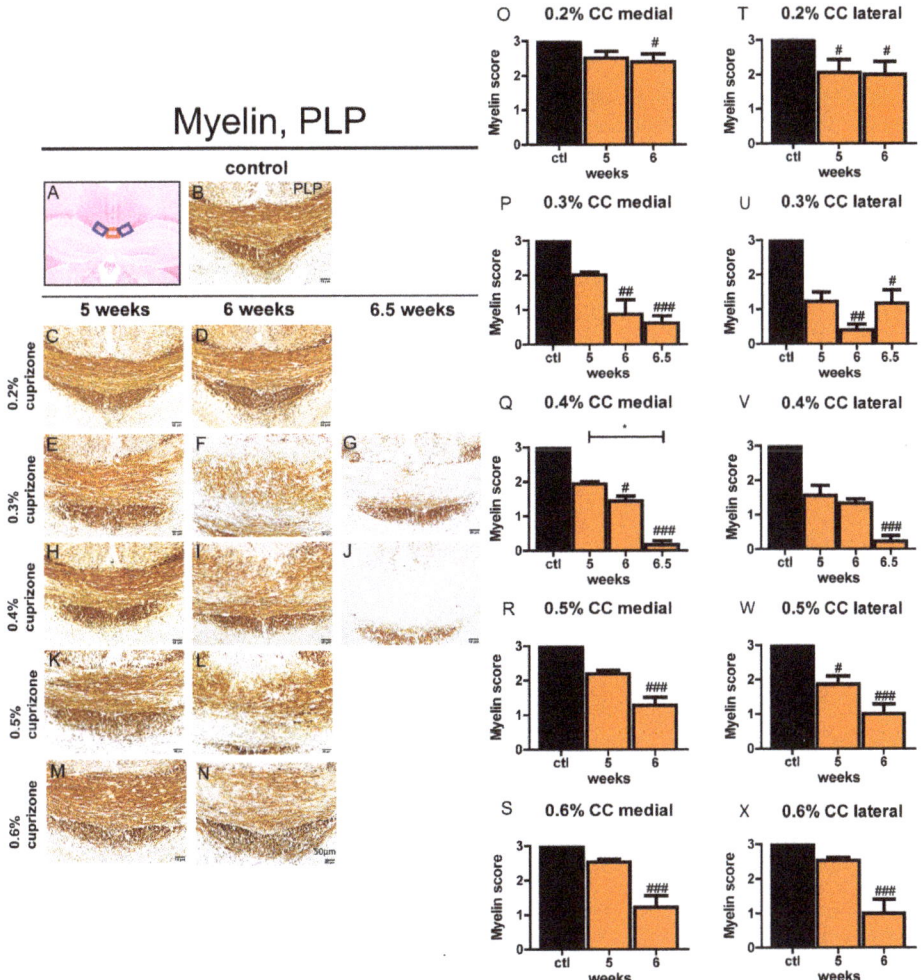

Figure 1. PLP loss during demyelination in the corpus callosum of aged mice. Hematoxylin and eosin (H & E)-stained control mouse brain (**A**) shows the areas of the corpus callosum that were analyzed (red box: medial part; blue boxes: lateral parts). Representative PLP-stained sections (**C–N**) show a decrease of PLP-positive myelin fibers during the course of demyelination in the central corpus callosum of aged mice after cuprizone treatment with different concentrations (0.2–0.6% cuprizone) for different feeding periods (5, 6, or 6.5 weeks). An exemplary picture (**B**) shows PLP staining in the midline of the corpus callosum of an age-matched control animal. A myelination score of 3 represents complete myelination, whereas a score of 0 represents complete demyelination. Graphs display the myelin score per time point and group in the midline (**O–S**) and in the lateral part of the corpus callosum (**T–X**) in aged animals. Bars represent mean + SEM. Significant effects between different investigated time points are indicated by asterisks and effects in comparison to control are indicated by hashmarks (*/# $p < 0.05$; **/## $p < 0.01$; ***/### $p < 0.001$). Ctl. = control; 5, 6, or 6.5 weeks = treatment period with cuprizone for respective duration. N = 5–6 animals per group.

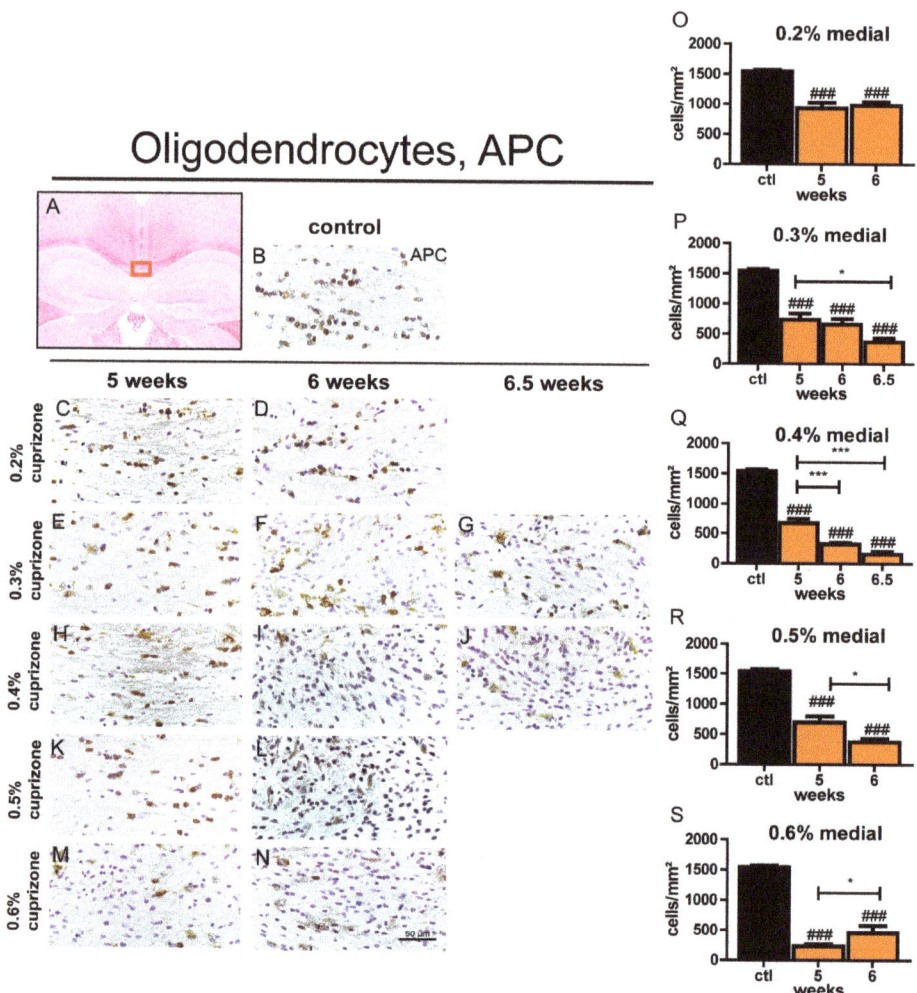

Figure 2. Depletion of adult oligodendrocytes in the midline of the corpus callosum in aged mice after different cuprizone feeding protocols. The outlined area (red box) shows the medial part of the corpus callosum which was investigated (**A**). Representative images from APC-stained sections (**C–N**) show the depletion of oligodendrocytes during the course of demyelination in the midline of the corpus callosum of aged mice after cuprizone treatment with different concentrations (0.2–0.6% cuprizone) for different time periods (5, 6, or 6.5 weeks). (**B**) shows a control brain section stained with APC. Graphs (**O–S**) represent numbers of APC-positive cells/mm^2 in the medial part of the corpus callosum in aged animals. Bars display mean + SEM. Significant effects between different investigated time points are indicated by asterisks and effects in comparison to control are indicated by hashmarks (*/# $p < 0.05$; **/## $p < 0.01$; ***/### $p < 0.001$). Ctl. = control; 5, 6, or 6.5 weeks = feeding period of cuprizone for respective duration. N = 5–6 animals per group.

3.4. Maximum Microglia Activation and Accumulation is Evident after 6.5 Weeks with 0.4% Cuprizone Treatment

To assess microglia reaction during cuprizone-induced demyelination in aged mice, the number of activated microglia was determined by RCA-1 staining. Iba-1 was used to quantify accumulation of the entire microglia population. Applying the feeding protocol of young mice with 0.2% cuprizone for 5 weeks resulted in a significant infiltration of Iba-1-positive cells (Figure S4) but only mild and not significant activation of these microglia was apparent compared to controls (Figure 3). Prolongation of cuprizone treatment to 6 weeks led to more pronounced activation of microglial cells in the midline of the corpus callosum (Figure 3). An increase of cuprizone dose (0.3–0.6%) led to a robust accumulation and activation of microglia already after 5 weeks of cuprizone feeding, and extending cuprizone treatment for an additional week enhanced these effects in most treatment groups (Figure 3 and Figure S4). Interestingly, the effect of dose increase between the 0.3% and 0.6% conditions on the amount and activation of microglia was limited. The maximum microglial activation and accumulation in the midline of the corpus callosum as judged by RCA-1 and Iba-1 immunopositive cells was actually seen after feeding 0.4% cuprizone for 6.5 weeks. In contrast, prolonging 0.3% cuprizone treatment to 6.5 weeks did not result in increased microglia activation or cell count (Figure 3 and Figure S4). The lateral parts of the corpus callosum exhibited a more pronounced increase of activated microglia after just 5 weeks of cuprizone feeding as compared to the medial part (Figure S5). Similar to the midline of the corpus callosum, there was no clear impact of increasing cuprizone concentrations on induction of microglia reaction, with feeding protocols containing 0.5% and 0.6% cuprizone even showing a tendency towards less pronounced microglial accumulation. The maximum amount of RCA-1 and Iba-1-positive cells in the lateral segments was also observed after feeding 0.4% cuprizone for 6.5 weeks (Figure S5).

3.5. The Extent of Astrocytosis is Independent of Duration and Dose of Cuprizone Treatment

The astrocyte response to cuprizone-induced demyelination in the corpus callosum of aged mice was examined by staining for GFAP. Feeding of cuprizone resulted in significantly increased numbers of GFAP-positive astrocytes in the midline and adjacent lateral segments of the corpus callosum in virtually all treatment groups compared to control animals (Figure 4 and Figure S5). No significant changes of the amount of GFAP-expressing cells were observed between the different treatment groups depending on feeding duration or cuprizone concentration. Similar trends in the astrocyte reaction were observed in the lateral part compared to the medial part of the corpus callosum (Figure S5).

3.6. Aged Mice Show Rapid Induction of Remyelination but Remyelination Remains Incomplete

After we established the best protocol for complete demyelination in the corpus callosum by feeding 0.4% cuprizone for 6.5 weeks, we investigated remyelination with this treatment regime. After removing cuprizone from the diet, remyelination was studied in the corpus callosum for up to 3.5 weeks. Remyelination in the medial and lateral parts of the corpus callosum was assessed by staining for the myelin proteins MBP and PLP. After the switch to normal chow, there was prompt and significant re-appearance of the myelin proteins PLP (Figure 5) and MBP (Figure S6) as early as 0.5 weeks after termination of cuprizone treatment (week 7). Interestingly, myelin staining with MBP remained unchanged after week 7 in the subsequently analyzed time points whereas PLP staining showed a further increase of myelin status at week 8 before reaching a plateau. Remarkably, even after 3.5 weeks of remyelination, expression of MBP and PLP myelin proteins did not reach the myelin status of control mice, but stagnated at a reduced level, representing partial myelination (Figure 5 and Figure S6). In contrast, young mice showed more advanced remyelination 1.5 weeks after termination of the cuprizone diet as visualized by MBP and PLP staining (Figure 5 and Figure S6) compared to aged mice. Remyelination in the lateral segments of the corpus callosum followed the same temporal pattern as in the midline area (Figure S9).

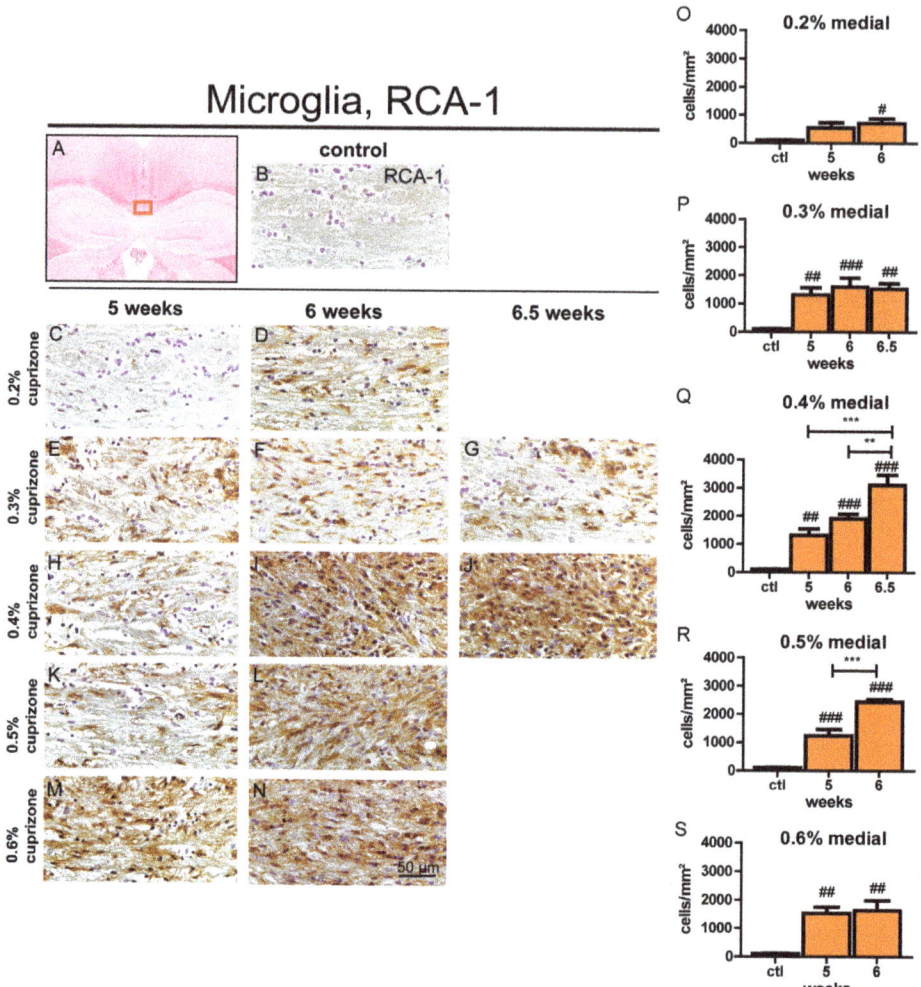

Figure 3. Activation of microglia in the central corpus callosum during cuprizone-induced demyelination in aged mice. The red box in (**A**) displays the medial section of the corpus callosum that was analyzed. Representative pictures (**C–N**) of RCA-1-stained brain sections show accumulation of activated microglia during the course of demyelination in the midline of the corpus callosum of aged mice after cuprizone treatment with various doses (0.2–0.6% cuprizone) for different feeding periods (5, 6, or 6.5 weeks). An exemplary brain section of a control animal stained for RCA-1 is shown in (**B**). Graphs depict the amount of RCA-1-positive cells/mm^2 per time point in the midline of the corpus callosum in aged animals (**O–S**). Bars represent mean + SEM. Effects between different investigated time points are indicated by asterisks and effects in comparison to control are indicated by hash marks (*/# $p < 0.05$; **/## $p < 0.01$; ***/### $p < 0.001$). Ctl. = control; 5, 6, or 6.5 weeks = feeding period of cuprizone for respective duration. N = 5–6 animals per group.

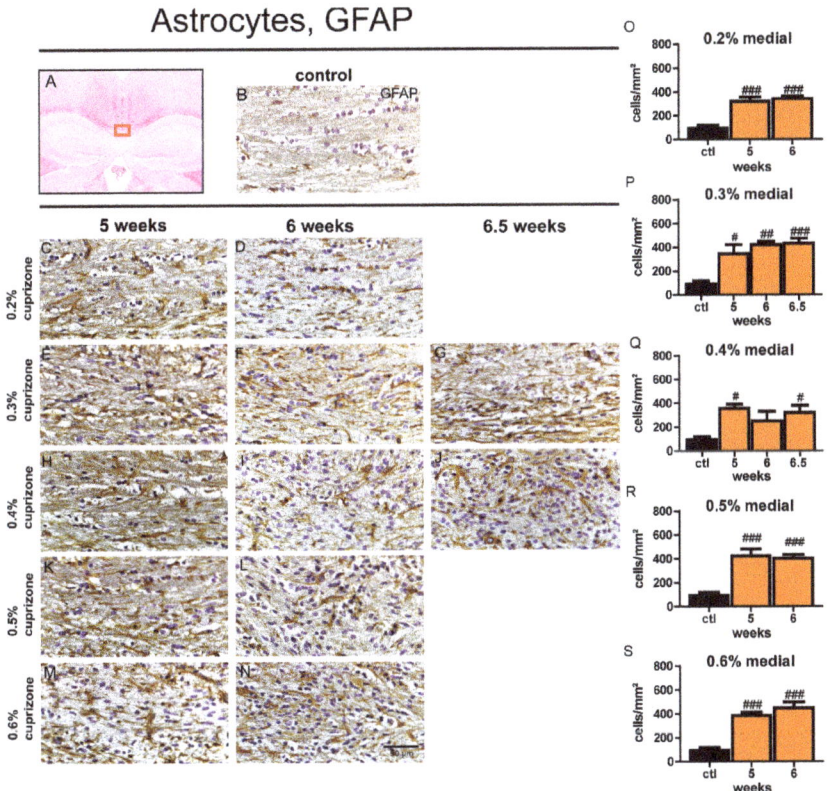

Figure 4. Astrocytosis in the medial corpus callosum of aged mice after different cuprizone treatment protocols. The boxed area represents the medial part of the corpus callosum which was examined (**A**). An exemplary picture shows a brain section of a control animal stained for GFAP (**B**). Representative images of GFAP-stained sections (**C–N**) depict astrocyte hypertrophy and hyperplasia during demyelination in the central corpus callosum of aged mice after cuprizone treatment with different concentrations (0.2–0.6% cuprizone) for different treatment periods (5, 6, or 6.5 weeks). Graphs show the number of GFAP-positive astrocytes/mm^2 in the midline of the corpus callosum in aged animals (**O–S**). Bars represent mean + SEM. Effects between different investigated time points are indicated by asterisks and effects in comparison to control are indicated by hashmarks (*/# $p < 0.05$; **/## $p < 0.01$; ***/### $p < 0.001$). Ctl. = control; 5, 6, or 6.5 weeks = feeding period of cuprizone for respective duration. N = 5–6 animals per group.

3.7. Repopulation of Oligodendrocytes in the Corpus Callosum during Remyelination is Less Efficient Compared to Young Mice

APC and Nogo-A, as markers for mature oligodendrocytes, were used to investigate the reappearance of oligodendrocytes in the corpus callosum after demyelination induced by feeding mice with 0.4% cuprizone for 6.5 weeks. A significant increase in the number of APC- and Nogo-A-positive cells in the corpus callosum of aged mice was already detected 0.5 weeks after cessation of cuprizone feeding at week 7 (Figure 6 and Figure S7). The density of oligodendrocytes further grew steadily during the remyelination observation period. After 3.5 weeks of remyelination, the amount of adult oligodendrocytes in the midline of the corpus callosum almost equaled the control level. In contrast, in young mice, the density of Nogo-A- and APC-positive cells reached the level of control animals at the latest after 1.5 weeks of remyelination with a trend of even exceeding baseline numbers of controls (Figure 6 and Figure S7). Thus, repopulation of the demyelinated corpus callosum with mature oligodendrocytes seemed to proceed more slowly in aged mice compared to young animals. It is noteworthy that the absolute amount of oligodendrocytes in the corpus callosum of aged mice was higher compared to young mice in the control group (Figure 6 and Figure S7). Re-appearance of mature oligodendrocytes in the lateral parts of the corpus callosum occurred in a similar manner to that of the midline, though the number of Nogo-A-positive cells did not reach the cell count in control mice (Figure S9).

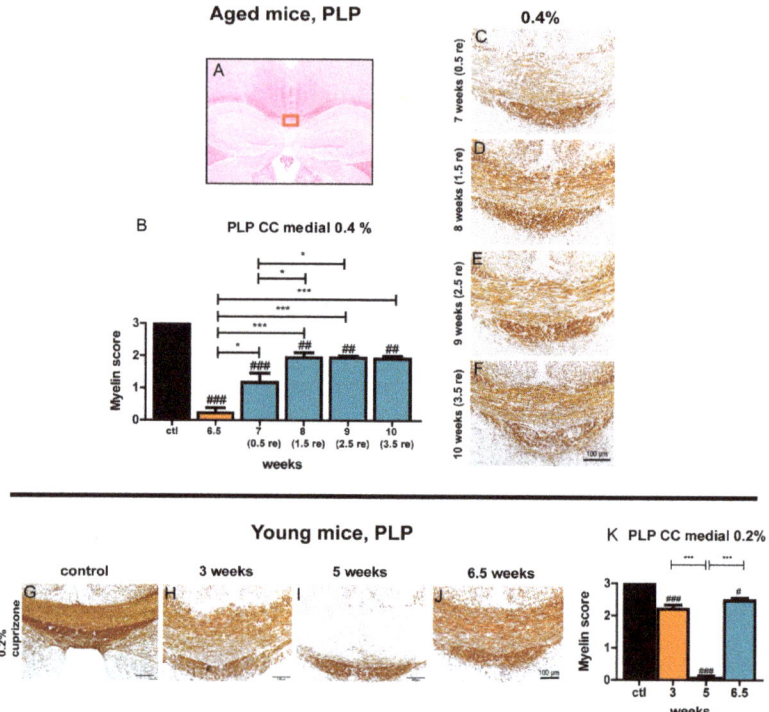

Figure 5. The marked area (red box) shows the medial part of the corpus callosum which was examined (**A**). (**B**) shows the myelin score for PLP in the midline of the corpus callosum in aged animals fed with 0.4% cuprizone for 6.5 weeks and subsequent remyelination (0.5, 1.5, 2.5, and 3.5 weeks after cessation of treatment with cuprizone). A score of 3 represents complete myelination, whereas a score of 0 represents complete demyelination. Representative PLP-stained sections (**C–F**) demonstrate the course of remyelination in aged mice. See Figure 1 for a representative image of a control animal and of demyelination after 0.4% cuprizone feeding for 6.5 weeks in aged mice. The myelin score for young mice treated with 0.2% cuprizone for 5 weeks and subsequent remyelination for 1.5 weeks is shown in **K**. Representative PLP-stained sections show the course of de- and remyelination in young mice (**G–J**). Bars display mean + SEM. Significant effects between different investigated time points are indicated by asterisks and effects in comparison to control are indicated by hashmarks (*/# $p < 0.05$; **/## $p < 0.01$; ***/### $p < 0.001$). Ctl. = control; 6.5 weeks = feeding period of 0.4% cuprizone in aged mice; 7 (0.5 re) weeks = 0.5 weeks of remyelination, 8 (1.5 re) weeks = 1.5 weeks of remyelination, 9 (2.5 re) weeks = 2.5 weeks of remyelination, 10 (3.5 re) weeks = 3.5 weeks of remyelination in aged mice; 3 and 5 weeks = feeding period of 0.2% cuprizone in young mice; 6.5 (1.5) weeks = 1.5 weeks of remyelination in young mice. N = 5–6 animals per group.

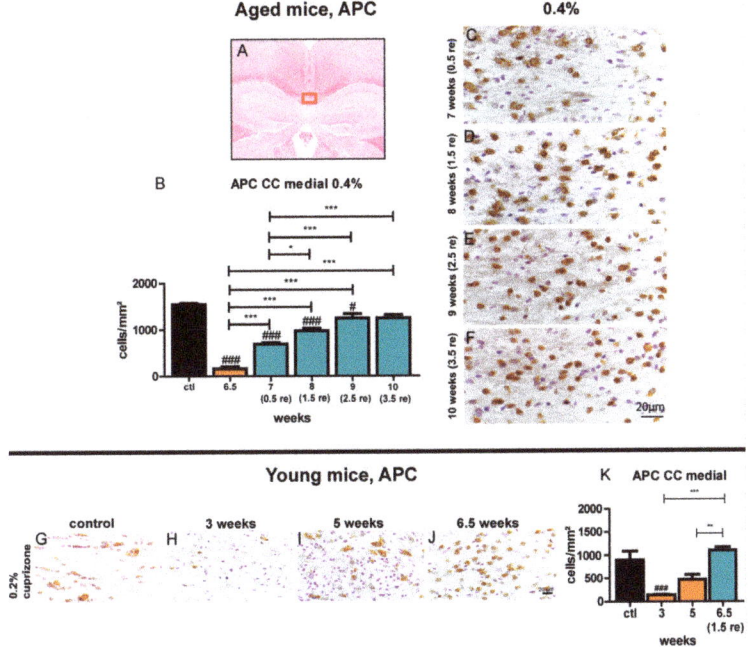

Figure 6. Repopulation of mature oligodendrocytes during remyelination in the medial corpus callosum of aged mice. The marked area (red box) in (**A**) shows the medial part of the corpus callosum that was investigated. Graphs display the number of APC-positive oligodendrocytes/mm^2 for the respective time points of demyelination and subsequent remyelination in aged mice fed for 6.5 weeks with 0.4% cuprizone (**B**) and young mice treated for 5 weeks with 0.2% cuprizone (**K**). See Figure 2 for representative sections of aged mice for control and demyelination after 0.4% cuprizone feeding for 6.5 weeks, respectively. Exemplary images show repopulation of APC-positive oligodendrocytes during the course of remyelination in the central corpus callosum of aged mice (**C–F**) and during de- and remyelination in young mice (**G–J**). Bars show mean + SEM. Significant effects between different investigated time points are indicated by asterisks and effects in comparison to control are indicated by hashmarks (*/# $p < 0.05$; **/## $p < 0.01$; ***/### $p < 0.001$). Ctl. = control; 6.5 weeks = feeding period of 0.4% cuprizone in aged mice; 7 (0.5 re) weeks = 0.5 weeks of remyelination, 8 (1.5 re) weeks = 1.5 weeks of remyelination, 9 (2.5 re) weeks = 2.5 weeks of remyelination, 10 (3.5 re) weeks = 3.5 weeks of remyelination in aged mice; 3 and 5 weeks = feeding period of 0.2% cuprizone in young mice; 6.5 (1.5) weeks = 1.5 weeks of remyelination in young mice. N = 5–6 animals per group.

3.8. Prolonged Activation of Microglia during the Recovery Period

Iba-1 and RCA-1 were used to quantify the degree of microglia cell accumulation and their activation status during remyelination. After a sharp rise of the amount of activated microglia was observed at 6.5 weeks of 0.4% cuprizone treatment, a swift and pronounced decrease of the number of RCA-1-positive activated microglia was apparent within the first days after cessation of cuprizone treatment (Figure 7). Interestingly and in contrast to the fast return of the elevated RCA-1-positive cell count in young mice towards control levels during remyelination, significantly elevated numbers of activated microglia persisted until week 8, and a trend towards an enhanced amount of these cells was obvious until the end of the observation period at week 10. The overall Iba-1-positive microglia population followed a similar temporal pattern compared to RCA-1-positive activated microglia (Figure S8). Additionally, the lateral segments of the corpus callosum displayed the same changes of microglia during remyelination in comparison to the processes observed in the medial part of the corpus callosum (Figure S9).

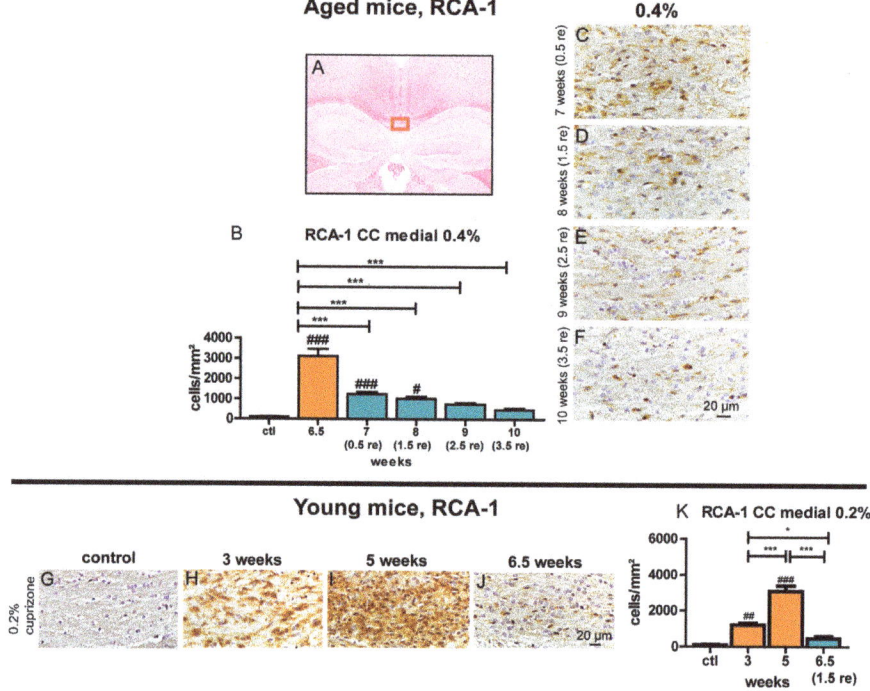

Figure 7. Delayed decrease of activated microglia during the course of remyelination in the medial corpus callosum of aged mice. The medial part of the corpus callosum that was analyzed is highlighted (**A**). Graphs show the amount of RCA-1-positive activated microglia/mm^2 for the respective time points of demyelination and subsequent remyelination in aged mice treated with 0.4% cuprizone for 6.5 weeks (**B**) and young mice fed with 0.2% cuprizone for 5 weeks (**K**). See Figure 3 for representative images of RCA-1 staining of aged mice for controls and demyelination after 0.4% cuprizone feeding for 6.5 weeks, respectively. Representative sections show the decrease of activated microglia populations during the course of remyelination in the central corpus callosum of aged mice (**C–F**) and the increase of activated microglia during demyelination in young mice plus a decrease during subsequent remyelination (**G–J**). Bars show mean + SEM. Significant effects between different investigated time points are indicated by asterisks and effects in comparison to control are indicated by hashmarks (*/# $p < 0.05$; **/## $p < 0.01$; ***/### $p < 0.001$). Ctl. = control; 6.5 weeks = feeding period of 0.4% cuprizone in aged mice; 7 (0.5 re) weeks = 0.5 weeks of remyelination, 8 (1.5 re) weeks = 1.5 weeks of remyelination, 9 (2.5 re) weeks = 2.5 weeks of remyelination, 10 (3.5 re) weeks = 3.5 weeks of remyelination in aged mice; 3 and 5 weeks = feeding period of 0.2% cuprizone in young mice; 6.5 (1.5) weeks = 1.5 weeks of remyelination in young mice. N = 5–6 animals per group.

3.9. Astrogliosis Remains Unchanged Despite Ongoing Remyelination

Staining for GFAP was used to determine astrocyte hypertrophy and hyperplasia during remyelination. At all investigated time points during the remyelination period, the number of GFAP-positive cells in the midline of the corpus callosum was significantly increased as compared to control (Figure 8). The extent of astrogliosis did not change significantly over the time course of remyelination and remained as high as at the point of maximum demyelination at 6.5 weeks.

Astrocytosis in the lateral segments of the corpus callosum followed the same trend as in the medial segment of the corpus callosum (Figure S9).

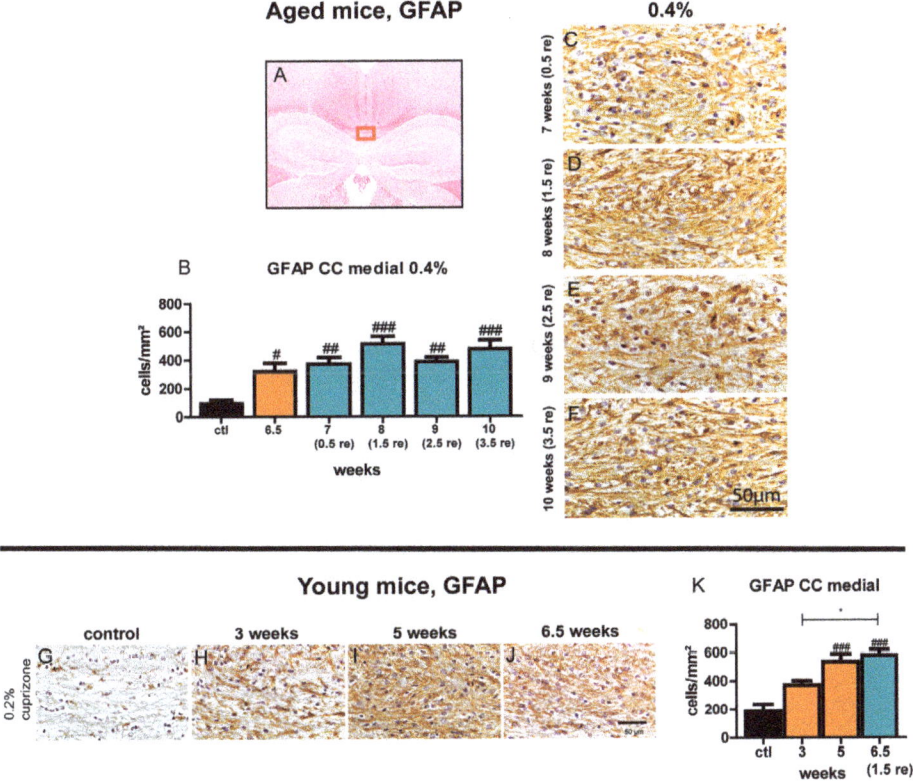

Figure 8. Persisting astrocytosis during remyelination in the midline of the corpus callosum of aged and young mice. The medial part of the corpus callosum that was investigated is marked (**A**). Graphs display the quantity of GFAP-positive astrocytes/mm^2 for the particular time points of demyelination and following remyelination in aged mice treated with 0.4% cuprizone for 6.5 weeks (**B**) and young mice fed with 0.2% cuprizone for 5 weeks (**K**). Representative sections of control and demyelination after 0.4% cuprizone feeding for 6.5 weeks in aged mice are shown in Figure 4. Exemplary sections show persistently elevated numbers of astrocytes during remyelination in aged mice (**C–F**) and during de- and remyelination in young mice (**G–J**). Bars show mean + SEM. Significant effects between different analyzed time points are indicated by asterisks and effects in comparison to control are indicated by hashmarks (*/# $p < 0.05$; **/## $p < 0.01$; ***/### $p < 0.001$). Ctl. = control; 6.5 weeks = feeding period of 0.4% cuprizone in aged mice; 7 (0.5 re) weeks = 0.5 weeks of remyelination, 8 (1.5 re) weeks = 1.5 weeks of remyelination, 9 (2.5 re) weeks = 2.5 weeks of remyelination, 10 (3.5 re) weeks = 3.5 weeks of remyelination in aged mice; 3 and 5 weeks = feeding period of 0.2% cuprizone in young mice; 6.5 (1.5) weeks = 1.5 weeks of remyelination in young mice. N = 5–6 animals per group.

3.10. Axonal Pathology Occurs during Cuprizone-Induced Demyelination in Aged Mice and Corresponds to Microglia Activation

In order to evaluate axonal damage and vesicular axonal transport disturbances during cuprizone-induced demyelination in aged mice, the amount of APP/Synaptophysin double positive spheroids was determined in the medial section of the corpus callosum as previously described [28]. Similar to the reported changes in young mice, the number of APP/Synaptophysin-positive bulbs increased dramatically during cuprizone-induced demyelination, reaching a peak after 6–6.5 weeks of 0.4% cuprizone feeding (Figure 9) and corresponding to the peak of microglia accumulation and activation in this model (Figure 3 and Figure S4). During remyelination, the numbers of APP/Synaptophysin double positive beads rapidly decreased, however, larger-sized spheroids were still present in low numbers suggesting permanent axonal dissection (Figure 9). Standard treatment protocol with 5 weeks as well as a prolonged feeding period of 6 weeks with 0.2% cuprizone did not lead to significant axonal damage (Figure 9).

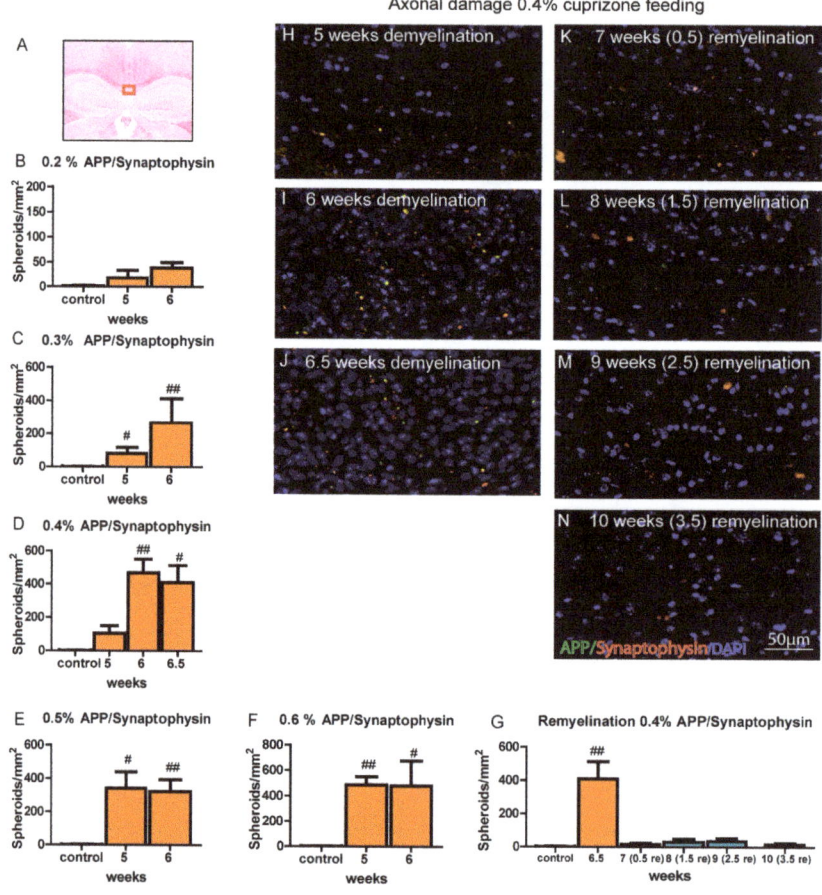

Figure 9. Axonal pathology during cuprizone-induced demyelination in aged mice. The medial part of the corpus callosum that was analyzed is highlighted (A). Graphs (B–G) represent number of APP/Synaptophysin double positive spheroids/mm^2 per time point and group in aged mice during different cuprizone treatments protocols. Bars show mean + SEM. Significant effects between different analyzed time points are indicated by asterisks and effects in comparison to control are indicated by hashmarks (*/# $p < 0.05$; **/## $p < 0.01$; ***/### $p < 0.001$). 6.5 weeks = feeding period of 0.4% cuprizone in aged mice; 7 (0.5 re) weeks = 0.5 weeks of remyelination, 8 (1.5 re) weeks = 1.5 weeks of remyelination, 9 (2.5 re) weeks = 2.5 weeks of remyelination, 10 (3.5 re) weeks = 3.5 weeks of remyelination in aged mice. N = 5–6 animals per group. Representative images show axonal damage/axonal transport disturbances during de- and remyelination in aged mice as depicted by the accumulation of pathological APP/Synaptophysin-positive spheroids in the central corpus callosum (H–N).

4. Discussion

Since remyelination is a highly effective regenerative process by which clinical disability can be prevented, development of remyelination-enhancing therapies for MS is an urgent medical need [36]. Therefore, the cuprizone mouse model represents a suitable approach to investigate remyelination failure and remyelination-promoting agents. However, the currently widely used cuprizone model is only well established in young (8–10 weeks old) mice displaying rapid and extensive remyelination [26] and thus does not reflect the situation of MS pathology in humans regarding age and remyelination efficiency. Therefore, we aimed to establish the cuprizone model in 6-month-old mice representing an aged, mature adult phenotype, corresponding to an adult age in humans in which MS is often diagnosed. Male C57BL6 mice were used since in these mice the cuprizone model is reliably implemented without interference of the hormonal cycle. The establishment of a standardized and optimized cuprizone treatment protocol for aged mice is particularly needed since widely varying cuprizone concentrations and feeding durations have been reported for aged mice with contradictory results [21–24].

We found that the standard cuprizone feeding protocol for young mice with 5 weeks 0.2% cuprizone was not sufficient to establish significant demyelination in aged mice. We show here that robust demyelination in aged mice is only up to a certain degree concentration-/dose-dependent and rather relies on a prolonged feeding duration, establishing 0.4% cuprizone for 6.5 weeks as the best cuprizone treatment protocol for mature adult (6 month) mice to achieve complete demyelination of the corpus callosum. This delayed progress of demyelination was not attributable to a single cell population. In contrast to young mice in which oligodendrocyte depletion and microglia accumulation precedes demyelination, in aged mice, the maximum degree of oligodendrocyte loss, microglia activation, and demyelination occurred simultaneously after 6.5 weeks of treatment with 0.4% cuprizone. This may be explained by a higher resistance of mature oligodendrocytes in aged animals against cuprizone-induced apoptosis on the one side and a reduced phagocytotic capacity of aged microglia resulting in delayed removal of myelin debris [18,37,38] on the other side. However, after demyelination was accomplished, prompt initiation of remyelination as judged by the re-expression of myelin markers accompanied by repopulation of the corpus callosum with oligodendrocytes was evident in aged mice. However, throughout the complete observation period of 3.5 weeks after withdrawal of cuprizone, myelination in the corpus callosum in aged mice remained diminished compared to control. This is in line with findings from ethidium bromide-induced focal demyelination in aged rats, in which remyelination was incomplete 4 weeks after lesion-induction [16]. A further increase in myelination over a longer remyelination period in our model is possible, however, there seemed to already be a stagnation of remyelination 1.5–2 weeks after cuprizone withdrawal. In accordance with remyelination remaining incomplete, re-appearance of mature oligodendrocytes in the corpus callosum was diminished and delayed compared to young mice. This finding is concordant with reports attributing the age-dependent decline of remyelination efficiency to a reduction of oligodendrocyte progenitor recruitment and differentiation [39]. Similar to the situation in young mice [28], axonal pathology was observed, accompanying the advancing degree of demyelination and microglia infiltration after 6 and 6.5 weeks of cuprizone treatment but rapidly improved during subsequent remyelination. Thus, this cuprizone protocol in aged mice displays important pathological hallmarks of human MS pathology [1].

Interestingly, after reaching a similar degree of activation and accumulation of microglia in the corpus callosum during demyelination compared to young mice, aged animals showed prolonged activation and an elevated cell count of microglia in the corpus callosum during the remyelination period. It is conceivable that this constitutes a reflection of the impaired ability of microglia in aged animals to resolve inflammation after demyelination [19]. One might speculate that microglia in aged mice do not represent a remyelination-supporting phenotype to the same extent as in young mice, e.g., by differently expressing pro-myelinating factors [40]. Furthermore, the phagocytosis activity may be diminished in aged microglia and thus may delay remyelination. Significant astrocytosis was observed throughout de- and remyelination and did not display significant changes over time. Since astrocytes are crucial for efficient remyelination after acute demyelination in young animals, e.g., by recruiting microglia and by producing pro-remyelinating factors [30,33], it stands to reason that astrocytes in aged mice are not as capable of creating a remyelination-supportive environment.

In summary, by comprehensively characterizing de- and remyelination in adult mature mice we established a reliable and feasible new protocol for the cuprizone model in which the remyelination capacity is impaired compared to young animals. This better represents the incomplete remyelination in human disease and allows for the study of the capacity of remyelinating agents.

Supplementary Materials: The following are available online at http://www.mdpi.com/2073-4409/9/4/945/s1; Figure S1. Experimental design, Figure S2. MBP loss in the corpus callosum of aged mice after different cuprizone treatment protocols, Figure S3. Depletion of NOGO-A-positive mature oligodendrocytes during demyelination in the midline of the corpus callosum of aged mice, Figure S4. Accumulation of microglia during demyelination in the medial corpus callosum of aged mice, Figure S5. Changes of different glia populations during demyelination in the lateral parts of the corpus callosum of aged mice, Figure S6. MBP re-expression during remyelination in the medial corpus callosum of aged mice, Figure S7. Repopulation of mature oligodendrocytes during remyelination in the central corpus callosum of aged mice, Figure S8. Decrease of microglia during the process of remyelination in the medial part of the corpus callosum of aged mice, Figure S9. Changes of myelin and glia cell populations during remyelination in the lateral parts of the corpus callosum in aged mice, Figure S10. Correlation of myelin changes and microglia reaction during de- and remyelination in aged mice.

Author Contributions: S.G., M.S., and V.G. planned the experiments. S.G., F.H., S.H., T.M.M., and V.G. performed the experiments. S.G., F.H., T.M.M., M.W.H., T.S., and V.G. analyzed the data. S.G., F.H., M.S., and V.G. drafted and wrote the manuscript. All authors read and approved the final version of the manuscript.

Funding: This research received no external funding.

Acknowledgments: The authors thank Ilona Cierpka-Leja and Sabine Lang for excellent technical support. This work is part of the doctoral thesis of Florian Henkel.

Conflicts of Interest: The authors declare no conflict of interest.

References

1. Lassmann, H. Multiple Sclerosis Pathology. *Cold Spring Harb. Perspect. Med.* **2018**, *8*, a028936. [CrossRef]
2. Smith, K.J.; Blakemore, W.F.; McDonald, W.I. Central remyelination restores secure conduction. *Nature* **1979**, *280*, 395–396. [CrossRef]
3. Duncan, I.D.; Brower, A.; Kondo, Y.; Curlee, J.F., Jr.; Schultz, R.D. Extensive remyelination of the CNS leads to functional recovery. *Proc. Natl. Acad. Sci. USA* **2009**, *106*, 6832–6836. [CrossRef]
4. Jeffery, N.D.; Blakemore, W.F. Locomotor deficits induced by experimental spinal cord demyelination are abolished by spontaneous remyelination. *Brain* **1997**, *120*, 27–37. [CrossRef]
5. Mei, F.; Lehmann-Horn, K.; Shen, Y.A.; Rankin, K.A.; Stebbins, K.J.; Lorrain, D.S.; Pekarek, K.; Sagan, A.S.; Xiao, L.; Teuscher, C.; et al. Accelerated remyelination during inflammatory demyelination prevents axonal loss and improves functional recovery. *Elife* **2016**, *5*, e18246. [CrossRef]
6. Irvine, K.A.; Blakemore, W.F. Remyelination protects axons from demyelination-associated axon degeneration. *Brain* **2008**, *131*, 1464–1477. [CrossRef]
7. Franklin, R.J.M.; Ffrench-Constant, C. Regenerating CNS myelin—from mechanisms to experimental medicines. *Nat. Rev. Neurosci.* **2017**, *18*, 753–769. [CrossRef]
8. Patrikios, P.; Stadelmann, C.; Kutzelnigg, A.; Rauschka, H.; Schmidbauer, M.; Laursen, H.; Sorensen, P.S.; Bruck, W.; Lucchinetti, C.; Lassmann, H. Remyelination is extensive in a subset of multiple sclerosis patients. *Brain* **2006**, *129*, 3165–3172. [CrossRef]
9. Goldschmidt, T.; Antel, J.; Konig, F.B.; Bruck, W.; Kuhlmann, T. Remyelination capacity of the MS brain decreases with disease chronicity. *Neurology* **2009**, *72*, 1914–1921. [CrossRef]
10. Skripuletz, T.; Manzel, A.; Gropengiesser, K.; Schafer, N.; Gudi, V.; Singh, V.; Salinas Tejedor, L.; Jorg, S.; Hammer, A.; Voss, E.; et al. Pivotal role of choline metabolites in remyelination. *Brain* **2015**, *138*, 398–413. [CrossRef]
11. Hiremath, M.M.; Saito, Y.; Knapp, G.W.; Ting, J.P.; Suzuki, K.; Matsushima, G.K. Microglial/macrophage accumulation during cuprizone-induced demyelination in C57BL/6 mice. *J. Neuroimmunol.* **1998**, *92*, 38–49. [CrossRef]

12. Skripuletz, T.; Gudi, V.; Hackstette, D.; Stangel, M. De- and remyelination in the CNS white and grey matter induced by cuprizone: The old, the new, and the unexpected. *Histol. Histopathol.* **2011**, *26*, 1585–1597. [CrossRef]
13. Flurkey, K.; Currer, J.M.; Harrison, D.E. Mouse Models in Aging Research. In *The Mouse in Biomedical Research*, 2nd ed.; Fox, J., Barthold, S., Davisson, M., Newcomer, C., Quimby, F., Smith, A., Eds.; Elsevier: New York, NY, USA, 2007; Volume 3, pp. 637–672.
14. Goodin, D.S. The epidemiology of multiple sclerosis: Insights to disease pathogenesis. *Handb. Clin. Neurol.* **2014**, *122*, 231–266. [CrossRef]
15. Dutta, S.; Sengupta, P. Men and mice: Relating their ages. *Life Sci.* **2016**, *152*, 244–248. [CrossRef]
16. Shields, S.A.; Gilson, J.M.; Blakemore, W.F.; Franklin, R.J. Remyelination occurs as extensively but more slowly in old rats compared to young rats following gliotoxin-induced CNS demyelination. *Glia* **1999**, *28*, 77–83. [CrossRef]
17. Chari, D.M.; Crang, A.J.; Blakemore, W.F. Decline in rate of colonization of oligodendrocyte progenitor cell (OPC)-depleted tissue by adult OPCs with age. *J. Neuropathol. Exp. Neurol.* **2003**, *62*, 908–916. [CrossRef]
18. Ruckh, J.M.; Zhao, J.W.; Shadrach, J.L.; van Wijngaarden, P.; Rao, T.N.; Wagers, A.J.; Franklin, R.J. Rejuvenation of regeneration in the aging central nervous system. *Cell Stem Cell* **2012**, *10*, 96–103. [CrossRef]
19. Cantuti-Castelvetri, L.; Fitzner, D.; Bosch-Queralt, M.; Weil, M.T.; Su, M.; Sen, P.; Ruhwedel, T.; Mitkovski, M.; Trendelenburg, G.; Lutjohann, D.; et al. Defective cholesterol clearance limits remyelination in the aged central nervous system. *Science* **2018**, *359*, 684–688. [CrossRef]
20. Neumann, B.; Baror, R.; Zhao, C.; Segel, M.; Dietmann, S.; Rawji, K.S.; Foerster, S.; McClain, C.R.; Chalut, K.; van Wijngaarden, P.; et al. Metformin Restores CNS Remyelination Capacity by Rejuvenating Aged Stem Cells. *Cell Stem Cell* **2019**, *25*, 473–485.e8. [CrossRef]
21. Blakemore, W.F. Remyelination of the superior cerebellar peduncle in old mice following demyelination induced by cuprizone. *J. Neurol. Sci.* **1974**, *22*, 121–126. [CrossRef]
22. Irvine, K.A.; Blakemore, W.F. Age increases axon loss associated with primary demyelination in cuprizone-induced demyelination in C57BL/6 mice. *J. Neuroimmunol.* **2006**, *175*, 69–76. [CrossRef]
23. Shen, S.; Sandoval, J.; Swiss, V.A.; Li, J.; Dupree, J.; Franklin, R.J.; Casaccia-Bonnefil, P. Age-dependent epigenetic control of differentiation inhibitors is critical for remyelination efficiency. *Nat. Neurosci.* **2008**, *11*, 1024–1034. [CrossRef]
24. Doucette, J.R.; Jiao, R.; Nazarali, A.J. Age-related and cuprizone-induced changes in myelin and transcription factor gene expression and in oligodendrocyte cell densities in the rostral corpus callosum of mice. *Cell Mol. Neurobiol.* **2010**, *30*, 607–629. [CrossRef]
25. Mason, J.L.; Jones, J.J.; Taniike, M.; Morell, P.; Suzuki, K.; Matsushima, G.K. Mature oligodendrocyte apoptosis precedes IGF-1 production and oligodendrocyte progenitor accumulation and differentiation during demyelination/remyelination. *J. Neurosci. Res.* **2000**, *61*, 251–262. [CrossRef]
26. Gudi, V.; Gingele, S.; Skripuletz, T.; Stangel, M. Glial response during cuprizone-induced de- and remyelination in the CNS: Lessons learned. *Front. Cell Neurosci.* **2014**, *8*, 73. [CrossRef]
27. Mahler, M.; Berard, M.; Feinstein, R.; Gallagher, A.; Illgen-Wilcke, B.; Pritchett-Corning, K.; Raspa, M. FELASA recommendations for the health monitoring of mouse, rat, hamster, guinea pig and rabbit colonies in breeding and experimental units. *Lab. Anim.* **2014**, *48*, 178–192. [CrossRef]
28. Gudi, V.; Gai, L.; Herder, V.; Tejedor, L.S.; Kipp, M.; Amor, S.; Suhs, K.W.; Hansmann, F.; Beineke, A.; Baumgartner, W.; et al. Synaptophysin Is a Reliable Marker for Axonal Damage. *J. Neuropathol. Exp. Neurol.* **2017**, *76*, 109–125. [CrossRef]
29. Gudi, V.; Moharregh-Khiabani, D.; Skripuletz, T.; Koutsoudaki, P.N.; Kotsiari, A.; Skuljec, J.; Trebst, C.; Stangel, M. Regional differences between grey and white matter in cuprizone induced demyelination. *Brain Res.* **2009**, *1283*, 127–138. [CrossRef]
30. Skripuletz, T.; Hackstette, D.; Bauer, K.; Gudi, V.; Pul, R.; Voss, E.; Berger, K.; Kipp, M.; Baumgartner, W.; Stangel, M. Astrocytes regulate myelin clearance through recruitment of microglia during cuprizone-induced demyelination. *Brain* **2013**, *136*, 147–167. [CrossRef]
31. Paxinos, G.; Franklin, K.B.J.; Franklin, K.B.J. *The mouse brain in stereotaxic coordinates*, 2nd ed.; Academic Press: San Diego, CA, USA, 2001.

32. Lindner, M.; Heine, S.; Haastert, K.; Garde, N.; Fokuhl, J.; Linsmeier, F.; Grothe, C.; Baumgartner, W.; Stangel, M. Sequential myelin protein expression during remyelination reveals fast and efficient repair after central nervous system demyelination. *Neuropathol. Appl. Neurobiol.* **2008**, *34*, 105–114. [CrossRef]
33. Gudi, V.; Skuljec, J.; Yildiz, O.; Frichert, K.; Skripuletz, T.; Moharregh-Khiabani, D.; Voss, E.; Wissel, K.; Wolter, S.; Stangel, M. Spatial and temporal profiles of growth factor expression during CNS demyelination reveal the dynamics of repair priming. *PLoS ONE* **2011**, *6*, e22623. [CrossRef]
34. Skuljec, J.; Gudi, V.; Ulrich, R.; Frichert, K.; Yildiz, O.; Pul, R.; Voss, E.V.; Wissel, K.; Baumgartner, W.; Stangel, M. Matrix metalloproteinases and their tissue inhibitors in cuprizone-induced demyelination and remyelination of brain white and gray matter. *J. Neuropathol. Exp. Neurol.* **2011**, *70*, 758–769. [CrossRef]
35. Acs, P.; Kipp, M.; Norkute, A.; Johann, S.; Clarner, T.; Braun, A.; Berente, Z.; Komoly, S.; Beyer, C. 17beta-estradiol and progesterone prevent cuprizone provoked demyelination of corpus callosum in male mice. *Glia* **2009**, *57*, 807–814. [CrossRef]
36. Stangel, M.; Kuhlmann, T.; Matthews, P.M.; Kilpatrick, T.J. Achievements and obstacles of remyelinating therapies in multiple sclerosis. *Nat. Rev. Neurol.* **2017**, *13*, 742–754. [CrossRef]
37. Gilson, J.; Blakemore, W.F. Failure of remyelination in areas of demyelination produced in the spinal cord of old rats. *Neuropathol. Appl. Neurobiol.* **1993**, *19*, 173–181. [CrossRef]
38. Natrajan, M.S.; de la Fuente, A.G.; Crawford, A.H.; Linehan, E.; Nunez, V.; Johnson, K.R.; Wu, T.; Fitzgerald, D.C.; Ricote, M.; Bielekova, B.; et al. Retinoid X receptor activation reverses age-related deficiencies in myelin debris phagocytosis and remyelination. *Brain* **2015**, *138*, 3581–3597. [CrossRef]
39. Sim, F.J.; Zhao, C.; Penderis, J.; Franklin, R.J. The age-related decrease in CNS remyelination efficiency is attributable to an impairment of both oligodendrocyte progenitor recruitment and differentiation. *J. Neurosci.* **2002**, *22*, 2451–2459. [CrossRef]
40. Hinks, G.L.; Franklin, R.J. Delayed changes in growth factor gene expression during slow remyelination in the CNS of aged rats. *Mol. Cell. Neurosci.* **2000**, *16*, 542–556. [CrossRef]

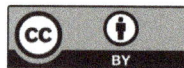

© 2020 by the authors. Licensee MDPI, Basel, Switzerland. This article is an open access article distributed under the terms and conditions of the Creative Commons Attribution (CC BY) license (http://creativecommons.org/licenses/by/4.0/).

MDPI
St. Alban-Anlage 66
4052 Basel
Switzerland
Tel. +41 61 683 77 34
Fax +41 61 302 89 18
www.mdpi.com

Cells Editorial Office
E-mail: cells@mdpi.com
www.mdpi.com/journal/cells

www.ingramcontent.com/pod-product-compliance
Lightning Source LLC
LaVergne TN
LVHW070052120526
838202LV00102B/2050